FITTING GUIDE
FOR RIGID AND SOFT CONTACT LENSES

A Practical Approach

HAROLD A. STEIN, *M.D., M.Sc (Ophth.), F.R.C.S. (C)*

Professor of Ophthalmology, University of Toronto, Toronto, Canada; Chief, Department of Ophthalmology, Scarborough General Hospital, Scarborough, Ontario; Attending Ophthalmologist, Mt. Sinai Hospital, Toronto, Ontario; Past President, Contact Lens Association of Ophthalmologists, New Orleans, Louisiana; Past President, Canadian Ophthalmological Society, Ottawa, Canada; Immediate Past President, Joint Commission on Allied Health Personnel in Ophthalmology, St. Paul, Minnesota; Director, Professional Continuing Education, Centennial College of Applied Arts, Toronto, Ontario

BERNARD J. SLATT, *M.D., F.R.C.S. (C)*

Associate Professor of Ophthalmology, University of Toronto, Toronto, Ontario; Attending Ophthalmologist, Mt. Sinai Hospital, Toronto, Ontario; Attending Ophthalmologist, Scarborough General Hospital, Scarborough, Ontario

RAYMOND M. STEIN, *M.D., F.R.C.S. (C)*

Lecturer, University of Toronto, Toronto, Canada
Attending Ophthalmologist, Scarborough General Hospital, Scarborough, Ontario; Attending Ophthalmologist, Mt. Sinai Hospital, Toronto; Commissioner, Joint Commission on Allied Health Personnel in Ophthalmology, St. Paul, Minnesota; Alumni, Mayo Clinic, Department of Ophthalmology, Rochester, Minnesota

THIRD EDITION

with 713 illustrations
including 48 illustrations in full color
and 18 in 2 color

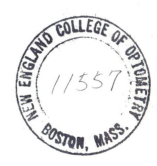

The C. V. Mosby Company

ST. LOUIS · BALTIMORE · PHILADELPHIA · TORONTO   1990

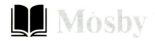

Editor: Eugenia A. Klein
Developmental editor: Kathryn H. Falk
Assistant editor: Ellen Baker Geisel
Production editor: Radhika Rao Gupta
Book design: Gail Morey Hudson

THIRD EDITION

The C.V. Mosby Company 11830 Westline Industrial Drive,
St. Louis, Missouri 63146

Library of Congress Cataloging in Publication Data

Stein, Harold A. (Harold Aaron), 1929-
    Fitting guide for rigid and soft contact lenses: a practical
approach/Harold A. Stein, Bernard J. Slatt, Raymond M. Stein. —
3rd ed.
        p.   cm.
    Bibliography: p.
    Includes index.
    ISBN 0-8016-5182-4
    1. Contact lenses.   I.   Slatt, Bernard J., 1934-   .   II.   Stein,
Raymond M.   III.   Title.
    [DNLM: 1.   Contact Lenses.   WW 355 S819f]
RE977.C6S73   1990
617.7'523—dc20
DNLM/DLC
for Library of Congress   89-12614
                                                                              CIP

GW/W/W   9   8   7   6   5   4   3   2   1

FOREWORD

Drs. Stein, Slatt, and Stein should be congratulated for the success of their practical clinical guide for the fitting of rigid and soft contact lenses, which is in its third edition. The major thrust of this book is to provide a step-by-step, concise clinical guide for contact lens fitting. This book is aimed at the clinician who wants to know how to fit a lens and deal with its problems without the heavy theoretic and scientific background of corneal and lens physiology and biochemistry.

Practitioners will find this approach direct and clear. The visual emphasis on photographs and drawings and the well-illustrated instructions make this book easy to understand.

In this enriched edition all aspects of rigid and soft lens fitting are covered meticulously, including the new modalities of gas-permeable lenses, extended-wear lenses, disposable lenses, and bifocal lenses. Controversial methods such as orthokeratology have also been dealt with.

Dr. Raymond Stein, a new author for this book, has expanded the areas of corneal and external disease with a number of new chapters.

Several contributing authors appear in this edition and have enhanced the value of this textbook.

Great care has been given to the strictly practical aspects of rigid and soft contact lens fitting. Without any doubt, this book should be profitable reading for the student learning contact lens fitting, as well as for the practitioner who needs help now and then with problem cases. The high standard of this book should be no surprise because Drs. Stein, Slatt, and Stein are the authors of *The ophthalmic assistant*, which is in its fifth edition and has become a classic text in its field.

This book is a must on the bookshelf of every contact lens fitter. I consider it a privilege to recommend without reservation this most useful and practical fitting guide for rigid and soft contact lenses.

G. Peter Halberg, M.D., F.A.C.S.

Chairman, International Contact Lens Council of Ophthalmology;
Professor of Clinical Ophthalmology, New York Medical College,
New York, New York

To
ANNE, CAROL, and NANCY
our wives, whose encouragement and
understanding made it possible
for us to enhance and enlarge
this third edition.

PREFACE

We welcome the opportunity to bring out this edition of the *Fitting Guide*. The first and second editions have been surpassed by so much advanced technology that they were on the verge of becoming collectors' items. Most new editions are strictly a matter of mending and pruning—correcting errors, updating, perhaps reorganizing material, adding some tables, diagrams, and photographs here and there—the work of a dilettante. Not so with this new edition. It required so much work that the pruning knife was insufficient as a tool—it required an axe.

The soft lens section was literally redone. Care systems have totally changed. We now recognize the importance of cleaning and the potential toxic and hypersensitivity reactions of these supposedly innocuous solutions. Soft lenses have lost weight and become trimmer. It seems as if they cannot get thin enough, especially in the quest for more oxygen permeability.

There are so many companies now making soft contact lenses that we decided to go generic, using examples where indicated. Also, the soft lens field has broadened immensely in the past years. Newer soft lenses come in a variety of polymers, with varying degrees of water content, tints, toric front and back surfaces, and variable central thicknesses. It meant new material and writing. Even the traditional sections of insertion and removal could not be salvaged because the newer hyperthin lenses easily collapse on a wet finger, and the taco test for determining which side of the lens is right has become a quaint oddity; it no longer works with most of these newer lenses.

The safety of extended-wear lenses has been challenged; the section has been upgraded and expanded in deference to their importance. The current thrust is to develop lenses with the greatest comfort, convenience, and safety. We stress safety for obvious reasons but also because

a patient may not know when these lenses are a hazard. The warning devices of reactive symptoms may be absent. Patients simply do not know when their corneas are slightly edematous and vascularized. The disposable lens has now become a reality along with systems of patient management.

Gas-permeable lenses have been emphasized in this edition because they have come out of adolescence into maturity. These lenses are now the prime lens of the rigid lens variety. In many areas of the world, gas-permeable lenses are preferred over soft lenses. Their role in an extended-wear function is just in its infancy.

Silicone lenses, both in the resin and elastomer form, are being relegated to the realm of antiquity except for special uses. We have had to take the axe to this chapter from the last edition.

Polymethylmethacrylate is looking more like a relic of the past. Gas-permeable lenses do the same job, but better. This discussion was pruned to indicate the material's shrinking prominence.

Bifocal lenses and the fitting of the presbyope have struggled along, but they now seem to be emerging as a practical reality. A number of new lenses has come to the foreground and is covered in this edition.

The lid is off the age ceiling on the use of contact lenses. Children a day old as well as their grandparents are being fitted with lenses. New instruments and techniques have been developed to adapt to the special needs of children.

This edition of *Fitting Guide* is really a new book. It has expanded from 32 chapters to 45 in the third edition. Only the intent remains the same: to provide clear, useful information to assist the fitter in the practical management of a contact lens practice. It is not an academic reference book. We have our bias toward certain lens designs and our own ways of treating trouble. Our personal preferences are revealed because we made no attempt to hide in the name of impartiality what we think works best. It is our editorial license and our duty to show our experience.

Canada has a unique situation in North America in the contact lens area. Unhampered by restrictions imposed by the FDA, we serve as the center of cross-winds blowing new and exciting products from Japan and Europe. In addition, our own Canadian contact lens industry coupled with Canada's status as the testing-ground for American manufacturers has brought exciting new products to us for clinical evaluation long before their market introduction in the United States. We are thankful to our vantage point for being privy to this rich experience in the contact lens field.

New sections by Drs. John F. Morgan, James Key III, Alan Mandelberg, Mathea Allansmith, Joshua Josephson, Robert Ross, Carole Mobley, and Keith W. Harrison have been added, in addition to revised chapters contributed by Dr. James Aquavella and Dr. J. Peter Halberg.

We are particularly indebted to the extensive critical review of the manuscript and the contribution of new concepts by Dr. Joshua Josephson. We are indebted to Keith Harrison for reviewing sections of the new manuscript. We are grateful to Mr. Norman Deer and Ms. Laurie Stein for the illustrations.

Harold A. Stein
Bernard J. Slatt
Raymond M. Stein

CONTRIBUTORS

MATHEA R. ALLANSMITH, M.D.

Associate Professor of Ophthalmology, Harvard Medical School Institute Scientist, Eye Research Institute, Boston, Massachusetts

JAMES V. AQUAVELLA, M.D., F.A.C.S.

Director, Department of Ophthalmology, Park Ridge Hospital; Medical Director, Rochester Eye Bank; Clinical Associate Professor of Ophthalmology, University of Rochester, Rochester, New York

JEAN-PIERRE CHARTRAND, M.D.

Department of Ophthalmology, Lakeshore General Hospital, Dorval, Quebec, Canada

PENNY COOK, M.O.C.L.A.

Optician; Certified Contact Lens Fitter, Toronto, Ontario, Canada

G. PETER HALBERG, M.D., F.A.C.S.

Chairman, International Contact Lens Council of Ophthalmologists, Professor of Clinical Ophthalmology, New York Medical College, New York, New York

KEITH W. HARRISON, M.O.C.L.A.

Lecturer and Instructor, Contact Lens Certification Program, Seneca College of Applied Arts and Technology, Willowdale, Ontario, Canada

JOSHUA E. JOSEPHSON, O.D., F.O.A.A.

Private Practice, Toronto, Ontario, Canada

JAMES E. KEY, M.D.

Clinical Assistant Professor, Baylor College of Medicine, Houston, Texas

ALAN I. MANDELBERG, M.D.

Attending Surgeon, Department of Ophthalmology, St. Joseph's Medical Center, Burbank, California; Assistant Clinical Professor, Department of Ophthalmology, University of Southern California

Medical Center, Los Angeles, California; Private Practice, North Hollywood, California

CSABA MARTONYI, F.O.P.S., C.O.P.R.A.

Associate Professor, Director of Ophthalmic Photography, W.K. Kellogg Eye Center, University of Michigan School of Medicine, Ann Arbor, Michigan

CAROLE L. MOBLEY, C.O.T., H.F.C.L.S.A., N.C.L.C.

Certified Ophthalmic Technician, Contact Lens Consultants, Houston, Texas

JOHN F. MORGAN, M.D., F.R.C.S. (C)

Professor, Faculty of Medicine, Queen's University of Kingston, Department of Ophthalmology, Hotel Dieu Hospital, Kingston, Ontario, Canada

ROBERT N. ROSS, Ph.D.

Staff Associate, Eye Research Institute, Boston, Massachusetts

BERNARD J. SLATT, M.D., F.R.C.S. (C)

Associate Professor of Ophthalmology, University of Toronto, Toronto; Attending Ophthalmologist, Mt. Sinai Hospital, Toronto; Attending Ophthalmologist, Scarborough General Hospital, Scarborough; Director, Association of Ophthalmic Assistants of Ontario; Board of Advisors, Toronto, Ontario

HAROLD A. STEIN, M.D., M.SC (Ophth.), F.R.C.S. (C)

Professor of Ophthalmology, University of Toronto, Toronto; Chief, Department of Ophthalmology, Scarborough General Hospital, Scarborough; Attending Ophthalmologist, Mt. Sinai Hospital, Toronto; Past President Contact Lens Association of Ophthalmologists, New Orleans, Louisiana; Past President, Canadian Opthalmological Society; Past President, Joint Commission on Allied Health Personnel in Ophthalmology, St. Paul, Minnesota; Director of Professional Continuing Education, Centennial College of Applied Arts, Toronto, Ontario

RAYMOND M. STEIN, M.D., F.R.C.S. (C)

Lecturer, University of Toronto, Toronto
Attending Ophthalmologist, Scarborough General Hospital, Scarborough, Ontario; Commissioner, Joint Commission on Allied Health Personnel in Ophthalmology, St. Paul, Minnesota; Alumni, Mayo Clinic, Department of Ophthalmology, Rochester, Minnesota; Past Corneal Fellow, Wills Eye Hospital, Philadelphia, Pennsylvania

CONTENTS

COLOR ATLAS

I. CORNEAL DISORDERS

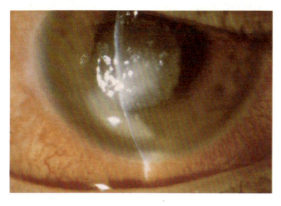

Plate 1. Corneal ulceration caused by *Pseudomonas aeruginosa*.

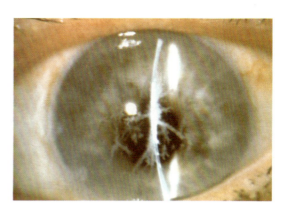

Plate 2. Granular corneal dystrophy.

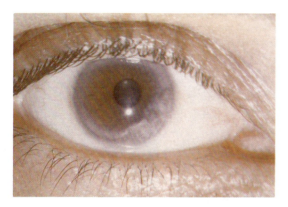

Plate 3. Terrien's marginal degeneration of the cornea.

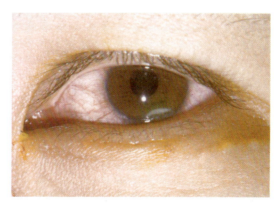

Plate 4. Marginal corneal erosion caused by *Staphylococcus aureus*.

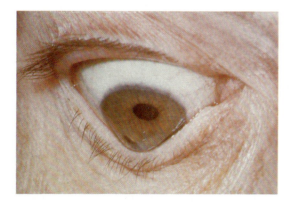

Plate 5. Advanced keratoconus. A cone-shaped deformity of the cornea with thinning of the cornea.

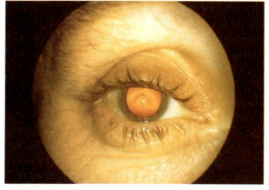

Plate 6. Keratoconus reflex. Retinal reflex as seen through a thin protruding cornea.

(**1** and **2**, Courtesy Mentor O & O Inc., Hingham, Mass.; **5** and **6**, Courtesy Dr. Dean Butcher, Australia.)

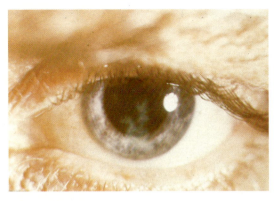

Plate 7. Herpes simplex dendritic ulcer. Fernlike projection on the epithelial surface of the cornea from herpes simplex of the cornea.

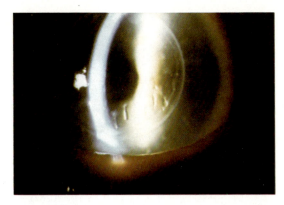

Plate 8. Filamentary keratitis covered by a therapeutic lens.

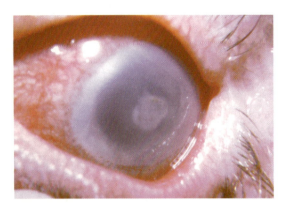

Plate 9. Fungal corneal ulcer leading to endophthalmitis.

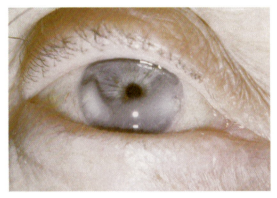

Plate 10. Band keratopathy of the cornea.

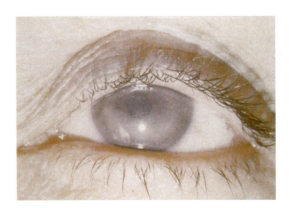

Plate 11. Fuchs' corneal dystrophy resulting in progressive decrease of vision and eventually bullous keratopathy.

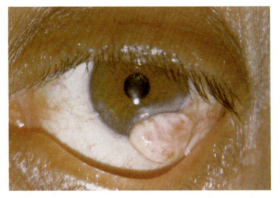

Plate 12. Large corneal dermoid requiring surgical removal before patient could wear contact lens.

(**7,** Courtesy Dr. Ira Abrahamson, Jr., Cincinnati, Ohio.)

II. EXTERNAL DISORDERS OF THE EYE AND EYELID

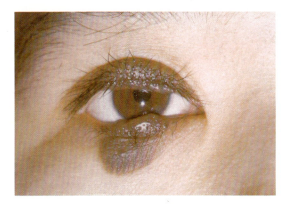

Plate 13. Kissing benign nevus of the upper and lower eyelid.

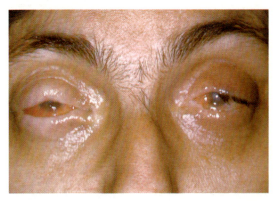

Plate 14. Advanced trachoma with diffuse scarring of the cornea and symblepharon and entropion.

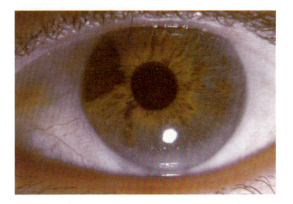

Plate 15. Melanoma of iris. A pigmented lesion of the iris.

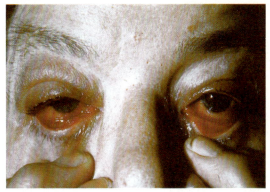

Plate 16. Acute bacterial conjunctivitis. Inflammation of the conjunctival lining caused by *Streptococcus.*

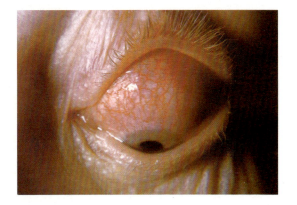

Plate 17. Scleritis. Nonbacterial inflammation of the sclera.

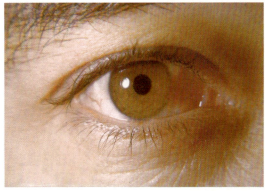

Plate 18. Pterygium. A triangular membrane extending from the conjunctiva over the cornea.

(**15** to **18** from Stein, H.A., and Slatt, B.J.: The ophthalmic assistant, ed. 4, St. Louis, 1983, The C.V. Mosby Co.)

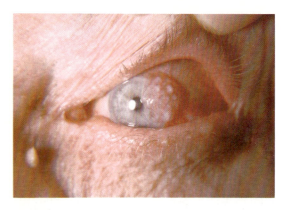

Plate 19. Squamous cell carcinoma of cornea. A cancer growth occurring at the limbus and invading the cornea.

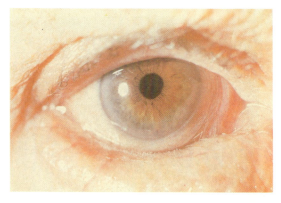

Plate 20. Spastic entropion. In-turning of the lower eyelid from spasm.

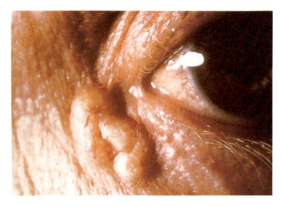

Plate 21. Basal cell carcinoma of eyelid (rodent ulcer), a neoplasm of the lower eyelid that is locally invasive.

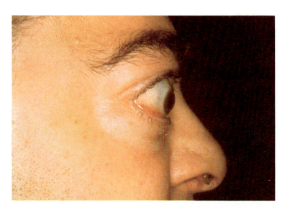

Plate 22. Thyroid exophthalmos. Note ocular protrusion and lid retraction.

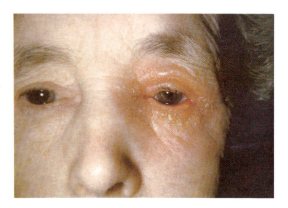

Plate 23. Allergic blepharodermatitis, a skin condition that resulted from atropine sensitivity.

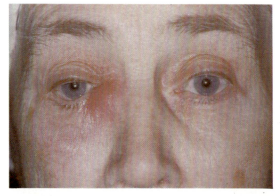

Plate 24. Acute dacryocystitis caused by obstruction of nasal lacrimal duct.

(**20,** Courtesy Dr. Ira Abrahamson, Jr., Cincinnati, Ohio; **19** and **21** to **23** from Stein, H.A., and Slatt, B.J.: The ophthalmic assistant, ed. 4, St. Louis, 1983, The C.V. Mosby Co.)

III. CONTACT LENS PROBLEMS

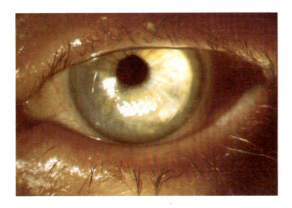

Plate 25. Plaque-like deposits on a soft lens.

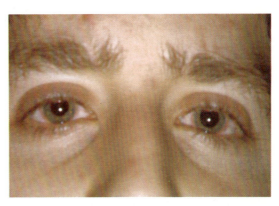

Plate 26. Allergic conjunctivitis occurring after the use of a soaking solution containing thimerosal.

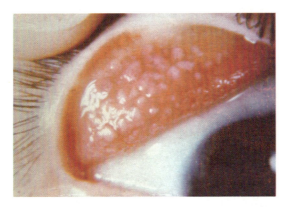

Plate 27. Giant papillary conjunctivitis in a patient wearing daily-wear soft contact lenses for 2 years.

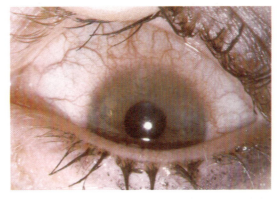

Plate 28. Vascular invasion superiorly in a patient wearing extended-wear contact lenses for 6 months without removal, cleaning, or monitoring.

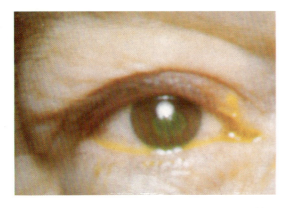

Plate 29. Overwear syndrome from acute corneal hypoxia after 12 hours of wear with PMMA rigid lenses. Denuding of the epithelium resulting in extreme pain, photophobia, and blurring of vision.

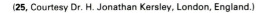

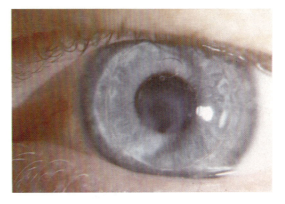

Plate 30. Keratoconus with central scarring. A rigid lens is shown partially decentered.

(**25,** Courtesy Dr. H. Jonathan Kersley, London, England.)

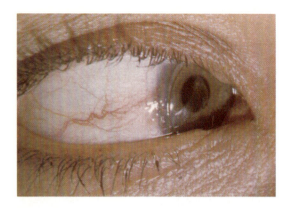

Plate 31. Staining at 3 and 9 o'clock positions in a patient wearing a small gas-permeable lens with thick edges. A large leash vessel has developed.

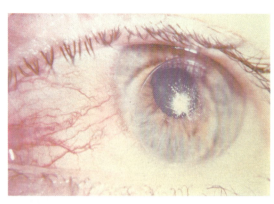

Plate 32. A partially decentered rigid lens leading to marginal erosion and vascularization.

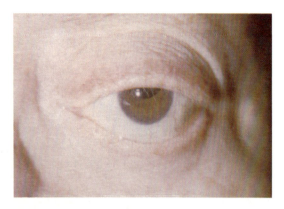

Plate 33. Scleral show below limbus caused by low-lying lower lid. This creates a dryness of the lower portion of a soft lens with resultant drying out of the lens and blurriness of vision.

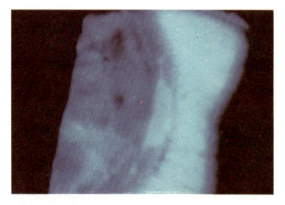

Plate 34. Marginal ulceration at the limbus caused by a decentered rigid lens on a toric cornea with constant indentation and necrosis of the underlying epithelium by the edge of the lens.

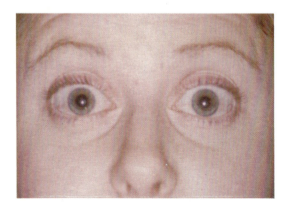

Plate 35. Staring effect of a new contact lens wearer. This may result in drying of the lens, blurring of vision, and 3 and 9 o'clock staining.

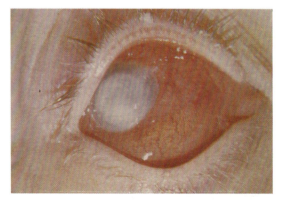

Plate 36. Endophthalmitis after finger-to-eye contamination of a daily soft lens wearer with *Pseudomonas aeruginosa*.

IV. SPECIAL INDICATIONS FOR CONTACT LENSES

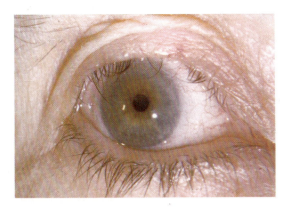

Plate 37. A plano high-water-content lens used for entropion after scarring from injury. The in-turned aberrant lashes are prevented from irritating the cornea.

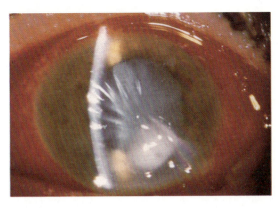

Plate 38. Penetrating corneal wound in which a therapeutic lens was used to restore integrity of the anterior chamber.

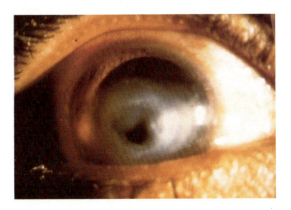

Plate 39. Lye burns with descemetocele. A therapeutic lens can prevent perforation.

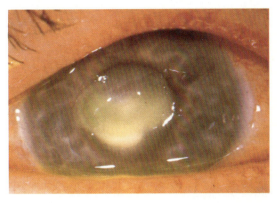

Plate 40. Necrotic metaherpetic corneal ulcer that failed to heal until a therapeutic lens was applied.

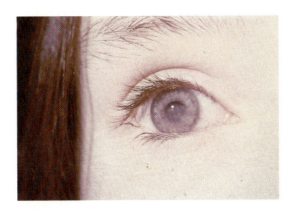

Plate 41. Riley-Day syndrome with necrotic corneal ulcer requiring a low-water-content, thin, extended-wear lens to maintain the corneal integrity.

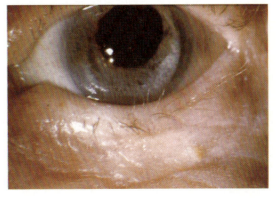

Plate 42. Aphakic extended-wear lens protecting against corneal irritation by trichiasis.

(**39,** Courtesy Dr. B. Bodner, Boston, and Syntex Ophthalmics, Inc., Phoenix, Arizona; **42,** courtesy Dr. H. Jonathan Kersley, London, England.)

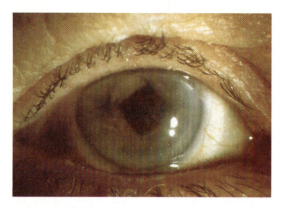

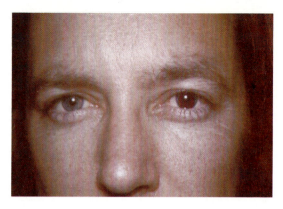

Plate 43. Bandage lens to give comfort to an eye with bullous keratopathy after intraocular lens insertion.

Plate 44. Red-dyed soft lens on one eye used to enhance color perception in a red-green–blind individual.

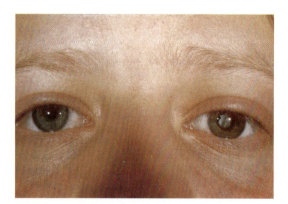

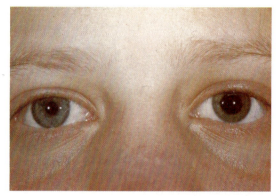

Plates 45 and 46. Inoperable cataract in which a colored therapeutic lens was applied for cosmetic advantage in a young child.

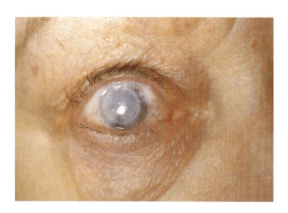

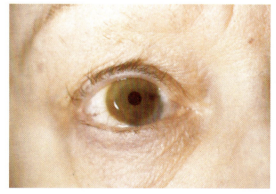

Plates 47 and 48. Cosmetic therapeutic lens used to mask an unsightly corneal graft.

(**45** and **48,** Courtesy Narcissus Foundation, San Francisco, California.)

PART ·I

FUNDAMENTALS

1▪ ANATOMY AND PHYSIOLOGY OF THE CORNEA

- ▪ Gross anatomy
- ▪ Microscopic anatomy and physiology
- ▪ Summary

Since contact lenses can cause anatomic and physiologic changes of the cornea, an understanding of the normal anatomy and physiology of the cornea is necessary for the contact lens fitter to better detect and understand pathophysiologic changes.

GROSS ANATOMY

The cornea is the transparent, avascular tissue that corresponds to the crystal of a watch. It has an elliptical anterior surface with average dimensions of 11 mm in the vertical plane and 12 mm in the horizontal plane (Fig. 1-1). The cornea is thinner centrally, averaging 0.56 mm, whereas the periphery measures approximately 1 mm in thickness (Fig. 1-2). Generally, there is an increase in corneal thickness with age.

The central one third of the cornea is almost spherical and is the optical zone. In the periphery the cornea becomes flatter, but the rate of flattening is not symmetrical. Flattening is more extensive nasally and superiorly than temporally

and inferiorly. This topography is important for contact lens fitting, because the keratometer is designed to measure only a small spherical area of the cornea, which is approximately 3.6 mm.

The corneal curvature also changes somewhat with aging. Generally, it is more spherical in

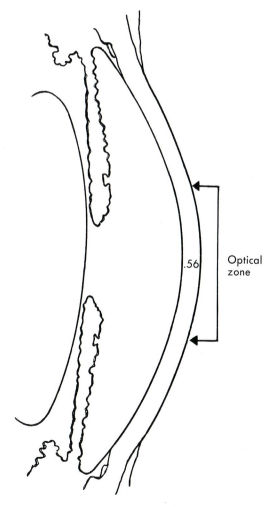

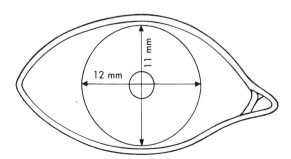

Fig 1-1 ▪ Anterior dimensions of the cornea.

Fig 1-2 ▪ The cornea is thinner centrally (0.56mm) and measures >1.0mm in the periphery.

infancy and changes to astigmatism with the rule during childhood and adolescence; it becomes more spherical in middle age and changes to astigmatism against the rule in the elderly.

MICROSCOPIC ANATOMY AND PHYSIOLOGY

The cornea may be separated into five layers (Fig. 1-3):
- 1/ Epithelium (and its basement membrane)
- 2/ Bowman's layer
- 3/ Stroma
- 4/ Descemet's membrane
- 5/ Endothelium

Corneal epithelium

Functions. The major functions of the corneal epithelium are:
- 1/ Providing a mechanical barrier to microorganisms and foreign matter.

- 2/ Maintaining a barrier to the diffusion of water and solutes.
- 3/ Creating a smooth, transparent optical surface to which the tear film can adsorb.

Structure. The epithelium consists of five to seven cell layers with three cell types: basal cells, wing cells, and superficial flattened cells (Fig. 1-4). The basal cells are the deepest layer and comprise a single layer of columnar cells that rest on the basement membrane. These cells are connected to the underlying basement membrane by hemidesmosomes. These focal spots consist of intracytoplasmic tonofilaments that extend through the basement membrane to the Bowman's layer. Any clinician who has attempted to remove a normal corneal epithelium with a moistened Q-tip or a scalpel blade appreciates the tenacity of the adhesion. The wing cells, of which there are two layers, and the superficial flattened cells, of which there are three layers, complete the epithelium. The multi-sided wing cells interdigitate with each other and adhere with large numbers of desmosomal attachments to the adjacent cell. These desmosomal attachments consist of tonofilaments that extend across the intercellular space from the plasma membrane of one cell to an adjacent cell. The most superifical cells are flat, overlapping squamous cells, similar to the most

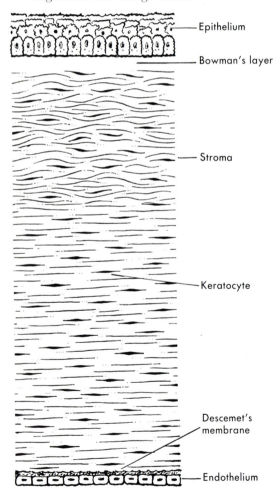

Fig 1-3 ■ The five layers of the cornea.

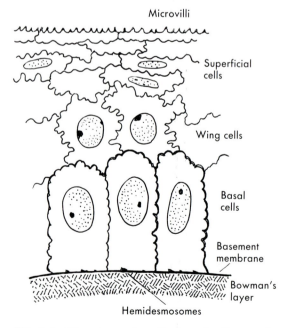

Fig 1-4 ■ The corneal epithelium to Bowman's layer.

superfical epithelial cells of the skin. Unlike these cells, however, normal corneal epithelium is not keratinized. The surface epithelial cells are uniform and smooth and have desmosomal intercellular attachments. In addition these surface cells are zippered together by zonulae occludentes (tight junctions), which encircle the cells and consist of adhesion of the two adjacent plasma membranes. This strong barrier blocks the penetration of most micro-organisms and prevents the flow of fluid and electrolytes from the tears to the stroma, which assists in keeping the corneal stroma in a state of relative dehydration.

By electron-microscopy the outer cell membranes of epithelial cells show fingerlike projections known as microvilli (Fig. 1-5). These microvilli project into the tear film and may trap tear fluid and thus prevent drying of the epithelial cells. There is a continuous migration of epithelial cells from the basal surface toward the tear film. Dividing basal cells become the wing-shaped cells that migrate superficially as flattened squamous cells and ultimately lose their attachments to the cornea and slough into the tear film. The corneal epithelium turns over about once a week.

Fluid can accumulate in the epithelium both intracellulary and extracellulary. Intracellular fluid expands the cells into round vesicles. The

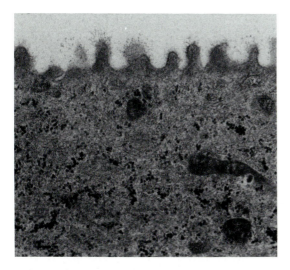

Fig 1-5 ■ Microvilli of the surface of the cornea; magnification × 36,600; (Courtesy Dr. Adolph I Cohen; from Moses RA and Hart WM: Adler's physiology of the eye, ed 8, St. Louis, 1987, The CV Mosby Co.)

extracellular fluid accumulates between the cells, which continue to remain attached by desmosomes. These pockets of fluid produce a microcystic texture, which is easily appreciated at the slitlamp, and act to diffract the light, which creates the halos that are described by patients with epithelial edema.

The basal cells of the epithelium are attached to the underlying basement membrane. If the basement membrane is damaged it can be regenerated by the epithelium. Abnormalities of the basement membrane appear most commonly in disorders such as recurrent corneal erosion, epithelial basement membrane dystrophy, and diabetes mellitus. Abnormal adhesion of the epithelium and abnormal secretion of basement membrane frequently result in surface irregularity with blurred vision and occasional painful erosions.

Metabolism of corneal epithelium. A contact lens resting on the cornea may interfere with the normal metabolic pathways and result in morphologic cell changes and corneal edema. An understanding of oxygen and nutrient delivery to the cornea provides the clinician with the background knowledge necessary to understand pathophysiologic changes.

Oxygen is provided to the epithelium via the precorneal tear film and to the endothelium and stroma from the aqueous humor. The primary metabolic substrate for the epithelial cells, keratocytes, and endothelium is glucose. It is provided to the stroma primarily from the aqueous humor via facilitated diffusion through the endothelium, and to the epithelium by passive diffusion through the stroma. The precorneal tear film and limbal vessels supply approximately 10% of total glucose; however, this pathway is not adequate for the maintenance of normal physiologic function of epithelial and stromal cells.

Oxygen dissolves in the tear film and diffuses into the cornea across the epithelium. Under normal conditions the cornea receives a satisfactory supply of oxygen. Hypoxia and resultant edema may result if there is less than 7 to 15 mm Hg partial pressure of oxygen in the tear film. Under normal conditions with the eyes open, the oxygen tension in tears is approximately 155 mm Hg. With the eyes closed, oxygen diffuses into the tears from the conjunctival capillaries and provides a pressure of 55 mm Hg. The oxygen diffuses across the epithelium through the stroma to the endothelium, which receives most of its required oxygen supply from the aqueous humor.

The epithelium uses glucose as a primary source of energy, and amino acids as building blocks, both of which diffuse from the aqueous humor across the endothelium and stroma. The tear film is of lesser importance in supplying nutrients because of the strong epithelial barrier that prevents their diffusion and because of the small amounts of glucose and amino acids in tears.

The epithelial cells store large quantities of glycogen that provide an energy reserve. Glycogen can be converted to glucose, which can be metabolized through two major pathways. The Krebs (tricarboxilic acid) cycle and the hexosemonophosphate shunt provide energy for metabolic functions. Under hypoxic conditions, as may occur with a tightly-fitted contact lens,

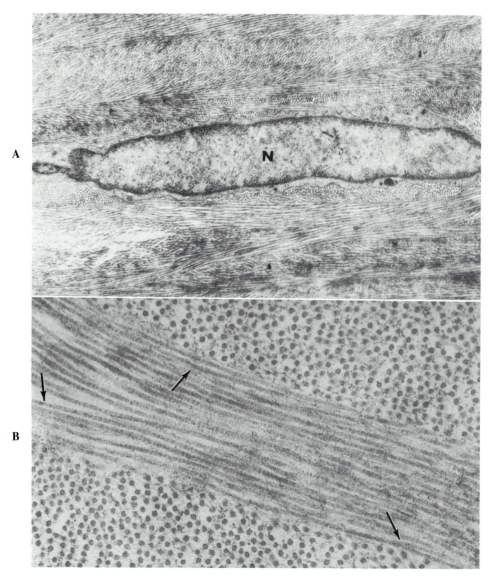

Fig 1-6 ■ **A,** Electron micrograph showing the nucleus, N, of a keratocyte and layers of corneal stromal collagen are seen from various angles; magnification × 9000; **B,** Higher magnification of stromal collagen, showing collagen fibrils cut on end and from side visible (arrows); magnification × 72,000; (Courtesy Dr. Jack Kayes; from Moses RA and Hart WM: Adler's physiology of the eye, ed 8, St. Louis, 1987, The CV Mosby Co.)

the epithelium can metabolize glucose anaerobically by way of the Embden-Meyerhof pathway. This results in the production of lactic acid with resultant corneal epithelial edema.

Bowman's layer and stroma

Functions. These layers perform three functions:

- They are transparent, so they allow the transmission of light;
- They maintain a fixed shape so that the cornea can function optically; and
- They protect the intra-ocular contents.

Bowman's layer

On the posterior side of the epithelial basement membrane lies Bowman's layer. By light microscopy this layer is seen as a relatively homogeneous, acellular sheet and in the past was referred to as Bowman's membrane. However, as seen by electron microscopy, this zone is a specialized layer resembling corneal stroma and is not a true membrane. It is a condensation of the superficial stroma, which consists of collagen fibrils. The layer cannot be detached from the stroma into which it imperceptibly blends. Unlike the epithelial basement membrane or Descemet's membrane it cannot be replaced, and so, following injury, it may become opacified by scar tissue. There are tiny perforations in Bowman's layer that permit passage of corneal nerves to the epithelium.

Stroma

The stroma, which constitutes about 90% of the corneal thickness, consists primarily of collagen fibers, a ground substance, and keratocytes. The collagen fibers of the corneal stroma are uniform and small, about 250 to 300 Å (Fig. 1-6). Bundles of collagen fibers constitute lamellae, which stretch from limbus to limbus. The collagen bundles in the anterior zone are small and are neither as clearly defined nor as regular in size and arrangement as those found in the posterior portion of the stroma. Lamellae cross each other at right angles in a regular fashion, and layers of lamellae run parallel to each other and to the surface of the cornea. The ground substance consists of keratin sulfate and chondroitin sulfate and fills all the space not occupied by the fibrils and cells in the corneal stroma. In swollen corneas the volume of the ground substance increases, but the individual

collagen fiber size does not change. The stroma also consists of keratocytes, which lie between the corneal lamellae and are capable of synthesizing collagen and mucoprotein. Other freely moving cells seen in the stroma include histiocytes, lymphocytes, and, occasionally, polymorphonuclear leukocytes. These cells are generally present in response to some abnormal condition, and there is some disagreement as to whether they can be seen in a normal healthy cornea.

Corneal transparency

The cornea is transparent; light makes its way through it with minimal interference (Fig. 1-7). Light waves are able to pass undisturbed through the cornea because of the relatively small diameter of the collagen fibrils and the narrow separation between the fibrils. An analogy may help to explain this phenomenon. A bowling ball thrown down a lane will not be deviated by specks of dust on the ground, but it will be thrown off its course if it encounters large potholes or if it collides with another ball. Similarly, the light waves passing through the cornea are undeviated by the small variations in the structures of the cornea.

Descemet's membrane

Descemet's membrane is produced by the endothelium. Its thickness increases with age. At birth it is approximately 3 to 4 μ; in adulthood it is approximately 10 to 12 μ. The anterior por-

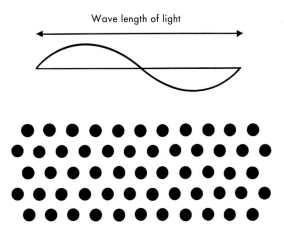

Wave length of light

Fig 1-7 ■ Cross-sectional view of fibrils arranged in lattice. Size of a wavelength of light shown above for comparison. (Modified from Maurice D: The physics of corneal transparency. In Duke-Elder S, editor: Transparency of the cornea, Oxford, 1960, Blackwell Scientific Publications Ltd.)

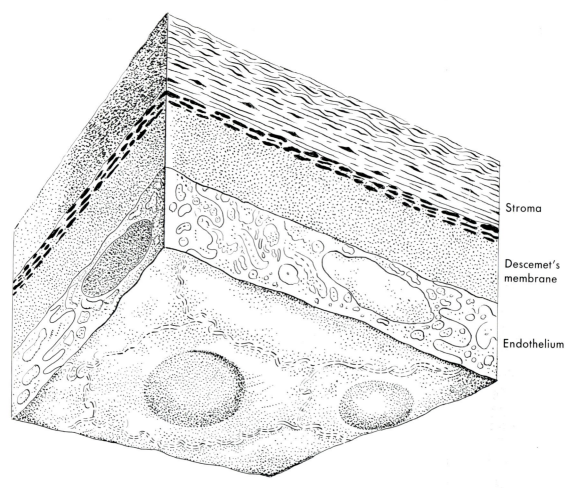

Stroma

Descemet's membrane

Endothelium

Fig 1-8 ■ Details of the inner portion of the cornea, including stroma, Descemet's membrane, and endothelium.

tion of the membrane, which is adherent to the stroma, is fibrous and banded, while the posterior portion, adjacent to the endothelial cells, is a more homogeneous, nonbanded granular material (Fig. 1-8). The anterior portion of Descemet's membrane is the "oldest" portion and therefore the earliest to be laid down during fetal life. In contrast, the posterior portion is the youngest portion of the membrane and the part in which new material is continuously being laid down.

In contrast to Bowman's layer, Descemet's membrane is easily detached from the stroma and it regenerates readily after injury. Excrescences or thickenings of Descemet's membrane may occur as a normal aging change in the peripheral cornea and are known as Hassall-Henle warts. These are considered abnormal when they occur in the central cornea (corneal guttata).

Endothelium

Functions. The corneal endothelium has a number of important functions. It functions as
- 1/a permeability barrier, allowing the diffusion of nutrients to the cornea, and as
- 2/a pump mechanism to maintain the cornea in a partially dehydrated state.

Structure. Lining the posterior surface of the cornea and forming the anterior boundary of the anterior aqueous chamber is a single layer of cells known as the corneal endothelium. The endothelial cells are flat and hexagonal and are in direct contact with the aqueous humor. This cell layer has limited, if any, reproductive capacity. The endothelial surface can be visualized and photographed *in vivo* with the clinical specular microscope.

Aging causes endothelial cell loss, and the remaining cells enlarge, reorganize, and migrate to maintain the intact monolayer so that Descemet's membrane remains completely covered. Therefore, endothelial cell density, expressed as cells per unit area, decreases with age. Similarly, cell loss from trauma, inflammation, or intra-ocular surgery is compensated for by increased cell size and decreased cell density. Although some cells enlarge in response to aging or disease, other cells remain the same size, so the original homogeneous endothelial population gradually becomes heterogeneous. The cell density at birth is approximately 3000 cells per mm^2 and generally decreases with age. However, one cannot look at an endothelial photograph and accurately predict an individual's age because there is often significant variation in cell density within various age groups.

The functional capacity of the endothelium does not correlate well with cell density. As the cells enlarge, they can maintain a functional capacity that keeps the cornea clear. However, as the cell density drops below 500 cells per mm^2, the functional reserve is minimal and corneal edema is likely to appear.

Maintenance of corneal transparency

The corneal stroma has a natural tendency to imbibe water because of two forces:
- 1/The intra-ocular pressure pushes the aqueous humor into the stroma; and
- 2/The glycosaminoglycans exert an osmotic pressure called the swelling pressure that pulls water into the stroma. Corneal transparency is maintained by the endothelium by counteracting this hydrophilic tendency by a pump function, which transports water out of the stroma, and by a barrier function, which decreases the flow of water into the stroma (Fig. 1-9).

The endothelial barrier is normally leaky to water; however, the leak rate normally equals the ability of the endothelium to pump water back out of the stroma. The stromal water content remains relatively constant at about 78% by weight and the corneal thickness remains relatively constant at approximately 0.56 mm.

The endothelial cells are attached to each other by a variety of junctions that do not form a tight barrier to the passage of small mole-

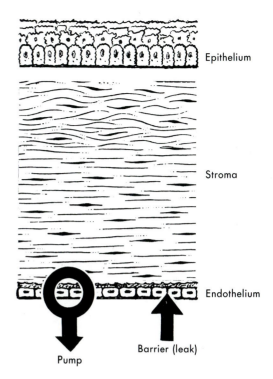

Fig 1-9 ■ Two endothelial functions that maintain corneal deturgescence: the leaky barrier and the metabolic pump. (Modified from Waring GO, Bourne WM, Edelhauser HF, and Kenyon KR: The corneal endothelium: normal and pathologic structure and function, Ophthalmology 89:531, 1982.)

cules and water, unlike the zonulae occludentes of the surface epithelial cells. This allows nutrients to freely penetrate the posterior layer of the cornea. The endothelial pump, an energy-dependent mechanism, results in ions being transported from the stroma to the aqueous humor, creating an osmotic gradient that draws water out of the stroma. This allows the stroma to maintain a partially dehydrated state that is necessary for the transmission of light to occur.

Corneal nerves

The cornea is richly supplied with sensory nerves. From 12 to 16 large, radially oriented nerve branches enter the cornea at the mid-stromal level at various clock positions around the limbus. The nerves travel in a radial fashion toward the center of the cornea; they branch horizontally and vertically, forming a dense subepithelial plexus beneath Bowman's layer. From this plexus, axonal extensions pass through Bowman's layer and into the epithelium to provide sensation (Fig. 1-10).

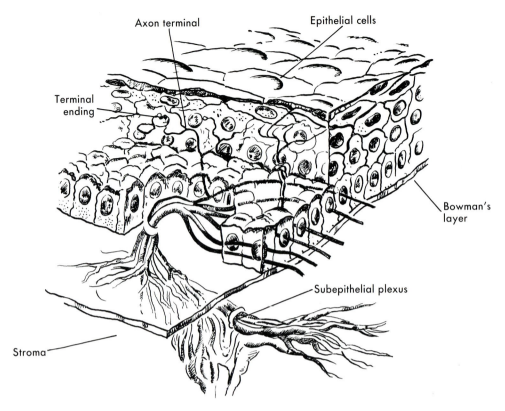

Fig 1-10 ■ Corneal nerves travel through the stroma, pierce Bowman's layer, and then supply sensation to the epithelium. (Modified from Rozsa AJ and Beuerman RW: Density and organization of free nerve endings in the corneal epithelium of the rabbit, Pain 14:105-120, 1981.)

The nerve fibers generally lose their myelin sheaths when they have traversed 1 to 2 mm from the limbus; thus in the periphery of the cornea they often can be seen as fairly thick fibrils.

The cornea is one of the most sensitive tissues of the body, and this sensitivity serves to protect it. It can be exquisitely painful when the nerve endings are exposed, as in corneal abrasions or ulcers.

Precorneal tear film

Functions. The tear film is vital for normal corneal function. It has a number of important roles. It

- 1/moistens and lubricates the anterior surface of the globe; it
- 2/provides a smooth optical surface, which allows a sharp image to be focused on the retina; it
- 3/removes desquamated corneal cells and bacteria; it

- 4/protects the cornea against infection, since it contains an enzyme called lysozyme that can destroy bacteria by acting on their cell·walls; it is the
- 5/main source of oxygen to the corneal epithelium; and it
- 6/provides a slight amount of nourishment to the corneal epithelium, although its glucose concentration is extremely low.

Structure. The anterior surface of the cornea is covered by the tear film, which is composed of three different layers (Fig. 1-11): an anterior lipid layer, a middle aqueous layer, and a posterior mucous layer. The average thickness of the precorneal tear film is 6.5 to 7.5 μ with the aqueous phase constituting the majority of the thickness.

The lipid layer is 0.1 μ thick and is secreted primarily by the meibomian glands located in the tarsal plates of the upper and lower lids. There are approximately 30 to 40 meibomian glands in the upper lid and 20 to 30 smaller

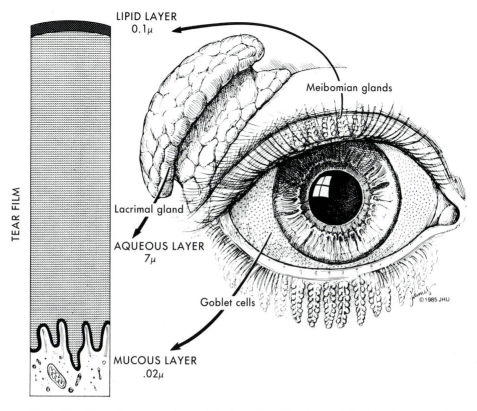

Fig 1-11 ■ Three-layer structure of the tear film. (Courtesy of Dr. AE Maumenee.)

glands in the lower lid. Each gland has an orifice that opens on the lid margin between the tarsal "gray line" and the mucocutaneous junction. The sebaceous glands of Zeis, located at the palpebral margin of the tarsus, and the apocrine glands of Moll, located at the roots of each eyelash, also secrete lipid that is incorporated into the tear film. The lipid layer increases the surface tension of the tear film and decreases its rate of evaporation.

The aqueous layer is 0.7 μ thick and is secreted by the main lacrimal glands and by the accessory glands of Krause and Wolfring. This is the largest component of the tear film and acts to prevent epithelial drying.

The main lacrimal gland provides reflex secretion. This secretion may be in response to a number of different stimuli:

- 1/ Physical irritation of the trigeminal nerve (V_1) fibers that originate from the conjunctiva, cornea, nasal mucosa, or eyelid margins;
- 2/ Psychogenic stimulation; and
- 3/ The effect of bright light on the retina.

The accessory glands of Krause and Wolfring

provide basic secretion. There is no known stimulus for basic tear secretion or specific innervation to the basic tear secretory glands. The glands of Krause comprise two-thirds of the accessory lacrimal glands and are located in the lateral part of the upper fornix proximal to the main lacrimal gland. A variable number of Krause glands are located in the lower fornix. The glands of Wolfring are located along the orbital margin of each tarsus.

The mucous layer is the thinnest; it is approximately 0.02 to 0.05 μ thick. It is secreted by the goblet cells of the conjunctiva and spreads directly over the microplicae of the corneal epithelial cells. This acts to decrease surface tension so that the aqueous component of the tears can spread over and adsorb to the epithelial surface and maintain an intact tear film for 15 to 25 seconds between blinks. Abnormalities of the mucin layer or the epithelial surface will cause the tear film to break up rapidly into dry spots after the resurfacing effect of a blink.

Since the tear film is hypertonic to the corneal stroma, it draws water out of the stroma osmotically. When evaporation of the tears during waking raises the osmolarity, more water is drawn out of the cornea, but when the osmolarity falls during sleep, less fluid is removed from the stroma. Therefore corneal thickness is greatest during eyelid closure.

Eyelid movement is important in tear film distribution. As the eyelids close in complete blink, the superior and inferior fornix are compressed by the force of the preseptal muscles—which are part of the orbicularis muscle—and the lids move toward each other with the upper lid moving over the largest distance and exerting force on the globe. This force clears the anterior surface of debris and expresses sections from the meibomian glands. The lower lid moves horizontally in a nasal direction and pushes tear fluid and debris toward the superior and inferior puncta. When the eyelids are opened, the tear film is redistributed in two steps. Initially, the upper lid pulls the aqueous phase of the tear film by capillary action; secondarily, the lipid layer spreads slowly and upward over the aqueous phase.

Abnormalities in the quantity or quality of the tear film (mucin, aqueous, or lipid layers) or problems with the blink response, which governs the distribution of tears, can create problems for the wearer of contact lenses.

SUMMARY

In this chapter, information on the normal anatomy and physiology of the cornea and tear film is presented. With this background information the contact lens fitter should be able to detect and understand pathophysiologic changes. Medical complications such as the ingrowth of vessels into the cornea, epithelial cysts, corneal edema, abrasions, and corneal ulcers will be discussed in detail in future chapters.

2 ▪ TERMINOLOGY*

- ▪ Types of lenses
- ▪ Design of lenses
- ▪ Rigid or hard lenses
- ▪ Soft lenses
- ▪ Contact lens problems
- ▪ Instrumentation
- ▪ Anatomic and surgical terminology of contact-related areas
- ▪ Glossary

Contact lens jargon is fundamental to following and understanding most of this text. We shall try to clarify the terminology used.

Contact lens refers to any lens that is placed on the surface of the cornea and sclera, either for *optical* purposes (improvement of visual acuity) or for *therapeutic* purposes (treatment of eye disorders).

TYPES OF LENSES

Scleral contact lenses are contact lenses that cover not only the cornea but also the conjunctiva overlying the sclera (Fig. 2-1, *A*). *Corneal contact lenses* are those lenses confined to the cornea (Fig. 2-1, *B*). *Semiscleral lenses* are those that bridge the limbus and lie partially on the conjunctival tissues overlying the sclera adjacent to the limbus (Fig. 2-1, *C*).

Lenses may be *rigid* or *soft* depending on the nature of the material composition. *Extended-wear* or *prolonged-wear lenses* are lenses that are worn for 24 hours or more. *Gas-permeable lenses* are lenses that permit the passage of oxygen and carbon dioxide. Although soft lenses do this, by convention the term *gas-permeable* is used only for rigid lenses. The term *rigid* is primarily a departure from the word *hard* that was

*This chapter reproduced in part from Stein H, Slatt B, and Stein HR: Ophthalmic terminology, ed 12, St Louis, 1988, The CV Mosby Co.

used for the polymethylmethacrylate (PMMA) lenses. *Cosmetic lens* is the term for a colored lens used to cover an unsightly blind eye; this term is sometimes applied to lenses that are used for nonpathologic conditions to enhance cosmetic appearance or as a substitute for spectacles. The lenses replacing spectacles should be referred to as corrective lenses. A *bandage lens* is a contact lens that is used over the cornea to protect the cornea from external influences and to permit healing of underlying corneal disorders. Soft lenses may be also classified according to whether they are *hydrophobic* (fear water) or *hydrophilic* (love water). Soft lenses are made of two different materials: the *hydrogel* and the *nonhydrogel* soft lenses.

DESIGN OF LENSES

The *base curve* of a lens is the curvature of the central portion of the back surface of a lens and is measured in millimeters of radius of an arc. This is the *central posterior curve (CPC)* or *posterior central curve (PCC)*.

The *primary base curve* and all other curvatures of a lens may be expressed in terms of millimeters of radius of curvature. It can also be expressed in diopters—a primary base curve of 43.24 D is equal to 7.8 mm and a 42 D base curve is equal to 8.0 mm radius (see Appendix B). The primary central posterior curve of a lens is designed to conform to the optic zone of the cornea.

The *optic zone* of a lens is the central zone that contains the refractive power and generally corresponds to the central corneal cap.

The *posterior zone* of a lens is the central zone that contains the refractive power and generally corresponds to the central corneal cap.

The *posterior apical radius (PAR)* refers to the radius of curvature of the back surface of a lens at its apex. This is the area of curvature that will conform to the front surface of the apex of

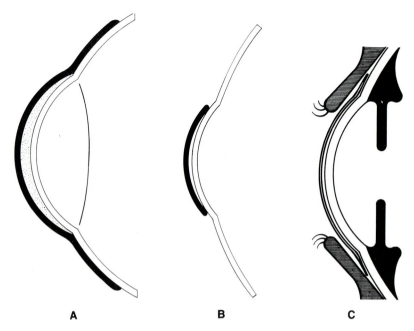

A   B   C

Fig 2-1 ■ A, Scleral contact lens. The contact lens fits over the cornea and sclera. **B,** Corneal contact lens. This is the typical position of the rigid lens. **C,** Semiscleral lens that bridges the limbus and lies partially on the conjunctival lining over the sclera: This is typical of the soft lens. (From Stein HA, Slatt BJ, and Stein RM: Manual of ophthalmic terminology, ed 2, St Louis, 1982, The CV Mosby Co.)

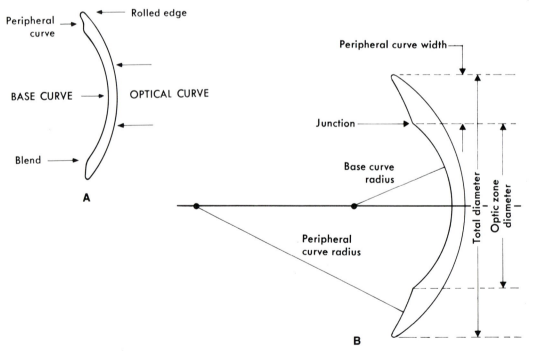

Fig 2-2 ■ A, Bicurve lens design indicating two curves, a primary base curve and a flatter peripheral curve with rolled edges to permit greater comfort. **B,** Same bicurve lens indicating the diameter of the peripheral curve. The combination of the two makes up the total diameter of the lens.

the cornea. This is particularly applicable to the Bausch & Lomb spin-cast Soflens, whose posterior curvature is not uniform. Lenses are labeled by the posterior radius at the apex of the lens.

When a base curve of a lens is said to be made steeper, this means that the posterior radius of curvature is decreased, for example, from 8.4 to 8.1 mm, so that the curvature is now steeper. When the base curve is said to be made flatter, it means that the posterior radius of curvature of the lens is increased, for example, from 8.4 to 8.7 mm, so that the curvature is now flatter.

Most rigid corneal lenses used today are either bicurve or tricurve. A *bicurve lens* has one base curve and one secondary curve (Fig. 2-2). A small lens is usually bicurve. An *intrapalpebral lens*, a lens that fits within the palpebral fissure limits, is bicurve. This type of lens is small and steep, with narrow peripheral curves of 0.2 mm and small diameters of 7.5 to 8.8 mm.

A *multicurve lens* has a base curve and three or more peripheral curves. A *tricurve lens* usu-ally has a large diameter (Fig. 2-3). A contour lens is basically a tricurve lens with a narrow intermediate curve. These latter lenses have an outer *peripheral posterior curve (PPC)* and one or more *intermediate posterior curves (IPC)*. At each junction of these curves there is a *junctional zone*. One can obtain smoothness of this junction by *blending* the zone to remove the sharp junctional line between zones.

Not every lens has a smooth spheric back surface. Some lenses have an *aspheric* or nonspheric back surface that is not of uniform radius but shaped like a parabola. The radius of curvature of these aspheric lenses must be measured at the apex or center of the lens; this measurement is called the *posterior apical radius (PAR)*.

Every contact lens has a diameter or *chord diameter*, which is the width or measurement from one edge of the lens to the opposite edge. Each of the curves referred to previously, the CPC, the PPC, and the IPC, also has its own *curve widths*.

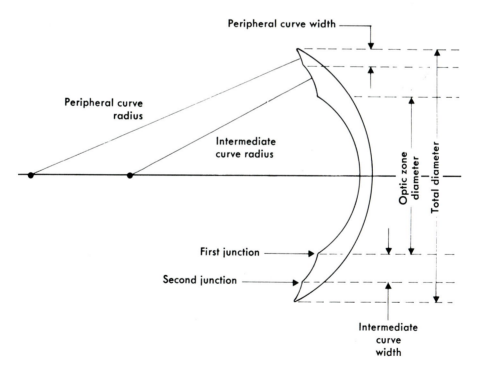

Fig 2-3 ■ A tricurve lens has two peripheral curve radii. The intermediate curve may be very narrow, as found in contour lenses. These lenses have large diameters—9.5 mm or greater—with an optic zone of 6.5 to 7.5 mm, which is just large enough to clear the maximum pupil diameter. The peripheral curves are slightly flatter than the base curves by 0.4 to 0.8 mm with a width of 1.3 mm. With a standard tricurve lens the intermediate curve is 1 mm flatter than the base curve. The peripheral curve is a standard 12.25 mm radius.

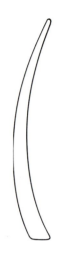

Fig 2-4 ■ Prism ballast to provide weight and stop rotation of a lens. (From Stein HA, Slatt BJ, and Stein RM: The ophthalmic assistant, ed 5, St Louis, 1987, The CV Mosby Co.)

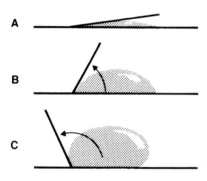

Fig 2-5 ■ The smaller the angle of contact (θ), the greater the spreading of a liquid over a solid. A hard lens is hydrophobic and has a 60-degree angle of contact with water. **A,** Low-wetting angle; **B,** Wetting angle of polymethylmethacrylate rigid lens; **C,** Large wetting angle with droplet of mercury.

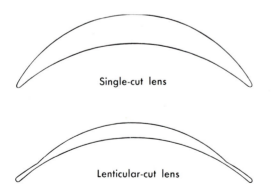

Single-cut lens

Lenticular-cut lens

Fig 2-6 ■ Single-cut and lenticular-cut lenses. (From Stein HA, Slatt BJ, and Stein RM: The ophthalmic assistant, ed 5, St Louis, 1983, The CV Mosby Co.)

The *central thickness* of a lens is the separation between the anterior and posterior surfaces at the geometric center of the lens. The higher the minus power, the thinner the center, whereas the higher the plus power, the thicker the center.

A *ballasted lens* is one that has a cross-sectional shape with a heavier base so that it becomes oriented inferiorly when the lens is worn. It is usually *prism ballasted* because of the use of a prism wedge to weight the lens (Fig. 2-4). A *truncated lens* is one that is cut off to form a horizontal base. The amputation of the lens is usually at the inferior pole of the lens, though superior and inferior truncations have been used. Truncation is frequently used to add stability to a soft toric lens.

The *back vertex power* of a lens refers to the effective power of lens measured from the back surface. The *wetting angle* of a lens is the angle that the edge of a bead of water makes with the surface of the plastic. The smaller the angle, the greater the wetting ability (Fig. 2-5).

Toric lenses or *toroid lenses*, derived from Latin *torus* meaning 'bulge' or 'cushion,' are lenses with different radii of curvature in each meridian. The meridians of the shortest and longest radii are called the *principal meridians* and differ by 90 degrees. These lenses are used to correct astigmatism.

A *front surface toric lens* has an anterior surface with two different radii but a posterior surface that is spheric. A *back surface toric lens* has a posterior surface that has two different radii and an anterior spheric surface. In a *bitoric* lens both the anterior and posterior surfaces have different radii.

Higher power plus lenses are often designed with a *lenticular bowl* or central area that has the appearance of an upside-down bowl-like lens sitting on the underlying lens (Fig. 2-6).

The *sagittal depth* or *height* of a lens is the distance between a flat surface and the back surface of the central portion of the lens. Thus for two lenses of the same diameter but of different sagittal depths, the lens of the greater sagittal depth would produce a greater "vaulting" of the lens and in effect would be steeper (Fig. 2-7). This is often referred to as the *sagittal vault*.

There are two important variables to understanding the mechanism of loosening or tightening a lens. These variables are the diameter and the radius of the lens. If the diameter is kept

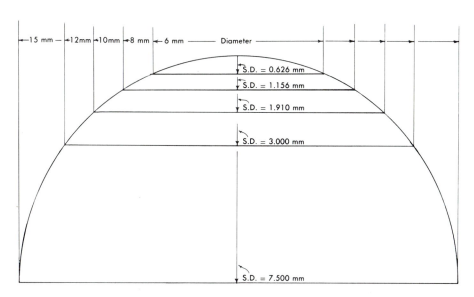

Fig 2-7 ■ A ball-bearing is divided into five sections of different diameters. Compare the varying sagittal depths (S.D.) of one section to another. (From Soper JW and Girard LJ: Designing the corneal lens. In Girard LJ, Soper JW, and Sampson WG, editors: Corneal contact lenses, ed 2, St Louis, 1970, The CV Mosby Co.)

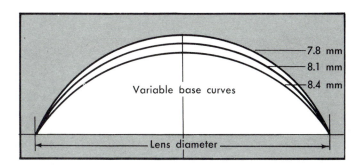

Fig 2-8 ■ If the diameter is held constant, when the radius of curvature is decreased from 8.4 to 7.8 mm, the sagittal height or vault of the lens is increased.

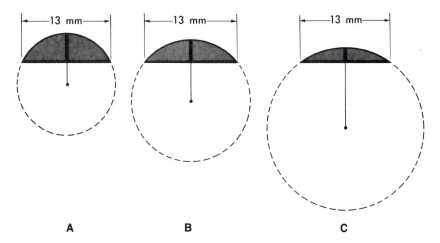

Fig 2-9 ■ **A, B, C,** Three circles of increasing length of radius. If the diameter of a given arc of the circle is kept constant, the sagittal height will decrease from A to C.

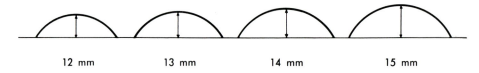

| 12 mm | 13 mm | 14 mm | 15 mm |

Fig 2-10 ■ When the radius is kept constant and the diameter increased, the sagittal height of the lens is increased and the lens becomes steeper.

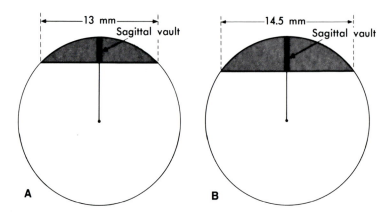

Fig 2-11 ■ If portions of two similar circles are cut off, each with a different diameter, portion B, with the larger 14.5 mm diameter will have a greater sagittal depth or vault than portion A with the smaller 13.0 diameter.

constant, with the radius being changed to a longer one, for example, from 7.8 to an 8.4 mm radius, the sagittal vault or sagittal height of the lens becomes shorter and the lens becomes flatter. The converse is also true (Figs. 2-8 and 2-9).

If the radius of the lens remains the same but the diameter is made larger, for example, from 13 to 15 mm, as occurs with soft lenses, the sagittal vault or sagittal height of the lens is increased and the lens becomes steeper. The converse is also true (Fig. 2-10).

For example, if we consider the lens as being part of a similar circle (Fig. 2-11) and we take two parts of the circle with different diameters, the portion of the circle with the larger diameter will have a greater sagittal vault.

RIGID OR HARD LENSES

Rigid or hard lenses may have a *standard*, or *thin*, thickness. They may be composed of a material made of *polymethylmethacrylate*, sometimes referred to as *PMMA*, a hard transparent plastic with a long history of acceptance. Currently, newer gas permeable materials such as *silicone acrylate* (a combination of silicone and PMMA) and *fluorocarbonate silicone acrylates* have added a new dimension to the contact lens field, within the category of rigid gas-permeable contact lenses.

Types of rigid lenses

The following are the main types of rigid corneal contact lenses. Moreover, each lens type can be modified by such features as lenticular bevels, prisms, fenestration, and truncation.

• *Spherical*. This is the most frequently fitted lens; it has spherical curves on both the anterior and posterior surfaces.

• *Front toric*. This is similar to the spherical lens except that the anterior surface has a cylinder ground onto it. It is used to correct residual (lenticula) astigmatism.

• *Back toric*. The cylinder is on the back surface only; this lens is used for high corneal astigmatism when unstable fit is a problem.

• *Bitoric*. This lens has a minus cylinder curve on the posterior surface and a plus cylinder on the anterior surface. It is used to fit highly cylindric corneas combined with residual astigmatism.

- *Bifocal*. This lens is used to correct presbyopia.
- *Cosmetic*. This is a laminated lens that has opaque iris imprint. It is used to cover disfigured corneas and to create a more acceptable pupil in some cases of aniridia and coloboma of the iris.
- *Aspheric*. This lens, which has a varying base curve, is used to match the anterior surface of an aspheric cornea.

Rigid lenses may be modified by *fenestration*, which is the drilling of one or more holes through the plastic. The lens may be *polished* or the edges refinished by the *Con-Lish method* or the *rag-wheel method*, or by use of a felt discpolisher. This is seldom necessary today because of the existence of gas-permeable contact lenses.

SOFT LENSES

Soft lenses are composed of hydrogel, which is a watery gel-like material. Soft lenses may be manufactured by the *spin-cast process*, which uses liquid material revolving in a given mold at a controlled speed and temperature to produce the resultant curvature, design, and power. Soft lenses may be lathe-cut by a machine lathe that is used to grind lens design, size, and power. Newer automated lathes make reproducibility very accurate and minimize labor costs. New molded lenses are also available today.

Most hydrogel soft lenses are made with HEMA, which stands for *hydroxyethylmethacrylate*, as their base ingredient but are often copolymerized with other materials. There are, however, other nonHEMA materials available such as glycerol methylmethacrylate.

CONTACT LENS PROBLEMS

When a lens or base curve is said to be made *steeper*, it means that the posterior radius of curvature is decreased. When a lens or base curve is said to be made *flatter*, it means the opposite, that the posterior radius of curvature is increased.

Decentration of lens indicates that the lens is sliding off center and may give rise to poor vision or *arcuate staining*, or both. Arcuate staining is arc-like staining in the periphery of the cornea. *Vertical striae* are small vertical lines in the cornea caused by folds in Descemet's membrane and are an early sign of cornea hypoxia. *Limbal compression* occurs with soft lenses that are too tight and cause pressure at the periphery of the

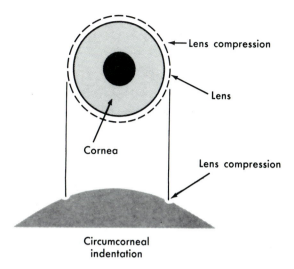

Fig 2-12 ■ The tight lens causes compression at the limbus.

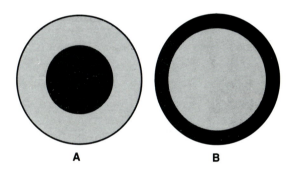

Fig 2-13 ■ **A,** Fluorescein pattern of a flat lens. Note absence of dye centrally. **B,** Fluorescein pattern of a steep lens. Note absence of dye at the periphery because of marginal touch. (From Stein HA, Slatt BJ, and Stein RM: The ophthalmic assistant, ed 5, St Louis, 1988, The CV Mosby Co.)

cornea (Fig. 2-12). *Fluorescein* is a dye used to analyze rigid lens problems because it mixes with the tear film and glows in the presence of ultraviolet light or cobalt blue light (Fig. 2-13).

Modulus is the resistance to change. The higher the modulus, the greater the resistance to change and the more likely the lens is to break; for example, a rubber lens is less likely to break than a glass lens, which has a higher modulus. On the other hand, a lens with greater modulus has less flexure and so provides greater optic performance.

INSTRUMENTATION

An *ophthalmometer* is an instrument designed to measure the radius of curvature of the cornea,

Fig 2-14 ■ **A,** Taking a K reading. **B,** The principle of the keratometer. The visual axis is aligned along the optic axis of the instrument so that the central front surface of the cornea reflects the mires of the keratometer. (**A** from Stein HA, Slatt BJ, and Stein RM: The ophthalmic assistant, ed 5, St Louis, 1988, The CV Mosby Co.)

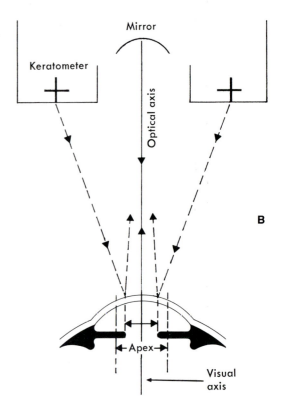

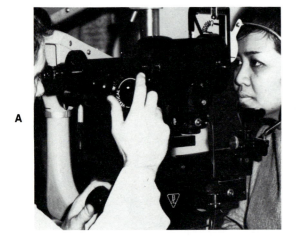

using the mirror effect of the cornea's front surface (Fig. 2-14). This instrument is most commonly referred to as a *keratometer*, the name originated by Bausch & Lomb from *kerato-,* meaning 'horn (cornea)' and *meter,* 'a measure.' The instrument measures a small portion of the *corneal cap* (Fig. 2-15), the central zone of the cornea, and the measurement is often called the *K reading.*

In *astigmatism with the rule* the vertical corneal meridian has the steepest curvature, whereas in *astigmatism against the rule* the horizontal meridian has the steepest curvature (Fig. 2-16).

In performing *keratometry* some authors record the flattest meridian first and the steepest meridian next so that a keratometer (K) value, for example, of 44.00 D × 46.000 D × 85, in-

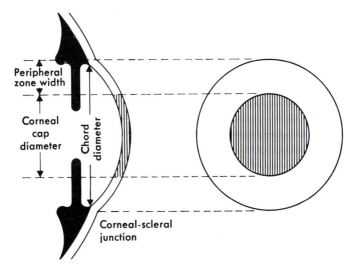

Fig 2-15 ■ Corneal cap, representing the theoretic spheric central zone of the cornea.

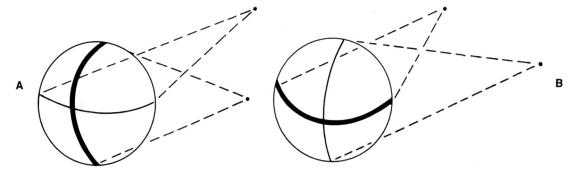

Fig 2-16 ■ A, Astigmatism with the rule. The vertical corneal meridian has the steepest curvature. **B,** Astigmatism against the rule. The horizontal meridian has the steepest curvature.

dicates that the horizontal meridian has a radius of 44.00 D and that the vertical meridian has a radius of 46.00 D with the axis at 85 degrees. Other authors prefer always to record the horizontal meridian first regardless of which is the flattest. This value may be expressed in either diopters or millimeters of radius. Table 2-1 gives a comparative value of the K reading in diopters and millimeters. Each 0.05 mm is equivalent to approximately 0.25 D, so that a 0.5 mm radius equals approximately 2.50 D. Expressed another way, each 1.00 D change in the K reading equals approximately a 0.2 mm radius change.

In lens work one usually first considers the flattest K reading. If the back surface of the lens is to be the same radius as K, this is referred to as "fitting on K." One may fit "steeper than K" as in rigid lens design or "flatter than K" as in soft lens design. In the latter situation the lens will have a posterior radius flatter than the flattest K reading.

The size of the *corneal cap* measured varies with the instrument used but is usually about 3.36 mm chord length. The *mires* of the ophthalmometer are the targets that are reflected back from the cornea (Fig. 2-17). The corneal cap is the central zone of the cornea and has a constant radius of curvature (Fig. 2-15) referred to as the *central posterior curve (CPC)*. The *peripheral* or *paracentral zone* of the cornea is the area surrounding the corneal cap and extending to the limbus. It has a much flatter curvature than does the central curve. The rate of flattening does not conform to a mathemetical progression; that is, the cornea is not a true ellipse; it is generally described as being aspheric.

The *topogometer* is a keratometer attachment with a movable light designed to localize the apical zone or corneal cap of the cornea to be measured by the keratometer. The limiting margin of the apical zone is determined by the points on the corneal surface where the radius of curvature of the cornea begins to flatten. The average diameter of the apical zone is about 6 mm.

Table 2-1 ■ Diopter-to-millimeter conversion

Keratometric reading (D)		Radius convex (mm)	Keratometric reading (D)		Radius convex (mm)	Keratometric reading (D)		Radius convex (mm)
47.75	=	7.07	45.00	=	7.50	42.25	=	8.00
47.50	=	7.11	44.75	=	7.55	42.00	=	8.04
47.25	=	7.14	44.50	=	7.59	41.75	=	8.08
47.00	=	7.18	44.25	=	7.63	41.50	=	8.13
46.75	=	7.22	44.00	=	7.67	41.25	=	8.18
46.50	=	7.26	43.75	=	7.72	41.00	=	8.23
46.25	=	7.30	43.50	=	7.76	40.75	=	8.28
46.00	=	7.34	43.25	=	7.80	40.50	=	8.33
45.75	=	7.38	43.00	=	7.85	40.25	=	8.39
45.50	=	7.42	42.75	=	7.90	40.00	=	8.44
45.25	=	7.46	42.50	=	7.95			

Courtesy Bausch & Lomb, Inc.

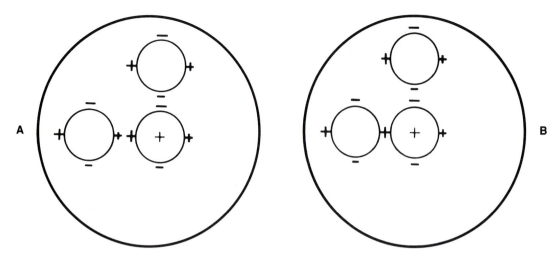

Fig 2-17 ■ Keratometer mires. **A,** Alignment of the mires for axis. **B,** Apposition of the plus mire to measure one meridian of corneal curvature. (From Stein HA, Slatt BJ, and Stein RM: The ophthalmic assistant, ed 5, St Louis, 1988, The CV Mosby Co.)

The topogometer can be used to measure corneal curvature values across multiple points of the cornea.

The *optic spherometer (radiuscope,* a term coined by the American Optical Company, sometimes called a radius gauge) is an instrument that measures the radius of curvature of a rigid contact lens. A *dial thickness gauge* is used to measure the thickness of a rigid contact lens.

A *profile analyzer* is an instrument used to assess the junctional zone blending of a hard lens (Fig. 2-18). A *shadowgraph* is an instrument that projects and magnifies a contact lens. It is used to examine defects in a lens and to determine measurements.

A *wet cell* or *hydrometric chamber* is used to retain a soft lens for evaluation and measurements of power and edge configuration (Fig. 2-

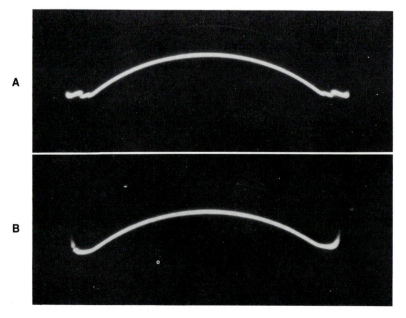

Fig 2-18 ■ **A,** Poorly finished transition zone as determined by the profile analyzer. **B,** Perfect transition zone with ski contour at its periphery.

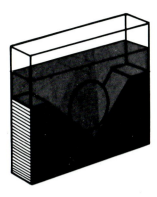

Fig 2-19 ■ Water cell used to measure power of a soft lens in the hydrated state. The soft lens is floated in normal saline solution and measured in a regular lensometer. (From Stein HA, Slatt BJ, and Stein RM: Manual of ophthalmic terminology, ed 2, St Louis, 1982, The CV Mosby Co.)

19). *Templates* are small elevated plastic domes of known radius of curvature for evaluation of base curves of soft lenses in a number of existing soft lens analyzers.

The *photokeratoscope* is an instrument that photographs the front surface of the eye and provides a permanent record of a large corneal area.

ANATOMIC AND SURGICAL TERMINOLOGY OF CONTACT-RELATED AREAS
Cornea

The cornea is a clear, transparent, structure with a brilliant, shiny surface. *Kerato-*, from Greek meaning 'horn,' is the prefix pertaining to the cornea. Ancient Greeks believed that the cornea resembled a thinly sliced horn of an animal.

When a cornea becomes cone shaped, the condition of *keratoconus*, or *conic cornea*, exists. If an inflammation *(-itis)* affects the cornea, it is called *keratitis*. A corneal transplant is referred to as a *keratoplasty*. A transplant may be penetrating, in which full-thickness layers of the cornea are replaced with a full-thickness layer from a donor, or a *lamellar section*, in which the outer two thirds of the cornea is replaced. *Refractive keratoplasty*, introduced by José Barraquer in 1949, refers to surgical procedures to modify corneal curvature and alter refractive errors. *Keratomileusis*, derived through Spanish from Greek words meaning 'cornea' and 'carving' *(mi-*

leusis), incorporates a lamellar section of the patient's own cornea layer in either a positive or negative fashion and is used to correct either myopic or hyperopic refractive errors. *Keratophakia* is a surgical alteration of the anterior radius of curvature of the cornea in which a positive lenticule *(phakos)* is cut from a fresh donor cornea and is incorporated within the patient's corneal stroma. This is presently being used to eliminate aphakic and hyperopic refractive errors. *Radial keratotomy* is a surgical procedure in which clocklike radial incisions are made into the cornea to flatten it centrally and correct myopic refractive errors. *Epikeratophakia* is a procedure designed and popularized by Kaufman, MacDonald and co-workers in which a lenticule of donor cornea is sutured at the margins to a patient's cornea that is denuded of epithelium. *Keratoprosthesis* is an artificial synthetic cornea, which is implanted into the corneal substance for visual rehabilitation in severely scarred corneas in almost blind eyes. It is usually of a plastic material, of hydrogel or polysulfur.

A surgical instrument used to open the anterior chamber by cutting the cornea is called a *keratome*, from *tomos* meaning 'a cutting.'

The *limbus* is the annular border between the clear cornea and the opaque scleral conjunctival area. Other anatomic areas of interest are depicted in Fig. 2-20.

Eyelids

The globe is covered externally by the eyelids to protect it from injury and excessive light and to spread a thin film of tears over the cornea. From *blepharo-*, Greek meaning 'eyelid,' we derive words such as *blepharoplasty*, referring to any plastic surgery performed on the eyelid, and *blepharoptosis*, drooping eyelids. The muscle that elevates the eyelid is the *levator palpebrae superioris*, from Latin *levator*, 'one that raises,' *palpebra*, 'eyelid,' and *superioris*, 'upper.' The triangular spaces at the junction of the upper and lower lids are called *canthi* from Greek *kanthos*, meaning 'angle.' (Fig. 2-21). These canthi are denoted by the terms *medial* or *lateral*, the former being close to the nasal bridge because it is toward the 'middle' of the head. A surgical procedure to correct defects in the canthus is called *canthoplasty*. To open the angle, the procedure of *canthotomy* is performed.

In the medial angle of the eyelids is the *carun-*

Sclera   Limbus

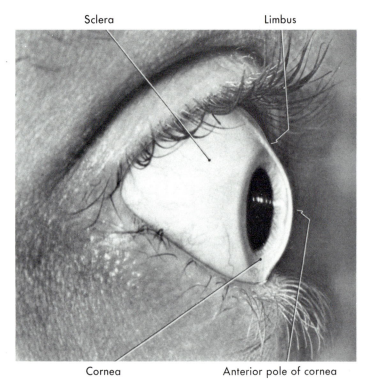

Cornea   Anterior pole of cornea

Fig 2-20 ■ The eye in side profile. (Courtesy Eastman Kodak Co., Rochester, NY.)

Orbital portion of lid ⎯   ⎯ Superior
                                                   palpebral furrow

Tarsal portion of lid ⎯

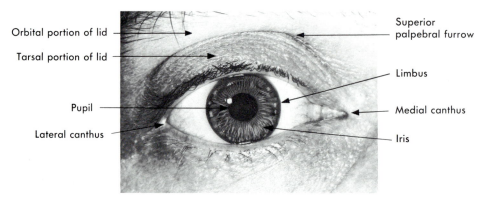

                                                ⎯ Limbus

Pupil ⎯   ⎯ Medial canthus

Lateral canthus ⎯   ⎯ Iris

Fig. 2-21 ■ Surface anatomy of the eye. (From Stein HA and Slatt BJ: The ophthalmic assistant, ed 5, St Louis, 1983, The CV Mosby Co.)

cle, from Latin meaning 'little piece of flesh,' because this is a fleshy mound on the eye (Fig. 2-22). Adjacent to it lies a fold, the *plica semilunaris* from Latin *plica*, 'a fold' and *semilunaris*, 'half-moon shaped,' because the tissue is folded over like a half-moon and was originally a remnant of the third eyelid as found in lower animals.

The eyelids have as part of their structure hard plates called *tarsi* from Greek *tarsos*, a term used by the ancient Greeks for a wickerwork frame or various flattened objects such as a flat basket, the sole of a foot, the rudder of a ship, the blades of oars, the stretched-out wing, and the edge of the eyelid. Because of the flatness of the eyelid, the term *tarsus* was applied to the fibrocartilaginous plate that is found in the eyelid, both upper and lower.

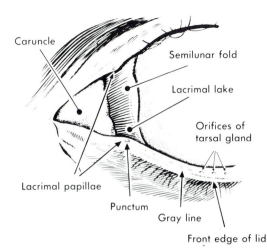

Caruncle

Semilunar fold

Lacrimal lake

Orifices of
tarsal gland

Lacrimal papillae

Punctum

Gray line

Front edge of lid

Fig 2-22 ■ Inner canthus, showing the semilunar fold and the caruncle. Normally the punctum is not visible unless the lower lid is depressed. (From Stein HA, Slatt BJ, and Stein RM: *The ophthalmic assistant*, ed 5, St Louis, 1988, The CV Mosby Co.)

Within the tarsal plate of the eyelid lie the *meibomian glands* named after Heinrich Meibom (1638-1700), who published the first accurate description of these secreting glands. A disorder of the glands gives rise to a *chalazion*, a word derived from Greek meaning 'little lump' or 'little hailstone' because of the similarity of this lump in the eyelid to the appearance of a hailstone.

Oxygen studies

Terminology pertaining to oxygen studies has taken an increasing importance in the contact lens literature because of the development of extended wear lenses and gas-permeable contact lenses. Investigators such as Miguel Refojo, Irving Fatt, Robert Mandell, Brian Holden, Richard Hill, and others have contributed significantly to our understanding in this area.

The oxygen transmission through a given material is a laboratory measurement, often referred to as the *DK value*, where *D* is the diffusion coefficient for oxygen movement in lens material and *K* is the solubility coefficient of oxygen in the material. It should be noted that a coefficient is a measure of a physical or chemical property that is constant for a system under specific conditions. The DK, or permeability, is characteristic of a given material obtained in a given condition at a given temperature in the laboratory only. The *oxygen flux* is the amount of oxygen that will pass through a given area of the material in a given amount of time driven by a given partial pressure difference of oxygen across the material. It is a function of the DK of the material, the lens thickness, and the pressure drop across the lens, ΔP.

$$\text{Oxygen flux} = \left(\frac{DK}{L}\right) \Delta P$$

L is the thickness of the central optical zone.

D is the diffusion coefficient for oxygen movement.

K is the solubility of oxygen in that material.

Low-flux materials. PMMA, HEMA, CAB, and some gas-permeable PMMA lenses.

Medium-flux plastics. Hard silicone, ultrathin or high-water-content hydrogels, silicone-organic copolymers.

High-flux materials. Pure silicone resins and elastomers, very high-water-content hydrogels and fluorocarbon silicone acrylate lenses.

When a lens is made thinner, more oxygen will pass through the material and so thickness becomes an important aspect of lens performance. The term *oxygen transmissibility* is used to indicate the oxygen permeability (DK) divided by the thickness of the lens, *L*, so that

$$DK/L = \text{oxygen transmissibility}$$

Of more meaningful and clinical importance is how much total oxygen passes through a lens and is permitted to reach the cornea. There are *in vivo* (in the living body) measurements. They involve the total lens and take into account not only the material but also the design of the lens. This measurement is called the EOP, or *equivalent oxygen performance*.

COMMENT. Water content alone does not ensure a high equivalent oxygen performance.

GLOSSARY

The following glossary provides some additional definitions and terms arranged alphabetically.

absorb: take in; soft lenses absorb water.

acid/alkali: two physical characteristics that neutralize each other. Solutions are made acid or alkali in order to perform specific functions.

annular bifocal contact: A lens with distance portion ground into the center of the lens and near ground into the periphery.

anoxia: a diminished supply of oxygen.

aphakic lenses: contact lenses designed for postcataract fitting.

apical zone of cornea: area of the central portion of the cornea with a constant radius of curvature. Sometimes called the corneal cap.

artificial tears: wetting agents for the cornea to supplement the loss of tear formation (methylcellulose, Liquifilm, and so on).

aspheric lens: a continuous lens with an elliptic or parabolic shape that has a flatter peripheral curvature.

bactericide: a chemical that disinfects and kills pathogenic organisms.

benzalkonium chloride: a preservative used in eye solutions because of its germicidal qualities.

binding: joining with as in protein-binding, when something joins with protein.

biocompatible: lenses that do not irritate the eye in any way are considerd to be biocompatible.

biomicroscopy: microscopic examination of the cornea, anterior chamber lens, and posterior chamber contents with a slitlamp (biomicroscope). The magnification is approximately 10 to 50 times.

bullous keratopathy: total swelling of the cornea with painful blister formation at the epithelial level, treated frequently with a therapeutic soft lens.

Burton lamp: an ultraviolet light used to excite the fluorescein dye that is used to analyze the fit of a rigid contact lens.

BUT: see *tear film breakup time* (BUT).

catalyst: an agent that produces a change in the rate of a reaction, as in the neutralization of hydrogen peroxide.

chord length: the straight-line measurement of the contact-lens diameter from edge to edge, distinguished from the slightly larger linear measurement of surface curvature.

chlorhexidine: a chemical used for disinfection.

chlorobutanol: an antimicrobial agent used in soaking solutions.

circumcorneal identation: circular depression caused by lens (Fig. 2-23).

circumcorneal injection: redness around the limbus of the eyes surrounding the cornea (Fig. 2-23).

compatible: lenses are tested to determine if they react with solutions used with them. If there is no reaction they are considered compatible.

conjunctivitis, giant papillary: see *giant papillary hypertrophy* (GPH).

contact lens blank: a sheet or rod of plastic, which may be methylmethacrylate or hydroxyethylmethacrylate or gas-permeable material used to make either hard or soft lenses.

contact lens wetting angle: the angle between the liquid and lens surface.

contaminant: something not wanted in a solution or on lenses, such as dirt and micro-organisms.

contour lens: a tricurve lens designed to conform to the curvature of the cornea, which flattens as it extends in the periphery.

copolymer: two or more chemicals that are combined to form a new chemical compound.

corneal cap: the apical zone or central zone of the cornea that has a constant area of curvature.

corneal diameter: the diameter of the cornea, usually taken along the horizontal meridian with a ruler, caliper, or reticule; see also *visible iris diameter*.

corneal edema: swelling of the cornea caused by hypoxia or insufficient oxygen.

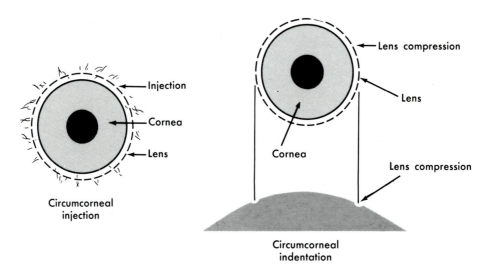

Fig 2-23 ■ Circumcorneal injection and circumcorneal indentation at the limbus. Notice considerable vascularity. (From Stein HA, Slatt BJ, and Stein RM: The ophthalmic assistant, ed 5, St Louis, 1988, The CV Mosby Co.)

dehydration: the drying out of a soft lens.

deturgescence, corneal: the state of relative dehydration maintained by the normal intact cornea that enables it to remain transparent.

diagnostic fitting set: a limited set of trial lenses used to gain a dynamic overview of the fit of a contact lens.

discoloration: a change in color of a contact lens.

disinfection: physical or chemical procedures that kill common pathogenic organisms but may permit some nonpathogenic organisms to survive.

DK value: A measure of the oxygen permeability through a given material where D is the diffusion coefficient for oxygen movement in the lens material and K is the solubility of oxygen in this material.

double slap-off lenses: sometimes called thick-thin lenses; the upper and lower portions of the lens are reduced in thickness so that when the lens is placed on the eye these portions lie under the upper and lower eyelids. The thin zones aid in stabilizing toric soft lenses.

dry spots: areas of drying as noted by absent areas of fluorescein-stained tear film on the cornea when the patient stares.

Dyer nomogram system of lens ordering: a simplified system of ordering PMMA rigid lenses based on clinical experience, corneal topometry, and charts of associated lens parameters.

EDTA: see *ethylenediamine tetraacetate*.

elasticity: the ability of a lens to stretch and return to the same configuration; lens memory.

endophthalmitis: an inflammation of the entire eye including the outer coats.

enzyme cleaner: a cleaning agent that acts on a soft lens by a digestion of protein.

epithelial edema: edema of the superficial layer of the cornea.

esthesiometer (Cochet-Bonnet): a device used to evaluate corneal sensitivity, consisting essentially of a nylon thread mounted in a handle so that its length may be varied and calibrated in milligrams of weight necessary to bend a given length of the thread when pressed against the cornea.

ethylenediamine tetraacetate (EDTA): a chemical used for disinfection.

eversion of the eyelid: the folding back of the eyelid on itself.

finished lens: a complete lens with anterior and posterior curves, a specified diameter, a designated peripheral curve, and edge design.

fitting set: a complete inventory of trial lenses of graduated powers and base curves.

flare: flutterings or fringing of lights, caused by a lens with an optic zone too small, a decentered lens, or an excessively loose lens.

flat cornea: a cornea with a K value less than 41 D.

fluid lens: power created by having a very convex or concave tear film; in most cases the power of the tear film is negligible because this layer is too thin (less than 0.02 mm) to have an appreciable effect on the power of the lens.

fluorescein: an organic compounds that is inert and used to stain the tear film for contact lens fitting and to assess the integrity of the cornea.

galilean telescope: a telescope with a minus ocular lens combined with a plus objective lens.

gas-permeable: lenses that allow gas to pass through the contact lens. The most important gas is oxygen.

germicide: a chemical, such as chlorhexidine, used for disinfection.

giant papillary hypertrophy (GPH): large elevated papules on the tarsal conjunctiva. Usually associated with soft lens wear but can occur with any contact lens. It is regarded as an autoimmune response to the patient's own protein. Also referred to as *giant papillary conjunctiva (GPC)*

GPC (giant papillary conjunctivitis): see *giant papillary hypertrophy*.

haptic: the part of a contact or intra-ocular lens that supports the optic portion and touches the peripheral portion of the cornea; the word indicates 'fastening, contact, sense of touch.' More widely used with intra-ocular lenses.

Harrison-Stein nomogram: a series of lens specifications for the initial prescribing of gas-permeable contact lens from silicone-PMMA material or fluoronated silicone acrylate material.

hydration: the process of adding water. Rinsing and storing solutions are good lens-hydrating agents.

hydrogen peroxide: a bactericide used for soft lenses.

hydrophilic: lenses that are wettable by water, that have an affinity for water.

hypoxia: low in oxygen.

hyprophobic: lenses that are not wettable by water.

hysteresis: phenomenon in which a lens, when subjected to stress, slowly changes its form.

keratitis: inflammation of the cornea.

keratoconjunctivitis sicca: drying of the cornea and conjunctiva.

keratomalacia: softening of the cornea.

Korb lens: a PMMA lens that is fitted in a position on the superior portion of the cornea, regardless of weight or power, and designed to move vertically over the cornea when blinking as if attached to the upper eyelid.

LD + 2: the longest diameter (LD) of the optic zone plus 2 mm (for the intermediate and peripheral curves) yields the diameter of a lens; determined by use of the topogometer.

lenticular lens: relatively large lens most suitable for large, flat eyes; consists of a central optic zone and a surrounding non-optic flange.

limbal zone: junction of the periphery of the cornea and the sclera.

loose lens: a contact lens with excessive movement; it can be caused by a lens that is too small in diameter, too thick, or too flat.

lubricate: to make slippery or smooth by applying a solution.

magnification: the ratio of image size to object size.

methylcellulose: a wetting agent.

micro-organisms: small living organisms such as bacteria and viruses that are seen only with the aid of a microscope.

microthin lens: a lens less than 0.10 mm in thickness.

minus carrier: a lens designed with an edge configuration similar to that of a minus lens that is thicker at its periphery; often used with high-plus lenses such as aphakic lenses.

monovision: single-vision contact lenses used for presbyopic people for whom the power of the lenses is such that one eye is used for distance vision and the other is used for near vision.

Morgan's dots: small discrete subepithelial cornea opacities resulting from corneal hypoxia.

nomogram: a table of precalculated mathematical values used to arrive at the specifications of a rigid lens design.

orthokeratology: the technique of flattening the cornea and thus correcting refractive errors by the use of a series of progressively flatter contact lenses.

overwearing syndrome: a misnomer for acute corneal hypoxia characterized by a latent interval after removal of the lens; extreme pain and congestion of lids, cornea, and conjunctiva are experienced. It is more common with rigid lenses.

oxygen flux: a measure of the amount of oxygen that will pass through a given area of material in a given unit of time.

oxygen permeability: the degree to which a lens permits the passage of oxygen across it. It depends on composition of the plastic (that is, silicone has excellent permeability, whereas PMMA has no permeability), the thickness of the lens, and its water content. It is often expressed as the DK value.

oxygen transmissibility: the ability of a lens to permeate oxygen to flow through the cornea. It is the oxygen permeability demanded by the thickness of the material.

pachometer, pachymeter: an instrument used to measure the thickness of the cornea and depth of the anterior chamber; the spelling "pachometer" is etymologically preferable to "pachymeter," a frequent usage.

pathogenic organism: an organism that causes disease.

photokeratoscope: an instrument designed to photograph annular rings of the cornea and to aid in making a contact lens that will contour to the cornea. The data are often fed to a computer for a readout for a lens design.

photophobia: sensitivity to light.

Placido's disc: a disc with concentric rings to determine the regularity of the cornea when its reflection is revealed on the corneal surface.

plano lens: a lens with zero power.

polymer: a chain of linked molecular units of dimension greater than 5 monomer units.

polymerization: the union of molecules of a compound to form larger molecules and a new compound.

polyvinyl alcohol: a wetting agent.

polyvinylpyrrolidone (PVP): a polymer often copolymerized with other plastics in hydrogel lenses.

preservative: a preservative is added to a solution to ensure that the solution remains sterile under normal conditions of use by destroying or inhibiting the multiplication of micro-organisms.

prism ballast lens: contact lens with based-down prism added inferiorly to improve the stability of the lens. Usually 1 to 1.5 D prism is added.

protein; mucins, lipids: substances found in tears. May be adsorbed to lenses and cause loss of clarity.

PVP: see *polyvinylpyrrolidone*.

quaternary ammonium chloride: known commonly as *quat*, it is a compond used for disinfecting contact lenses.

residual astigmatism: the astigmatism present after corneal astigmatism has been nullified by a contact lens. It is usually created by the lens of the eye.

retro-illumination: light is focused on deeper structures such as the iris, while the microscope is adjusted to study the cornea; best method of showing fine corneal edema.

Schirmer test: measures normal tear secretion; the ability of the eye to wet in 5 minutes 15 mm of a 5×35 mm strip of filter paper.

scratched lens: a defect in the lens surface consisting of a groove and ridge.

semifinished blank: a contact lens blank in which the posteior curve of the contact lens has been fabricated.

semifinished lens: a polished lens with an anterior and a posterior curvature.

soaking solution: a solution designed to keep a lens moist and free from contamination.

Soper lens: a rigid lens designed by Joseph Soper with a steep central posterior curve to accommodate large cones of keratoconus (Fig. 2-24).

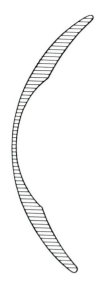

Fig 2-24 ■ Soper cone lens for keratoconus. There is a steep central posterior curve and a much flatter flange surrounding it. (From Stein HA and Slatt BJ: The ophthalmic assistant, ed 5, St Louis, 1983, The CV Mosby Co.)

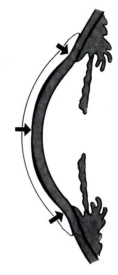

Fig 2-25 ■ Three-point touch—a normally fitting soft lens will rest lightly at the apex and at the periphery of the cornea.

spectacle blur: blurred vision that lasts for 30 minutes or longer after a rigid lens is removed and spectacles are used.

specular reflection: a reflection from a mirror surface, such as the back of the cornea.

spheric equivalent: It is the spheric power of the lens plus half the cylindric power. It represents the dioptric power of a cylindric or spherocylindric lens from the vertex to the plane of the circle of least confusion (the midpoint of the interval of Sturm).

SPK: see *superficial punctate keratitis*.

stable vision: visual acuity that does not fluctuate.

sterilization: a method to ensure the complete death of all forms of bacteria, fungi, and spores.

stippling: dotlike staining of the cornea.

superficial punctate keratitis (SPK): diffuse stippling of the cornea of multiple causes.

surfactant: a cleaner that acts on the surface of a contact lens.

taco test: a test whereby one can determine that a soft contact lens is not inside out by grasping the lens near its apex and folding it so that the edge will roll in like a Mexican taco if it is not everted. The test is not effective with ultrathin hydrogel lenses.

tear film breakup time (BUT): an evaluation of tear quality; the tear film will normally break up in 10 to 30 seconds and show dry spots. Any dry spot that appears in less than 10 seconds is pathologic.

tears: a composite of secretions from lacrimal glands, accessory glands of Kraus and Wolfring, mucin-secreting goblet cells of the conjunctiva, meibomian-secreting tarsal glands, and oil-secreting glands of Teis.

thermal disinfection: disinfection of a lens by heat.

thickness of a lens: the measurement of the center of a lens; a variable that depends on the posterior vertex power, the central base curve, the index of refraction of the lens material, and the lens diameter.

thimerosal (Merthiolate): a mercurial agent used for disinfection and found in contact lens' solutions.

three and nine o'clock staining: erosion of the cornea at the 3 and 9 o'clock positions; seen usually in patients wearing rigid lenses.

three-point touch: a lens that rests on the sclera and on the center of the cornea (Fig. 2-25).

tight lens: a lens that has minimal or no movement.

transitional zone: that area of the cornea between the apical zone and the limbal zone.

Trantas's dots: small peripheral limbal infiltrations caused by delayed hypersensitivity, as seen in vernal conjunctivitis.

truncation: a design feature used in toric lenses to reduce lens rotation by the cutting off of a peripheral portion of the lens to conform with the lower lid border.

ulceration of the cornea: a large defect in the cornea that may be caused by hypoxia, trauma, or infection.

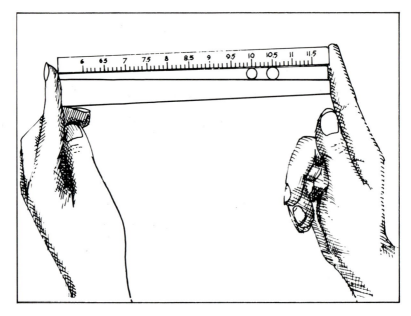

Fig 2-26 ■ V-groove diameter gauge. The lens is inserted at the widest opening and allowed to slide to its position of rest, where the diameter reading is obtained.

V-groove gauge: a ruler measure with a groove to measure the diameter of a rigid lens (Fig. 2-26).

vascularization: increased blood vessels occurring in a cornea.

VID: see *visible iris diameter*.

visible iris diameter (VID): a term that represents the iris diameter and aids in selecting the initial lens; often used in place of the term *corneal diameter*.

warpage: a permanent bending of a rigid lens. May also refer to a semipermanent altering of the corneal curvature.

wet storage: the use of soaking solution to store rigid contact lenses.

wetting solution: solutions that increase the spreading or wettability of liquids on the plastic contact lens by converting the surface of a lens from a hydrophobic to a hydrophilic surface.

X-CHROM lens: a red contact lens designed to aid the person with partial red-green color blindness.

xerophthalmia: a state of dryness of the eyes; conjunctivitis with atrophy and absent fluid discharge that produces a dry, lusterless condition of the eyeball.

xerosis: dying and keratinization of the tissues, usually the conjunctiva, seen most clearly when stained with rose bengal stain.

3 ▪ ASSESSMENT OF THE PROSPECTIVE CONTACT LENS WEARER

- ▪ General considerations
- ▪ The eyelids
- ▪ Tear film assessment
- ▪ Tear deficiency—an analysis to consider before fitting
- ▪ Role of blinking
- ▪ Corneal disorders that should be identified
- ▪ Assessment of a new lens wearer
- ▪ Slitlamp assessment
- ▪ When to refit

GENERAL CONSIDERATIONS

Contact lens fitters tend to be cornea oriented. They look to the cornea for guidance in their base curve, optic zone, and diameter. In fact, they only look at a small segment of the cornea, that is the apical spheric portion called the *corneal cap*. In the fitting with this type of approach the K measurements along with the refraction are sent to the laboratory, and a lens is made. Surprisingly enough, this method works a high percentage of the time. However, if a fitter wants better results and enjoys the pride of doing excellent work, there are a few other variables that must be considered—the eyelids, blinking patterns, tear film, and the general health of the eye and cornea.

The most neglected areas are the tear film and its layers and components. A poor or inadequate tear film will ruin the best of efforts. Blinking is also important, especially with a rigid lens. The full blink response provides tear exchange (venting) and moves the lens to sustain centration.

THE EYELIDS

The lids have to be studied. If the lids are tight, a rotational force may be exerted on the lens or the lens may be drawn up to ride high. Also the lid configuration determines the size of the palpebral fissure opening, which in turn has a direct influence on the size of the palpebral fissure. A small palpebral fissure may preclude the use of a large lens. A retracted lid may cause lid impact, and a lid with ptosis may not move the lens sufficiently to cause a tear exchange.

The inside tarsal surface has to be inspected. Any lens including rigid lenses can cause giant papillary conjunctivitis, an autoimmune inflammatory condition combined with foreign body irritation of the upper tarsal conjunctival surface. Some persons have this problem before they wear lenses, and the condition becomes aggravated by the lens. These persons may have vernal catarrhal or atopic allergies and may be poor candidates for contact lenses.

The lower lid may be important. If a truncated lens is used, the lower lid cannot be too close to the margin of truncation because it will displace the lens upward or, more commonly, tip the lateral side of the lens in a clockwise rotational manner. The lower lid orientation, be it oblique, S shaped, low, or lax, is especially significant in the use of bifocal toric lenses.

TEAR FILM ASSESSMENT

The tear film is vital. Not only does it provide oxygen exchange as the lens is moved, but it also passes lysozyme, an antibacterial enzyme that inhibits bacterial proliferation.

Patients with a tear deficiency are more prone to infections and often cannot be fit comfortably with lenses. Ideally each patient should have the following:
1. A rose bengal test to stain areas of devitalized tissue.
2. A Schirmer test with and without a local anesthetic. Wetting of the paper strip 10 mm within 5 minutes is considered satisfactory.
3. BUT (tear film breakup time). Disruption of

the tear film without blinking in less than 10 seconds is considered unsatisfactory.

4. Corneal assessment for erosions. If the dryness is severe enough to cause pitting of the corneal epithelium, rigid lenses should not be used. Not only is there a greater risk of infection but a portal of entry is also created. Associated findings that do not augur well for the contact lens patient include blepharitis and chronic conjunctivitis.

Serious problems can be anticipated. Suspect dry eye cases in menopausal women, women on birth-control pills, and patients with various forms of arthritis. Also normal tear production may be hampered by drugs taken orally such as antihistamines, belladonna derivatives, and some tranquilizers.

Contamination of the tear film may be patient-induced by rubbing of the eyes with dirty fingers or be a consequence of high bacterial skin and conjunctival flora as found in acne rosacea.

COMMENT. Contact lenses, whether rigid or soft, by themselves do not cause an increase in the normal pathogens found in the eye. The contamination, if active, is usually external from dirty cases, dirty fingers, and so on. A higher conjunctival bacterial count may be encountered in acne rosacea, seborrhea, and ordinary acne. If such patients suffer from recurrent blepharoconjunctivitis or have recurrent hordeolum, they may be poor candidates for lenses.

TEAR DEFICIENCY—AN ANALYSIS TO CONSIDER BEFORE FITTING

The most common type of dry eye situation clinically found is *keratoconjunctivitis sicca*. In this condition there is a loss of the aqueous component of tears from the lacrimal gland.

Diseases commonly associated with tear deficiency include

Rheumatoid arthritis
Lupus erythematosus
Periarteritis nodosa
Sjögren's syndrome (keratoconjunctivitis sicca)—dry eyes, dry mouth, and arthritis

Other causes include

Drugs such as belladonna derivatives
Menopause—hormonal changes

Normal tears are secreted at a low level—1 microliter per minute. The water-soluble components include proteins, inorganic salts, glu-

cose, and oxygen. Aqueous tears form the *middle layer* of the tear film. This component is secreted by the lacrimal gland (Fig. 3-1).

The *top layer* is a *lipid film* over the aqueous layer. It is an oily layer secreted by the meibomian glands. Its function is to prevent evaporation of the tear film. Deficiencies in this section of the layer are rare.

The *inner layer* is the *mucin film* obtained as a secretion of the goblet cells of the conjunctiva. Its purpose is to change the corneal epithelial hydrophobic surface to a hydrophilic surface upon which aqueous tears can spread. Mucin deficiency can be encountered in the following:

Stevens-Johnson disease
Ocular pemphigoid
Alkali burns

Signs of dry eyes:

Viscous mucous strands
Superficial epithelial erosions highlighted with rose bengal or fluorescein

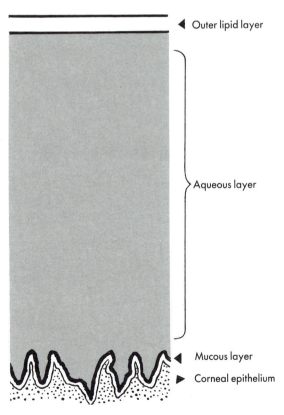

◄ Outer lipid layer

> Aqueous layer

◄ Mucous layer
► Corneal epithelium

Fig 3-1 ■ Three-layer structure of the tear film. (From Stein HA, Slatt BJ, and Stein RM: The ophthalmic assistant, ed 4, St Louis, 1983, The CV Mosby Co.)

Increased BUT (tear film breakup time), less than 10 seconds

Increased incidence of infection in terms of chronic conjunctivitis and blepharitis. These complications occur because of a loss of the normal antibacterial tear substances, lysozyme, β-lactam, and lactoferrin.

Positive Schirmer's test, wetting less than 5 mm after a piece of filter paper is placed into the lower conjunctival sac in a nonanesthetized eye for 5 minutes.

People with dry eyes or relatively dry eyes may make poor candidates for any contact lens. In a marginally dry eye a thin soft lens or a high water content soft lens with supplementary artificial tear drops can be used. Frequently a rigid lens works better in dry eye cases. This paradox occurs because the soft hydrated lens may cause an osmotic shift of fluid into the soft lens, making the tear film even drier.

ROLE OF BLINKING

Poor blinking habits can make a well-fitted lens create as many symptoms as an ill-fitted one. The front surface of the lens becomes misty because of drying and lack of polishing by the lids, vision suffers, and in addition the lens does not move properly. The tear film under the lens becomes stagnant and corneal edema ensues. Such a situation can create mild symptoms of burning and photophobia or create such distress that continued wear of the lens is intolerable.

An equally disturbing event occurs when a patient does not have a full and upward Bell's response. In such a person, the eyes do not roll up and out. Instead, the eyes may not move or actually roll slightly downward. If the lids are not totally closed with sleep, the exposed corneas may show signs of dryness or desiccation. Such a person frequently wakes up in the morning with a grittiness in the eyes. Poor blinkers and people with a paradoxical Bell's response should not be wearing rigid lenses.

A normal blink is executed by the pretarsal fibers of the orbicular muscle. It is an automatic reflex movement. It should be distinguished from voluntary lid closure, which requires the action of the pretarsal, preseptal, and orbital segments of the orbicular muscle. The latter is a much stronger action and is accompanied by Bell's phenomenon. Patients with blinking problems are frequently instructed in voluntary lid-closure movements when it is the light pretarsal-mediated blink that must be restored to normal.

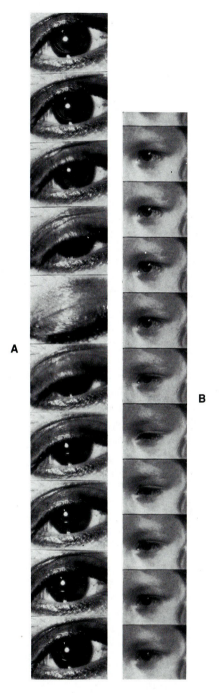

A

B

Fig 3-2 ■ **A,** Movement of the lens with blinking. The lens is initially depressed, then elevated, and then gently drops to a central position. **B,** Incomplete blink. The lid is never fully depressed. It halts its downward progression at the margin of the lens. (From Girard LJ, editor: Corneal contact lenses, St Louis, 1970, The CV Mosby Co.)

COMMENT. If blinking exercises are done, the second and third fingers should be placed just on the skin beyond the lateral canthus. Contraction of the underlying orbital segment of the orbicularis muscle should *not* be felt. With voluntary lid closure this muscle contraction can easily be felt.

The normal blink rate is quite variable. Approximately 15 to 18 blinks per minute is normal. Each blink lasts 0.3 seconds. The rate is higher for men than for women and is also increased with emotional outbursts or anxiety states. With a poor or tired blinker, the rate may go down as much as 60%. This occurs frequently with reading, driving, or watching computer screens during the full working day. Persons who have jobs that fatigue the normal blink response are best fitted with gas-permeable lenses, which do not depend heavily on blinking to relieve corneal hypoxia.

Types of blink activity with lens wearers

Partial blink. A partial blink is an incomplete blink in which the inferior half of the cornea remains exposed (Fig. 3-2).

Lid flutter. Lid flutter is a repressed blink. This typical habit appears in the apprehensive patient who tilts the head back, retracts the lids, and merely flutters the lids.

Normal blink. At first the lens is depressed by the descending lid. After full lid closure the lens rises as the lid elevates. Once the lid has achieved its full height the lens makes a slight gravitational movement downward.

Common findings with poor blink habits

The following are often found in persons with poor blink habits:

1. Low-riding lenses
2. Three and 9 o'clock staining (Fig. 3-3)
3. Corneal edema (Fig. 3-4)
4. Greasy or dry lenses with crystalline deposits

CORNEAL DISORDERS THAT SHOULD BE IDENTIFIED

The contact lens fitter should recognize and document any pre-existing corneal disorders before deciding whether a patient can be fitted with contact lenses. Certain conditions predispose patients to having problems with wearing contact lenses. By careful examination tech-

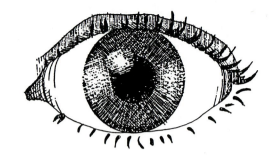

Fig 3-3 ■ Three and nine o'clock staining resulting from inadequate blinking.

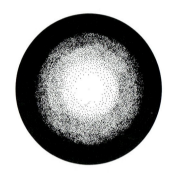

Fig. 3-4 ■ Corneal edema with a poor blink response. There is tear stagnation and little lens movement.

niques and an understanding of these conditions the clinician can prevent potential problems.

Corneal epithelial changes

The use of fluorescein or the rose-bengal test can detect superficial changes in the corneal epithelium. As noted previously, a punctate keratitis can be seen in patients with dry eyes and predisposes them to an increased risk of infection with the use of contact lens wear. In addition, patients with blepharitis may have a punctate keratitis, usually of the inferior cornea, that can lead to redness and photophobia with and without contact lens wear. In patients with blepharitis if an aggressive treatment program is initiated and there is a significant improvement in the lids and the corneal changes resolve, then they can be fitted with contact lenses and monitored closely. Treatment of blepharitis may include the use of lid scrubs using Q-tips and a mild shampoo, an antibiotic ointment at bedtime, and the frequent use of lubricating drops.

Abnormal wetting of the cornea can be seen in patients with old corneal scars from herpes simplex, trauma, etc. Although the scarring is in the corneal stroma there is usually an irregularity in contour to the corneal surface that may result in abnormal wetting and punctate corneal changes. If these patients are to be fitted with a contact lens it is important that the punctate changes resolve with frequent lubrication prior to lens wear.

Anterior basement membrane dystrophy is a relatively common condition that is generally not a contraindication to contact lens wear. Map-like changes, fingerlines, or microcysts can be detected in the corneal epithelium. With the use of fluorescein there is rapid tear break-up overlying these areas. The condition is caused by abnormal production and location of the epithelial basement membrane. Sheets of basement membrane can be found in an abnormal location within the corneal epithelium. Epithelial cells can degenerate beneath this abnormal basement membrane creating microcysts. Although most patients with this condition are asymptomatic, problems with corneal erosions can occur.

Corneal stromal changes

Documentation of the extent of the limbal vessels should be made in all patients who are potential lens wearers. The vessels do not ordinarily extend into the cornea as end vessels but tend to loop back toward the conjunctival side. If the patient has worn contact lenses, especially soft lenses, previously, neovascularization is not uncommonly seen. The vessels extending farther than 2.0 mm into the cornea is a contraindication to the fitting of contact lenses because of the potential for progressive neovascularization and scarring.

Corneal opacities from old scars or hereditary dystrophies can have a variety of appearances and are not considered contraindications to contact lens wear. The findings of an eye with keratoconus may include a cone-shaped cornea, thinning often in a central location, an iron ring (Fleischer ring) located in the epithelium and surrounding the base of the cone, striae or vertical lines in the deep stroma, and scarring in Bowman's layer. In early cases these findings may not be evident but the keratometry readings may show some distortion and irregularity of the mires, which is suggestive of keratoconus. Contact lenses provide these patients with improved vision because the rigid lens replaces the astigmatic and irregular cornea as the main refracting surface.

Corneal endothelial changes

Although the slit-lamp technique of specular reflection can enable one to observe the corneal endothelium, abnormalities in these cells are usually best appreciated with the specular microscope. Abnormalities in the number, shape, or size of the cells can be determined by careful evaluation of the endothelial photographs. Changes in the endothelium occur with all types of contact lenses and may be related to stress from hypoxia. There are currently no guidelines on whether patients with an abnormal endothelium should be fitted with contact lenses. Because of this lack of information, routine specular microscopy is currently not performed.

ASSESSMENT OF A NEW LENS WEARER
History

In the beginning, there will be many adaptive symptoms, such as flare, sensitivity to light, and tearing. These symptoms should be temporary and last no longer than 1 to 2 weeks.

Adaptive symptoms and those of a poor fit should not be confused with one another. Poor fittings will augment the normal conditioning to a rigid lens. If the patient complains of the lens falling out or being displaced on the sclera, the lenses are too loose. This problem will not get better with time. The patient may also have difficulty removing the lenses. Aphakic persons do because their lids are often loose and floppy. New young patients may also have trouble because of normal anxiety and clumsiness in learning a new procedure. However, the lenses may be too tight. Adaptive symptoms must be separated from those of an ill-fitting lens. The former improves with time; the latter does not. If a patient is not making satisfactory progress, a reassessment is in order.

Visual acuity with lenses

Vision should be corrected for near distance since many persons with myopia, though content with their distance acuity, experience difficulty with reading. This is particularly true for myopic persons who are over 35 years of age.

The vertex distance must be considered in the refraction, especially with refractive errors greater than about 4 diopters. An over-refraction of the lens will usually show that more plus is needed for high hyperopic errors and less minus is required for high myopic refractive errors.

If this adjustment is not made, the hyperope will be undercorrected and the myope overcorrected, and significant problems with reading will occur in both.

If the vision is not adequate, the following difficulties may be present:
1. The lens may not be centered.
2. The sagittal vault of the lens may be too great, and so a plus lens effect is created. Excess pooling of fluorescein may be present.
3. Tearing may be excessive, and so the lens may slide around too much.
4. The lenses may be switched. In the early days of contact lens wear, anything could happen.

Manifest refraction over lenses

Frequently 0.50 D of myopia will be found and is an acceptable consequence of mild corneal edema. Greater changes should require a re-evaluation of fit. Residual astigmatism may be increased. Amounts of 0.50 D are very common and can be ignored. Excessive residual astigmatism may require a change in power equal to the spheric equivalent or an anterior toric lens.

Astigmatism of magnitude 1.00 to 5.00 diopters can be fitted with large-diameter spheric gas-permeable lenses. This rule only applies if the cornea is the source of the astigmatism, that is, has toric curvatures in which the radius of curvature in one meridian is greater than in the other.

On the other hand, residual astigmatism, the astigmatism that is generated from the lens of the eye, should not be treated with a spheric lens. One can choose a front-surface toric soft lens (which we prefer) or a front-surface toric rigid lens.

An important cause of residual astigmatism is warping of a lens. Flexure of a lens may also contribute to residual astigmatism. This effect primarily occurs with thin small rigid lenses and the softer gas-permeable lenses. If residual astigmatism is against the rule and the corneal toricity is with the rule, residual astigmatism is reduced. If the residual astigmatism is against the rule and the corneal toricity is also against the rule, the astigmatism is increased and a lens should not be used.

Lens position and movement

The lens should center over the apical zone of the cornea. The lens should move easily with a blink—first down, then upward as the lid is raised, and then gently downward as the lens drops by gravity to a central position. The lens movements should be fluid and smooth. A lens that drops quickly or moves upward in a jerky fashion does not fit properly. With ocular rotations the lens may lag 1 or 2 mm against the movement of the eye. The lag should not carry the lens over the limbus.

SLITLAMP ASSESSMENT

The contact lens fitter must be skilled in the use of a slit-lamp in order to properly assess the fitting characteristics of a lens and to recognize and manage contact lens-related problems. The importance of being able to use the various slit-lamp techniques cannot be overemphasized.

Sclerotic scatter (Fig. 3-5)

Sclerotic scatter is the best way to detect gross edema. The beam, directed at a wide angle at the periphery of the cornea, causes the area of

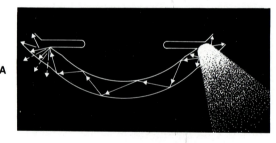

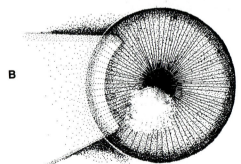

Fig 3-5 ■ A, Corneal edema can be detected grossly by angling the beam of the slitlamp 45 to 60 degrees at the limbus. **B,** Specular reflection. The internal reflection of light through the cornea makes the central edema stand out as a grey haze. The cornea is used as a fiber-optic channel.

corneal edema to stand out as a gray patch in relief at the center of the cornea.

Retro-illumination

This technique uses reflection from a diffusing surface as a secondary source of illumination for examination of a more anterior structure. For example, a light may be bounced from the iris or fundus to illuminate the cornea. The directed light beam should be laterally displaced so that it does not fall directly on the object of regard. This is the best method of showing microcystic edema in the corneal epithelium (Fig. 3-6).

Direct illumination

Direct illumination depends on passing an intense beam of light through a relatively transparent media and observing the scattered light against a dark background. It permits accurate determination of the depth of a lesion. With high magnification, beneath a contact lens one can detect corneal complications that include a superficial punctate keratopathy, erosions, abrasions, ulcers, and sterile infiltrates. Direct illumination is also good for inspection of the lens to reveal scratches, edge chips, and so on.

Specular reflection

Specular reflection is the most difficult technique to learn. The mirror-like reflection from a surface is used so that individual cells of the corneal endothelium can be visualized. In order to see the specular reflection, the angle between the illumination beam and the observation path is critical. For this reason the effect is seen only monocularly. With high magnification, one can focus on the endothelium and adjust the angle of the slit beam so that visualization is possible. The shape, size, and number of endothelial cells can thus be appreciated.

Fluorescein evaluation of rigid lenses

Fluorescein evaluation using a Burton ultraviolet light or the cobalt blue filter of the slitlamp, using a wide beam for an overview, and using a fine slitlamp beam and high magnification for detailed assessment of the tear film is a difficult assessment to make. The appearance of a normal fluorescein pattern depends on whether the lens is fitted on K, is a toric lens, is flatter than K, or steeper than K. A normal pattern is a variable picture depending on the lens used. For instance, a normal fluorescein pattern with a smaller thin lens can be considered steep with a conventional lens. The variability of "normal" fluorescein patterns is such that many fitters do not use it to assess fitting. Once the normal appearance becomes standardized for a given lens, the fluorescein test can yield interesting information on the corneal fit.

Serial keratometry

In serial keratometry (with the lens removed) K readings do not alter more than 0.50 D from well-fitting lenses. A cornea that varies from 42.50/42.75 to 43.50/43.75 D shows signs of steepening. This usually indicates that corneal edema is occurring and is usually caused by a tight lens. During adaptation the horizontal meridian may increase appreciably, and the vertical meridian often decreases, sometimes staying the same, sometimes increasing, but usually increasing less than the horizontal. In the long-term wearer there is often a sharp reduction of the K reading in the horizontal meridian, mean-

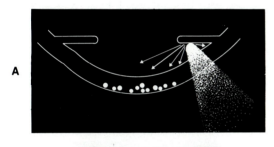

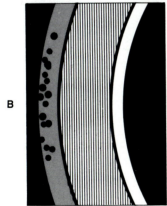

Fig 3-6 ■ **A,** Fine corneal edema. This is best appreciated through retro-illumination. **B,** The corneal epithelium has a stippled appearance.

ing that it has become much flatter. There is usually a slight reduction in the K reading in the vertical meridian. There is seldom an increase (steepening) in this meridian.

In the new patient there is a change from K readings of 42.50 D × 180/42.75 D × 90 to 45.75/42.00 D (flatter in vertical). This is often a result of a lens decentered in vertical meridian.

A change on a mildly astigmatic cornea 42.50 D × 180/44.50 D × 90 to 42.75/43.75 D × 90 (if a spheric lens is being worn) would be considered normal and would be caused by a slight molding of the cornea by the lens.

WHEN TO REFIT

The patient who requires a refit should be treated as a new patient. The lenses should be removed, the tear film assessed, the K readings redone, and the spectacle correction re-evaluated.

Most patients who requires a refit have symptoms such as burning, poor vision, decreased tolerance for the lenses, increased awareness of the lenses, and so on. However, there are patients who are asymptomatic and require a refit. These patients tolerate poorly fitted rigid lenses. They may be indifferent to grossly ill-fitting lenses such as a lens that is too tight (the less the movement, the better they feel), too low (the blink rate is reduced to ameliorate lid impact), corneal edema or erosions (the sensation of the cornea is reduced), 3 and 9 o'clock staining (extensive marginal erosions with episcleritis may cause episcleral redness without pain), and decentered lenses that roll with each blink in a clockwise or counterclockwise manner.

These patients with quiet or minimal symptoms require a refit before an ill-fitted lens turns into a corneal complication. The general assessment should be the same. The problem in the past has been when to refit.

Ideally one should refit the cornea when the K readings are stable and the refraction unchanged. This may take a day, a week, or even months. Until the corneas become stable, the patient is not allowed to wear the lenses. Glasses must be purchased, a task that by itself takes time and leaves the person functionally blind until they are made. The arrival of glasses is hardly a joyful event in a lens wearer's life. Vi-

sion and its attendant distortions through thick spectacle lenses are intolerable to the pampered lens wearer. Moreover there is the added grief that is caused by change. The corneal curvature and the refraction change daily as the edema recedes, but the power of the spectacles remains the same. This solution is hardly ideal.

The most expedient line of attack is to fit the patient immediately with gas-permeable lenses or alternatively to use soft lenses with high oxygen performance until the cornea is stabilized. At least the patient can wear a contact lens while the corneas return to their original shape. Then changes in the lens can be made as changes in the contour of the cornea occur.

Before refitting patients, many practitioners wait 48 hours while the corneas begin to return to their original shape and reduction of edema takes place. The patient is asked to accept a weekend of extremely poor vision that creates no inconvenience at work. This 48-hour rule of thumb has been shown to be useful but somewhat unrealistic.

These corneal and refractive changes move in the direction of flatter K readings in the primary meridian and less minus refractive error for a period of 3 to 4 days before they reverse or stabilize. Therefore any K readings taken 48 hours or later after lens removal will give values that are erroneous and certainly not so good as those taken immediately after lens removal.

With current gas-permeable lenses, it is no longer necessary for the patient to have to give up rigid lenses suddenly. The newer high DK lenses can be fitted based on old K readings because of the high oxygen permeability of the lenses. The K readings will gradually return to normal.

COMMENT. Induced corneal toricity is quite unpredictable. It can last hours, days, or months or become permanent. At times the corneal astigmatism is irregular, and so spectacles will not suffice as a bridge before stability ensues. Soft lenses may not be adequate, especially if the sphere is a low power (−3 or less) and the corneal astigmatism is greater than 1.50 diopters. The best solution is high-DK gas-permeable lenses. Such lenses require no waiting time, yield the best acuity, and may be changed when the cornea regains its integrity.

4 ▪ EXAMINATION OF THE ANTERIOR OCULAR SURFACE AND TEAR FILM

Joshua E. Josephson

- ▪ *Tear component assessment categories*
- ▪ *The structure and dynamics of tear film*
  - ▪ *Tear flow assessment*
  - ▪ *Tear spreading / stability / wettability*
  - ▪ *Resident tear volume*
  - ▪ *Evaluation of the anterior surface of the lipid layer*
  - ▪ *The condition of the ocular surface*
  - ▪ *The presence of debris in tear film*
  - ▪ *An assessment of tear viscosity*
- ▪ *Other conditions associated with dry eyes*
- ▪ *The role of blinking*
- ▪ *Assessing the blink characteristics*

The integrity of the anterior ocular surface and the quality and adequacy of the pre-ocular tear film are critical factors in determining the suitability of an individual for contact lens wear. Tear film quality and quantity play a major role in the length of time that contact lenses can be worn comfortably and the rate at which deposits build up on contact lens surfaces. Certainly, tear quality, quantity, and the condition of the ocular surface are important considerations for whether contact lenses should be fitted at all, the potential lens-wearing time, and the type of lens required (rigid or hydrogel). The tear film is a medium for exchange that provides oxygen and nutrients to the ocular surface. Tears also play a role in the immunology of the ocular surface and in facilitating the removal of ocular surface debris, sloughed exfoliated cells, and metabolites.

Based on the evaluation of the tear film and ocular surface, practitioners can exercise clinical judgment. For example, the patient diagnosed as having a "marginally dry eye" (as opposed to a pathologically dry eye) may be a suitable candidate for daily wear lenses but certainly would be contraindicated for extended wear lenses.

Another example is the patient who has reasonably good tear quality but significantly reduced tear quantity. This patient might be suitable for social or full day wear hydrogel lenses, but might be quite unsuited for wearing rigid contact lenses. This is because an adequate tear volume is necessary to fill the potential space between the peripheral curves of the rigid contact lens and the cornea, so that during the interblink interval, a stable tear layer is formed adjacent to the marginal tear meniscus at the edge of the lens (Figs. 4-1 and 4-2). This will reduce the tendency for the peripheral desiccation that occurs as a result of rapid thinning of the tear film in the tear meniscus at the lens edge, during the interblink interval.

The major questions that practitioners must consider when examining the tear film are what is adequate, and how adequacy should be determined. This chapter will concern itself with

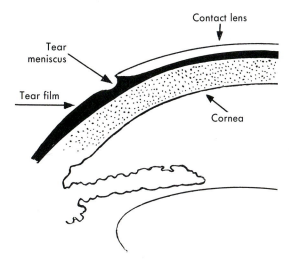

Fig 4-1 ▪ The tear meniscus profile of the edge of a hard contact lens. (After D. Korb)

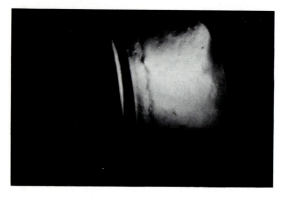

Fig 4-2 ■ The tear meniscus at the edge of a hard contact lens (frontal view).

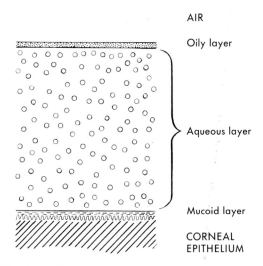

Fig 4-3 ■ The three-layered tear film with anterior oily layer, middle aqueous layer, and inner mucoid layer. (After Wolff, 1949.)

tests or observations that can be performed easily in a practitioner's office without the need for special laboratory equipment.

TEAR COMPONENT ASSESSMENT CATEGORIES
1) Tear flow assessment

   a) Schirmer tear test
   b) Hypofluorescence

2) Tear spreading/stability/wettability

   a) Tear film break-up time
   b) Evaluation of the anterior surface of the lipid layer

3) Resident tear volume

   a) Speed of the black line formation
   b) Saturation (height) of the tear meniscus

4) Evaluation of the anterior surface of the lipid layer
5) The condition of the ocular surface

   a) Staining after sequential instillations of fluorescein (sequential staining)
   b) Rose bengal staining
   c) Observations of the ocular surface with specular reflection

6) The presence of debris in the tear film
7) An assessment of tear viscosity

These tests and observations make up the group of clinical observations and procedures that can be used for assessing the adequacy of the tear film and its relationship with the ocular

surface in prospective contact lens patients. A poor result in only one test does not necessarily contraindicate the patient for contact lens wear. Usually, a poor result in two or more test categories would be clinically more significant. Obviously, an abnormally low or poor result on most tests would virtually contraindicate an individual for contact lens wear.

Diagnostic laboratory tests of tear chemistry that are not included in the above list are evaluations of the secretory IgA, IgG, lysozyme, a tear protein profile, the elisa technique, and others. Also, dye dilution tests for tear flow have not been included because they are complex and not easily usable as part of routine clinical test procedures. It is important to understand the structure and dynamics of the tear film before performing these clinical tests.

THE STRUCTURE AND DYNAMICS OF TEAR FILM

Wolff first proposed that tear film consists of three discrete layers (Fig. 4-3): a thin anterior surface lipid layer; a thick middle aqueous layer composed of water, inorganic salts, and proteins, which accounts for approximately 99% of the tear film thickness, and a thin inner mucous layer.

Another current theory suggests that the tear film may have only two layers; an anterior lipid layer and an aqueous glycoprotein solution with increasing viscosity towards the corneal surface,

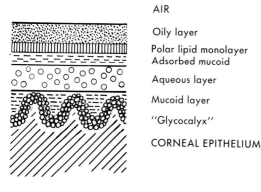

AIR

Oily layer

Polar lipid monolayer
Adsorbed mucoid

Aqueous layer

Mucoid layer

"Glycocalyx"

CORNEAL EPITHELIUM

Fig 4-4 ■ The six-layer tear film model (From Tiffany J: J Brit Cont Lens Assoc, 1988.)

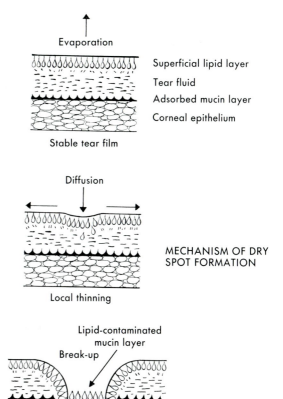

Evaporation

Superficial lipid layer

Tear fluid

Adsorbed mucin layer

Corneal epithelium

Stable tear film

Diffusion

MECHANISM OF DRY SPOT FORMATION

Local thinning

Lipid-contaminated mucin layer

Break-up

Dry spot formed by receding tears

Fig 4-5 ■ The mechanism for dry spot formation (After Holly FJ: Int Ophthalmol Clin 20(3):171, 1980.)

where the tear film becomes a highly hydrated semi-solid gel.

Also recently, Tiffany presented a six-layer model of the tear film: an anterior oily layer; a polar lipid layer; an adsorbed mucoid layer; an aqueous layer, a mucoid layer, and the *glycocalyx*, which is the mucopolysaccharide complex presented at the anterior surface of the cornea by the surface microvilli (Fig. 4-4). He suggests that the stabilizing actions of the tear film include lipid interaction with macromolecules to lower overall surface energy, lipid occlusion that reduces tear evaporation, a meibomian lipid barrier to delay entry of the highly polar skin surface lipids, and mucous viscosity, which slows the disruption of tear film and the interaction of tears at the epithelial surface. He suggests that contact lenses may disturb some of these stabilizing interactions. This suggestion has been supported experimentally by the observations of Hill, Martin, Cederstaff and Tomlinson, Korb, Guillon, and others.

In the healthy eye, the tear film covers the exposed cornea and bulbar/conjunctival surface. According to Mishima, the tear meniscus at the margin of the upper and lower lids contains a reservoir of tears that accounts for 70% to 80% of the tear volume at the ocular surface.

Holly has described the effect of blinking on the tear film. After blinking, when the lids begin to open, the upper lid initiates the spreading of the compressed lipid layer, which has an affinity for the upper lid margin. As the lipids spread, the aqueous is dragged upward by the spreading lipid layer from the inferior tear meniscus. This blink action has been reported to occur in Caucasians on an average of once every 4 to 6 seconds. In between blinks, no significant motion

occurs in the pre-ocular tear film except for a flow of aqueous towards the tear menisci and on to the nasal puncta.

The tear film remains stable for 10 to 30 seconds and then regional thinning occurs. In these areas, some lipid migrates to the mucoid glycocalyx, forming an unstable dry area of tear film break-up (Figs. 4-5 and 4-6). This will eventually initiate lid closure (blinking) where the lipid contaminated mucin is sheared away and rolled up into a thread-like form by the action of the upper lid margin on the cornea during lid closure. This also causes the redistribution of mucin over the ocular surface, and then, as the eyelids open again, the pre-ocular tear layer is reformed and the whole process is repeated.

Tear flow assessment

Schirmer tear test. Although the Schirmer tear test has been widely used, its validity and re-

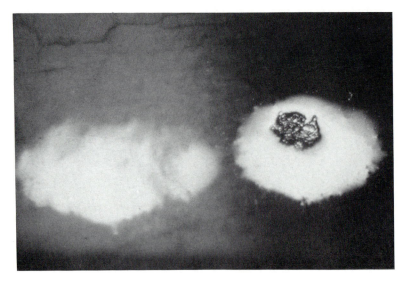

Fig 4-6 ■ A dry spot on the inferior cornea.

producibility is still controversial. For example, Shapiro and Merin found a mean schirmer value of 33.1 mm in 880 healthy eyes; however, the standard of deviation was 33.2 mm.

The procedure is to fold a strip of 5 × 35 mm filter paper at the notch located near one end. The short section is placed approximately one third of the way in from the outer canthus in the inferior palpebral conjunctiva so that the long portion beyond the notch rests against the lid margin. It is important that the strip be located in a temporal position so that when the lower lid kicks inward during blinking, contact with the limbal region, which may cause excess ocular irritation and reflex tearing, is avoided. During this procedure, the patient should continuously look upward (Fig. 4-7). It is preferable that the room be dimly illuminated. The patient should be reminded to blink normally and whenever necessary.

Typically, a length of strip wetting between 15 to 20 mm is considered normal. An eighty year old might wet a section of the strip that is one fifth of the length of a section of that of a twenty year old. A very high volume of tears, noted by the wetting of the complete strip or of most of the strip, may not be valid. An extremely low volume, noted by a very small area of strip coverage (0-4 mm), is usually valid. Because of the reported lack of reproducibility, Schirmer strip results should be repeated at the same time on a second day.

Hypofluorescence. When fluorescein is instilled for this procedure a minimal amount must be instilled, preferably with a liquid-saturated, fluorescein-impregnated strip. It is important to use the lowest possible illumination with the slit-lamp, filtered through a colbalt blue filter. It is helpful to use a fluorescence enhancement filter in front of the microscope, such as a Kodak wratten #12 gelatin filter. The slit-lamp illumination should be oblique to the ocular surface so as to minimize reflex tearing.

When a patient has normal tear flow, any hypofluorescence will quickly change to normal fluorescence after approximately three to five quick blinks. However, in an individual with reduced tear flow, normal fluorescence may not be observed until after 1 minute, or even much longer. In the course of making this observation an error can occur if an excessive amount of fluorescein is instilled.

Other tests for the evaluation of tear flow. Other tests not included that may be used to evaluate tear flow are the dye dilution test, the Cotton Thread Test, and the Kurihashi Thread Test. The subjectivity of the dye dilution test and the need for standardization from practitioner to practitioner has limited its usefulness as a routine test. In North America, the lack of commercial availability and regional distribution of the materials required for the Cotton Thread Test and the Kurihashi Thread Test have prevented them from being used routinely.

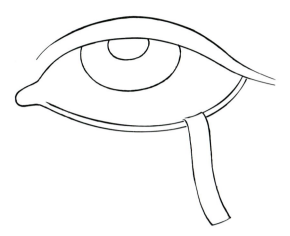

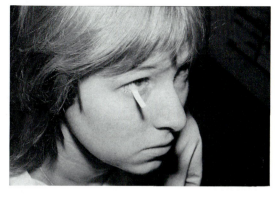

Fig 4-7 ■ The correct position of the Schirmer tear strip. The Schirmer strip is placed on the lower lid, one third in from the lateral canthus. The procedure is performed while the patient looks upward and blinks normally.

Tear spreading/stability/wettability

The tear film break up time (BUT) has been used as an index of tear film integrity and stability. Nevertheless, instilling fluorescein is an invasive technique and thus the tear film break-up time value has remained a controversial parameter.

Tear film break-up time (BUT). The tear film break-up time has been defined as the time between a complete blink and the appearance of the first randomly distributed dry spot. After fluorescein is instilled, the tear film should be illuminated by light filtered through a cobalt blue filter. The tear film should be observed through the biomicroscope (filtered by a Kodak wratten #12 fluorescence enhancement filter) until a "dry" spot appears, i.e., a dark area that seems to interrupt the uniformly yellow-green fluorescein-stained tear film (Fig. 4-8). The break-up time value is typically measured in seconds and the area of the break up is recorded (i.e., superior tear meniscus region, etc.) Since the tear film is typically more stable over the central cornea than in the superior and inferior regions (because of the proximity of the tear menisci) tear film stability is best assessed within a central 6 mm area. This technique helps to improve the reliability and reproducibility of this observation.

Norn believes that the tear film break-up time is quite useful in ophthalmologic practice as a unique parameter that indicates the stability of the tear film. However, Holly has reported that the coefficient of variation for BUT is 30% and that its reproducibility and value are dependent on the methods of observation used. In addition, he believes that the instillation of fluorescein dye, especially with preservatives, may increase the speed of the tear film break-up. Vanley, Leopold, and Gregg have reported that tear film break-up time is inconclusive in the diagnosis of dry eye syndrome and that it is not reproducible within normal limits. However, Forst and Andrews, Henriquez, et al., have reported that patients presenting BUT values of less than 10 seconds show clear signs of contact lens intolerance. Therefore, they feel that the BUT test is a relevant preliminary test in contact-lens fittings.

Non-invasive assessment of tear film break-up time and stability. To increase the accuracy and reproducibility of tear film break-up time

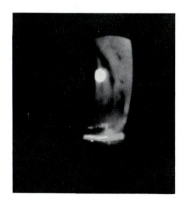

Fig 4-8 ■ Tear film break-up. (Courtesy of Dr. D. Korb.)

information, Mengher and Bron developed a non-invasive method of assessment of tear film stability. Their instrument consists of a hemispheric bowl attached to the apex of a monocular or binocular slitlamp microscope at the objective lens plane. A grid of white lines and a matte black background is inscribed on the inner surface of the bowl. The pattern inside the bowl appears in the form of a cross-hatching.

When projected onto the open eye and viewed as an image reflected from the tear film surface, the pattern of white lines appears as a rectangular grid projected onto the cornea. An intact tear film produces a regular image of the grid inscribed on the bowl. Loss of tear film integrity or stability produces distortions and/or discontinuities in the reflected image characteristic of tear film break-up or instability. The elapsed time, measured in seconds between the last complete blink and the first random discontinuity of the tear film, is taken to be the non-invasive break-up time (NIBUT). This value is then used as a measure of tear film stability.

Guillon has developed a more portable clinically practical instrument that is useful in assessing the non-invasive BUT (see Section C: Evaluation of the Anterior Surface of the Lipid Layer).

These non-invasive techniques provide an alternative to the use of fluorescein in the assessment of the precorneal tear film stability. The non-invasive break-up values of normal subjects are higher than the values obtained using the fluorescein instillation method. Guillon and Guillon have observed a binomial distribution in normals, with groupings at 15 seconds and 45 seconds. Therefore, it is conceivable that those inherent properties responsible for tear film stability are altered following the instillation of fluorescein.

Evaluation of the anterior surface of the lipid layer. The primary source of the lipid layer is the meibomian glands of the upper and lower lids. Meibomian gland dysfunction has been associated with dry eye symptoms and contact lens intolerance (Korb and Henriquez). The glands of Zeiss and Mol make a small contribution to the lipid layer. Tiffany reported that the lipid layer forms a duplex layer in which there are predominantly low polarity lipids (cholesterol esters) and, in much lesser concentrations, high polarity lipids (triglycerides, free fatty acids, and phospholipids).

Hamano et al. first reported a technique for evaluating the anterior surface of the tear film lipid layer, using a bio-differential interference microscope. However, the expense and lack of availability of the specialized equipment make its use impractical for private practitioners.

Josephson, and also Guillon, have developed clinically practical, simple slit-lamp techniques for observing, documenting, and recording the integrity and appearance of the anterior surface of the pre-ocular tear film lipid layer (see Section 4: Evaluation of the Anterior Surface of the Lipid Layer). These techniques render the anterior surface of the tear film visible without the instillation of any agents, and are substantial refinements of the original technique suggested earlier by Wolff and later by McDonald. The specular reflection from the anterior surface of the tear film can be evaluated with a slit-lamp biomicroscope using dim, oblique illumination. Recording can be documented by either 35 mm camera or video tape (Fig. 4-9).

Guillon's later technique uses a patented instrument to view the undisturbed tear film. Guillon reports that this instrument can also measure the non-invasive break-up time. The instrument projects a diffuse cold light source that is reflected by the anterior surface of the tear film.

The device (Fig. 4-10) consists of an illumi-

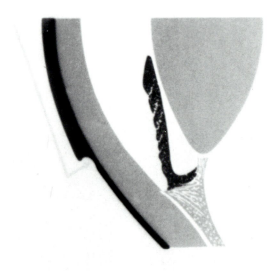

Fig 4-9 ■ Instrumentation for 35 mm and video photography. (From Josephson JE: Appearance of the preocular tear film lipid layer. Am J Optom Physiol Opt 60(11):1983.)

nation system with a ring-shaped cathode tube fitted over a hemispheric inner reflecting surface, which is coated a brilliant white. The cold light source is used to avoid drying the tear film when the instrument is held in close proximity to the eye. This reflecting surface acts as a secondary light source illuminating the tear surface. A central aperture in the hemispheric shell allows observation of the ocular or tear surface. A supplementary plus 12 or plus 14 diopter lens placed in the observation aperture can bring the tear surface under close observation and focus. The dimension and shape of the cup are chosen to maximize the area of the tear film observed (8 to 10 mm) and to allow easy observation with or without the biomicroscope.

Hamano first classified the appearance of the specular reflection of the pre-ocular tear film lipid layer as marmoreal (Fig. 4-11), amorphous, and flow or wavy (Fig. 4-12). Guillon has asso-

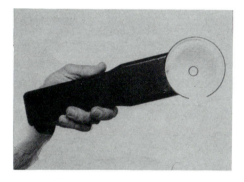

Fig 4-10 ■ Guillon's device for observing the anterior surface of the tear film. (Courtesy of Dr. Jean-Pierre Guillon.)

ciated the marmoreal pattern with potential drying problems. Guillon has also associated the flow or wave pattern with a stable tear film. He believes that patients who present the wave pattern are acceptable candidates for contact lens fitting. He has also reported that patients who present an amorphous pattern have a highly stable tear film, and that such patients are usually good candidates for contact lenses, although they occasionally have greasing problems because of the high volume of lipids present.

Some patients present a combination of patterns. Josephson has reported that specific patterns are not always repeatable in the same patient from visit to visit. Therefore, one should not automatically assume any clinical implications for contact lens wearers from a single observation.

The ability to observe and record the specular reflections from the surface of the pre-ocular tear film can be quite useful. When the lipid layer is thick enough (minimum: 120 nanometers) it begins to present colored patterns. In some patients, a wide range of colors, particularly third-order interference colors has been associated by Josephson and Guillon with contact lens deposit problems. McCulley and Sciallis have described the foamy appearance and prominent colored interference patterns observed in association with meibomian keratoconjunctivitis or low-grade meibomitis. The presence of certain organisms that hydrolyze the lipids in the orifices of the meibomian glands, causes the lipids that contribute to the lipid layer to become soluble. This destabilization of the lipid layer frequently

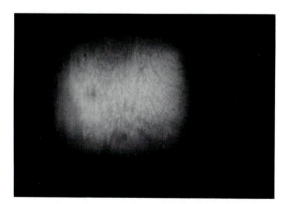

Fig 4-11 ■ Marmoreal pattern of the lipid layer.

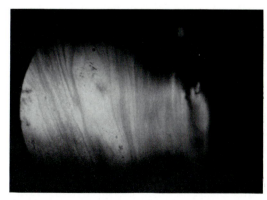

Fig 4-12 ■ Flow pattern of the lipid layer. (From Josephson JE: Appearance of the preocular tear film lipid layer. Am J Optom Physiol Opt 60(11):1983.)

causes the formation of foam along the lower lid margins and the temporal canthae (Fig. 4-13). The presence of foam has also been associated with an increased blink rate and with contact lens intolerance (Korb and Herman). The amount of foam can also depend on the frequency and intensity of blinking. After a period of ocular irritation, the presence of foam is usually an expected result and may have less to do with meibomitis. An unstable lipid layer has been associated with symptoms of dryness when the lipid layer appears grey, entirely without color and appears broken up into "islands" of lipid (Josephson; Fig. 4-14). This appearance of the lipid layer in association with symptoms of dryness may be compared to the normally smooth, stable, and intact appearance of the lipid layer.

Sebaceous gland dysfunction and meibomitis have been associated with chronic blepharitis. The associated abnormality of tear film function may be a result of increased secretion of polar lipids, particularly free fatty acids that may contaminate the tear film and hasten break up, thereby reducing the ability of the tear film to maintain a stable, uniformly wet surface on the anterior surface of the cornea, which increases the symptoms of dryness.

Resident tear volume

Speed of the black line formation. Following the instillation of fluorescein, the tear film may be disrupted, and blinking will redistribute the tear film until an equilibrium of the tear film thickness is re-established over the ocular surface. At this point, usually after one minute or approximately 12 blinks, one may examine the appearance of the fluorescein-stained tear layer adjacent to the upper and lower tear menisci, at the lid margins. Immediately following a blink, the tear meniscus begins to draw tears away from the adjacent ocular surface. Within a short period of time, typically within 10 to 12 seconds, a dark area will become visible in the shallowest area of the tear film that is adjacent to the tear meniscus. This dark area where the tear film is at its thinnest has been referred to as the "black line". It is observed adjacent to and follows the distribution of the tear meniscus

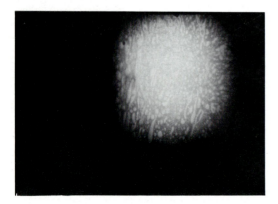

Fig 4-13 ▪ Foam along the lower lid margin.

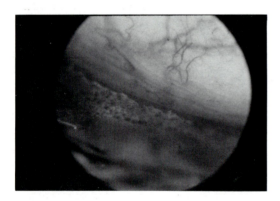

Fig 4-14 ▪ An unstable lipid layer. (From Josephson JE: Appearance of the preocular tear film lipid layer. Am J Optom Physiol Opt 60(11):1983.)

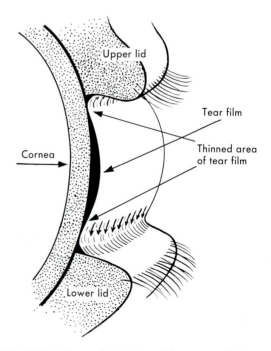

Fig 4-15 ▪ The redistribution of the pre-ocular tear film after blinking. The black line forms in the thinned area. (Courtesy Dr. Frank Holly.)

along the lid margins (Fig. 4-15). In individuals where the black line forms in less than five seconds, the tear volume should be considered lower than normal.

Saturation (height) of the tear meniscus. The observation of the volume of tears present in the tear meniscus at the margin of the upper and lower lids has been used by clinicians to assess resident tear volume. Mishima reported that approximately three quarters of the tear volume is contained in the tear menisci at the margin of the upper and lower lids. When the height of the meniscus on the lower lid margin is less than 0.1 mm, this measurement is considered to be lower than normal and has been described as a relatively unsaturated tear meniscus (Holly, Guillon and Guillon). Lamberts has expressed the view that since several ocular anatomic factors can play a role in the height of the meniscus, absolute measurements of the height of the meniscus can result in erroneous interpretations of a dry eye. The volume of tears within the tear meniscus can also be assessed after the instil-

lation of fluorescein and an interval of approximately 1½ to 2 minutes during which the patient is requested to blink normally. The fluorescein helps to make the meniscus more visible. The meniscus is easily visible when observed with the slitlamp using minimal illumination, a cobalt blue filter, and a fluorescence enhancement Kodak wratten yellow #12 filter placed in front of the microscope (Fig. 4-16). In my opinion, when the meniscus is so thin as to appear like a fine line (Fig. 4-17), it is a significantly unsaturated tear meniscus (provided that the lid margins are congruent with the ocular surface). Clinically, I find this information useful in helping to predict the "marginally dry eyed" patient.

Evaluation of the anterior surface of the lipid layer

Perhaps the most practical clinical method for observing the anterior surface of the lipid layer is by using the biomicroscope and employing specular reflection from the anterior surface. The least illumination possible from the slitlamp should be used to minimize reflex tearing and to avoid disruption of the lipid layer. The specular reflection is usually largest and most visible over the bulbar conjunctiva near the temporal border of the limbus (Fig. 4-18). The reflection of the cornea may also be used.

Fig. 4-19 shows the best positions for the slitlamp light and the microscope for observing the right eye. Once the desired specular reflection is located, the magnification should be increased to the maximum while maintaining the reflection

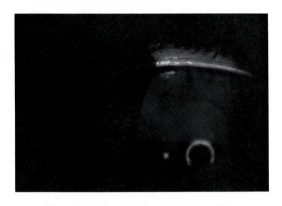

Fig 4-16 ■ An adequate tear meniscus.

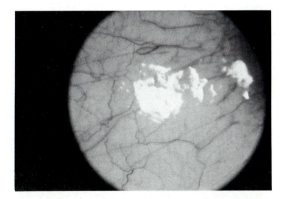

Fig 4-18 ■ The specular reflection from the lipid layer of the pre-ocular tear film, over the bulbar conjunctiva. (From Josephson JE: Appearance of the preocular tear film lipid layer. Am J Optom Physiol Opt 60(11):883,1983.)

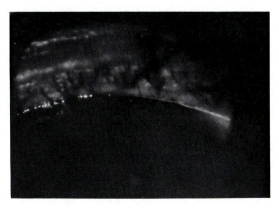

Fig 4-17 ■ An unsaturated tear meniscus.

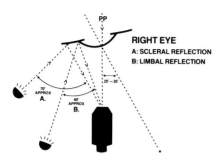

RIGHT EYE
A: SCLERAL REFLECTION
B: LIMBAL REFLECTION

Fig 4-19 ■ The schematic for observing and recording the specular reflection from the lipid layer. (From Josephson JE: Appearance of the preocular tear film lipid layer. Am J Optom Physiol Opt 60(11):883,1983.)

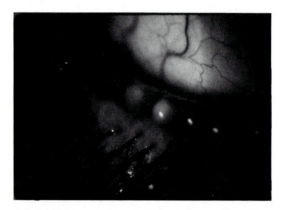

Fig 4-20 ■ A cloudy secretion expressed from the meibomian glands, induced by digital squeezing of the lid margins.

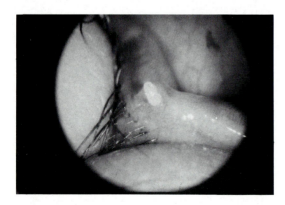

Fig 4-21 ■ Inspissated material expressed from the meibomian glands by digital squeezing of the lid margin.

within the field of view. The patient should be instructed to blink whenever necessary.

However, the best technique for observing a very large area of the ocular surface is to use the device developed by Guillon and Guillon (see Section 2C: Evaluation of the Anterior Surface of the Lipid Layer).

The role of the meibomian glands. The meibomian glands are the primary source of lipids contributing to the lipid layer of the pre-ocular tear film. The gland structure can be assessed by infra-red photography, to determine gland atrophy. Applying pressure on the glands by folding and gently squeezing the lids near the lid margins should reveal a clear, baby oil-like secretion. Less normal secretions may be cloudy (Fig. 4-20) or inspissated (Fig. 4-21). Sometimes very little secretion is produced, despite hard digital pressure or squeezing, which often results in slight pouting of the gland orifices. When there is minimal or no secretion, or when only inspissated material is produced, these conditions may predict possible dry eye symptoms and/or contact lens intolerance.

The condition of the ocular surface

Sequential instillations of fluorescein (sequential staining). Fluorescein staining in humans has been investigated by Norn, Korb and Exford, Korb and Herman, and Josephson and Caffery.

Korb and Herman associated significant staining after the sequential instillation of fluorescein with contact lens intolerance.

Josephson and Caffery have explored the possibility that this staining phenomenon is associated with normal corneal epithelial physiology in some individuals, and is somewhat variable over time both diurnally and over one month.

Fluorescein is widely used in both research and practice. It does not form chemical bonds with cellular components (Ehrlich) but diffuses through the intercellular spaces of tissues that permit its passage. Fluorescein will not penetrate the corneal epithelium unless spaces exist that are large enough to allow the fluorescein molecule to penetrate between intact surface epithelial cells. This situation can occur when the epithelium is damaged or, hypothetically, if the normal arrangement of cells from the basement membrane epithelium towards the epithelial surface is disrupted by abnormal cell growth.

There are several procedures that can be used for instillation of fluorescein. Liquid fluorescein can be instilled, one drop every three minutes for a period of 15 minutes, or a fluorescein-impregnated strip can be moistened with preservative-free saline solution and instilled by the application of the liquid on the tip of the strip to the superior bulbar conjunctiva while the patient looks down, or to the inferior cul-de-sac while the patient looks upward. The ocular surface should be observed after the first instillation of fluorescein once the patient has blinked 5 or 6 times, and after the final instillation of fluorescein, and compared. Any significant staining (Fig. 4-22) that occurs may be considered a possible contraindication for successful wearing of contact lenses, particularly if the staining result is severe (Korb and Herman).

Fluorescein penetration can be enhanced by the preliminary instillation of a single drop of a commercial preparation called proparacaine hydrochloride (Josephson and Caffery).

Rose bengal staining. Rose bengal is a true vital stain that binds strongly and selectively to cellular components (Schirmer and Sjögren). It particularly stains dead cells with an intense red color, while cells that are merely devitalized are stained a weaker color (Norn). In marginally dry eyes, the conjunctival surface may stain in a discrete punctate fashion, whereas in the pathologically dry eye there is typically a more dense confluent staining with a uniformly intense red color. Typically, the adjacent triangular sections of the exposed bulbar conjunctiva, nasally and temporally, will stain.

The procedure is to instill one drop of 1% rose bengal into the conjunctival sac. After the patient blinks 3 to 6 times and the excess dye has been washed away by the tears, the eye is examined with the slitlamp, using white light.

The grading of the color intensity is arbitrary; however, different systems have been suggested, such as those of Holm, Von Bijsterveld, and Norn.

Observations of the ocular surface with specular reflection. We have found it useful to observe the conjunctival and limbal surface with specular reflection when examining patients for contact lens suitability. Typically, in marginally dry and in more severely dry eyes, the conjunctival surface will present a granular, irregular appearance (Fig. 4-23). Frequently, this surface will stain after sequential instillations of fluorescein, or after a single instillation of rose bengal, typically in a punctate fashion where the condition is mild, and in a more severe fashion with dense areas of confluent staining in more severe cases of dry eye.

The presence of debris in tear film

There is more debris in the tear film in dry eyes (Norn). This debris primarily consists of mucous threads, but in more pathologic conditions may consist of exfoliated cells and other matter. Since we are considering patients with relatively healthy eyes, the presence of debris will often be less than obvious. Probably the best location to look for the presence of debris is the marginal tear meniscus on the lower lid margin (see Fig. 4-5).

An assessment of tear viscosity

Tear viscosity plays a role in the movement of tears between the contact lens and the ocular

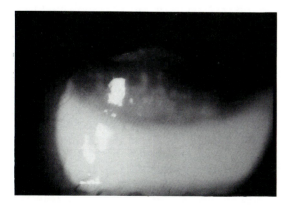

Fig 4-22 ■ Staining of the inferior cornea observed only after sequential instillations of fluorescein, seen on a healthy eye that has never worn contact lenses.

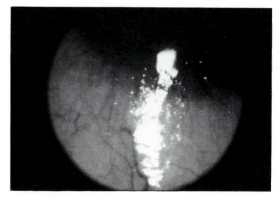

Fig 4-23 ■ An irregular (granular) appearance of the specular reflection of the tear film over the bulbar conjunctiva.

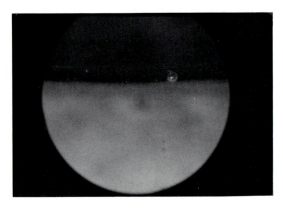

Fig 4-24 ■ A "particle" (bubble) in the tear meniscus.

surface in both soft and hard lens wear. Thus, the "tear pump" action can be adversely affected by highly viscous tears. Flushing of debris in the eye of a patient with a marginally dry eye may be inadequate when the tears are highly viscous.

To assess tear viscosity by observation, Terry and Hill described a technique where they examined the inferior tear meniscus with the slit-lamp, using minimal illumination (to prevent reflex tearing) and a small beam diameter that only illuminated the area under immediate observation. The patient was asked to look straight ahead and to blink normally while being observed. In the tear prism (meniscus) one can see such superficial particles as bubbles (Fig. 4-24), and deeper in the tear prism, small clumps of debris. When the patient blinks, these particles move towards the nasal puncta. With careful observation it is possible to compare the movement of these particles. A grading system from 1 to 5 is used, with 5 representing highly watery tears and 1 representing the most viscous tears. When the superficial and deep particles move swiftly towards the puncta at virtually the same speed, the grading of viscosity is 5. When both the superficial and deep particles are virtually immobile, the grading of viscosity is 1. However, when the superficial particles move more slowly than the deep particles, the viscosity could be graded 3.

OTHER CONDITIONS ASSOCIATED WITH DRY EYES

In some women, menopause may be associated with ocular dryness. Arthritis, lupus, erythematosus, and Sjögren's syndrome are systemic conditions that are also associated with dryness.

Marginal blepharitis may be associated with abnormal tear film function and should be resolved prior to fitting a patient with contact lenses. Often, routine prophylactic lid hygiene can be effective with certain conditions.

Many drugs such as decongestants, diuretics, and some tranquilizers may adversely affect tear film quality or quantity.

THE ROLE OF BLINKING

Poor blinking habits can adversely affect not only a potentially well-fitting lens, but also the performance of both soft and hard contact lenses. Incomplete or infrequent blinking often can cause soft lenses to become dry and their surface can become somewhat hydrophobic and coated with a deposit. The rate of deposition may increase (Lowther) and the quality of vision may be adversely affected. Frequently, truck drivers and individuals working on computers have a reduced blink rate and more often suffer from variable vision or reduced visual quality because of the infrequent blink rate and the resultant adverse effects of increasing deposits on the contact lens' surface. These individuals may also experience increased symptoms of dryness.

ASSESSING THE BLINK CHARACTERISTICS

It is important to examine the patient's blink characteristics prior to fitting him with contact lenses. Patients who do not close their lids completely during blinking, often presenting with anywhere from 10% to 50% closure, should not be considered suitable for rigid contact lens wear unless they are fitted with a lid attachment design that remains stable superiorly between blinks. In addition, if such patients are being fitted with a hydrogel lens, it is important that they be reminded about their blinking habits. They should routinely use enzyme cleaners at least once every six days to minimize protein build-up on the anterior lens surface. Often, individuals with a partial or infrequent blink, if fitted with rigid lenses, will present with low-riding lenses and 3 and 9 o'clock staining (peripheral desiccation).

The very infrequent blinker is contraindicated for any kind of contact lens wear. Any patient who does not have a blink rate of one blink every fifteen to twenty seconds should only consider soft contact lenses for social use, provided that he has a tear film that is otherwise adequate.

5 ▪ PATIENT SELECTION: FINDING THE RIGHT LENS FOR THE RIGHT PATIENT

- ▪ *Safety of contact lenses*
- ▪ *Patient selection*
- ▪ *Rigid lenses*
- ▪ *Gas-permeable lenses*
- ▪ *Soft lenses*
- ▪ *Comment*
- ▪ *Lenses for special situations*

Is the PMMA hard lens obsolete?

Do the newer soft lens designs and materials yield satisfactory visual performance?

Is gas permeability a feature that should be part of any lens—rigid or soft?

Which lenses are more likely to get dislodged from the eye, or spoiled, or damaged?

Are contact lenses dangerous in some occupations?

SAFETY OF CONTACT LENSES

Safety is a most important consideration. A properly fitting individually biocompatible contact lens that transmits sufficient oxygen should not cause any damage to the cornea regardless of the lens choice. However, in the real world there are many instances of transient corneal damage ranging from induced acute hypoxia to corneal abrasions. Loss of corneal regularity, asymmetric astigmatism, corneal vascularization, and endophthalmitis have been reported with both rigid and soft lenses.

Many occupations preclude the wearing of any type of contact lens. These involve welders, miners, construction workers, and people engaged in sand blasting or drilling. These are jobs in which the environment is inimical to the integrity of the cornea because of radiation, dust, high-velocity foreign bodies, vapors, or fumes.

The patient's hands may offer clues for his or her suitability for lenses. Many workers such as plumbers, furniture dyers, and automobile mechanics never get their hands perfectly clean. Their hands, palms, and nails at the best of times are etched with dirt and oil. The skin is tough and hard and could not ever handle a lens without damaging or contaminating it.

A patient with poor hygiene is also a poor candidate. In most studies, the patient's lack of hygiene has been the most common factor in injury to the eye by a contact lens. If the pa-

Currently there is an extraordinarily large number of types of contact lenses. In addition to the classic rigid (PMMA) lenses and hydrogel (soft) lenses, there are gas-permeable lenses made with the addition of silicone (polyorganosiloxane), called the silicone acrylates, silicone resins, silicone elastomers, cellulose acetate butrate and styrene, and the currently popular fluorocarbonated silicone acrylate, and the pure fluorocarbon lens.

New soft lens designs have also increased. There are soft lenses for presbyopia, toric lenses for astigmatism, tinted lenses, and lenses that can be retained in the eye for over 24 hours without needing to be removed (extended-wear lenses). With this variety, the choice becomes more difficult. Soft lens usage, which grew exponentially during the 1970s at the expense of the hard lens, is now being challenged by the gas-permeable rigid lenses.

The patient must be fitted with the appropriate lens. The question of which lens to choose is perhaps the fitter's most important decision. Does one go for the short-term reward and choose a soft lens because it meets with early and rapid patient acceptance or does one consider a rigid gas-permeable lens, which may be superior in the long term? Questions to be answered in this chapter include the following:

tient's teeth, hands, and face are dirty or his hair is unkempt, one can assume that the lenses will be carelessly maintained. A rigid lens can injure a cornea by either causing mechanical compression or creating tiny punctate erosions because of hypoxia. If the lens is contaminated or the conjunctiva infected, this small portal of entry allows bacteria to penetrate the cornea and create a corneal ulcer. The most common sources of contamination are dirty hands or wet, dirty cases, which permit *Pseudomonas aeruginosa* to grow. These accidents are common. In 1 year, approximately 8000 eyes were damaged from improper rigid lens wear. Ninety percent of the damage was reversible, but there was some severe sequelae including total loss of the eye.

A soft lens cannot damage the cornea by abrasion because of its supple nature. However, it has a tendency to collect protein from the tear film. This protein is an excellent culture medium. Bacteria adhere to a lens that is coated with protein. It is particularly common to see these protein-based infections with aphakic soft lenses and extended wear lenses. Serious corneal ulcers and endophthalmitis have been shown to occur with the improper use of soft lenses. In the past few years, the resulting corneal ulcerations in extended wear contact lens patients has reached such proportions that many doctors have condemned the use of extended wear lenses.

Aphakic people produce a smaller quantity of tears than younger people do and so protein deposition is more likely to occur. Also, elderly patients produce a smaller amount of lysozyme, which is a normal antibacterial enzyme in tears, which raises the possibility of infections in people with a depleted tear function. In the elderly, because of changes in tear composition, there may be also an increase in mineralization of the lens.

PATIENT SELECTION

The cosmetic lens patient with a healthy eye and intact adequate tear film has a 90% chance of being successfully fitted with a contact lens (in regard to the full spectrum of lens designs, materials, and support systems). Patients with the best prognosis for successful fitting are those who fit the following criteria:

Best age group: 13 to 38 years of age.
Women > men.

Refractive error, > -1.50 D, $> +1.50$ D.
K reading, 41.00 to 46.00 D.
BUTs > 15 seconds.
Cornea with no significant sequential staining.
Good tear flow by Schirmer test.
Regular corneas–no scarring or distortion of corneal mires.
Regular low astigmatism, $< +1.50$ D.
Good lid position with no scleral show.
Adequate manual dexterity.

Those patients with a reduced prognosis for successful fitting are the following:

Those who are going on a trip and need a lens fitted in 7 days. Do not oblige unless you are prepared to handle an emergency call from Bermuda. In addition, this could be construed as professional negligence, since it is not ideally in the patient's best interest.
Smokers of pipes, cigars, or cigarettes.
Sloppy and careless persons.
Those who are chronically anxious or under anxiety during the time of the contact lens fit.
Those myopic patients who are about to become presbyopic.
Those who are poorly motivated, e.g.:
Spouse wants him or her to wear lenses
Purchaser of a "party lens"
Those who have small refractive errors, less than −1.00 diopters.
Those who incur occupational hazards, such as hair dressers, truck drivers, and factory workers in chemical environments.
Those with excessive fears, such as being terrified of having anything touch their eyes.
Patients with strabismus or ptosis because a contact lens may make them look worse.
Those with ocular allergies, chronic blepharitis, arthritis, and exophthalmos.
Those who work or live in an acid- or alkaline-fume environment.
Avoid the 5 *D*'s—the dirty, the drunk, the diseased, the disabled, the dumb.

Medical factors that may reduce probability of wearing contact lenses

Skin disease. These particularly include seborrhea, psoriasis, and neurodermatitis, as well as chronic blepharitis from any atopic skin conditions. Swollen, inflamed lid margins significantly reduce progress for good patient comfort. The threshold for discomfort will be lower, and the debris from the lids will act as an irritant. In addition, the meibomian gland secretions become abnormal, thus affecting the stability of the tear film. The lens may be greasy and filmy, covered by sebaceous discharge from the irritated meibomian glands.

Dry eyes. This syndrome may include either individual dry spots or combinations of them on the cornea, aqueous deficiency, mucin deficiency, lipid deficiency, and extreme xerosis with conspicuous erosions of the cornea.

A Schirmer test should be done on each patient; the cornea should be observed for dry spots and a rose bengal test done to illustrate devitalized tissue.

Systemic drugs. Drugs for gastric ulcers (atropine-like drugs) may reduce tear flow and artificially create dry spots. Birth control pills may

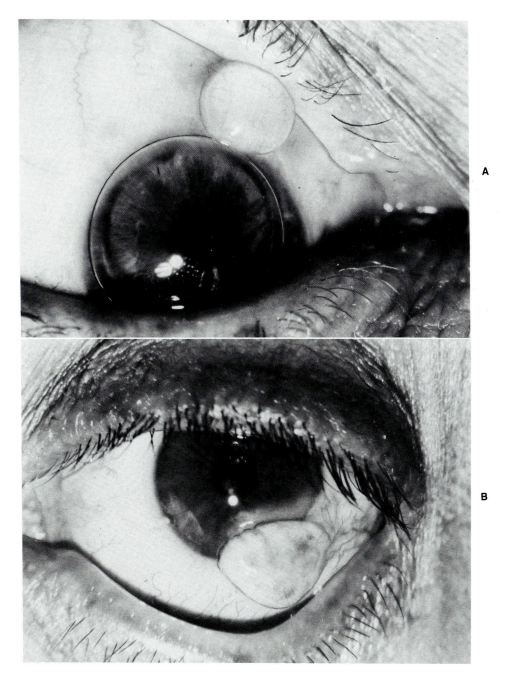

Fig 5-1 ■ **A,** Large cystic bleb occurring after glaucoma filtration procedure that would interfere with contact lens movement. **B,** Large limbal dermoid that should be surgically removed to permit the wearing of a contact lens.

cause rigid lenses to be intolerable and soft lenses to be rapidly covered with protein debris. Diazepam (Valium) and other tranquilizers have no direct effect on the cornea or tear film. But anxious patients requiring medication of this nature may be difficult to fit.

Handling problems. Usually problems with handling are obvious. Patients with arthritis of the hands, a parkinsonian-like tremor, and psoriasis of skin or nails make poor contact lens candidates. However, patients with dirty fingernails should also be rejected. The most common cause of corneal ulcers with soft lens wearers is poor hygiene, specifically dirty lens cases that grow *Pseudomonas aeruginosa*.

Corneal disease. Recurrent corneal erosion, corneal dystrophy of any kind, corneal scarring with dry spots of the cornea, old vernal conjunctivitis or trachoma, and any disease that results in a vascularized cornea may contraindicate wearing contact lenses.

Allergies. Lesions of the limbus such as dermoid cysts may require surgical removal before lens wear (Fig. 5-1). A history of hay fever, drug reaction, or atopic skin reactions to cosmetics or perfumes may be a warning to a later sensitivity to preservatives in contact lens solutions or the formation of giant papillary conjunctivitis. Allergic reactions to the plastics of a contact lens have not been proved to be a factor in these atopic reactions.

Corneal warpage and corneal anesthesia. Some PMMA rigid lens wearers may develop corneal warpage because of corneal hypoxia. Before the development of the gas-permeable lenses, the fitter usually required the patient to abstain from wearing contact lenses until the warpage was corrected. The newer lenses make this abstinence period unnecessary because one can fit patients with gas-permeable lenses and provide functional restoration of vision while the keratometric mires are restored to their baseline measurements.

A patient may have 20/20 vision, comfort, and total freedom of any symptoms and still develop a toric cornea. Look at the cornea at least once a year without the lenses to ensure that an induced toricity has not occurred.

PMMA lenses usually will result in corneal desensitization. There is a linear relationship with wear. The sensitivity may be measured with the Cochet-Bonnet hair test (Fig. 5-2).

The monocular patient. The monocular patient should be treated with special concern. If

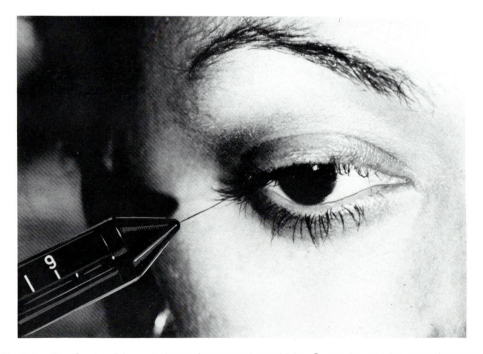

Fig 5-2 ■ The Cochet-Bonnet hair test for corneal sensitivity. Corneal sensation may decrease with oxygen deprivation after long-term use of rigid lenses that do not permit sufficient oxygen transfer.

the patient is a monocular lens wearer, that is, aphakia or anisometropia prevails, the person must be drilled about the ocular emergencies that can arise. A corneal abrasion in a monocular patient is a blinding event.

Pregnancy and menopause. Pregnancy, menopause, and birth-control medication cause a disruption in the normal hormonal balance. The sequelae are poorly understood, but the quality of the tear film and the integrity of the cornea is possibly altered during these states. Rigid lenses are rejected more easily than soft lenses, and it is certainly inadvisable to begin lens wearing during an endocrine flux.

COMMENT. We have observed a greater tendency for protein deposition on soft lenses during late pregnancy and lactation.

Diabetes. Patients with stable diabetes may be fitted with contact lenses. Those with unstable diabetes, which are mainly juvenile in grouping, should not be fitted. With a volatile blood glucose, a stable refraction may be difficult to obtain.

Thyroid disease with exophthalmos. Only a soft lens should be considered because the retracted upper and lower lid will dislodge a smaller, rigid lens. However, even a soft lens may create variable vision if the blink rate is infrequent and the excursions of the lid are incomplete. Drying of the lens may occur, and the lens may become proteinized (Fig. 5-3).

COMMENT. Before fitting any thyroid patient, make sure the lids cover the cornea with light lid closure during blinking and sleep.

If there are dry spots of the cornea or inferior keratitis from exposure, a low-water-content soft lens may be attempted, supplemented with additional artificial tears. Low-water-content lenses create less water demand from the cornea than high-water-content lenses do and

appear to perform better for dry eyes, but in dry environments the opposite is true.

These patients should be followed closely because 30% in our hands do poorly whatever lens or method is chosen. Contact lenses tend to dry because of incomplete or infrequent blinking.

Special indications

Nystagmus. Patients with congenital grade III nystagmus in which the eyes are oscillating all the time and patients with a significant refractive error with any congenital nystagmus may profit from contact lenses because the lenses move with the eye. Contact lenses may significantly improve visual acuity and also result in the lowering of the degree and amplitude of nystagmus.

Ocular albinism. A cosmetic contact lens with clear aperture but darkly tinted in the periphery may be very helpful against the glare effects that an albino suffers. The improvement in visual acuity is minimal because of the foveal aplasia found in this condition.

Aniridia. This refers to those patients who are born without an iris or those who have had the iris removed because of surgery or trauma. Most patients with congenital aniridia have cataracts, gross nystagmus, and foveal aplasia. They are much more comfortable with tinted cosmetic contact lenses because they lack any iris development.

Previously fitted patient. It is always a challenge to fit a person who has failed in the past to wear lenses. However, the new fitter should attempt to obtain the history of the previous fits. It may conserve time because the same errors do not have to be repeated and it might yield some insight into the patient's personality and problems. A refitting may require only a change of solutions. Check the patient's method of handling, use of cleaners, and storage and rinsing solutions. If the problem is corneal edema go to a gas-permeable lens, rigid or soft. Try to solve the problem. It can be the fit, an inappropriate lens design, the wrong choice of plastics, or poor quality control from the laboratory. Resolve the technical problems before you attribute the poor fit to a lack of patient resolve.

COMMENT. Never speak in a derogatory way about another or previous fitter. The total circumstance may not be known, and the criticism may be unfair. Also, no one has complete success with all patients. Anyone can make an error or omission.

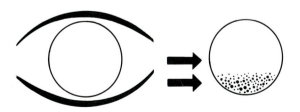

Fig 5-3 ■ Thyroid disease with exophthalmos. Incomplete blinking results in inferior keratopathy or drying of the surface of a soft contact lens because of exposure.

Psychiatric illness. The frequency of anxiety cannot be accurately gauged because there is no serum factor to reveal its presence. Seriously ill people are frequently on medications to control anxiety, depression, or manic-depressive states. Patients with psychiatric distress should be screened but not necessarily discouraged from wearing lenses. If contact lenses can significantly improve vision or cosmetic appearance, the benefits to the patient must be assessed individually. If the mental health of the person is so marginal that the physician has to be concerned over the hygiene and consistency to regulations of contact lens care, this type of individual should be ruled out as a candidate.

In many instances, the distress of a person may be temporary and the fittings should be postponed. Postpartum depression, depression after the death of a spouse or after a divorce, anxiety about a new job or before examinations at school, or financial pressures may cause a temporary lowering of threshold to pain. It is not within the scope of an eye practitioner to make a valid psychiatric assessment. But there are features to lend suspicion to a given case: history of taking mood-elevating or -depressing drugs; a history of admittance to a psychiatric institution; a desire to wear contact lenses that are perceived to be unreasonable; a person with a low refractive error (-0.75 sphere) who barely uses spectacles; or a person who will not or cannot submit to an applanation tonometer test, a Schirmer test, or even a proper slitlamp examination. Such a person will show excessive blepharospasm or light sensitivity. Also any person who has unrealistic attitudes toward wearing lenses, such as a person who wants extended wear lenses because they are so easy to wear and require a cleaning only twice a year, should be carefully screened.

COMMENT. It is important to note that the initial wearing of contact lenses may be anxiety-ridden. Many patients fear their dexterity will not be sufficient to get the lenses in or out, or the lenses will become trapped in or on the eye, or the pain will be excessive, or they are endeavoring to do something that can cause permanent damage to their eyes. These people are normal and rational and show the same fear as a novice skier who looking down from a hill asks himself, "Will I make it or not?" This is normal self-doubt. It is only when these normal, guarded feelings are excessive that a fitter has to be suspicious that he or she has embarked upon a task that will not be rewarding to both patient and physician.

RIGID LENSES

The rigid PMMA lens still has a small place in the contact lens fitter's armamentarium. It possesses two important qualities: durability and high visual performance.

Durability. The rigid PMMA lens is resistant to scratches and to breakage, especially at the edge; it does not become easily defaced with either lipids or protein adhering to its surface. As a result this lens lasts longer. Most types of PMMA lenses can be modified and blended, and their diameters can be reduced with office modification equipment. Surface scratches can be removed by polishing.

COMMENT. It is common to see rigid PMMA lenses survive 5 years or more, but rare for a soft lens.

High visual performance. The PMMA rigid lens and the gas-permeable rigid lens still offer one of the best visual performances although this is not necessarily true with toric corneas greater than 3.00 diopters when rigid PMMA lenses are used.

Good vision is constant and not subject to the variability that often plagues the soft lens wearer. Qualitatively, the optics are better. Even though a rigid lens wearer and a soft lens wearer may achieve 20/20 vision, the rigid lens wearer appears to "see better." Many rigid lens wearers who have been switched to soft lenses dislike the quality of soft lens vision, even though the visual numbers of both are 20/20. A reduction in contrast sensitivity is believed to be the reason for this discrepancy.

The PMMA lens has some serious faults. It has no permeability and can cause acute and chronic corneal hypoxia. It is the least comfortable lens and is more prone to cause ocular irritation in the face of wind, sun, dust, and debris. It is inadequate for the poor blinker and the person who reads all day and whose blink rate deteriorates after hours of doing close work. It is difficult for anyone who works outdoors to wear the rigid lens. Finally, a PMMA lens in spheric form does not center well in conventional diameters (7.8 to 8.2 mm) if significant corneal asigmatism is present (>2.00 diopters).

GAS-PERMEABLE LENSES

Gas-permeable lenses include the CAB lens, silicone-acrylate polymers, polystyrene materials, and the fluorocarbonated silicone acrylates. These lenses do not depend entirely on blinking for oxygenation through the tear film because they transmit oxygen through the material itself to reach the cornea. Because of their oxygen permeability, they can be made larger, thus providing more stability and better centration. They can be made to rise high enough to allow the upper lid to cover the superior edge of the lens to prevent lid impact and blink inhibition. The ability of the lids to blink without engaging the upper edge of the lens also makes the lens more comfortable than any comparable PMMA lens. Today it is the rigid lens of choice.

If vision is vital, a rigid lens with or without permeability may be the best choice. For architects, designers, and engineers, the rigid lens performance can be counted upon to give a consistent visual result.

COMMENT. Gas-permeable rigid lenses can cover up to 4 diopters of astigmatism when a large-diameter ($>$9.2 mm) spheric lens is used.

Ease in handling. For the bilateral aphake, a rigid lens may be the best choice. The aphakic person can feel the lens, a fact not true for one wearing a soft lens.

Lens removal is also easier for the aphakic person dealing with a rigid lens. One can remove the lens indirectly by using the lids or by a suction-cup device, or, when in distress, by a touch of honey on the fingertip.

Cost. Rigid lenses are less expensive than gas-permeable soft lenses, can be cleaned and polished easily, have a low maintenance cost, and can be modified in the office. Also rigid lenses last longer than other contact lenses and cost less to replace. On the other hand, a rigid lens is more likely to be lost because it is smaller, and it can be more readily dislodged from the eye because it is not a good lens when one is playing hockey.

Astigmatism correction. In lower spheric errors of refraction, a rigid lens is best. If the correction is -2.00 D $+$ 1.00 D $\times$ 90, a conventional soft lens will yield poor visual results. The ratio of cylinder to sphere should not exceed 1:4 with an outside maximum of 1.50 diopters of astigmatism tolerated for a spheric soft lens.

Toric soft lenses are available, but they are more difficult to fit, do not give visual results comparable to a rigid lens, and are technically difficult in cases of oblique astigmatism or with patients with tight lids.

Gas-permeable lenses are very helpful with any kind of astigmatism, especially at high levels of 4 to 5 diopters, which can be covered with a spheric lens.

A gas-permeable lens is preferred for the following situations.

Rigid lens dropouts. These people with either chronic corneal hypoxia or molding changes in the cornea induced by the wearing of a rigid lens can be *immediately fitted* with gas-permeable lenses. The corneal edema will eventually disappear on wearing such a lens. The old practice of wearing glasses until K readings stabilized or the refraction returned to normal is no longer necessary. The gas-permeable lens fills this void.

Keratoconus. The excellent optics of a gas-permeable lens and its ability to negate the effects of irregular corneal astigmatism make it the lens of choice for patients with keratoconus. The epithelium of the conic cornea is not likely to be healthy. It may be flattened, thinned, atrophic, or scarred. A gas-permeable lens provides sufficient oxygen to this atrophic layer of cells to keep it free of hypoxic complications.

Gas-permeable lenses require less frequent lens changes and are more comfortable for keratoconus patients. It should be the lens of choice. If it doesn't work, a soft lens carrier with a piggyback gas-permeable lens is the second best choice.

COMMENT. Gas permeability refers to the physical properties of the plastic; any lens design can be used.

Excessive spectacle blur. With gas-permeable lenses, spectacle blur is minimal because of the absence of central corneal hypoxia with resulting edema. With the patient who wants to read after the lenses have been removed for the night, this feature is very handy.

COMMENT. Spectacle blur caused by corneal edema is relieved with gas-permeable lenses. Spectacle blur caused by aberrations of a thick lens (about 6.00 D or greater) will not be altered with gas-permeable contact lenses.

Patients who are susceptible to flare

The optic zone of a standard PMMA lens is often too small to encompass the pupil. This is

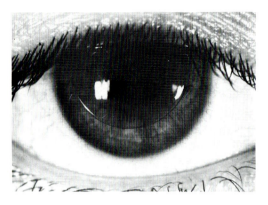

Fig 5-4 ■ The silicone-acrylate contact lens is gas-permeable. It may be fitted larger than conventional rigid lenses. Notice that the upper eyelid margin is covering the upper portion of the contact lens. (From Stein HA and Slatt BJ: The ophthalmic assistant, ed 5, St Louis, 1988, The CV Mosby Co.)

especially true for young blue-eyed myopic people with large pupils who drive in dim illumination. The small thin PMMA lenses are fitted tight but are not sufficient in size to counter the effects of a larger pupil.

The newer gas-permeable lens, because of its larger size, can have a larger optic zone than a PMMA lens has and is usually of sufficient size to eliminate flare, which is the sunburst effect around a light.

Rigid lens discomfort

The gas-permeable lens is a remedy for people with rigid lens discomfort who want rigid lens optics (Fig. 5-4). The lens is more comfortable for several reasons.

> The upper edge of the lens does not engage the upper lid and lies under the eyelid.
> The lens is stable and centers well.
> The movement of the lens with blinking is less than that of a smaller PMMA rigid lens.
> The cornea is well supplied with oxygen directly, and so the patient does not experience a burning sensation when the blink rate is likely to be reduced. This is likely to occur with prolonged reading, sewing, driving, and doing visual work that results in fatigue.

Soft lens dropouts

Some patients do not like soft lenses. Their vision may not be crisp because of astigmatism, they may be more prone to giant papillary conjunctivitis, or they may not like the care systems of a soft lens.

The gas-permeable lens provides a good bridge to better vision.

SOFT LENSES

A soft lens is preferred in the following situations and for the characteristics mentioned.

Rapid adaptation

A soft lens is recommended for people who require rapid adaptation; frequently a soft lens is comfortable 10 minutes after first being inserted and can be worn easily from the first day. Rapid adaptation is an important factor for people who are busy with work or study.

Comfort

For patients with a lowered threshold of discomfort, the soft lens is the only answer. Many who are rigid lens dropouts are quite content with soft lenses.

Low refractive errors

A soft lens is preferred for patients with low refractive errors of −1.50 diopters or less. With these persons the motivation to adapt to the continuous daily wear of rigid lenses is not sufficient. As a result, the comfort of soft lenses combined with the ability to wear the lenses intermittently offers a distinct advantage.

Inability to wear rigid lenses

A soft lens is preferable for persons unable to wear rigid lenses for many reasons: (1) intolerance because of pregnancy, (2) a bad experience with an overwear reaction, (3) induced astigmatism and spectacle blur created by rigid lens, corneal molding, (4) difficulty in maintaining a rigid wearing schedule, (5) excessive photophobia and glare, and (6) intolerance to sun, wind, and dust. A soft lens protects the eye and does not leave it vulnerable to exposure.

Athletes

Especially in body-contact sports such as hockey, basketball, and football a soft lens is less likely to be dislodged because it follows the eye closely on movement. In tennis the soft lens is less likely to drop when the eyes are raised for the serve, and in gymnastics the soft lens is less likely to pop out.

Safety

For the industrial worker who is working on dangerous machinery a soft lens is far less likely to be dislodged or decentered. The private pilot is better off with a soft lens, which is less likely to pop out of an eye or momentarily slide off the center of the eye.

Eye safety

The soft lens is less likely to cause a portal of entry in the cornea for bacteria or other pathogens by creating a cornea abrasion or ulcer. Corneal edema is minimal with an ill-fitting soft lens as compared to an ill-fitting hard lens.

COMMENT. Factory workers, patients who are working with chemicals, construction workers, furniture refinishers, and others are contraindicated for soft lens wear because of the dangers of toxic environmental vapors.

Children

Children who require contact lenses because of aniridia, amblyopia therapy, albinism, or congenital nystagmus should wear soft lenses. The soft lens is more comfortable and safer in these instances and, over the long haul, is less likely to abrade the eye. Also it is more suitable for sports or for play in a dusty atmosphere.

Swimming

Because of recent reports of contamination in swimming pools by *Pseudomonas auroganesa* and Acanthomoeba, swimming while wearing contact lenses is contraindicated. Corneal disasters have resulted from contamination in hot tubs, oceans, lakes, and pools in patients wearing soft contact lenses. Swimmers wearing hard lenses are likely to lose their lenses unless they wear scuba masks or swim goggles.

Intermittent wear

Persons who wear contact lenses infrequently, such as public speakers, athletes, or actors, prefer a soft lens to a rigid lens. These individuals desire a lens only for social occasions, sports activities, or their work on stage. The soft lens can be used just for such purposes. The cornea adapts quickly to its presence and does not require a buildup of wearing time. Also, most soft lenses do not create significant corneal edema or spectacle blur, and as a result the shift back to glasses can be achieved smoothly and without any visual disability.

Nystagmus

Soft lenses may significantly improve vision in patients with nystagmus because the lens tracks with the eye of the patient. Vision is not distorted by the parallax effect that occurs when glasses are worn or by the disturbing movement of the rigid lens during blinking.

Wide palpebral fissures

In patients with thyroid disease or congenitally wide eyelids, the soft lens can be ordered in a larger size so that the margin of the lid is less likely to engage the edge of the lens.

COMMENT

As a practitioner you cannot select your patients, but you can select your lenses. Be realistic and flexible. If a patient has tight lids and oblique astigmatism and wants soft lenses, outline the pitfalls of such a choice. Do not let the patient dictate the choice of lens you prescribe because he or she will hold you responsible if the device does not work.

Also of importance is the quality control of the lenses. If a laboratory makes a poor gas-permeable lens with thick or fragile edges, it would be inadvisable to use them. Thick edges lead to lid gap, 3 to 9 o'clock staining, red eyes, symptoms of dryness, and an unhappy patient.

Patient selection is perhaps the most important aspect of effective successful contact lens fitting. The public perception of a given lens may be inaccurate. For example, common misconceptions are that soft lenses grow fungi when worn, rigid lenses are hard to wear, or that gas-permeable lenses are semisoft. It is up to the fitter to educate the patients.

LENSES FOR SPECIAL SITUATIONS
Airline personnel

Commercial airlines generally frown upon the use of contact lenses by air-flight personnel, particularly by pilots and copilots. Airline and commercial transport pilots are not allowed to wear lenses in case of a loss of lens from a windblast or from spontaneous ejection of the lenses. A soft lens can't be extruded easily, but it can be decentered or dehydrated in the dry environment of the plane's cabin. Even if vision was lost only momentarily, it would risk the safety of the plane and its crew and passengers. Also airplane air tends to be quite dry. When evaporation occurs, the soft lens loses its smooth contours and its surface becomes wavy. However, at times exceptions are made and monocular aphakic pilots are allowed to wear a single contact lens.

Flight attendants are usually allowed to wear

contact lenses if their unaided vision is 20/100. This proviso is added so that the attendant can function without contact lenses if need be. Anyone can get a foreign body like debris or a hard particle of mascara under a lens. The rule is wise. The other requirement is that the person must show an ability to wear the lenses for the duration of the flight intended.

COMMENT. Unfortunately, occasionally a contact-lens scam occurs. Young men intent on being pilots have their eyes "normalized" by orthokeratology. The prospective pilot can pass the test and see 20/20 without glasses or contacts. He neglects telling anyone that he still needs a retainer lens to sustain his refractive status. We have seen a few cases of such a nature.

Athletes

Much has been said about the use of contact lenses for sports. They are certainly of value in tennis, squash, racquet ball, skiing, basketball, or football.

The contact lens offers no protection for the eye. If eye injury is a distinct possibility, eye guards must be used in addition to the contact lenses. Protection of this nature is mandatory for football, hockey, and squash where the incidence of ocular injury is high.

Most professional athletes are required to have a spare pair of lenses available in case of loss or displacement of lenses. The National Basketball Association frowns on 7-foot giants groping on the floor, feeling for a lost 8.5 mm lens.

Most eye professionals believe that the athlete is better served by contact lenses. Visual acuity for distance is better for the high myope, and the athlete does not have to endure restrictions of visual field and distortions of a thick lens system. However, before becoming evangelic about the merits of contact lenses for athletes, let us remember that Reggie Jackson, Billie Jean King, and Arthur Ashe did quite well in their respective sports while wearing spectacles.

Skiers at times can get epithelial edema while wearing their lenses. Because of the coldness of the environment, the oxygen needs of the corneal epithelium are low. The lenses feel quite comfortable. The tint on the lenses may make the skier feel well enough to go skiing without protective goggles, but this can be a mistake because the skier may be exposed to an intense ultraviolet burn from the direct and reflected sun rays.

Swimmers have to be careful with contact lenses. If swim goggles are used, they are rarely watertight and the lens may become dislodged or contaminated by the water. Goggles for swimming do not handle the moisture well and "fog up." They do not offer protection against infection, inflammation, or decreased vision. They do offer some protection against lens loss. Lenses should not be worn for diving or water skiing because the risk of losing one's lenses is quite high, as is the risk of corneal infection.

6 ▪ CONTACT LENS' MANUFACTURING

Joshua E. Josephson

Until recently, contact lens manufacturing technology had remained rather stagnant. Plastic produced in sheets or in tube molds was cut into buttons. All manufacturers, with the exception of Bausch and Lomb, used simple single-axis lathes to produce the front power curve and the posterior base curve of the finished lenses from these buttons. The surfaces of these unfinished lenses were then polished. Peripheral curves were added to the posterior surface with single-axis spinning tools; the edges were then finished and polished (Fig. 6-1).

Today, the major manufacturers use very sophisticated lathes with highly refined computer-aided manufacturing from computerized designs (Fig. 6-2). This technique of numerical-control positioning of the cutting tool is commonly known as CAD-CAM (computer-aided design—computer-aided manufacturing). Some of these lathes are capable of adding the posterior surface peripheral curves as part of the base curve lathe-cutting process. Even more recently, dual axis lathes have been used (University Optics; Fig. 6-3) for cutting the curves of lens' surfaces. These techniques can be so refined that very little polishing is required for the finished surfaces. Manufacturers, such as University Optics and Wesley-Jessen isolate their lathes from environmental vibration influences, using air-bearing technology in order to further improve the precision of lens manufacturing.

The material batch is the first concern when quality control and reproducibility of soft contact lenses is considered. The material must be consistent and of high quality; otherwise, with hydrogel lenses, the swell factor (the expansion that takes place when a lens absorbs water after being manufactured in the hard state) will not be consistent and errors will be introduced into the final product. With rigid lens materials, the quality of the batch can affect the base curve stability, lens durability, and optical quality.

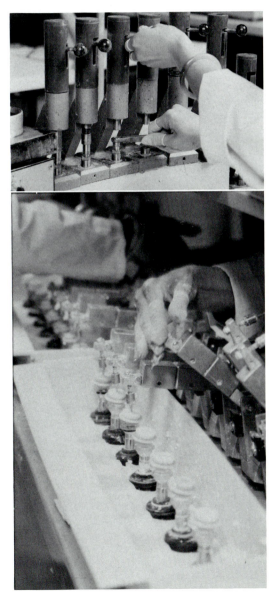

Fig 6-1 ▪ Automated surface polishing machines. (Courtesy Ciba Vision, Inc, Atlanta Ga.)

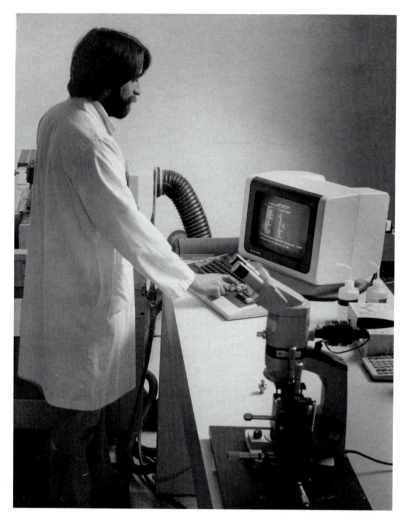

Fig 6-2 ■ CAD-CAM technology. (Courtesy University Optics, Largo, Fla.)

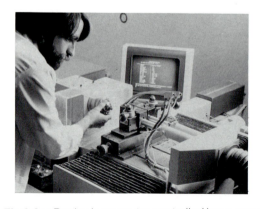

Fig 6-3 ■ Dual axis computer-controlled laser scanning system of lathing. (Courtesy University Optics, Largo, Fla.)

Some companies, such as the Menicon Company and Bausch & Lomb, make their own monomers to ensure lens reproducibility.

In order to improve reproducibility and reduce costs, several companies have developed hydrogel lens-molding technology. Bausch & Lomb licensed spin-cast technology from Hydron and refined the spin-cast process originally developed by Czech scientists, Otto Wichterle and V. Lim (Fig. 6-4). In this process the liquid monomer is injected into an optical quality mold as it is spinning. The liquid monomer is polymerized as the spinning mold shapes the front surface of the lens (Fig. 6-5). More recently, Bausch & Lomb developed a technology based on spin-cast molding, known as Reverse Process III, whereby the front surface is produced in the

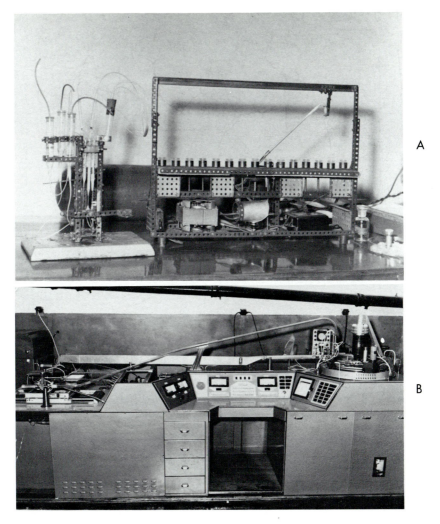

Fig 6-4 ■ **A,** The original fitting and spinning machines (erector set) the precursor of spin-casting technology, developed by Otto Wichterle and associates at the Prague Institute, Czechoslovakia, circa 1964. (Courtesy Martin M Pollack, Allergan Hydron, Inc, Syosset, NY.) **B,** The first production spin-cast machine, developed at the Prague Institute, Czechoslovakia, circa 1966. (Courtesy Martin M Pollack, Allergan Hydron, Inc, Syosset, NY.)

spin-casting process and the back surface is generated by computer-controlled lathing. Other companies, like Hydron and Cooper, for example, refined the technology of cast-molding lenses by injecting liquid monomers between two optical quality molds (Fig. 6-6). New proprietary polymerization technologies have helped to improve the quality of contact lens parameters. The Vistakon disposable contact lens is manufactured by cast-molding in a fully hydrated state by a process known as *stabilized soft molding* (SSM). In this process, finished lenses are less subject to the dry lens hydration distortion seen when hydrogel lenses are lathed in the dry state and then hydrated. Also, variations in dimension are not magnified during the typical 20% to 60% swelling that occurs upon hydration of most hydrophilic contact lenses. Molding technology has also been used for rigid gas-permeable contact lenses. Paragon Optical has developed the technique of injection-molding modified PMMA material into a button and then casting their contact lens material inside the button posterior surface radii (base curve and peripheral curves). This technique, known as *cast radius molding* (Figs. 6-7 to 6-9)

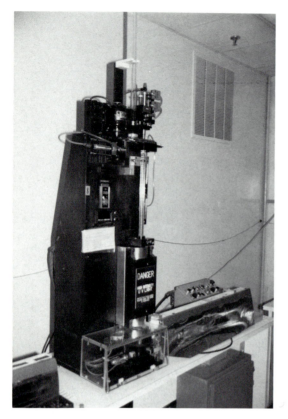

Fig 6-5 ■ Current spin-cast technology. (Courtesy Allergan Hydron, Inc, Syosset, NY.)

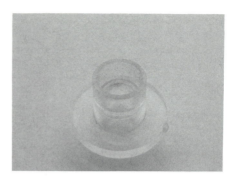

Fig 6-6 ■ A plastic mold for cast radius molding. (Courtesy Ultrasoft Laboratories, Vancouver, Canada.)

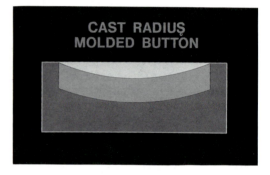

CAST RADIUS
MOLDED BUTTON

Fig 6-7 ■ Schematic of cross-section of cast radius molded button. (Courtesy Paragon Optical, Mesa, Ariz.)

is reported to increase the reproducibility and stability of the finished product, in addition to improving the optical quality.

Wesley-Jessen has improved toric lens axis accuracy and reproducibility by developing a method of moving an unfinished toric lens from one machine to another. This process is known as *transfer blocking methodology* and it can consistently place the design elements of a lens to within 0.0127 mm of its intended position. This system eliminates the need for an operator to visually align the lens for axis position.

New technologies have been developed to monitor lens quality and reproducibility more closely. Both these are major concerns of the manufacturer and the busy practitioner. One of the newest devices that has been applied to contact lens manufacturing is the laser. University Optics was first to use this device for monitoring the surface parameters of the Alges[R] bifocal contact lens. A laser is projected onto the surface

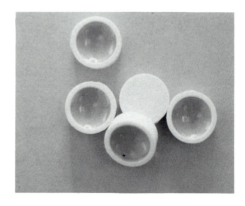

Fig 6-8 ■ Cast molds for contact lenses.

of the contact lens during the lathing process. The computerized optical feedback ensures very close tolerances during production (see Figure 6-3). Surface accuracy is ultimately confirmed after manufacturing. The surfaces are checked by mounting the lens in a specially designed

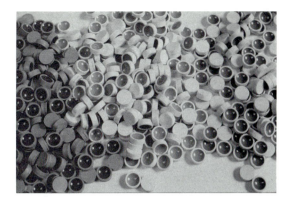

Fig 6-9 ■ Cast radius molded buttons. (Courtesy Paragon Optical, Mesa, Ariz.)

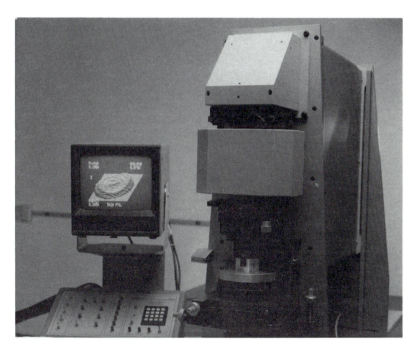

Fig 6-10 ■ Laser interferometer used in measuring surface quality and parameters of a contact lens. (Courtesy University Optics, Largo, Fla.)

Fig 6-11 ■ CRT output of device shown in Fig. 6-12. (Courtesy University Optics, Largo, Fla.)

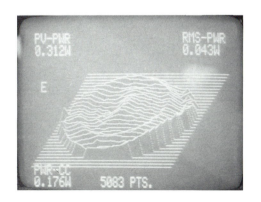

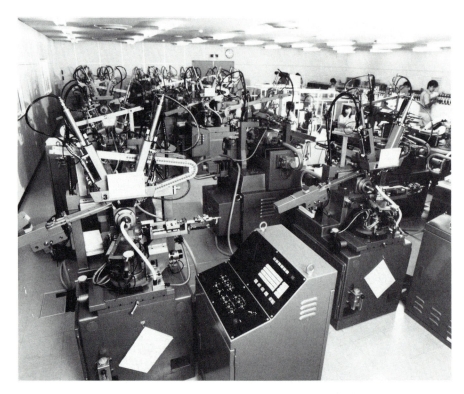

Fig 6-12 ■ Robot technology used in highly automated production line. (Courtesy the Menicon Company, Nagoya, Japan.)

laser interferometer. The surface of the lens is scanned and the information is processed, producing an image on a television monitor (CRT) that has been reported to reveal inaccuracies as small as ten to fifteen nanometers in size (Figs. 6-10 to 6-12).

Robotic technology has been used, especially by the Menicon Company (Figure 6-12), in the processing and transferring of raw materials (plastics, liquids, monomers, or buttons) to finishing machines. The finished product may be received, packaged, labelled, and forwarded to the shipping department without significant human effort.

The evolution of manufacturing technology over the past 20 years has made possible the most advanced lens designs available, such as ultrathin lens construction, thin edges, torics, and new bifocals. In addition, the cost of contact lenses in "real dollars" compared to the cost of the PMMA lenses made 25 years ago, has been dramatically reduced by the new technology and efficiency in lens production. This new manufacturing technology should lead to further developments that were previously not possible.

PART II

BASIC FITTING: AN APPROACH TO LENS-FITTING FOR THE STUDENT AND SMALL-VOLUME FITTER

7 ■ *SOFT LENSES*

Characteristics, Advantages, and Disadvantages

■ *History*
■ *Characteristics*
■ *Advantages*
■ *Disadvantages*
■ *Thin and ultrathin soft lenses*

There are two basic types of lenses considered to be soft lenses: (1) the *hydrophilic* (sometimes referred to as *hydrogel) lens*, which owes its softness to its ability to absorb and bind water, and (2) the *silicone soft lens*, which owes its softness to the intrinsic property of the rubbery material from which it is made. The silicone lens is fast becoming obsolete and is used primarily in cases of pediatric aphakia. It has not survived the test of time; not only was the lens troublesome but, in some cases, the main problem was one of breakdown of the lens surface, which led to poor wetting and deposit formation. In this chapter emphasis will be placed on the hydrophilic hydrogel soft lenses, which have gained widespread popularity and are readily available, reliable, and a proven entity. These may be divided into HEMA lenses and non-HEMA lenses.

HISTORY

It is always interesting and informative to learn from the past, and so it is with soft hydrogel contact lenses, which have had a major impact in the world, not only for their correction of refractive errors for cosmetic purposes, but also for their contribution to the management of aphakia and the treatment of disease states of the eye by use of the bandage lens.

In 1960 two young New York lawyers established a company with the unique function of promoting patent exchanges between corporations. Their specialty was combing through the dusty corporate files for idle patents and setting up licensing agreements with other companies interested in putting the dormant ideas to use. They achieved a measure of success, and their clients included du Pont de Nemours, Chrysler Corporation, Swift & Company, and Thiocol Chemical Corporation.

In 1965 the men who had established the National Patent Development Corporation suddenly dissolved their patent law business. They had uncovered a patent with so many exciting possibilities that they decided to pick up a license themselves. In effect, they became their own client, abandoning their role as middlemen.

The new material was a plastic they called "hydron." It was developed by Dr. Otto Wichterle, head of the Institute of Macromolecular Chemistry of the Czechoslovakian National Academy of Science and a leading expert on polymer chemistry, and by Dr. Drahoslav Lim. The new material appeared to be like other plastics in that it was a hard transparent substance that could be cut, ground, or molded into a variety of shapes. However, when placed in water or an aqueous solution, the tough, rigid plastic became soft and pliable. In its wet form it could be bent between the fingers until the edges met or could be easily turned inside out; yet it would snap back into its original shape quickly. When allowed to dry, the supple water-logged material became dry as a cornflake and crushed to a powdery dust if smashed. The substance was subjected to rigorous biologic tests and was found to be inert and fully compatible with human tissue. One of its spectacular properties was that although highly elastic when wet, it remained strong and able to hold its shape (Fig. 7-1).

The plastic is *hydroxyethylmethacrylate (HEMA)*, a plastic polymer with the remarkable

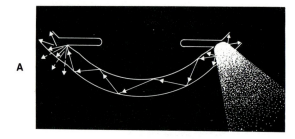

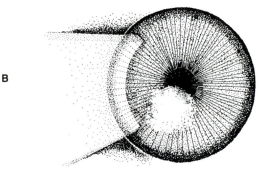

Fig 7-1 ■ **A,** Corneal edema can be detected grossly by angling the beam of the slitlamp 45 to 60 degrees at the limbus. **B,** Specular reflection. The internal reflection of light through the cornea makes the central edema stand out as a gray haze. The cornea is used as a fiber-optic channel.

ability to absorb water molecules. Chemically, the polymer consists of a three-dimensional network of hydroxyethylmethacrylate chains crosslinked with ethylene glycol dimethacrylate molecules about once every 200 monomer units. As the water is introduced to the plastic, it swells into a soft mass with surprisingly good mechanical strength, complete transparency (97%), and the ability to retain its shape and dimensions when equilibrated in fluid.

Over the years, many modifications of the plastic were introduced, new polymers added, and new lens' designs created. Five hard years of improvements and clincial trials were conducted on the soft lens before the Federal Drug Administration (which considered the lens a drug) approved the lens as a safe prosthetic device of good optic quality. The FDA's caution, after the thalidomide tragedies, was understandable. Both the public and the practitioner needed protection. In the first phase of research the soft lens was tested on laboratory animals to ensure that it was nontoxic; later it was given to selected practitioners and independent research workers for clinical trials on humans.

Many laboratories, most notably Griffin Laboratories, began experimenting with soft plastics. Griffin's soft lens received its initial impetus as an optic bandage to be used over diseased corneas. Dr. Herbert Kaufman spearheaded the program. He found that many diseased and damaged corneas healed best under a soft lens, and thus it emerged as an exciting therapeutic device. As for tolerance, many of his patients wore their lenses 24 hours a day for months without any detrimental changes in their eyes.

It soon became apparent that the soft lens was an innovation of major importance with widespread application, not only as an instrument for treating diseased corneas, but also as a superior contact lens. In the early stages, however, the therapeutic possibilities of soft lenses overshadowed any other consideration, since it appears that these lenses would replace many conventional treatments for external diseases of the eye.

As the number of soft lens companies expanded throughout the world, a search for newer and better lens designs and lens plastics resulted in some companies emphasizing and developing research activities directed toward correcting astigmatism with soft lenses, developing bifocal soft lenses, and tinting soft lenses for cosmetic purposes. Ultrathin and high-water-content lenses have opened up the realm of extended wear, although not without shortcomings. In the manufacturing area, the emphasis has been on automated and semi-automated systems to produce a soft contact lens.

COMMENT. There are over 60 major companies in North America making contact lenses. When one considers that the technology of the material and its application were developed in just over 25 years, it becomes evident that refinement of these lenses makes broad application possible.

CHARACTERISTICS
Durability

Many soft lenses can be stretched but are durable and have a "memory" to return to their original size and shape (Fig. 7-2). Some soft lenses, however, do not have a memory and will not go back; they can be ruined.

Size

The soft lens is tolerated in a size larger than the cornea for optimum centering and stability. Its large size lying under the eyelid margins permits the lid margins to glide over its surface (Fig.

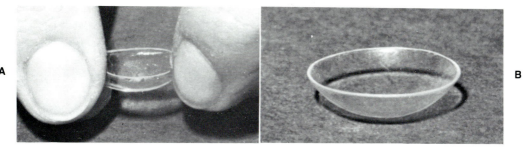

Fig 7-2 ■ **A,** The soft lens is sturdy despite its flexible quality. It can be stretched, dried, or crumpled, and still retain its integrity. **B,** After stretching, the hydrophilic lens retains its "memory" and returns to its original shape. (From Stein HA and Slatt BJ: The ophthalmic assistant, ed 5, St Louis, 1988, The CV Mosby Co.)

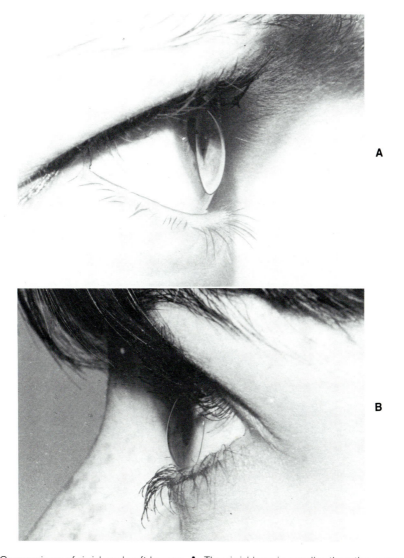

Fig 7-3 ■ Comparison of rigid and soft lenses. **A,** The rigid lens is smaller than the cornea and can be easily dislodged with the edge of the lid. **B,** The soft lens is larger than the cornea, hugs the eye tightly, and seldom is displaced even during contact sports. (From Stein HA and Slatt BJ: The ophthalmic assistant, ed 5, St Louis, 1988, The CV Mosby Co.)

7-3) without impinging on the edges of the lens. This is one of the secrets of soft lens comfort. Interestingly enough, a small, 9 mm soft lens has all the initial discomfort of a hard lens because of the irritation of the edge against the lid margin.

Ability to contour to the eye

The softness of the lens permits the lens to contour itself to the shape of the eye. This is especially true of ultrathin lenses.

Composition

Hydrogel soft lenses are made of different polymers but most are basically hydroxyethyl-methacrylate (HEMA) cross-linked with ethylene glycol dimethacrylate (EDMA). These may be copolymerized with polyvinylpyrrolidone (PVP) to achieve a greater water absorption. A few (non-HEMA) soft lenses are made without HEMA as a constituent, and a few manufactured lenses have methyl methacrylate added for firmness. Glycerin combined with PMMA is also used.

Water absorption

Hydrogel lenses absorb water in varying degrees to provide a water content of 25% to 85%. The less the water content, the more resistant the lens is to damage and the closer its behavior is to the rigid lens. The higher the water content, generally the more fragile the lens, but there is a proportional increase in the oxygen trasmission.

Flexibility

Hydrophilic lenses are hard and brittle when dry but become so soft and flexible when fully hydrated that they can be folded (Fig. 7-4).

Pore structure

Soft lenses have a very small pore structure with a variation in the size of the small openings. These pores are so small that they do not permit the larger molecules of bacteria or fungi to penetrate an intact lens (Fig. 7-5). They can, however, lodge on the surface of a soft lens. A damaged lens that has a superficial abrasion may be contaminated by bacteria or fungi.

Wetting angle

The wetting angle in hydrophilic lenses can be grossly misleading because it depends a great deal on the technique of measurement, the manufacturing process, and the type of hydrophilic material used. It does not appear to be dependent on the water content of the soft lens itself.

Oxygen transmission

A full discussion of soft lens oxygen transmission is covered in Chapter 33 concerning extended wear, in which oxygen transmission is more critical. Suffice it to say that if a lens is made one half as thick, the oxygen transmission will double. Also, if the water content of a lens is raised by 10%, the oxygen transmission will double. There is little tear exchange under a soft lens with each blink (4% to 6%) as compared to a rigid lens (40% to 50%), and so one is depen-

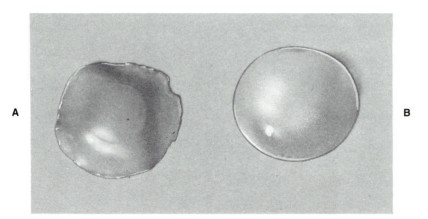

Fig 7-4 ■ A hydrophilic lens becomes hard and brittle like a cornflake when dry as in **A** but becomes soft and flexible when fully hydrated as in **B**. The great danger to the lens in the dry state is chipping.

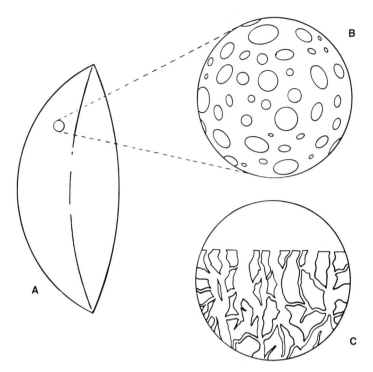

Fig 7-5 ■ A, Pore structure of a soft lens. **B** is an artist's drawing of a small section of a soft lens. **C** represents a single pore showing the irregular size of each opening into the lens substance. The pore structure is sufficiently small to prevent penetration of bacteria. (Courtesy Barnes-Hind Pharmaceuticals, Inc, Sunnyvale, Calif.)

dent on through-the-lens oxygen transmission to prevent corneal hypoxia. Although these lenses are more fragile, the ultrathin type of high-water-content lenses provides better corneal physiologic performance.

COMMENT. The soft lens is much more comfortable than the rigid lens because of its soft qualities, its ability to flex on blinking, the minimal movement of the lens, and particularly its large size, which has its edge lying under the upper and lower eyelids.

The pore structure of the soft lens is extremely small, being less than 3 nm, whereas the smallest bacterium is about 220 nm, and too large to invade the lens. Drugs, vapors, and chemicals, however, will penetrate the soft lens. This factor is important in the use of the soft lens in a smog environment and in fume-exposure industries. It may be important to discourage its use in persons who have occupations in which they are exposed to a high concentration of vapors.

ADVANTAGES

The soft lens has the following advantages:

Comfort

The soft lens is comfortable because the lens fits under both eyelid margins, flexes with each blink, and is soft (Fig. 7-6). It permits some oxygen to reach the cornea.

Rapid adaptation

It is easy for the wearer to build up an all-day wearing schedule in just a few days.

Spectacle blur uncommon

After removal of the lenses the wearer can see as well with spectacles. Spectacle blur is uncommon because of the diffuse nature of any corneal edema, which spreads evenly over the entire cornea and does not alter its radius (Fig. 7-7).

Intermittent wear

The soft lens does not require a rigid daily wearing schedule. The individual can choose to wear the lens only at certain times, such as during the evening or on holidays.

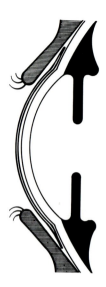

Fig 7-6 ■ Soft lens fits under the eyelid margins. This accounts for its comfort factor.

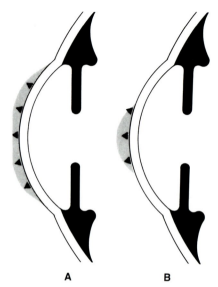

Fig 7-7 ■ The soft lens in **A** produces a diffuse area of corneal edema that does not alter the radius of curvature of the cornea and does not cause spectacle blur. In **B** the rigid lens produces a discrete type of corneal edema, confined to the corneal cap, which does cause spectacle blur because it produces a radical steepening of the corneal curvature.

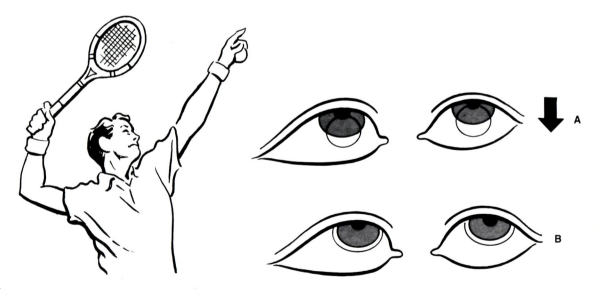

Fig 7-8 ■ **A,** With rigid lenses the lenses drop when the tennis player moves his eyes up to hit the ball. **B,** Soft lenses move with the eye and show only minimal lag.

Minimal lens loss

Because of the large size and minimal movement of soft lens, lens loss is reduced considerably. The lens is not ejected by a blink because the lid margin does not touch the edge. Lens loss is further minimized on lens removal because one has to pinch and hold the lens rather than pop it out as in the removal of a rigid lens. The soft lens is difficult to dislodge and makes an ideal sports lens (Fig. 7-8).

COMMENT. Although lens loss is reduced, the wear and tear on the soft lens is considerably increased; consequently statistics show a much higher replacement requirement for the soft lens. A soft lens becomes spoiled by protein deposition in its surface, which reduces comfort, visual acuity, and durability.

Minimal overwear reaction leading to acute corneal hypoxia

Because of its soft nature and its ability to create an oxygen-tear pump mechanism by flexing with each blink, this lens creates minimal overwear reactions (Fig. 7-9). In addition, oxygen can permeate through the soft lens, particularly if the lens is made very thin.

Less flare and photophobia

Because only minimal movement on the cornea occurs, there is less irritation of the corneal epithelium. The soft hydrated material of hydrophilic lenses is more compatible with the delicate tissues of the cornea. The generous size of the optic zone because of the large diameters of the soft lenses means that the pupil is always

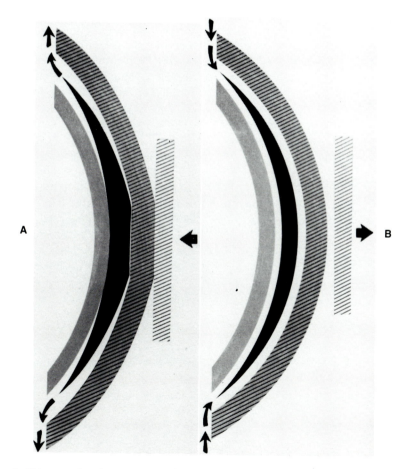

Fig 7-9 ■ **A,** Diagram showing pressure of upper lid being transmitted to soft lens with collapse of interface area. **B,** Diagram showing reformation of interface area after removal of upper lid pressure. (From Aquavella JV: In Gasset AR and Kaufman HE, editors: Soft contact lens, St Louis, 1972, The CV Mosby Co.)

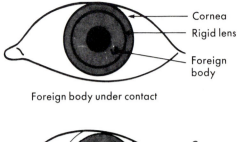

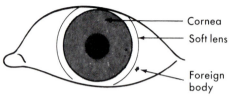

Foreign body under contact

Fig 7-10 ■ The rigid lens permits foreign particles to enter under the lens, whereas the soft lens tends to prevent the tracking of foreign bodies under it by its scleral impingement and minimum movement.

covered, even in dim illumination, a situation that minimizes flare.

Corneal protection

Because of its large size, the soft lens can protect the entire cornea from exposure and from debris getting under the lens (Fig. 7-10).

Alternative for rigid lens dropouts

Sensitive persons who are unable to tolerate the rigid lens can often find comfort with the soft lens.

Excellent cosmetic lens

These lenses are virtually invisible to the observer.

Ideal for infants and children

Because of the comfort feature and the larger sizes available with soft lenses, the lens loss factor can be minimized. Thus soft lenses are ideal for small infants and children.

DISADVANTAGES

The soft lens has the following disadvantages:

Astigmatism

Astigmatism is not readily corrected or covered by conventional soft lenses and even less with ultrathin lenses. The soft lens contours itself to the eye, and corneal astigmatism fre-

quently remains uncorrected. This feature becomes clinically more significant in the lower powers but is not significant in the higher refractive powers. For example, -3.00 D -2.5 D $\times$ 180 is difficult to mask with the soft lens, whereas in the higher powers, for example, -9.00 D -2.5 D $\times$ 180, the astigmatic error may be less significant and better tolerated, even though left uncorrected by the soft lens. The reason is that patients with high refractive errors, that is, -8.00 or more diopters, may have macular problems and many see only 20/25 at best. A drop of one or two lines on the chart in these cases is tolerated.

Many optical firms claim that their soft lenses mask a certain amount of astigmatism. Depending on the lens thickness only about one third to one half of the corneal astigmatism is corrected. We have found that this is highly unpredictable and that often none of the astigmatism is obliterated. However, there is a toric soft lens that provides the fitter an opportunity to correct both corneal and residual astigmatism. Toric lens should be fitted when the astigmatism is 1.00 D or greater. These lenses are discussed in Chapter 29.

Poor vision

In addition to faulty vision because of uncorrected astigmatic errors, poor vision may result from an improperly fitted soft lens. Fluctuating vision may result if the lens is fitted too steeply so that it vaults the central cornea, because as the patient blinks the center of the lens is compressed by the eyelid and so it "irons out" the lens on the cornea. If the lens is fitted too flat, it may become decentered or it may move excessively during a blink, resulting in faulty vision. Union is worse after a blink if the lens is too loose.

The soft lens may become partially dehydrated under certain conditions of low humidity, such as indoors during the heating season and in air-conditioned rooms, especially for patients who are partial or infrequent blinkers or who produce an inadequate volume of tears.

Patients with insufficient tears are not good candidates for soft lenses. The hydrophilic lens demands water, and if it is not satisfied by adequate tears, the thickness and consequently the optic properties of the lens will change. Patients with excess tears may also have faulty vision because the lens may move about excessively. This is a problem for patients with ocular allergies.

Proper respiration is provided to the cornea through the tears by the pumping action created during blinking. This is a two-stage action: (1) During blinking the lens flexes inward, pumping the tears from the small vaulted areas in the intermediate areas across the cornea and out under the lens edge. (2) As the blink is completed, the lens recovers its shape, creating a lowered pressure area under the vault of the lens and thus sucking in fresh tears under the lens. This pumping action produces tear exchange so that proper oxygen is provided to the cornea. This is the most important reason for obtaining a proper fit with a proper cornea-lens relationship.

Allergic patients with excess mucus production will quickly form tacky deposits on the front surface of the lens, resulting in excessive blink-induced lens excursions.

COMMENT. The drier the eye, the harder the lens should be to offset the shift of tears into the lens to provide osmotic balance.

Lack of durability

Frequent handling may cause the soft lens to form a tiny crack and eventually to split. Rough handling or improper removal with a sharp fingernail can also cause a tear or scratch in the lens (Fig. 7-11). The edges may become roughened or damaged with time; occasionally the lenses become yellow and rigid with time. At times yellowing may be a result of aging from boiling or disinfecting, or it may be a result of epinephrine-like compounds, protein, or impurities gathering in its substance. Even with the best of care, a daily wear lens has a limited lifespan. On the average, this has been about 2 years for most of our patients. Annual or bian-

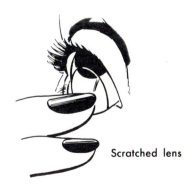

Scratched lens

Fig 7-11 ■ Scratch in a soft lens from a sharp fingernail.

nual replacement of all lenses would greatly reduce lens wear–related problems.

COMMENT. Nasal sprays frequently contain epinephrine-like drugs, which can discolor a lens. Hair sprays cause vacuoles and punctate opacities in the lens.

Faulty duplication

Quality control on replacement of a lens is most important. Manufacturing processes for lenses must be extremely rigidly controlled so that if a lens is lost, it can be replaced with an exact duplicate. This exact duplication is dependent on the reliability of the manufacturer both in fabricating the lens and in checking its quality. Unlike those for rigid lenses, many parameters such as water content and edge design cannot be verified by the practitioner.

COMMENT. Spin-cast lenses as a group provide better quality control than lathe-cut lenses do.

Precipitates and protein buildup

With long-term wear, precipitates occur in the lens and protein and lipids accumulate on the surface (Fig. 7-12). Although special cleaning and protein-removing agents are available, one must rigidly adhere to their use to eliminate precipitates and protein buildup and preserve the life of the lens. If protein is left present in the lens, fine stippling and even microcystic changes can occur in the cornea. Lens solution preservatives will cling readily and build up on the lens surface, inducing a toxic reaction.

COMMENT. Protein precipitates can make the lens uncomfortable, make it lose some permeability features, change its shape to become steeper with resultant pseudomyopia, form a nidus for infection or hypersensitivity reactions, and add weight to it or alter its fitting. A happy soft lens wearer is a person with no protein on the lenses.

Impossible modifications

Although a soft lens can be dehydrated to the dry state, it does not form a regular shape in the dry state so modifications are not possible.

Lens disinfection

The routine of disinfecting must be rigidly adhered to, or infection may occur. This applies whether the lenses sit in the drawer during illness or vacations or when there is a respite back to glasses.

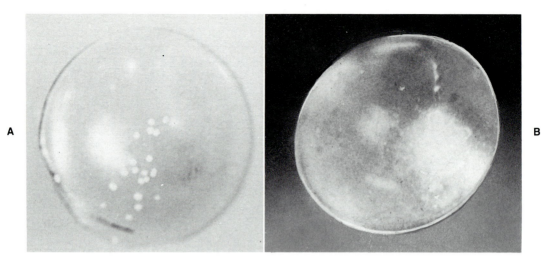

Fig 7-12 ■ **A,** Deposits on a soft lens. **B,** Protein buildup on a soft lens will vary with the duration of wear, the method of sterilization, and the tear composition and concentration of individual patients. (From Stein HA, Slatt BJ, and Cook P: Manual of ophthalmic terminology, St Louis, 1987, The CV Mosby Co.)

Both the boiling method and chemical method of disinfection have their advantages and drawbacks. In any event rigid adherence to disinfection procedures is most important both for the practitioner who keeps an inventory and for the patient who wears the lenses only occasionally. Fungus growth has been reported occasionally, as has bacterial contamination of the lenses. However, widespread infection of the eye is clincally rare. Because soft lenses can be scratched and damaged more easily and consequently can be penetrated by infectious organisms, they are theoretically more dangerous than hard lenses. In clinical practice, however, this does not seem to be a real problem, and patients with soft lenses do not seem to have any higher incidence of corneal or conjunctival inflammatory conditions than people wearing rigid lenses do. One source of soft lens contamination results from human neglect. Patients neglect to boil their lenses as instructed or neglect to use fresh solutions daily for disinfection. Unlike that for rigid lenses, it is unwise to recommend a duplicate pair of soft lenses because the patient usually neglects the disinfection routine required of soft lenses. If the spare set is not opened and the vial is intact, there is no risk of infection. Once the vial is opened, fungus contamination will occur if the storage solutions are not changed regularly (Fig. 7-13).

THIN AND ULTRATHIN SOFT LENSES

A major technologic change in soft lens manufacture has been the development of the thin and ultrathin soft lenses with center thicknesses of less than 0.1 mm and even as thin as 0.025 mm for conventional lenses and 0.0005 mm for special lenses.

The advantages and disadvantages of these thinner soft lenses are outlined in Table 7-1. Of

Table 7-1 ■ Thin and ultrathin soft lenses

Advantages	Disadvantages
1. Initial comfort and rapid adaptation	1. Exaggerated dehydrating in a dry environment
2. Higher oxygen permeability	2. More difficult to handle
3. Decreased incidence of overwear	3. More easily damaged
4. Can be fitted tighter for stable vision during sport activities	4. No masking of corneal astigmatism resulting in poorer quality of vision
5. Alternative for highly sensitive individuals	
6. Reduced risk of corneal warpage	

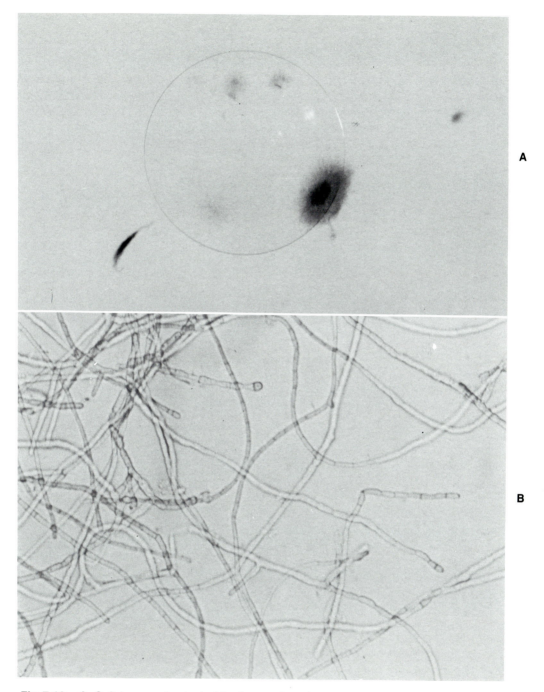

Fig 7-13 ■ A, Soft lens contaminated by fungus from improper daily sterilization routine. **B,** Mycelium of *Cladosporium* identified from soft lens in **A.**

importance is the fact that these lenses provide exceptional initial comfort. Being thin, they provide some diffusion of oxygen and minimize corneal edema formation from hypoxia. Because of their oxygen permeability characteristics, these lenses may be fitted slightly tighter than regular soft lenses and hence produce more stable vision; thus they are useful for sporting activities.

One of the disadvantages of thin and ultrathin lenses is the fact that they are harder to handle and require more patience by the fitter and patient in instruction. They also have an exaggerated dehydration effect in dry environments. These lenses may become damaged more easily and may also not mask as much astigmatism as regular soft lenses do and thus may give a poor quality of vision in those with corneal astigmatism.

COMMENT. The advantages of the soft lens are its excellent comfort, rapid adaptation, and the ability of the wearer to wear the lens intermittently without adhering to a rigid wearing sched-

ule. We have found the soft lens ideal for men and women who are active in sports, for the elderly, and for many persons who are not strongly motivated to persist with the rigorous daily wearing schedule often required of hard lenses. On the other hand, soft lenses are not as durable, require more care and attention to cleaning and disinfecting, and have a greater maintenance cost factor.

8 ▪ OFFICE EVALUATION AND VERIFICATION OF SOFT LENSES

- ▪ General inspection
- ▪ Diameter
- ▪ Base curve
- ▪ Power
- ▪ Optic qualities of the plastic

What type of lens verification should be performed on soft lenses in the office of the average fitter? Unlike rigid lenses, soft lenses have a somewhat limited verification procedure insofar as parameters such as water content, base curve, and peripheral curve measurements cannot be easily obtained by the average fitter. In this situation the fitter must trust the manufacturer.

However, there are certain minimum procedures that we have found worthwhile in evaluating a soft contact lens to ensure a high standard of quality. These procedures are most helpful in ensuring the continuing quality of the product and also in explaining some of the problems that too often we assume are caused by poorly selected lenses clinically when in reality they are caused by poorly manufactured lenses. Also there are occasions when one reviews patients whose files are unobtainable and one wishes to have on hand as many of the contact lens specifications as possible.

GENERAL INSPECTION

Using a monocular magnifying lens or the slitlamp (biomicroscope), the lens should be evaluated for discoloration, protein buildup, nicks, and ruffled edges. The lens should be viewed against a black background in which the light beam of the slitlamp can be gradually spread over the lens' surface. One can also project light through a wet cell that contains the lens and has a black background.

DIAMETER

By viewing the lens with the monocular magnifier with a reticule or gauge, both the overall diameter and the optic zone can be measured (Figs. 8-1 and 8-2). There is available a special monocular magnifier with gauge that permits the

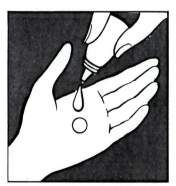
Fill lens with saline

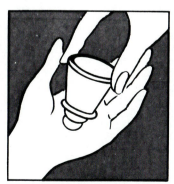
Touch loupe to lens, forcing out excess saline

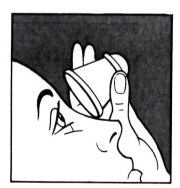
Look toward light source for inspection

Fig 8-1 ▪ Viewing the soft lens with a monocular magnifier.

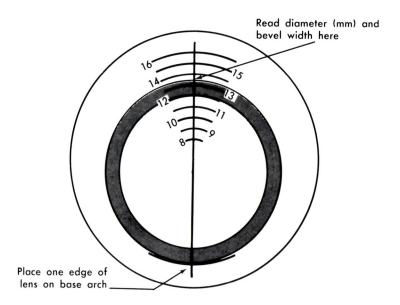

Fig 8-2 ■ Obtaining the diameter measurement of a soft lens with a monocular magnifier.

soft lens to contour itself to the magnifier. One edge of the lens is placed along the base arch of the grid and the opposite arch is used to measure the diameter.

BASE CURVE

The base curve may be measured on plastic templates of known radius (Fig. 8-3). A central bubble indicates that the lens is too steep for the template and that the lens must be moved to a flatter template (Fig. 8-4). If there is edge stand-off, the lens should be moved to a steeper template of known radius. We have not found the template method to be a truly exact measure of the base curve because the lens will often accommodate to two or more of the templates of different radii and seem to be a good fit in each instance.

The template method is also dependent on the relationship of the diameter of the lens and the diameter of the template that corresponds to the sagittal height of the lens.

Template measurement is even less accurate when one is measuring ultrathin lenses.

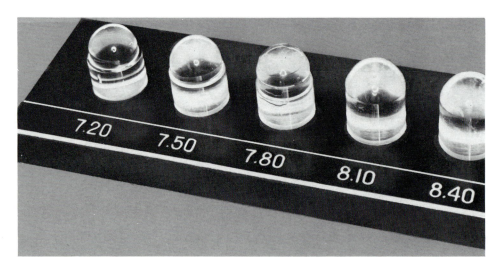

Fig 8-3 ■ Plastic templates of known radii can be used to determine the base curve of a lathe-cut soft lens.

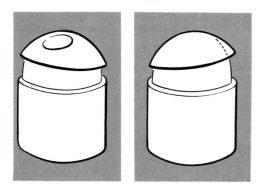

Fig 8-4 ■ Use of the template to measure the base curve of a soft lens. The lens on the left has a bubble under the center, indicating that the lens is too steep for the template. The lens on the right has edge stand-off, indicating that the lens is too flat for the template. (From Stein HA and Slatt BJ: The ophthalmic assistant, ed 4, St Louis, 1983, The CV Mosby Co.)

One instrument, the Soft Lens Analyzer (Hydrovue, Inc., Richmond, California) was developed to measure the base curve of hydrogel lenses. In addition, it measures diameter and center thickness and provides close surface and edge inspection on soft lense and on rigid lenses (Fig. 8-5). It may be used to show patients some problems with existing lenses such as surface defects.

Because hydrogel lenses all contain some percentage of water, accurate measurement is best attained in the hydrated state. The Soft Lens Analyzer provides a wet cell in which the lens is immersed in saline solution. The lens is then measured against a series of hemispheric standards with known radii from 7.6 to 9.8 mm in 0.2 mm increments. A beam of light is projected through and around the lens positioned on the standard. This image is projected onto a small built-in screen at 15 magnification. The operator determines the base curve based on the lens-bearing relationship to the standard on which it is centered (Fig. 8-6). This system for measuring the base curve of a lens is applicable to all lathed lenses. It fails to take into consideration the diameter of the lens in relation to the diameter of the template. There is no reliable office system for measuring the base curve of spin-cast lenses because of their thinness and asphericity.

There is available a soft lens radius gauge that measures the central posterior radius of a soft lens in the hydrated state. Other sophisticated

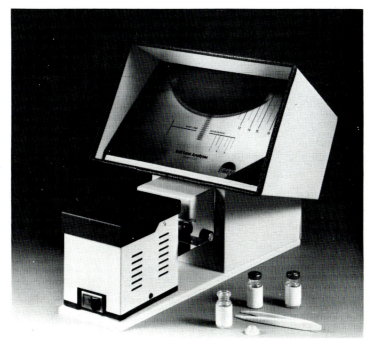

Fig 8-5 ■ The Soft Lens Analyzer. (Courtesy Hydrovue, Inc., Richmond, Calif.) (From Stein HA and Slatt BJ: The ophthalmic assistant, ed 4, St Louis, 1983, The CV Mosby Co.)

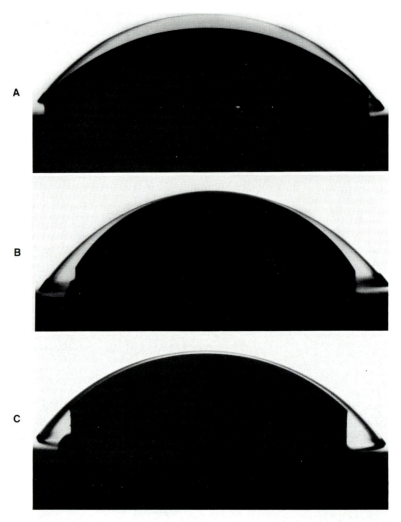

Fig 8-6 ■ **A,** Peripheral touch and apical vault or lens too steep. **B,** Apical touch and peripheral flare or lens too flat. **C,** Alignment: proper fit for accurate base-curve determination. (Courtesy Hydrovue, Inc., Richmond, Calif.) (From Stein HA and Slatt BJ: The ophthalmic assistant, ed 4, St Louis, 1983, The CV Mosby Co.)

wet cell radiuscopes are available, but these may be too expensive for the average fitter.

POWER

To measure the refractive power of the lens, one should clean and gently blot the lens dry for a few seconds with lint-free tissue or chamois (Fig. 8-7) and then hold the lens in the lensometer with the concave surface against the lens stop. Some manufacturers determine the power with the convex surface against the lens stop. Therefore, it is important to check which side has been chosen. Care must be taken when the lens is being blotted. If it is too dry, the power reading will be less accurate.

The Nikon lensometer is ideal because it is able to measure the lens by resting it rather than pinching it because of the horizontal positioning of the lens (Fig. 8-8). One may use a water cell described by Maurice Poster, to which normal saline has been added (Fig. 8-9). The lens floats freely with the finger held over the opening of the water cell. The water cell is placed in the lensometer with the concave side of the lens away from the observer and the lens power is measured. By multiplying the lensometer reading by the factor four, one can compute the refractive power of the lens. This is a somewhat cumbersome and not totally reliable method, since there is considerable error in the water-cell method of determining power. The power can vary with the thickness of the plastic, which varies from high plus to low minus. In our experience the lensometer method has been faster and more reliable than the water-cell method.

OPTIC QUALITIES OF THE PLASTIC

Occasionally soft lenses are manufactured with stress lines in the lens or with an irregular anterior surface. Their quality can be assessed with a hand magnifier or with the retinoscope. In a lens with poor surface optic properties the retinoscopy reflex appears either irregular or decentered. In many cases the faulty or irregular reflex is caused by improper fitting. This is most commonly seen with lenses that are too tight and stretched out on the eye.

Positioning a retinoscope with a +1.50 diopter lens over the contact lens is an easy way to detect lens protein. The lens protein or debris

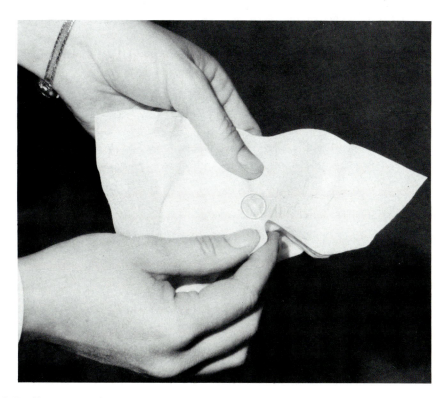

Fig 8-7 ■ To measure the power of a soft lens, clean and gently blot the lens dry with lint-free tissue before evaluating the power with a lensometer.

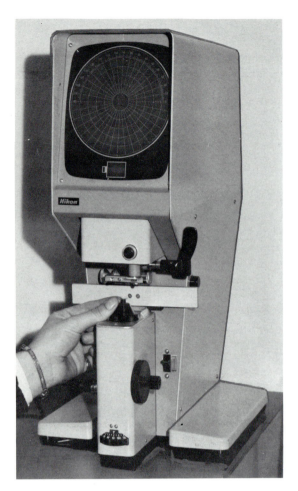

Fig 8-8 ■ Nikon lensometer used to measure the power of a soft lens.

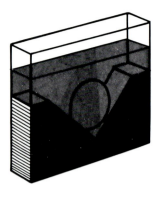

Fig 8-9 ■ Water cell used to measure power of a soft lens in the hydrated state. The soft lens is floated in normal saline and measured in a lensometer.

(lipids and minerals) stand out as clumps on ground glass. Using a wet cell with a large aperture lens is another good way to detect poor surface optics or debris on the lens.

COMMENT. An important advantage of having the equipment and being able to verify soft contact lenses is that the practitioner will be in a better position to evaluate lens changes that may occur with time and thus can solve clinical contact lens problems of the patient. Not uncommonly, chips and nicks will appear, deposits will accumulate, or the lens may change its parameter and become steeper, or occasionally, flatter. We have seen lenses steepen because of aging and deposit formation. We have seen lenses flatten from vigorous hand cleaning with loss of the material's shape retention.

It is important to note that verification of a soft lens is not up to the standards of a rigid lens. One must accept the water content as an article of faith. Base-curve measurement is not precise. The blend on the lathe-cut lens defies projection. A thickness gauge that is reliable still needs an inventor, and flexibility and tensile strength (durometer factor) cannot be gauged by the practitioner.

9 ▪ GENERAL GUIDELINES FOR FITTING SOFT LENSES

- General principles
- Basic guidelines for fitting
- Evaluating a properly fitting lens
- Inventory versus diagnostic lenses

This chapter is written to provide basic principles and guidelines in the fitting of soft contact lenses. Manufacturers' specific instructions should be followed for any particular lens because each company has its own base curves and diameters. For economic reasons companies have standardized dimensions for lenses that are available from that company. Custom-ordering individual soft lenses has not been as commercially workable an undertaking as has been custom-ordering rigid lenses that are manufactured by small laboratories.

This chapter provides guidelines in principles for considering small-diameter versus large-diameter lenses, thin versus standard-thickness lenses, spheric lenses versus toric-designed soft lenses and the percentage of water content. We shall provide some rationale for what manufacturers have incorporated in their individual manuals.

GENERAL PRINCIPLES

Theoretically, all soft lenses, regardless of power, size, or manufacturer, are ideally fitted to obtain three-point touch. They should parallel the superior and inferior sclera and the corneal apex (Fig. 9-1). Rigid polymethylmethacrylate (PMMA) lenses, of smaller diameter, are usually fitted either on K, flatter than K, or steeper than K to increase tear exchange, minimize the bearing area, and still permit tear exchange. In contrast, soft hydrophilic lenses are usually fitted larger than the corneal diameter to maintain centration and stability. Because of the large di-

ameter of these soft lenses, they should be fitted appreciably flatter than the flattest K of the cornea. Lens diameter and base curve are directly related. To arrive at essentially the same fit, the base curve of the lens selected should be flattened as the lens diameter is increased. For example, a 12 to 13 mm diameter lens is usually fitted approximately 2.00 to 3.00 D flatter than K, whereas a 14 to 15 mm diameter lens will have to be fitted approximately 3.00 to 5.00 D flatter than K. Expressed another way, if the diameter of a soft lens is increased, the lens becomes tighter, and one may lengthen the radius of the base curve to make the lens flatter.

Peripheral stability*

The preceding discussion does not consider the fact that the flexibility of the soft lens causes the lens to conform to the shape of the eye to a varying degree. The periphery of the lens tends to flare outward into a flatter curvature than the central posterior portion. Some means must be provided to achieve peripheral adherence or the lens will simply roll up at the edges and thus be unstable on the eye.

One way to stabilize the periphery is to fabricate a hemispheric lens with a thin edge whose flexibility enables it to achieve paralimbal alignment. This design is usually referred to as a *monocurve* because the curvature is constant over the entire posterior surface. Lenses with this configuration are usually of a 13.0-mm chord length and undergo minimal peripheral flattening on the typical eye. With corneas of average size (12.5 mm to 13.0 mm), these lenses are

*From Stein HA, Slatt BJ, Stein RM, and Feldman GL: Fitting soft contact lenses. In Duane, Thomas D and Jaeger Edward A, editors: Clinical Ophthalmology, Philadelphia, 1988, JB Lippincott.

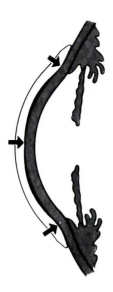

Fig 9-1 ■ Three-point touch—a normally-fitting soft lens will rest lightly at the apex and at the periphery of the cornea.

actually corneal and have a secondary bearing surface on the paracentral cornea instead of on the sclera. This design concept works well with corneas of average size and shape but can cause problems in the atypical fitting situations discussed later in this chapter. Moreover, such a design is dependent on uniformity of size, thickness, and base curve to achieve reproducible fitting characteristics. These minor criticisms do not detract from the utility of the monocurve configuration. Problems, when they occur, can be readily resolved with other designs, including alternatives offered by the two laboratories that use the monocurve design.

Another way to achieve peripheral stability is to use a bevel that is an added curve in the periphery that rests on the sclera. The posterior peripheral bevel with a radius of curvature is flatter than the base curve of the lens. Most manufacturers use a posterior peripheral bevel whose radius of curvature is 12.5 mm to 13.0 mm so as to provide alignment on the average sclera. The bevel thus becomes a secondary bearing surface for the lens, causing the periphery of the lens to remain in contact with the sclera rather than to roll away from it.

With atypical scleras, the stabilizing effect of the posterior peripheral bevel may not be achieved and the edge of the lens tends to roll away from the sclera. This geometric incompatibility can be controlled by decreasing the lens

size to minimize the adverse effect of the sclera. However, such cases will occur rarely if the fitter pays close attention to lens size considerations.

Lens designs and properties

Differences in lens design and in the properties of the various polymers from which soft lenses are made may affect the way in which they have to be fitted. Some differences that should be considered include the following.

Material considerations. Most hydrogel lenses consist of HEMA (hydroxyethylmethacrylate) or HEMA combined with PVP (polyvinylpyrrolidone). When PVP is added, it enhances the water-carrying component of the plastic but may cause some yellowing with repeated boiling or age. A few manufacturers add methyl methacrylate (MMA), which gives more firmness. Those that have this property are often slightly more rigid and perhaps more durable than the other materials.

Soft lenses that contain methyl methacrylate have some firmness and will usually vault over the elliptic periphery of the cornea (Fig. 9-2). This vaulting may create a minus tear layer and result in slightly more plus power required in the final prescription.

Type of posterior curvature. All lathe-cut lenses have spheric posterior curves in contrast to the spin-cast lens, which uses an elliptic posterior curve.

Posterior peripheral curve width. For lenses of the same diameter and the same base curve, the wider the peripheral curve, the looser the lens will fit.

Anterior surface construction. Single-cut lenses may fit differently from those with a lenticular construction because of the effects of lid action on the anterior periphery of the lenses. The carrier radius and carrier width of lenticular lenses also affect the fit of the lens.

Water content. Lenses of appreciably higher water content are usually less durable than those of lower water content but permit greater oxygen diffusion through the plastic than standard lenses of similar thickness.

In general, the lower the water content, the more durable the lens. The water content of various polymers will vary with the manufacturer of the lens. However, lenses of the same water content from different manufacturers may be more or less durable, depending on the properties of the polymers from which the lenses are

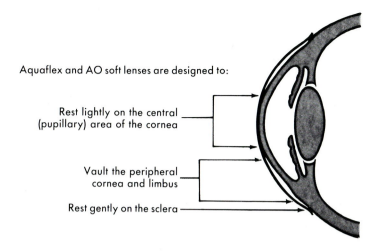

Aquaflex and AO soft lenses are designed to:

Rest lightly on the central
(pupillary) area of the cornea

Vault the peripheral
cornea and limbus

Rest gently on the sclera

Fig 9-2 ■ Lenses containing polymethylmethacrylate wrap around entire central pupillary area of the cornea and vault the peripheral area of the cornea.

made. Also, we have found that the higher the water content, the greater is the tendency for protein to be deposited on the lens.

Lens thickness. Soft hydrogel lenses may be divided into standard-thickness, thin, and ultrathin lenses. The thinner the lens, the more oxygen is transferred across the lens material and consequently the tighter the lens may be fit because tear exchange and lens movement are not so crucial.

Oxygen permeability. The thinner the lens, the greater the oxygen transmissibility. Also, for lenses of equal thickness, the higher the water content, the greater the oxygen transmissibility. Increasing oxygen permeability may be effected by increasing the water content of the lens or decreasing the thickness.

Many lens-design and polymer variations mentioned previously are interrelated. Some of these relationships include the following.

Lens weight. The weight of a lens is influenced by its thickness and water content. Polymers with higher water content are usually structurally weaker than those of lower water content and require lenses of greater thickness. The increased gravitational pull on a heavier lens such as an aphakic lens has to be offset by the use of a larger diameter.

Lens rigidity. The rigidity or stiffness of a lens is a function of its thickness, its water content, and the unique properties of the polymer from which it is made. (One way to understand the concept of rigidity is to visualize a very large rigid lens fitted much flatter than K. This lens

would tend to rock excessively on the corneal apex because of its excessive rigidity, whereas a soft lens would tend to wrap itself around the corneal apex to varying degrees, depending on the degree of rigidity that it possesses.) Soft lenses of greater rigidity have to be fitted more precisely (and flatter) than those possessing a lesser amount of rigidity. However, rigidity is not really an apt term to describe a soft lens; *flexibility* or *drape* would be more descriptive.

Edge considerations. How comfortable a soft lens is depends on the manufacturing quality of the edge and the edge design. If the edge is too thick, it will cause discomfort, and if it is too thin, it will cause nicking and tearing. A fine balance between these two extremes is arrived at by each manufacturer and varies with the durability of the material.

BASIC GUIDELINES FOR FITTING

Because of the many variables and interrelationships involved, the fit achieved with a certain diameter and base curve from one lens manufacturer may be considerably different from the fit that results from a lens with the same parameters obtained from another manufacturer. Therefore it is strongly recommended that the fitting guidelines supplied by each manufacturer be followed in the fitting of its lenses.

The following basic guidelines, however, apply to the fitting of all soft lenses:

1. A normal-fitting soft lens theoretically should show three-point touch, with touch at the corneal apex and the periphery. This

is ideal but difficult to demonstrate because fluorescein is usually not used. However, high molecular weight fluorescein can be used.

2. Hydrogel lenses are usually fitted as large as or larger than the diameter of the cornea and the diameter ranges in size from 12 to 15 mm.

3. Small corneas often require smaller diameters and consequently steeper base curves, whereas larger corneas are fitted with larger lenses and flatter base curves. The shape of the patient's eye should determine the size of the lens. Corneal size can be measured with a metric ruler at the slitlamp to within +/− 0.50 mm. The size of the palpebral fissure also plays a role. For example, the Oriental eye usually has a smaller palpebral fissure and is smaller than the Caucasian eye and will often require a smaller lens.

4. Soft lenses are generally fitted flatter than the flattest K; usually about 2.00 to 3.00 D flatter (approximately 0.4 to 0.6 mm) for the smaller lenses and 3.00 to 5.00 D flatter (approximately 0.6 to 1.0 mm) for the larger lenses.

   There are two important variables in understanding the mechanism of loosening or tightening a lens. These are the *lens diameter* and the *lens radius*.

5. Lens diameter and lens radius are inversely related. If one increases the diameter of the lens (e.g., from 12.5 to 13.5), one increases the sagittal height of a contact lens and so the lens will be tighter on a given cornea. If one decreases the radius or base curve of a contact lens (e.g., from 8.4 to 7.8 mm), one also increases the sagittal height and so the lens will be tighter on the same cornea

(Fig. 9-3). Thus, some manufacturers maintain a constant diameter of their lenses but change the base-curve radius, whereas others feature a change in the diameter but keep the radius controlled. One should understand this relationship of sagittal height to both radius and diameter.

Most fitters are not used to working with sagittal values but are more comfortable with K values, base curve radii, and diameters. The sagittal values should, however, be understood in principle.

6. One may change the fit of a lathe-cut lens by varying the lens diameter, lens radius, or both (Fig. 9-4). It has been mathematically established that the change in lens vault (sagittal-height difference) for a 0.3 mm change in lens radius is approximately equal to a change of 0.5 mm in lens diameter (Fig. 9-5). Knowledge of this relationship (0.3 mm radius change = 0.5 mm diameter change) permits maintenance of the same vault through selective changes of either lens radius, lens diameter, or both.

   The system of fitting lenses is designed to reduce the complications inherent in having so many different lens diameter/lens radius combinations by standardizing the lens diameter.

7. Lenses should be fitted flatter if: the palpebral fissures are large; the corneal diameter is large; the water content is low; the lens is less flexible; the lens is thick in diameter; and the lens has poor oxygen permeability.

   One may determine increased steepness or flatness from Table 9-1, which shows the relationship of diameter to radius (sagittal values). To loosen a lathe-cut lens, one may

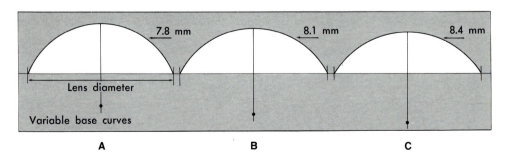

Fig 9-3 ■ All three lenses have a constant diameter. The radii of lenses **B** and **C** have been increased by 0.3 mm so that the lenses have a smaller sagittal height and are therefore flatter.

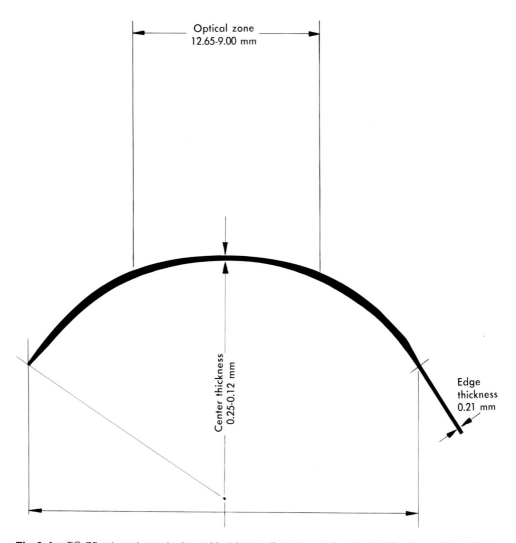

Fig 9-4 ■ TC 75 minus lens design with 14 mm diameter and wet specifications. (From Stein HA and Harrison KW: In Hartstein J, editor: Extended wear contact lenses for aphakia and myopia, St Louis, 1982, The CV Mosby Co.)

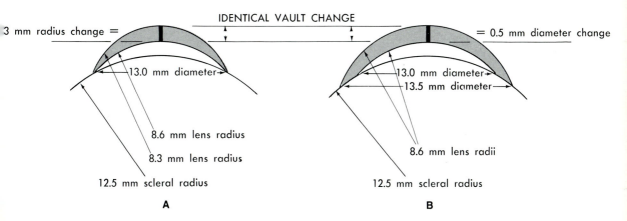

Fig 9-5 ■ By decreasing the radius 0.3 mm as in **A** or by increasing the diameter 0.5 mm as in **B,** there is an identical change in the vault of the lens.

Table 9-1 ■ Sagittal relationship of various base curves and diameters

Diameter	Radius	Diameter	Radius
Flatter		14.0	8.1
12.0	8.7	13.0	7.2
12.0	8.1	14.5	8.4
12.5	8.7	13.5	7.5
12.0	8.4	15.0	8.7
12.5	8.4	14.0	7.8
12.5	8.1	14.5	8.1
12.5	7.8	15.0	8.4
12.0	7.8	15.5	8.7
13.0	8.7	13.5	7.2
13.0	8.4	14.0	7.5
13.5	8.7	14.5	7.8
13.0	8.1	15.0	8.1
13.5	8.4	15.5	8.4
14.0	8.7	14.0	7.2
13.0	7.8	14.5	7.5
13.5	8.1	15.0	7.8
14.0	8.4	15.5	8.1
13.0	7.5	15.0	7.5
14.5	8.7	15.5	7.8
13.5	7.8	**Steeper**	

fit smaller diameters in 0.5 mm steps or increase the radius in 0.2 to 0.3 mm steps.

8. The lower the water content of the lens, the less the build-up of precipitates and protein deposits. The higher the water content, the more the lens absorbs deposits.

9. The lower the water content of the lens, the more durable the lens. The higher the water content, the more fragile the lens.

10. With low-water-content soft lenses we have seen the painful overwear syndrome with corneal epithelial loss that is seen with rigid lenses. One must guard against advising a too rapid acceleration of the wearing schedule for the initial few weeks with low-water-content soft lenses.

11. The thinner the lens, the greater the oxygen transmission to the cornea.

12. Ultrathin lenses provide greater initial comfort than standard-thickness lenses.

13. Thin and ultrathin lenses can be fitted tighter and with less movement than standard-thickness lenses. This eliminates wrinkling of the lens, which may result in fluctuating vision.

14. Hazy vision caused by oxygen deprivation may occur from wearing a thick lens either centrally, as in the case of high-plus lenses,

or in the periphery, as in the case of high-minus lenses.

15. Contact lens decentration can be caused by tight eyelids, large corneas, against-the rule astigmatism, or asymmetric corneal topography.

16. Spheric soft lenses will not mask large amounts of corneal astigmatism. In general, astigmatism over 1.00 D requires correction by toric soft lenses, rigid lenses, or even spectacles.

17. With soft lenses, conventional fluorescein cannot be used to study tear exchange because it permeates the lens. High molecular weight fluorescein can be used, but it is no more effective than an evaluation of tear exchange by noting the movement of the lens.

18. Heavier lenses usually have to be fitted larger than usual. The lens weight is influenced by its thickness and water content. Higher water content polymers are usually weaker than those of lower water content and require lenses of greater thickness. The increased gravitational pull on a heavier lens has to be offset by the use of a larger diameter.

19. The flexibility of a lens is a function of its thickness, its water content, and the unique properties of the polymer of which it is made.

20. When fitting soft lenses, one should aim at fitting the flattest possible lens that will provide good clear vision, center well, and have no effect on the corneal integrity.

21. The practitioner is forced to buy all soft lenses blindly, since there are no convenient and reliable inexpensive office measures available for checking lens thickness, water content, lens weight, lens flexibility, and peripheral and base curves. Also, faults in the plastic may be impossible to detect on first examination and may only appear as problems occur with the lens.

22. Retinoscopy:* For some unexplained reason, most fitters avoid using the retinoscope to evaluate the fit of the lens; yet it is by far the most sensitive indicator of a marginally tight lens. Its value becomes readily appar-

---

*From Stein HA, Slatt BJ, Stein RM, and Feldman GL: Fitting soft contact lenses. In Duane TD and Jaeger EA, editors: Clinical ophthalmology, Philadelphia, 1988, JB Lippincott.

ent when the way in which a soft lens fits the eye is considered. If the geometry of the lens matches that of the eye, there is an area of alignment over the apex with a very thin, plano underlying tear layer. Soft lenses work by giving this area of the cornea a new, regular, refracting surface, and therefore this apical alignment is mandatory to provide good visual function.

A lens that is too tight lacks apical alignment and has a tendency to lift away from the apex. When this occurs, the radius of curvature of the lens at the apex changes and elicits an adverse effect on visual acuity. The retinoscope is so sensitive to this response that it will display a distortion in the central part of the reflex regardless of whether the spot or the streak retinoscope is used. It is not necessary to use a + 1.50-D lens, because we are concerned only with the quality of the reflex and not with a

retinoscopic refraction to determine emmetropia. It is axiomatic that good visual acuity is consistent with a sharp, clear retinoscopic reflex because only then is the optical system in optimal condition. Thus, a lens that does not fit properly also fails to perform optically in the desired manner.

The retinoscope is probably the best device to determine minimal protein on a lens. A lack of symmetry in the reflex with or without scattered opacities is frequently the earliest sign of protein debris.

23. It should be noted that for the Bausch & Lomb spin-cast series the inside *posterior apical radius* (PAR) changes as the power becomes steeper in units, approximately 0.05 mm for a 0.25 D increase in minus power. Thus large changes in power will change the fitting characteristics (Fig. 9-6). This is not true of lathe-cut lenses.

24. The less material on the eye, the better. Fit

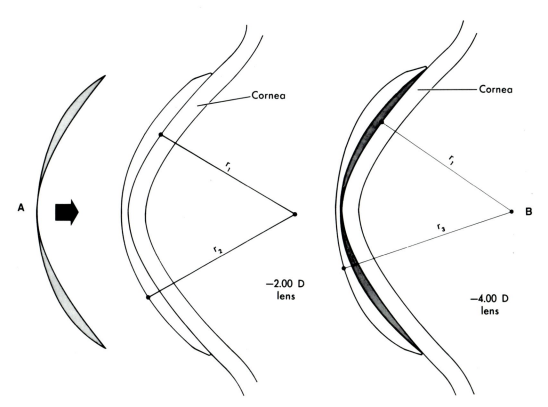

Fig 9-6 ■ **A,** r_1 = corneal radius; r_2 = new anterior surface radius, which has a flatter curve than that of the cornea. **B,** When additional plastic is added to the periphery to create a − 4.00 D power lens, the new anterior radius r_3 has a still flatter curve because of the flexible nature of the material that is placed in the periphery. The fit will vary with the power of the lens. (Courtesy Bausch & Lomb, Inc.)

the smallest, thinnest lens that will provide a good fit, good comfort, and a good physiologic response.

25. The flatter the cornea, the larger the diameter of the lens required to give the lens a stable fit and prevent decentration.

26. The drier the eye, the lower the water content of the lens required. A higher water content lens creates an osmotic shift from the tear film into the lens, which makes the surface of the cornea even drier.

27. The pore structure of a soft lens is 4 nm. The smallest size structure visible today is the herpes simplex virus, which is 15 nm. Thus bacteria and viruses usually do not penetrate an intact lens.

28. There is only half the tear film thickness behind the thin and ultrathin lenses as compared to standard-thickness lenses; hence there is less opportunity for tear exchange with metabolic products and debris, and there is more chance for red eyes to occur.

29. In fitting larger lenses, there is less movement because of greater surface adhesion of a larger lens and less lid impact with larger lenses, and thus less movement.

COMMENT. Because there are no effective quality controls for soft lenses, the lens on the cornea becomes the best tool for a fitting guide, albeit a pragmatic one. Some fitters do not even bother with K readings. The fitting is then based on centration, visual acuity, lens movement, and lens stability with eye movement. K readings do not add much science to the art of fitting a soft lens; they are merely a guide.

EVALUATING A PROPERLY FITTING LENS

Criteria for evaluating a properly fitting soft lens include the following (see also pp. 99 to 105 for a more detailed discussion).

Movement*

The lens should move with each blink and with rotation of the eye. An incomplete blink will cause poor movement, which has nothing to do with the dynamics of the lens on the eye. Following movements are slow (e.g., following

---

*From Stein HA, Slatt BJ, Stein RM, and Feldman GL: Fitting soft contact lenses. In Duane TD and Jaeger EA, editors: Clinical ophthalmology, Philadelphia, 1988, JB Lippincott.

a finger). In such a test, the lens may have enough drag to stay on the cornea. Test with fast movement—a saccade—in which the patient looks from one finger to the other, and note the position of the lens.

Passive movement of the lens should also be tested. With the lens in place, the index finger is placed under the lower lid and the lens is gently nudged. With this gentle pressure, displacement of the lens upward should occur. If it does not, the lens is probably too tight.

A lens that fits correctly should show about 0.5 to 1 mm of lag as the eye is turned up or to the side. Subtle differences in movements are best detected by having the patient look up and blink. The amplitude of movement depends on the lens size and its average thickness. A soft lens that moves excessively (more than 1 mm with each blink) is too flat; a soft lens that moves less than 0.5 mm with each blink is too steep and will limit tear exchange. Ultrathin lenses may be fitted with less movement because some oxygen passes through the lens.

Centration

A normal-fitting lens should completely cover the cornea. If a lens is slightly decentered, the fit is acceptable provided that the edge of the lens opposite the direction of decentration continues to cover the cornea. Uncovered corneal areas will often show corneal irritation and staining.

A soft lens that becomes decentered is usually too flat or too small. To correct this problem, select a lens with a larger diameter. It will usually reduce the flatness of the lens and improve corneal coverage.

The size of the lens diameter also differs when comparing small lenses with large lenses. If the lens is 1.0 mm to 1.5 mm larger than the visible iris diameter (VID), it should completely cover the cornea while the eye is in primary gaze. Failure to do so will result in arcuate staining of the paracentral cornea. If a larger lens is to be fitted, it should be at least 2.0 mm to 3.0 mm larger than the cornea and at no point should the edge of the lens be closer than 1.0 mm from the limbus while the eye is in primary gaze. Encroachment of the edge onto the limbal area will result in chronic injection, peripheral staining, and a high potential for the formation of a neovascular pannus.

Many fitters make the mistake of attempting

to improve centration through the use of a steeper base curve. However, the disadvantage of this is that the patient ends up with a tight lens. A far better approach is to use a larger lens with an appropriate base curve, being careful to select a lens that also has a larger optic zone.

The fitter should remember that the geometric and visual axes of the eye do not always correspond. In some cases, the corneal apex can be sufficiently decentered so as to affect the centration of a small lens over it, resulting in poor visual acuity. It is not unusual to see the reverse situation in which a lens centers perfectly over a centrally located corneal apex, but the patient obtains poor acuity without evidence of residual astigmatism, which does not improve with over-refraction. In both situations, poor vision results because both axes are not contained within the optic zone of the lens. Thus, in addition to parametric changes, the fitter should consider an alternative that provides for a larger optic zone.

Occasionally, the lens may be centered at the time of the fitting, but a month later, the lens may be decentered. What has occurred?

Protein may have accumulated on the lens and changed its shape and fitting characteristics.

The lens may have settled—especially if there was axial vaulting. The lens can become decentered and tight in the new position if the sagittal vault is excessive. Reduce diameter or make the lens flatter.

The lens may have become displaced upward. This is especially true in high myopes. If there is giant papillary conjunctivitis, the cobblestone surface of the tarsal surface of the conjunctiva may pull the lens upward.

The lens may have dropped. This tends to occur in high myopes, especially aphakes. This is because of the weight of the lens and indicates that a smaller lens is required.

The cornea may be edematous and the lens may no longer fit.

Vision. For the fit to be acceptable, vision must be clear and constant before, during, and after blinking. Fluctuating vision is a symptom of a marginal or improper fit.

Relationship of lens power to refractive error. Soft lenses should rest on the corneal apex and may create a small minus-powered tear layer by standing away from the cornea peripheral to the apex (Fig. 9-7). This relationship has to be corrected by the addition of plus power to the final prescription (in the range from +0.12 to +0.50 D). This correction is in contrast to that of rigid lenses, which usually vault the corneal apex and create a plus tear layer, requiring the addition of −0.25 to −0.50 D to the final prescription

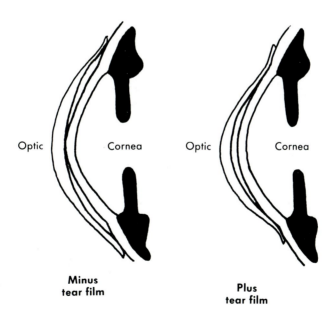

Minus tear film   **Plus tear film**

Fig 9-7 ■ Minus and plus tear film. A tear film is created between the contact lens and cornea. This tear film may balance as either a minus lens or a plus lens and may alter the end point of the refractive change.

of a hard lens. Therefore one way to determine whether a soft lens is seated properly on or is vaulting the corneal apex is to compare the refractive error to the final lens prescription.

The following simple rules are presented for hydrogel lenses for myopic refractive errors: (1) If the final lens prescription is more myopic than (or at least the same as) the refractive error, apical contact is being made and vision will probably be satisfactory. (2) If the final lens prescription is not as strong as (more plus than) the refractive error, the lens is probably vaulting the corneal apex and creating a plus tear film, and the patient will probably demonstrate variable vision (Fig. 9-7).

Aphakic lenticular lenses, because they are thick, may touch at the apex of the cornea but stand away paracentrally and thus create a minus tear film. Hence an aphakic lens may require more of an increase in plus power than one would expect.

Fitting. When fitting soft lenses, one should aim at fitting the flattest possible lens that will provide good clear vision, center well, and have no effect on the corneal integrity.

COMMENT. "The best way to fit a contact lens is to use a given lens." Place a lens of known parameters on the eye, evaluate the fit, and when the correct fit is achieved, over-refract to determine the final lens power.

INVENTORY VERSUS DIAGNOSTIC LENSES

Soft lenses may be fitted in one of two ways:
1. from an inventory of lenses by selection of the proper lens that gives the best fit and the best visual acuity, or
2. from a diagnostic trial set of standard diameters and base curves to obtain the proper fitting dimensions. One can then over-refract to obtain the correct lens power and order the final lens. This requires the fitter to be able not only to fit a lens but also to refract over the trial lens. It is almost impossible to predict how a soft lens will perform on an eye until it has been tested. The

only foolproof method for the fitting of a soft lens is to apply a contact lens to the eye for evaluation of its performance.

With rigid lenses most practitioners know that the effects of lid action on the front surface and lens periphery may be different on lenses of greatly different powers. Most of us have had the experience of determining the fit of a person with high myopia with a −3.00 D diagnostic lens and then finding that the higher-powered minus lens that was ordered rode high or moved excessively. The same principle applies to soft lenses, though to a somewhat lesser degree. Therefore to ensure that the soft lens ordered will fit in the same manner as the diagnostic lens used, it is desirable that the lens power of the diagnostic lens be reasonably close (within 2.00 or at most 3.00 D) of the refractive error. Thus the inventory method is a more desirable method of fitting.

If one fits from inventory, it is important to set up some form of an inventroy control system so that when a lens is dispensed from stock it will be marked off on the master list and a replacement lens will be ordered to fill the depleted inventory. A number of systems are available from the manufacturers. It is important however to reorder a lens to the inventory set once it is dispensed to keep the inventory intact.

Of great importance is the care and disinfection of the inventory set of soft lenses. At least once a week, the lenses should be disinfected to prevent not only bacterial contamination but also fungal contamination.

COMMENT. For an inventory a high-volume practice is required. With the ever-changing advances in contact lens technology, one should not be married to a single laboratory or given lens. It is important to be able to change one's entire inventory every 3 months just to be flexible and remain current. For low-volume practices a small diagnostic fitting set is the best choice. Do not accumulate obsolete lenses. If an inventory is kept, the rate of utilization can be best checked if a computer is used for inventory control.

10 ▪ *FITTING METHODS FOR SOFT LENSES*

There is really no formula that can predict that a certain lens will give a tight fit and another will give a loose fit. In our guidelines for fitting we have had to fall back on generalizations and hope that these will not be taken as dogma to be followed without deviation. The topography of each cornea, even with standard measurements, will often vary. The quality control check by the manufacturer of soft lenses is almost impossible to assess by the fitter. Factors such as lid adherence and thickness of the tear film cannot be quantitatively evaluated. Each point we have tried to make must be viewed and analyzed in reference to one's own fitting experience.

Standard fluorescein cannot be used with soft lenses. Early corneal edema may be not only too small but also too diffuse to detect. Consequently the evaluation of the fit of a soft lens is dependent largely on certain characteristics of lens behavior, determined by its positioning and movement on the eye and by the final vision obtained.

Fitters today are in a fortunate position because they can choose from among a variety of materials with different amounts of hydration, thickness, durability, size, design, and cost. As a result they can provide the lens that performs best for an individual patient.

Lens selection may be based on one of three methods: (1) selection of soft lenses based on probable corneoscleral profiles in which one may select a lens diameter based on the horizontal iris diameter and observe how the lens performs on a given eye, (2) selection of a soft lens with a posterior radius of curvature based on K readings of the cornea determined by actual measurement of the cornea, and (3) selection of a soft lens based on the sagittal value of the lens, which requires the K reading of the cornea and takes into account not only the posterior radius of the lens curvature but also the diameter of the lens.

Each manufacturer has its own fitting method depending on the diameter and base curves that the company makes available. The following is an outline of a universal system that appears to be applicable to most soft lens fitting. Specialized types of fitting for aphakia and toric soft lenses are discussed in the chapters specific to these areas (Chapters 29 and 32).

BASIC FITTING METHOD

1. Record the K readings and convert to millimeters.
2. Measure the corneal diameter in millimeters. The initial lens diameter to be selected should be 0.5 to 2 mm larger than this measurement. There is no set rule. This is a decision that should be based on clinical experience combined with the diameters made available by the manufacturers.
3. Determine the spheric power required: change the refraction prescription to minus cylinders and use the spheric equivalent of the cylinder if the cylinder is greater than 0.50 D. Add this to the sphere to determine the initial lens power. Compensate this for vertex distance; for example:

$$-5.50 + 1.00 \times 90$$
$$\text{change to } -4.50 - 1.00 \times 180$$

Add ½ of cylinder (0.50) to sphere so that power = -5.00. Look up in the vertex table; so -5.00 at a spectacle vertex of 12 mm becomes −4.75 at the corneal plane. Power selection is −4.75.

4. If using a trial set, select a suitable trial lens with a base curve of 0.4 to 0.6 mm (2.00 to 3.00 D) flatter than the flattest K in the smaller diameter lenses (12 to 13 mm) and 0.6 to 1 mm (3.00 to 5.00 D) flatter in the large diameter lenses (14 to 15 mm).

   Evaluate the fit of the lens according to the criteria just outlined for a normal fit (see below).

   Perform an over-refraction on a properly fitted lens.

   Order the lens of appropriate power, base curve, and diameter or select it from the lens inventory.

   Re-evaluate the fit and the vision.

5. If using an inventory set, repeat steps 1, 2, and 3 above. Over-refract with ±0.25 sphere lenses to refine the power requirements after the lens has become stabilized.

Helpful hints to fitting

Keratometric readings should always be made, primarily (a) to compare at a later date in case the corneal measurements change, (b) to detect whether any astigmatic error is corneal or lenticular in origin, and (c) to use as a guideline for selecting the initial base curve of the lens.

One should measure the visible iris diameter (VID) by using a number of methods such as a pupillary gauge, a reticule in a slitlamp objective lens, a rule held toward the cornea, or a draftsman's caliper with blunted points, or by the application and centering of a trial soft lens of known chord diameter. The P-D Gauge manufactured by Essilor (Paris, France) is an excellent instrument for measuring the visible iris diameter.

The best method of all is by using a contact

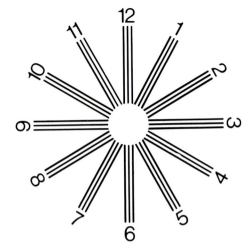

Fig 10-1 ■ Astigmatic clock, which can be used to determine poor vision caused by residual astigmatism. Once detected, a different type of lens can be selected. This test can save considerable chair time.

lens of known diameter. Place the lens on the eye and allow it to settle for 15 to 20 minutes to equilibrate with tears. Then check the diameter on the slitlamp so that the lens fully covers the cornea, centers well, and shows satisfactory movement.

Soft lenses are best fitted from a complete inventory set where an instant fit can be achieved and the patient instructed and able to wear the lenses that day. Alternatively, for those with low-volume practices, diagnostic trial lens sets may be used to determine the optimum lens diameter.

Our usual procedure for standard thickness lenses is to use as flat a base curve as possible and satisfy our previously mentioned criteria. Ultrathin lenses can be fitted slightly steeper because of their oxygen-transmission properties.

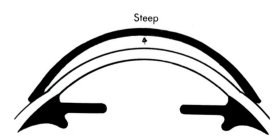

Fig 10-2 ■ Cross section of a steep lens showing absent touch centrally.

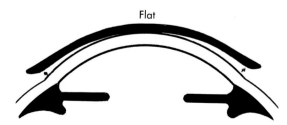

Fig 10-3 ■ Cross section demonstrating a flat lens with edge stand-off.

Decentration of a lens may be caused by tight eyelids, large corneas, astigmatism against the rule, or asymmetric corneal topography.

The astigmatic clock is helpful in lens fitting (Fig. 10-1). After the patient has the initial or second-choice lens fitted, he or she is asked to look at the clock. If some lines are considerably more predominant, this indicates that the problem is residual astigmatism, which cannot be overcome with changes in soft lenses. A considerable amount of chair time can be saved if one switches to the central type of lenses.

FITTING EVALUATION
Normal fit

A soft lens should be fitted with what is known as *three-point touch*. The lens should parallel the superior and inferior sclera as well as the corneal apex. When the lens rests only on the superior and inferior sclera and vaults the corneal apex, the lens is too steep (Fig. 10-2). If the lens rests on the corneal apex and the edges stand off from the sclera, the lens is too flat (Fig. 10-3).

All soft lenses, regardless of power, size, or manufacturer, should be fitted to obtain this three-point touch (Fig. 10-4).

A well-fitted lens will show six basic qualities: good centration, adequate movement, stable vision, a crisp retinoscopic reflex, clear undistorted keratometry mires, and clear end-point over-refraction.

Good centration. The lens will center itself easily after insertion in the eye. After the patient blinks, it will not show more rim of lens on one side of the cornea than on the other side. Lens decentration requires refitting with either a steeper base curve or a larger diameter (Fig. 10-5). In some cases a shift to a flatter lens will be necessary.

A decentered spin-cast lens that persists in decentering after trial with a different and larger series will necessitate a change either to a thinner spin-cast lens or to a lathe-cut lens for stabilization and proper fit. Spin-cast lenses result in more centering difficulties than do lathe-cut lenses because of the smaller size, the aspheric shape of the posterior surface of the lens, or the design of the lens periphery.

Adequate movement. A standard-thickness lens may show movement of 0.5 to 1 mm on upward gaze after a blink, and it should show no greater movement on lateral gaze. If the lens is equilibrated with tears and does not move, the person should be switched to a lens with a flatter base curve (Fig. 10-6, *A*). If the lens moves excessively, a lens with a steeper base curve (Fig. 10-7) series or one with a larger diameter should be substituted (Fig. 10-6, *C* and *D*).

The thinner series of soft lenses are fitted with slightly less movement than a standard-thickness lens needs. Thus lenses of a thinner series may be fitted with 0.5 mm movements or less. This prevents a wrinkling effect that can be

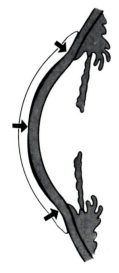

Fig 10-4 ■ Three-point touch—a normally fitting soft lens will rest lightly at the apex and at the periphery of the cornea.

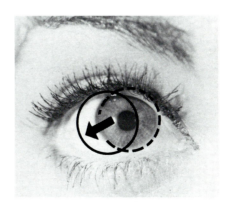

Fig 10-5 ■ Decentration of a soft lens. The lens slides temporally and down. (From Stein HS, Slatt BJ, and Stein RM: Ophthalmic assistant, ed 5, St Louis, 1988, The CV Mosby Co.)

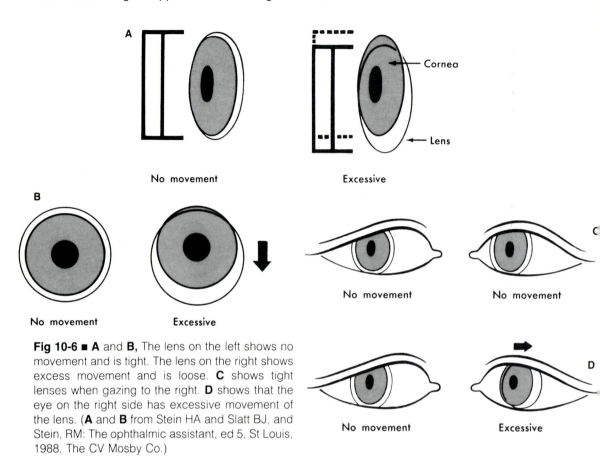

Fig 10-6 ■ **A** and **B,** The lens on the left shows no movement and is tight. The lens on the right shows excess movement and is loose. **C** shows tight lenses when gazing to the right. **D** shows that the eye on the right side has excessive movement of the lens. (**A** and **B** from Stein HA and Slatt BJ, and Stein, RM: The ophthalmic assistant, ed 5, St Louis, 1988, The CV Mosby Co.)

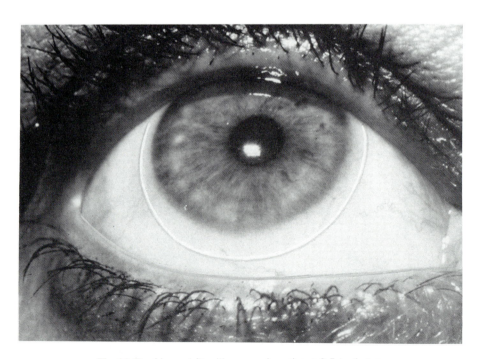

Fig 10-7 ■ Normal fit with excursion about 0.5 to 1 mm.

produced by looser thin lens. Also one may successfully fit these lenses slightly tighter than standard-thickness lenses because thin lenses provide sufficient oxygen transmission to ensure corneal integrity.

The slitlamp is invaluable for evaluation of proper movement. Fit should be evaluated while the patient looks straight ahead, upward, and laterally. The patient should be asked to blink under slit-lamp observation. Evaluation should be made clinically as to whether the movement is excessive, negligible, or adequate.

Stable vision. When the patient blinks, the vision should remain equally clear before and during the blink and visual acuity should be as sharp as possible (Fig. 10-8). If trial-set lenses are used for fit evaluation, an over-refraction should be performed.

If visual acuity is not adequately sharp after changing the lenses or holding over low-plus or low-minus lenses, we have found it useful to have the patient view an astigmatic clock. If some of the clock lines are significantly blurred, residual astigmatism is present and vision cannot

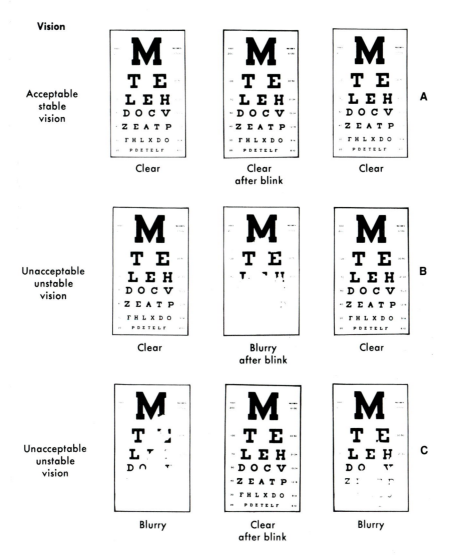

Fig 10-8 ■ **A,** Acceptable stable vision. Vision is clear at first, clears immediately after blinking, and remains clear when not blinking. **B,** Unacceptable unstable vision that occurs when a lens is too loose because of the sliding effect of the lens after blinking. **C,** Unacceptable unstable vision that occurs when a lens is too tight. Vision is unclear at first but clears after blinking because of the flattening effect of the eyelids on a steep lens at the apex of the cornea.

be improved any further with conventional soft lenses. Variable vision initially may be caused by a lens that is either too loose or too tight. If the fit is found to be adequate and the patient still complains of fluctuating vision, factors such as dryness of the eye or the environment, lack of blinking, or excess mucus secretions must be considered as causes.

COMMENT. Normally, blinking may be reduced while driving and reading. The patient should be warned of soft-lens variable vision. It is easily reduced by a series of blinks or artificial tears.

Crisp retinoscopic reflex. As confirmatory evidence of a good fit, the retinoscope, streak, or spot is flashed in all meridians while the patient blinks. When the patient is adequately fitted, the retinoscopic flex will be sharp and crisp as

if no lens were in place, both before and after blinking (Fig. 10-9, *A*). If the lens is steep, there will be a spreading of the streak centrally in the rest position, which will clear after a blink because of ironing out of the apical vault (Fig. 10-9, *C*). If the lens is flat, it may ride low, a position that can be detected by retinoscopy, or the retinoscopic shadow may be blurry immediately after a blink (Fig. 10-9, *B*).

Even though residual astigmatism may be detected, if the fit is adequate the reflexes will remain sharp and clear when there is an adequate fit.

COMMENT. Occasionally the lens may have poor surface optics and, even though the fit is adequate, the retinoscopic reflex will not be sharp. A poor surface optic figure in a new lens is caused by uneven hydration, flaws in the plas-

Retinoscope reflexes

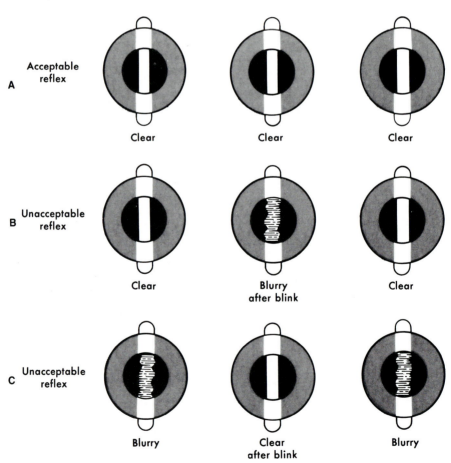

Fig 10-9 ■ A, Acceptable retinoscopic reflex when lens fits well. **B,** Unacceptable retinoscopic reflex when lens is too loose. **C,** Unacceptable retinoscopic reflex when lens is too tight.

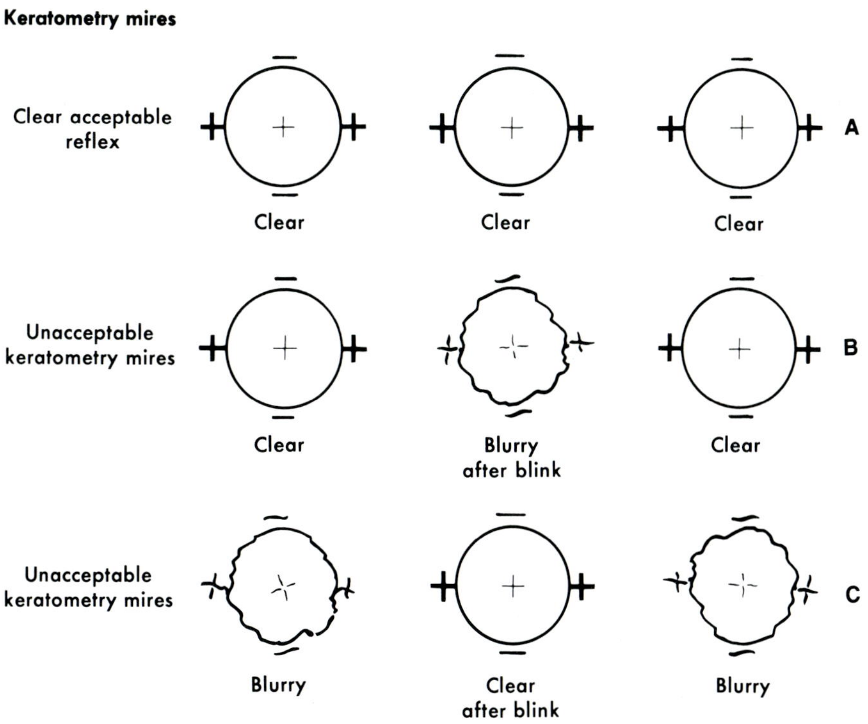

Keratometry mires

Clear acceptable reflex	Clear	Clear	Clear	**A**

Unacceptable keratometry mires	Clear	Blurry after blink	Clear	**B**

Unacceptable keratometry mires	Blurry	Clear after blink	Blurry	**C**

Fig 10-10 ■ **A,** Clear mire reflexes when the lens fits well. **B,** Unacceptable mire reflexes when the lens is too loose. **C,** Unacceptable mire reflexes when the lens is tight.

tic, a poor polishing. In a worn lens this may be a result of protein, lipid, or mineral deposits.

Clear, undistorted keratometry mires. The mires that are reflected from the keratometer while the person is wearing the soft lens will often indicate if the fit is adequate. With the correct fit, the mires of the keratometer should not be distorted either before or after a blink (Fig. 10-10, *A*). If the mires are blurred, the patient should blink several times; if the mires are still distorted, the lens should be changed (Fig. 10-10, *B* and *C*).

COMMENT. Keratometry is a valuable and simple test to perform for final evaluation after centration, vision, and movement have been analyzed. It will act as a check on the other parameters that have been evaluated. Occasionally the mires will be blurred because of surface mucus or dehydration. When this occurs, blinking will usually restore the anterior surface to a normal luster if the problem is not one of fitting. Any blurring of the mires or irregular patterns are indicative of a poorly fitted lens, which may give rise to potential fitting problems. Occasionally blurring may be caused by a poor surface figure

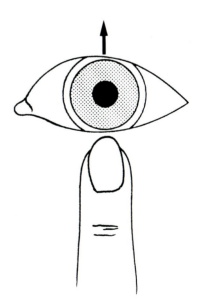

Fig 10-11 ■ By pressing gently on the lower eyelid, the lens should be able to be shifted. If not, the lens is too tight.

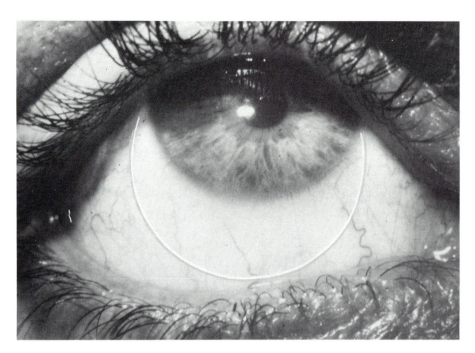

Fig 10-12 ■ Loose lens indicated by lag on upward gaze.

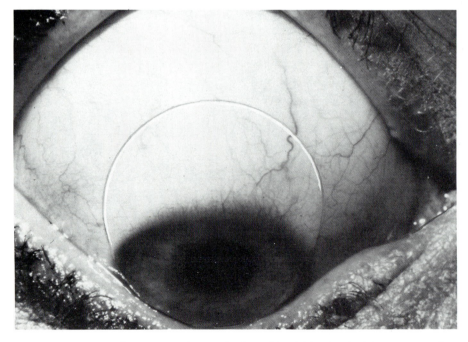

Fig 10-13 ■ Loose lens. On downward gaze the lens rides high. A valuable test to confirm the fitting of a soft lens.

in the lens, a drying out of the lens surface, or mucous debris.

Dr. Josh Josephson has pointed out an additional method of evaluating the fit of a soft lens. While viewing the eye with the slitlamp, one can press gently on the lower lid toward the globe and against the edge of the lens (Fig. 10-11). If an acceptable fit has been achieved, the lens will show a slight edge lift-off after it is digitally moved across the limbus. If the lift-off is excessive, the lens is too flat. If the lens does not lift off from the globe at all, it is probably too tight. This is referred to as the *edge-lift effect*.

Loose fit

Symptoms and signs of a loose lens. The following indicate that the fit of a lens is loose:
1. Variable vision, clear at first but poor after blinking (Fig. 10-8, *B*)
2. Excess awareness of the lens
3. Poor centering
4. Excess movement (Figs. 10-6, *A, B,* and *D,* 10-12, and 10-13)
5. Edge stand-off (Fig. 10-14)
6. Lens falling out of the eye
7. Bubble under the lens edge (Fig. 10-15, *B*)
8. Keratometry showing clear mires at first that blur after a blink and then clear (Fig. 10-10, *B*)
9. Retinoscopy that is clear at first but blurs after blinking (Fig. 10-9, *B*)

A loose lens may show movement of 2 to 4 mm on downward excursions and may even slide off the cornea entirely on lateral movement (Fig. 10-6, *B*). The vision is often clear at first but may decrease by two or three lines after a blink, though it may recover quickly. In an extremely loose lens the edge may roll out the so-called edge and stand-off and the lens may fall out of the eye on a blink because of contact of the lids with the rolled-out edge. Because it may require a few minutes before edge stand-off appears in a loose lens, it is best to allow 15 to 20 minutes before completion of the evaluation of fit.

COMMENT. A valuable test for a loose lens is to have the patient look down. If the lens floats high, it should be considered loose (Fig. 10-12).

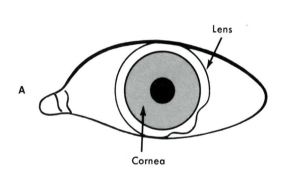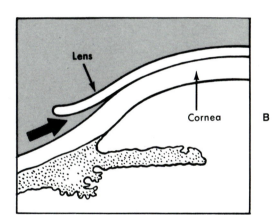

Fig 10-14 ■ Loose lens with edge stand-off. **A,** Edge lifting off the scleral rim; **B,** Schematic side view interpretation of the edge lift-off of a loose lens.

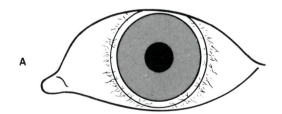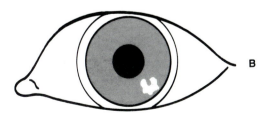

Fig 10-15 ■ **A,** Circumcorneal injection; **B,** bubble under a loose soft lens.

Correction of a loose lens. The following steps should be taken to correct a loose lens:
1. For a lathe-cut lens, switch to a lens with a steeper base curve or a larger lens diameter.
2. For Bausch & Lomb spin-cast lenses, switch to a series of a larger diameter.

COMMENT. It is therefore necessary because of the thinness and asphericity of the Bausch & Lomb lenses that they be fitted according to the *horizontal visible iris diameter* (HVID). The initial lens chosen should be 1 mm larger than the HVID.

With lathe-cut lenses one can switch to a radius steeper in 0.2 to 0.3 mm steps or increase the diameter 0.5 mm up to a lens size of 15 mm in diameter. Both methods will tighten the lens and decrease lens movement. It is preferable to fit the patient initially with a loose lens and make it tighter until the lens of choice is determined. This should be the flattest lens possible that fulfills all the criteria of a good fit.

Tight fit

Symptoms and signs of a tight lens. The following indicate a lens that is tight-fitting:
1. Fluctuating vision that clears immediately after blinking (Fig. 10-8, *C*)
2. Initially comfortable but increasingly uncomfortable as the day progresses
3. Circumcorneal injection, or redness around the circumference of the cornea (Fig. 10-16, *A*)
4. Circumcorneal indentation—the conjunctiva is compressed at the limbus and there is a ditchlike depression that obstructs the normal flow of the vessels (Fig. 10-16, *B*)
5. Absent or minimal movement after a blink (Figs. 10-2 and 10-17)
6. Keratometry with lens in place that shows distorted mires before a blink, which clear immediately after blinking (Fig. 10-10, *C*)
7. Retinoscope reflex that may be fuzzy at first and may clear momentarily after a blink (Fig. 10-9, *C*)

If the lens is too steep, there is no touch at the apex because of apical vaulting. Vision is improved immediately after a blink because the eyelid on a blink "irons out" the soft lens and compresses the lens against the apex of the cornea. The patient's only complaint may be fluctuating vision, which may be momentary but annoying.

It may take several days of wearing time before circumlimbal injection and indentation occurs. This is a late sign of a tight lens. Lenses, however, should be changed before this has had a chance to occur. Complaints of a burning sensation may precede limbal compression and are an indication of a tight lens. The uncomfortable feeling caused by a tight lens may take several hours or days to appear.

We have noted that some lenses that are well fitted at the beginning gradually change their parameters and tighten up months later. This

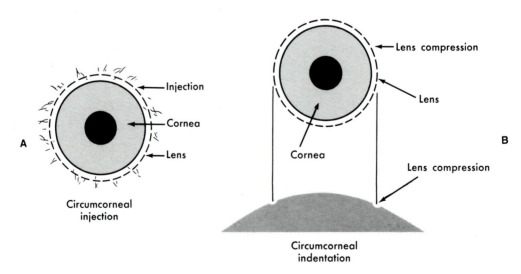

Fig 10-16 ■ **A,** Circumcorneal injection. Note the considerable vascularity at the limbus. **B,** Circumcorneal indentation. The tight lens compresses the peripheral limbal tissues.

may be caused in part by alteration in the plastic by the chemical disinfection process or by the accumulation of denatured protein. This should be taken into consideration at every examination.

If the lens is very tight, the patient or the practitioner may have difficulty removing it.

There have been instances of the epithelium being denuded on removal. If removal is difficult, saline drops should be added before removal is attempted.

Exceptions to the rule. A tight lens may show excessive movement and may ride low and behave like a loose lens. When the lens is made

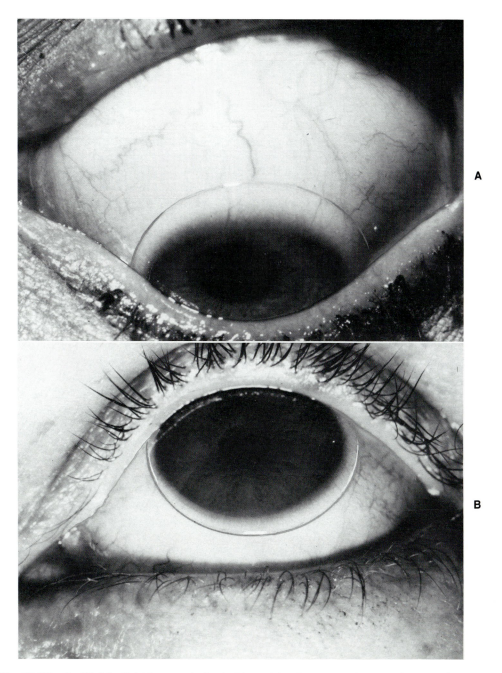

Fig 10-17 ■ A, Slightly tight lens as indicated by minimal movement up on downward gaze. **B,** Tight soft lens. Note the lack of lag on upward gaze and indentation in perilimbal area.

tighter, it may move even more than before. The reason is that there is no longer three-point touch (apex and periphery) but only touch at the periphery so that the lens loses some of its normal capillary attraction to the cornea. Thus the degree of movement alone is not sufficient to determine whether the lens is loose or tight.

A steep lens, like a flat lens, may decenter low because of increased lid action on blinking resulting from lack of touch of the lens at the apex of the cornea. A steep lens frequently decenters downward and nasally because of the direction of the lid action. The obicularis muscle is anchored medially so that on blinking the lid shifts to the nasal side.

Correction of a tight lens. The following steps should be taken to correct a tight lens:
1. Switch to a flatter lens.
2. For spin-cast Bausch & Lomb series lenses, switch to a smaller diameter series or a thinner lens.
3. For lathed lenses, switch to a flatter base curve or reduce the diameter of the lens.

A reduction in the diameter of a lens or flattening the base curve will reduce the apical vault of the lens; as a result the lens apex will be closer to and will rest lightly on the apex of the cornea. Unlike with rigid lenses, fenestration is not a solution for soft lenses because bacteria and fungus invasion can occur when a portal of entry is created in the lens substance. Although it is theoretically possible to dehydrate carefully an existing soft lens for modification, it is not practical from a financial point of view. It is easier and less expensive to fabricate a new lens.

A lens may behave like a tight lens if blinking is infrequent or incomplete.

HELPFUL HINTS ON FITTING

1. If rigid methyl methacrylate lenses have been worn, it is essential that stabilization of the keratometry mires occurs before a soft lens evaluation is made. The cornea may require several weeks or even months to resume a stable topography. This can be shown by two repeatable refractions and K readings.

    A thin, oxygen-permeable soft lens should be used as a temporary lens until the refraction or K readings are stable.
2. Peripheral arcuate abrasion of the cornea, which can cause moderate to severe discomfort, may be caused by an eccentrically po-

sitioned, small soft lens. It can be overcome by choosing a larger or steeper lens.

At times the problem of decentration is best handled if one switches to a lathe-cut lens.
3. If a particular lens appears too loose and the next lens is too steep, try another lens of the same specification as the original lens. Occasionally lenses have been found to be incorrectly labeled.
4. The importance of blinking, especially while one is reading and driving, should be stressed. Alteration in the blink rate is the most common cause of late afternoon variable vision. This is especially true if one has to read a great deal on one's job and if one works in a relatively dry office environment.
5. A measure of the visible iris diameter with a gauge or ruler may be helpful in selecting a lens of the proper diameter, particularly if the cornea is unusually large.
6. Keratometer mires should be rechecked over the lens to make sure that they are not distorted.
7. When a lens is placed on the eye, it may take a few minutes before edge stand-off occurs and the lens shows characteristics of appearing loose. Always wait 15 to 20 minutes before completing an evaluation of the fit.
8. The configuration of the lids and the size of the palpebral aperture are very important in determining the size of the lens required. Wide palpebral fissures such as those that may occur with lid retraction of hyperthyroidism or congenitally prominent eyes may require larger lenses. The small palpebral fissures and the small corneal diameters of Orientals usually require smaller diameter lenses than normal.

    Tight lids can cause traction and make the lens move excessively with a blink. It can ruin a good toric lens fit.
9. The elliptic curve of the back surface of the Bausch & Lomb spin-cast lens, however, makes it more difficult to predict the initial performance of the lens.
10. Clinically it is important to work always in the same direction from a looser to a tighter fit, starting with a loose lens and working toward a lens of proper fit. As previously indicated, one may tighten lathe-cut lenses by steepening the base curve in 0.3 mm

steps or by increasing the diameter in 0.5 mm steps. Alternatively one may loosen lenses by flattening the base curve in 0.3 mm steps or by decreasing the diameter in 0.5 mm steps.

11. In those instances where larger or smaller diameter lenses are not readily available and changing the base curve does not produce the desired effect, it may be necessary to switch to a manufacturer that can custom grind the desired lens.

12. With the low-water-content soft lenses, an acceptable fit is one that affords considerable movement compared to that of other soft lens materials. Even a soft lens fit that would normally appear sloppy is acceptable in the case of a low-water-content lens.

13. The posterior surface of a spin-cast lens is aspheric throughout the extent of the back surface. The central portion is virtually spheric and it is this surface that provides the power of the lens. It is towards the periphery that the lens becomes aspheric. With lathe-cut lenses, the curvature of the anterior surface differs from that of the posterior surface. The anterior surface varies according to the power that is desired. The power of the lens with a spin-cast lens, the curvature of the front surface provides positive power. The back surface, which varies with each series, provides the negative power. Resolution of powers between the front and the back surface yields the final optical power. In the case of a spin-cast lens, the diameter is usually 14.5 mm with the optical portion being 8.66 mm. With the lathe-cut lens, the overall diameter varies but usually is 14 mm, with the optical portion being 8.5 mm. All lenses now have a median diameter that falls between the range of 13.5 to 14.5 mm.

14. Because the posterior surface of a spin-cast lens is aspheric, the traditional K readings and their relationship to the base curve are not applicable to spin-cast lenses. The basic fitting system depends on measurement of the horizontal visible iris diameter and selection of a suitable diameter of lens with proper power. The numerical suffix on the label denotes the lens diameter. A label ending in 4 is 14.5 mm in diameter, a 3 is 13.5 in diameter, and the absence of a number is 12.5 mm in diameter.

    Minus-power contact lenses are available in nine primary series. The O series lens is the thinnest lens presently available; it has a thickness of 0.035 mm.

15. The slitlamp is invaluable in detecting many of the foregoing criteria for a good fit. Attention should be paid to bubbles under the lens or scleral indentation indicating a steep fit and one in which a flatter base curve should be selected.

16. Drs. Hikaru Hamano and Hideaki Kawabe of Japan have shown that the base curve of a lens decreases within 5 to 10 minutes after a lens is inserted and then becomes stable. Thus one should always permit the patient to wait at least 15 to 20 minutes before assessing the fit.

    A thick soft lens can cause changes in the endothelium in 1 day. If vision is impaired, switch to a much thinner lens to avoid minimal corneal edema.

17. Discomfort can arise even with thin soft lenses. They may be so low that movement with a blink is excessive. They may be slightly decentered so that a rim of cornea is exposed. The eyes may be moderately dry, and the thin lens may exaggerate the condition to become symptomatic. The lens may be turned inside out, and that position not be recognized.

11. *HANDLING OF SOFT LENSES*

Insertion, Removal, and Wearing

- *Insertion and removal technique*
- *Taco test*
- *Helpful hints on patient instruction*
- *Wearing schedule and follow-up*

INSERTION AND REMOVAL TECHNIQUE

The technique for insertion and removal of soft lenses is different from that of conventional rigid lenses. The soft lens is inserted onto the lower part of the sclera and gently pushed onto the cornea with the lower eyelid. When soft lenses are being removed, it is generally recommended that the patient slide the lens down with the index finger to the lower part of the sclera and then pinch off the lens.

Insertion by the practitioner

The following technique is used for lens insertion by the practitioner:

1. Keep fingernails short at all times.
2. Wash and rinse hands thoroughly to remove all traces of soap; dry them with a lint-free towel. Avoid using oils and hand creams on hands before handling the lens.
3. Remove the right lens from the vial or case. Lenses that have been soaked in a germicide must be rinsed thoroughly with normal saline solution. A preservative-free saline (unit dose or spray can) may be preferable to a saline containing chemical preservative. Do not touch the inside lens surface after rinsing.
4. Place the lens on the tip of the index finger, concave side up. Have the patient look straight ahead. Stand to the right of the patient and retract the lower lid with your middle finger (Fig. 11-1). If patient is blinking constantly, hold upper lid with middle finger of other hand.
5. Have the patient look up and stare at a point on the ceiling. Be sure that the head is firmly against a head rest. Roll the lens onto the lower white of the eye and express the air buddle. Swirling the lens momentarily on the lateral part of the sclera also helps to make the lens comfortable by introducing tears under the lens and thereby replacing the saline along the lens with the patient's own tears.
6. Have the patient close his or her eyes and lightly massage the closed lid to help center the lens.
7. Repeat the same procedure for the left lens.

COMMENT. If the eye feels irritable after insertion of the lens on the cornea, slide the lens on the conjunctiva and swirl it around to permit tears to flow under the lens and take on the tonicity of the tears before centering again on the more sensitive cornea.

If the patient blinks his eyes frequently and forcefully or has sustained closure, it may be easier to fold the lens and insert it on the temporal conjunctiva rather than on the lower part of the eye.

With thin lenses, permit the lens to dry on the finger for a moment before insertion. Be sure the finger itself is relatively dry or the lens will stick to the finger (Fig. 11-2).

Removal by the practitioner

The following technique is used for lens removal by the practitioner:

1. Wash hands before removal as before insertion.
2. Be sure that the lens is on the cornea before attempting removal.
3. Have the patient look up. Place the middle finger on the lower eyelid, and touch the edge of the lens with the forefinger.
4. While the patient is looking up, slide the lens

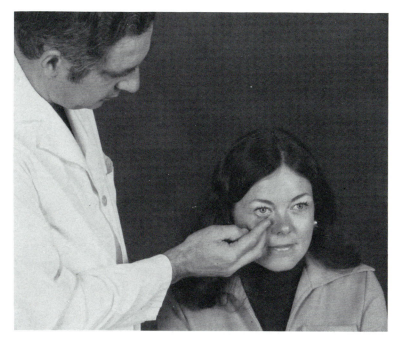

Fig 11-1 ■ Insertion of lens by practitioner. The middle finger retracts the lower lid while the contact lens is gently applied with the index finger to the lower conjunctiva.

down onto the lower conjunctiva of the eye. Bring the thumb over and compress the lens lightly between the thumb and the index finger so that the lens folds and comes off easily.

COMMENT. If the patient is apprehensive and makes the application of a lens difficult because

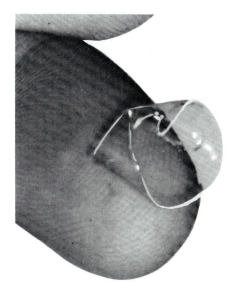

Fig 11-2 ■ An ultrathin lens is more difficult to insert unless permitted to dehydrate.

of blepharospasm, have him open his mouth. It is difficult to squeeze the lids shut with the mouth wide open.

Insertion by the patient

The following technique is used for lens insertion by the patient:

1. Keep fingernails short. Wash hands carefully with soap that does not contain cold cream and dry them. (It is important that the hands be carefully scrubbed and that all traces of makeup or nicotine be removed; otherwise, these will be transferred onto the lens.)
2. Take the lens out of the vial, preferably by pouring the contents of the vial into the palm of the hand. Alternatively, one can use forceps but lenses are often damaged by this method.
3. Rinse with saline and shake off excess.
4. Place the lens on the tip of the index finger of the dominant hand.
5. While looking up, retract the lower lid with the middle finger and apply the lens to the lower part of the eye (Fig. 11-3, *A*).
6. Express any air, remove the index finger, and then slowly release the lower lid.
7. Close the eyes and gently massage the lids to help center the lens (Fig. 11-3, *B*).

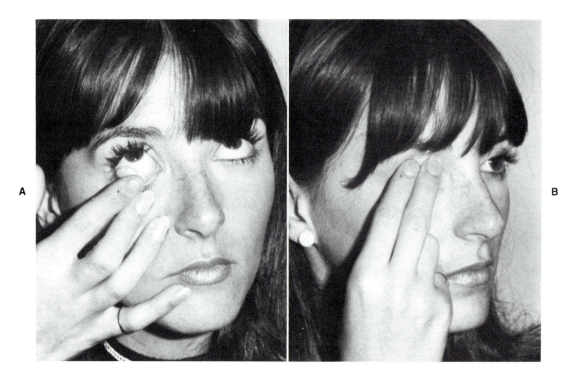

Fig 11-3 ■ A, Inserting the soft lens. **B,** Centering the lens through the closed eyelid. (From Stein HA and Slatt BJ: The ophthalmic assistant, ed 4, St Louis, 1983, The CV Mosby Co.)

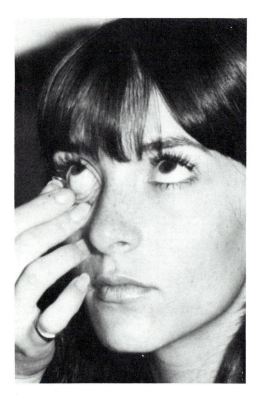

Fig 11-4 ■ Removing the lens. The lens is gently pinched between the thumb and forefinger. (From Stein HA and Slatt BJ: The ophthalmic assistant, ed 4, St Louis, 1983, The CV Mosby Co.)

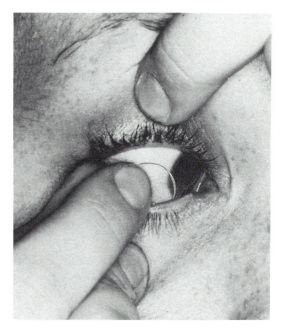

Fig 11-5 ■ An alternate method of removal is to slide the lens to the temporal portion of the globe and fold it off or else use light pressure on the lids at the upper and lower edges of the lens to flex the lens to permit the eyelids to blink the lens out.

8. Cover the other eye and focus to make sure that the lens is centered.
9. Repeat the same procedure for the left lens.
   COMMENT. The ultrathin transparent lenses are difficult to see and feel. A tinted lens aids in the visual identification of the lens.

Clinical experience has shown that the thin edge of a high-plus lenticular lens, an ultrathin lens or a high-water-content lens may sometimes tend to fold over while it is being placed on the patient's eye. This difficulty may be reduced if the lens is held on the patient's finger for about 10 to 20 seconds before placement, thus allowing drying to occur and the edge to stabilize. It may also be necessary to hold the upper lid in order to offset some of the blink reflex.

Removal by the patient

The following technique is used for lens removal by the patient:
1. Check each eye's vision separately by covering the opposite eye to be sure that the lens is in place on the cornea.
2. Wash hands and rinse thoroughly.
3. Look upward. Retract the lower lid with the middle finger and place the index fingertip on the lower half of the lens.
4. Slide the lens down to the white of the eye.
5. Compress the lens between the thumb and the index finger so that air breaks the suction under the lens. Remove the lens from the eye (Fig. 11-4).
6. Prepare the lens for cleaning and sterilizing according to the recommendation of the manufacturer and the practitioner.
7. Alternative method of removal: (1) Look nasally and slide the lens to the outermost portion of the eye before removal (Fig. 11-5), and (2) use the thumb to press the lower lid up and the index figner against the upper lid edge. By flexing the edges and blinking, one can make the lens come out and can grasp it by the thumb and forefinger.

Elderly patients may have difficulty in placing, removing, and handling lenses. Normally if this problem cannot be overcome by in-office training, the patient should not receive the lens. Often, however, another person—a spouse, daughter, or son—may be taught to place, remove, and handle the lenses for the patient. The same is true with children who are being fitted with hydrophilic lenses. Insertion devices are available for the soft lens, but we have not found

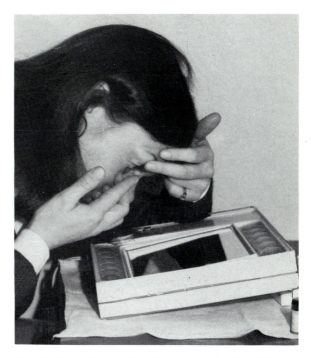

Fig 11-6 ■ A large mirror is a helpful adjunct in insertion of a lens.

them to be very helpful on a prolonged basis. The patient must learn to handle his own lenses directly. See Fig. 11-6.

For those females who resist cutting their nails, we have occasionally resorted to the use of rubber finger cots in the insertion and removal procedure (Fig. 11-7).

Dr. Thomas Spring of Melbourne, Australia, has suggested the use of a sterile finger cot to minimize contamination from fingers. Finger contamination in America has not been a serious problem, but it may apply in other parts of the world.

COMMENT. One of the advantages of extended-wear lenses is that lens-handling is drastically reduced. But persons who wear such lenses do not have a lesser frequency of infection. In fact, the frequency of serious infection is increased. Lens-handling is probably overrated as a cause of infection in contact-lens wearers.

TACO TEST

Before insertion of lenses by either practitioner or patient, one should be sure that the lens is not inside out. One can verify this by gently folding the lens between the thumb and forefin-

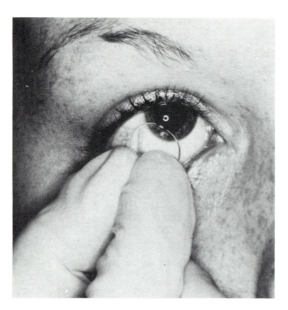

Fig 11-7 ■ Finger cots can be used for those who persistently scratch their lenses or who resist cutting their fingernails.

ger. The edges should point inward and look like a Mexican taco with the edges touching. When the edges roll out rather than in, like an inverted wartime helmet, the lens is inside out and must be reversed (Fig. 11-8). It is important that the lens be grasped and folded near its apex rather than at its edges. Grasping the lens near the edges may give a false and unreliable result. This

test does not appear to work well with the very large lathe-cut lenses.

HELPFUL HINTS ON PATIENT INSTRUCTION

1. Show an audiovisual training film and give instruction booklets to patients before instruction (Fig. 11-9).
2. Do not rush patients. They have spent their lives keeping things out of their eyes, and it is a worrisome experience to put anything in them.
3. Be patient during instruction. No session should last longer than 1 hour.
4. If patients cannot master insertion and removal on the first day, do not keep them there until they can, otherwise, they will become nervous and tense and the eye will become irritated. Have them return another day for further instruction. If they are allowed to take their lenses home before they feel confident handling them, a high percentage of patients will stop wearing their lenses.
5. Carefully explain the importance of hygiene and care. Patients who have received good instructions in the beginning will have fewer problems.
6. Explain that lenses may be extremely difficult to find in the bottle or lens container and that the container should be emptied into the palm of the hand (Fig. 11-10).

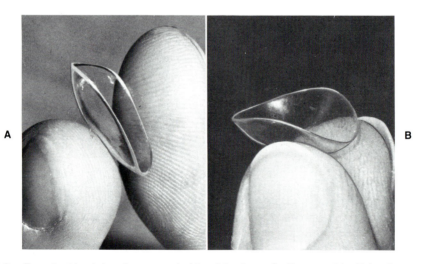

A   B

Fig 11-8 ■ Taco test to determine correct side of the lens. **A,** Correct side. Edge is erect and points slightly inward. **B,** Edge appears to fold back on the finger, indicating that the lens is inside out and must be reversed. (From Stein HA and Slatt BJ: The ophthalmic assistant, ed 4, St Louis, 1983, The CV Mosby Co.)

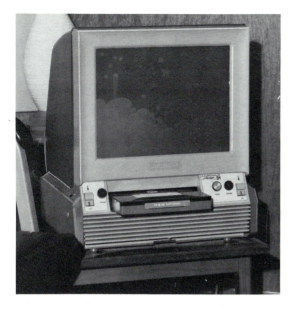

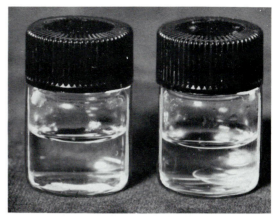

Fig 11-10 ■ Two bottles. The bottle on the right contains a soft lens. It is often impossible for the patient to identify the presence of the lens in the bottle. The bottle should be emptied in the palm of the hand.

Fig 11-9 ■ Audiovisual equipment is helpful in patient instruction.

7. Emphasize that great care should be observed by the patients to avoid switching lenses by placing them in the wrong container.

8. Lenses should be immersed in solution to avoid closing the case lid on them.

9. When inserting the lenses for the first time, have the patients rest their heads on the headrest. Nervous patients will back away as the practitioner comes close to the eye.

10. If patients are extremely nervous, pull the lids apart without inserting the lens to relax the patients and get them used to the feel of the lids being pulled apart. Tell patients that lens awareness may be present initially on the lower lids but will disappear shortly.

11. When the soft lens is applied and stings, it is helpful to slide the lens from the cornea onto the outer part of the sclera and rub gently to get the patient's own tears under the lens. This makes the lens isotonic with the tears, resulting in greater comfort. We have called this technique the *scleral swirl*.

12. If a patient's eyes are red while wearing soft lenses, remove lenses and stain the eye with fluorescein, checking for staining, stippling, or any interference with corneal metabolism or breaks in the corneal epithelium. Do not re-insert lenses for at least 1 hour after fluorescein is used because the residual fluorescein may stain the lens.

13. Always remember that problems of corneal irritation are often caused by a sensitivity to the cleaning and storing saline solutions used, and, in particular, to thimerosal, which is used as a preservative in contact lens solutions. If using a hydrogen peroxide system, make sure that the lenses have been completely neutralized.

14. If hydrogen peroxide is used, make sure that the patient is fully aware of the importance of proper neutralization.

15. Outline a conservative wearing schedule for the patient to follow.

16. Explain the various systems available for disinfecting lenses and explain why a particular one is being recommended and the reasons why patients should not change systems on their own.

17. Carefully instruct patients (1) not to use any over-the-counter eye medication or lens-cleaning solutions, and (2) not to switch from disinfecting by chemicals to boiling, without advice from the practitioner.

18. Avoid fitting patients who have abnormal hand or fingernail problems (Fig. 11-11).

19. Avoid moist-heat disinfection with anything but the recommended saline solution. Some preserved saline solutions have an adverse effect on lenses.

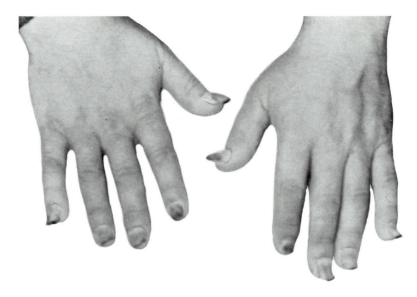

Fig 11-11 ■ Onychogryposis of fingernails, which makes insertion and removal of lenses virtually impossible.

20. If make-up is to be worn, it should be applied after the lenses have been inserted.

WEARING SCHEDULE AND FOLLOW-UP

Soft lenses that are well manufactured, are polished, and have good edge design can be worn for a considerably longer period the first day than was initially realized. Each manufacturer outlines its own protocol, which usually tends to be somewhat conservative. As new lens' designs and new soft lenses with better oxygen performance appear, routines will naturally have to be modified. We can only offer as a guideline our present protocol for standard-thickness and toric soft lenses. The wearing time may be increased considerably for ultrathin and higher-water-content lenses.

The first day the patient may wear the soft lenses for 4 hours. The wearing time may be increased 2 hours daily until an all-day wearing schedule is achieved. Persons with hyperopia, including those with aphakia, should have a somewhat reduced wearing time on the first day because of the greater central thickness of the lens. Three hours is a safe initial wearing time for these persons.

Many practitioners recommend a more rapid wearing schedule in which the patient wears the lenses for 4 or more hours the first day, removes the lenses for 1 hour, and then wears the lenses again for 4 or more hours. The wearing time increases by 2 hours daily with a 1-hour break period. Occasionally we have found patients whose cornea has not tolerated such a lengthy contact the first few days with standard-thickness and low water content lenses. Also, inexperienced lens-wearers sometimes have difficulty with the extra insertion and removal procedure that is required for this schedule.

Full wearing time is an individual variation, and some persons may develop diffuse corneal edema in 10 to 12 hours or sooner. They may not be able to tolerate a soft lens beyond this time even when extremely thin lenses are provided.

Acquired astigmatism with changes in K values has been noted in over 80% of soft lens wearers who wear their standard lenses continuously for more than 12 hours a day. The degree of astigmatism induced is minor, and most fitters do not limit their soft lens wearing time to 12 hours a day. In the fully adapted lens wearer, full daily wearing time is advocated especially with the newer oxygen-permeable soft lenses. Induced astigmatism should and can be monitored with follow-up K readings. One has to pay attention to the quality of the mires and to the change in the radius of curvature. The mires may be blurred or distorted and the valves unchanged. This condition would indicate the start of alterations in corneal topography.

The patient should return to the office for follow-up in 1 week and then at 2-week intervals for three visits. During these visits the fit of the lenses should be evaluated and lens changes made if required. This follow-up procedure is usually adequate for the majority of myopic soft lens wearers.

The appearance of any constriction at the limbus or vessels that begins to invade deeply into the cornea, or of any reduction in movement should be noted and the lens changed to a flatter lens.

Conventional standard-thickness soft lenses should not be worn during sleep. The absence of blinking results in absent tear exchange, insufficient oxygen, and consequently, corneal anoxia (see Chapter 31). The development of higher O_2-permeable polymers and thinner lens designs may make it possible to accelerate adaptation. However, we still prefer a gradual build-up period for all lens-wearers. We adhere to this philosophy in an effort to eliminate any early reactions associated with lens overwear.

12 ▪ *CARE SYSTEMS FOR SOFT LENSES*

- ▪ *Cleaning agents*
- ▪ *Methods of cleaning*
- ▪ *Disinfection of soft lenses*
- ▪ *Rinsing solutions*
- ▪ *Lubricating/rewetting and rehydrating solutions*
- ▪ *Role of preservatives*
- ▪ *Selecting the correct care system*
- ▪ *Switching from one system to another*
- ▪ *Conclusion*

The formation of deposits on contact lenses is almost inevitable. Factors that influence deposit formation include the lens material, the patient's tear characteristics, the wearing time, and the lens care system used. Patient compliance to the lens care system is of major importance. Discomfort problems are frequently associated with deposit formation as is lens awareness and reduced vision.

A wide variety of products is presently available for contact lens care. This large number of available products frequently causes confusion for the practitioner and the public. This section discusses some basic principles and rationales for various cleaning, disinfecting, and rinsing solutions. Whenever changes are made in the care system, one must be fully aware of the interactions of products and the nature of possible adverse reactions. One must also keep in mind the efficacy of the product in cleaning the lens

and in its ability to disinfect. Thus there must be guidelines and rationales for a systemic method of selecting an appropriate effective hydrogel care system for a given person or type of lens. We shall attempt to outline these.

Available care products fall into six categories of function:
1. Cleaning agents
2. Disinfecting solutions—chemical and thermal
3. Rinsing solutions
4. Lubricating-rewetting-cleaning eye drops
5. Special weekly cleaning methods
6. Cases and devices.

There is a variety of available products to be discussed. Although reference may be made to specific trade names, this has been done to illustrate and clarify and does not necessarily constitute any endorsement by us.

CLEANING AGENTS

Soft lenses worn over a period of time gradually become coated and cloudy. This cloudiness not only interferes with clarity of vision but also acts as an irritant, making the patient uncomfortable. The coating may also cause adverse tissue responses. The cloudiness is usually related to surface debris consisting of protein, inorganic films, mucins, lipids, and minerals (Fig. 12-1).

Surface debris on the lens may be diffuse, mottled, or concentrated in one area. It may be

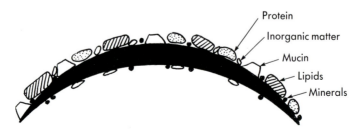

Protein

Inorganic matter

Mucin

Lipids

Minerals

Fig 12-1 ▪ Common deposits on the surface of a contact lens.

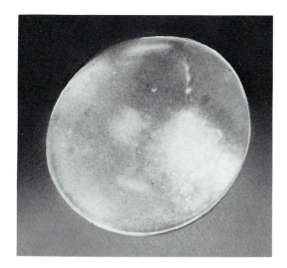

Fig 12-2 ■ Protein buildup on a soft lens will vary with the duration of wear, the method of disinfection, and the nature of the tears of the wearer.

a mixture of protein with lipid or calcium deposits. It is more common in persons with relative tear deficiency or with high serum cholesterol levels. Micro-organisms usually adhere tenaciously to the deposit, which forms a film around the organism. The most common deposits are proteins and lipids (Fig. 12-2). However, there are many extrinsic factors that contribute to lens spoilage. Unclean fingers may transfer grease, dirt, mascara, eyeliner, nicotine, or lipstick, and, most importantly, bacteria. Face powder or environmental dust as well as toxic fumes may also affect the lens surface. Blinking causes the palpebral conjunctiva to rub over the deposit up to 15,000 to 25,000 times

per day, depositing mucin from the goblet cells and perhaps exposing the tarsal conjunctiva to an immunologic response to the coating on the surface of the lens.

The buildup of protein, lipids, and minerals on the lens may result in the following:
1. A decrease in vision
2. A red and irritable eye
3. An increase in the mass of the lens, which may affect the fit of the lens
4. A change in the parameter of the lens, which may cause the lens to tighten
5. A decrease in the oxygen transmission of the lens
6. An increase in the protein antigen factor on the lens, which may in turn cause:
   a. Giant papillary hypertrophy of the conjunctiva
   b. Corneal and bulbar conjunctival inflammatory response

The net effect of these changes is to make the lens uncomfortable and the vision blurry.

Allansmith and Fowler have shown that surface deposits extend over 50% of a hydrogel lens within 5 minutes after the soft lens is worn and over 90% of the lens after 8 hours.

Because some coating occurs within 30 minutes, it is quite likely that it may be necessary for coating to occur. Perhaps mucinous coating is necessary to reduce the wetting angle of the plastic and to permit greater comfort and enhanced vision. With time, however, the coating becomes plaque-like and produces problems as described above.

Kleist has demonstrated that the thermal method of disinfection produces an incidence higher than usual of most deposits except cal-

Table 12-1 ■ Incidence of common deposits on 370 lenses with deposits

Type of deposit	Incidence		
	Overall (%)	Cold regimen (%)	Heat regimen (%)
Abrasions	25	28	22
Protein films	19	14	24
Pigment	25	9	38
Micro-organisms	10	4	28, unpreserved saline
			11, preserved saline
Inorganic films	10.5	5.9	14.4
Rust-colored spots	13	7	18
Lens calculi	13	13	13
Calcium carbonate	9.5	16	4
Calcium phosphate	4.6	9	1
Mercurial origin	10.5	5	21, preserved saline

From Kleist F: Deposits, International Contact Lens Clinics, May-June, 1979.

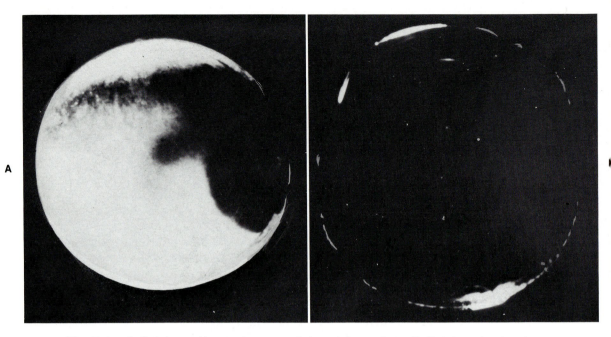

A

Fig 12-3 ■ A, Soft lens with protein accumulation of the surface. **B,** Soft lens that has been routinely cleaned with cleaning agents.

cium, which appears higher with chemical disinfection (Table 12-1). We have also found deposits to be more frequent with the thermal method of disinfection than with chemical disinfection. The heat tends to denature or coagulate the proteinaceous material on the surface of the lens. In a retrospective study, Josephson found that the rate of replacement almost doubled in switching patients from chemical to thermal disinfection. The exception to this rule is white crystalline deposits, which occur less frequently with the thermal system.

Protein buildup is now believed to be a form of denatured lysozyme, a normal antibacterial enzyme found in tears (Fig. 12-3). Almost all soft-lens wearers eventually will develop this protein buildup, but it will vary with the type of soft-lens material, the duration of time that the lenses are worn, the nature of the tears of each individual, and the method and efficiency of cleaning.

Small amounts of protein buildup can be detected more easily if the lens is removed from the eye, allowed to partially dehydrate, and then held against a black background with oblique light from a slitlamp. If the protein buildup is excessive, a reasonable assessment can be obtained when one examines the lens on the eye

with the slitlamp. Even modest amounts may be detected by intense scrutiny.

Unfortunately there are no methods to ensure that an adequate cleaning has been done by the patients when they take their lenses home.

Deposits may be studied by immunofluorescence, visible and ultraviolet spectroscopy, and various forms of histochemical stains. Immunofluorescence techniques provide qualitative information about protein deposition. Spectroscopy identifies types of discoloration and chemicals in the lens. Staining demonstrates the presence of protein and lipids. Scanning electron-microscopy and electron-microprobe techniques identify inorganic ions. The phase-contrast microscope allows very subtle deposits to be seen without altering the lens. These procedures are beyond the reach of most contact-lens' clinicians but research continues to be conducted. Allansmith and Fowler have shown that the deposits on daily wear soft lenses show peaks and valleys whereas the deposits on extended wear lenses are diffusely coated with a relatively even smooth surface (Fig. 12-4). In effect, these deposits on extended wear lenses may be more innocuous because they provide a smooth refracting surface on the lens, which may be less traumatic for the tarsal conjunctiva. Allansmith

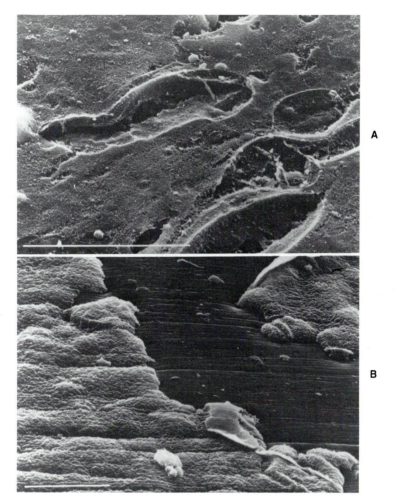

Fig 12-4 ■ **A,** Electron-microscopy photograph showing coating on an extended-wear lens being relatively flat. **B,** Coating on a daily-wear lens revealing large valleys and bare areas of a contact lens after cleaning. (Courtesy Mathea Allansmith and Sherry Fowler, Boston.)

believes that the peaks and valleys' coating on daily wear soft contact lenses are attributable to repeated rubbing away of a portion of the plaques on the surface of the contact lenses, whereas with extended wear soft lenses the deposits are not cleaned frequently and build up as a flat coating.

METHODS OF CLEANING

There are three distinct types of soft-lens cleaners—surface-acting, oxidative, and enzyme cleaners. Added to this is the use of ultrasound, which can help speed up the cleaning process. These cleaners can be further broken up into daily and weekly categories (Tables 12-2 and 12-3).

Surface-acting (surfactant) cleaners

Surfactants mobilize, emulsify, and solubilize most of the adhered daily accumulation of proteins, lipids, and minerals from the surface of a lens during a day of wear (Fig. 12-5). Bacteria adhere to the surface of lens deposits, and surfactants facilitate disinfection by reducing microbial contamination on the lens surface.

The surfactant agent is usually a high molecular weight to prevent molecules from entering the pores of the lens. Surfactants act to lower

Table 12-2 ■ Daily cleaners

Manufacturer	Solution	Preservative
Alcon	Opti-Clean	Thimerosal
	Opti-Clean II	Edetate Disodium 0.1%, Polyquad 0.01%
	Preflex for Sensitive Eyes	Sorbic Acid
Allergan Optical	LC-65	Thimerosal
	Lens Clear	Sorbic Acid
	Lens Plus Daily Cleaner	None
Barnes-Hind	Soft-Mate Daily Cleaning Solution	Thimerosal
	Soft-Mate p.s. Daily Cleaner	Potassium Sorbate 0.13%
	Soft-Mate Daily Cleaning Solution II	Potassium Sorbate 0.13%
Bausch & Lomb	Bausch & Lomb Daily Cleaner	Thimerosal
	Bausch & Lomb Sensitive Eyes Daily Cleaner	Sorbic Acid 0.25%
Blairex	Duracare	Thimerosal
Charter Laboratories	Charter Cleaning Solution for Sensitive Eyes	Sorbic Acid
Ciba Vision	Ciba Vision Cleaner	Sorbic Acid
CooperVision	Pliagel	Sorbic Acid 0.25%, Edetate Disodium 0.5%
	Miraflow	None
Ross Laboratories	Murine Contact Lens Cleaner	Sorbic Acid
Sherman Laboratories	Sof/ProClean	Sorbic Acid
Strieter Laboratories	Sof/Clens	Sorbic Acid

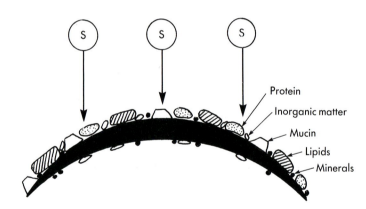

Fig 12-5 ■ Action of surfactant on a lens surface is to mobilize, emulsify, and solubilize the deposits on a lens.

Table 12-3 ■ Protein removers (weekly cleaners)

Manufacturer	Solution	Preservative
Alcon	Opti-zyme	Pancreatin
	Encymatic Cleaner for Extended Wear	Pancreatin
Allergan	Allergan Enzymatic Contact Lens Cleaner	Stabilized Papain
	Extenzyme Protein Cleaner	Stabilized Papain
	Ultrazyme Enzymatic Cleaner	Subtilisin A
Barnes-Hind	Soft-Mate Weekly Cleaner	Thimerosal 0.001%, Edetate disodium 0.1%
	Soft-Mate Protein Remover Solution	None
Bausch & Lomb	ReNu Thermal Enzymatic Cleaner	Subtilisin A
	ReNu Effervescent Enzymatic Cleaner	Subtilisin A

surface tension of the lens-water interface. Surfactant-cleaner formulations also contain a chelating agent that binds metal ions. Some surfactant cleaners are hypertonic with the purpose of drawing out or absorbing material from within the lens. Other surfactant formulations lower or raise pH so as to maximize protein removal. Examples of these are Softmate and Pliagel. Miraflow incorporates isopropryl alcohol added to Pliagel to remove lipids and protein. Miraflow is the only non-aqueous solution and incorporates isopropyl alcohol added to Pliagel to remove lipids and protein.

Some surfactants are anionic or negatively charged, which means that they react with cations such as magnesium or calcium and precipitate these ions out. These cleaners can be used for any type of soft lens, rigid lens, CAB, gas-permeable rigid lens, or silicone lens. One cleaner, Opti-Clean II (Polyclens), contains large molecule granules that shear the deposits from the lens surface without any adverse effects on the surface.

COMMENT. All surfactants should be thoroughly rinsed. Otherwise stinging, burning, conjunctival hyperemia, and keratoconjunctivitis may occur.

We have found the use of Miraflow, which is 20% isopropyl alcohol added to Pliagel, a better surfactant cleaner than Pliagel alone. It must be washed off by thorough rinsing and the lens soaked or the residual alcohol on the lens surface can cause corneal insult.

Boyd and Korb have advocated the use of commercial salt made into a paste and used twice weekly for cleaning of a hydrogel lens. This salt mush has an excellent abrasive effect in removing surface coating. Other practitioners have recommended the use of baby shampoo, baking soda, and water on the lens surface for at least 20 seconds. Allansmith believes that the mechanical action of rubbing a lens is just as effective as the surfactant.

Method of use of surfactants. The hands are carefully washed with a soap without cream, oils, or perfume, and rinsed well. A drop or two of a surface-acting solution is placed on the lens, which is held concave side up in the palm of the hand (Fig. 12-6). The lens is rubbed lightly with the ball of the finger for at least 20 seconds. The palm should be fully open so that the skin is stretched firm. The patient should press the lens into the palm while rubbing so that the palm

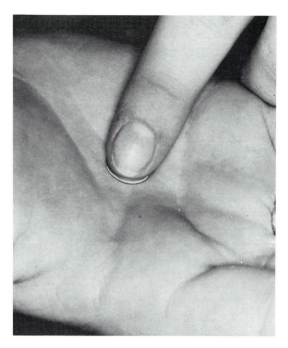

Fig 12-6 ■ The lens is rubbed in the palm of the hand with a surfacting soft lens cleaner.

just begins to blanch. The lens is inverted and cleaned in the same manner. The lens is rinsed well with preserved saline solution or distilled water. While rinsing, the patient rubs the lens until it feels clean. This should be a daily routine. Any unrinsed residue can produce a film by itself, and so careful rinsing of the surfactant cleaner is important.

Surfactants are special agents that have hydrophilic and lipophilic (lipid-loving) characteristics within the same molecule. These molecules can attach themselves to a variety of soils typically found in all contact lenses (e.g., proteins, lipids, mucins, cosmetics, and environmental soils). By finger-rubbing, these soils are softened, loosened, and easily removed.

Alternatively, a cleaning device (e.g., Barnes-Hind Hydromat II) may be used with the surfactant cleaner (Table 12-4).

LC 65 (Allergan). This chemical compound was initially introduced as a rigid-lens cleaner. It has been modified to perform as a surface-acting agent for both soft and rigid lenses.

Opti-Clean II (Polyclens). This (Alcon, Forth Worth, Texas) is a broad-spectrum universal contact lens cleaner that may be used to reduce deposit formation on all rigid and soft contact

Table 12-4 ■ Daily cleaning products

Product name	Active ingredient(s)	Lens type	Company
Opti-Clean	S/P+	H/GP/C	Alcon
Preflex	S		
LC-65	S	H/GP/C	Allergan
Lens Clear	S	H	
Lens Plus	S	H	
Easy Cleaner/GP	S	GP/C	
SoftMate	S	H	Barnes-Hind
GP Cleaner	S	GP/C	
Titan	S	C	
Daily Cleaner	S	H	Bausch & Lomb
Concentrated Cleaner		GP	
Cleaner	S	H	Ciba Vision
Miraflow	S/I	H/C	
Murine	S	H	Ross
Boston	S	GP	Polymer Technology
Pliagel	S	H	Wesley-Jessen

CODE
S = Surfactant   C = Conventional Hard Lenses
P = Particles   H = Hydrophilic Soft Lenses
I = Isopropyl Alcohol   GP = Gas-Permeable Lenses

lenses. This cleaner is composed of a surfactant with high-molecular-weight polymer beads. These beads act by actually shearing off many deposits from the contact lens' surface without damaging it. The cleaner is a milky suspension preserved with Polyquad (Opti-Clean II) or thimerosal and EDTA. It is compatible with both heat and chemical disinfecting regimens. It is effective when used for 20 seconds on each side and may minimize the necessity for using enzyme cleaners or weekly cleaners. For sensitive eyes, Preflex, which contains sorbic acid as the preservative, is recommended.

COMMENT. Clinical studies that we have performed indicate that Opti-Clean II (Polyclens) can facilitate the removal of protein as well as lipids and minerals in most instances. It is the first cleaner in which a high-molecular-weight polymeric bead has been introduced in a surfactant for the mechanical shearing of surface bonds of protein and lipids. In our detailed study of 25 patients (49 eyes) followed for 1 year, 95% to 97% of the lenses remained clear. Most of them did not require the use of an enzyme cleaner. The product has a milky color and is slightly granular, which aids the patient in thorough rinsing of the cleaner before lens insertion. However, during clinical studies, one patient inserted the lens daily without rinsing and suffered no corneal insult except a mild stinging and feeling of grittiness. All individuals found this product comfortable when it was used as directed.

Oxidative agents

The oxidative agents are used to remove bound deposits. By a combination of heat, oxidation, and large swings in the pH and osmolarity, these agents degrade pigment and discolor lenses. A large shift in pH and osmolarity stresses the lens. This may crack some deposits on the lens surface, which may irreversibly damage the lens by oxidation of the hydroxyl group. This may result in an alteration of the lens parameters and the fitting characteristics of the lens. Monoclens, Ren-O-Gel, Lipofin, and hydrogen peroxide fall into this group of oxidative agents.

Lipofin. Although not available in North America, Lipofin is used in many parts of the world. It is an inorganic electrolyte with oxygen-releasing action. The released oxygen breaks down organic material by oxidation into smaller components, which become readily soluble. Dr. John DeCarle has described a modified use in which one sixth of a packet is dissolved in 120 ml of water and the lens is boiled in a basket of this solution for 10 minutes. Lipofin works best between 45° and 60° C. It then remains in the solution for 1½ hours and is removed and disinfected in a disinfecting solution for 2 hours before the lens is worn. Lipofin was originally used for Permalens when the lens became uncomfortable. It has been shown to have germicidal and viricidal properties as well as cleaning ability.

Enzyme cleaners

The forerunner of the enzyme cleaner group has been papain, a proteolytic enzyme used in meat tenderizers and derived from the fruit of the tropical melon tree. Papain acts on peptide linkages in protein. When used properly and regularly, it retards protein deposit formation on the lens and removes some previously formed protein deposits from the surface of a lens. Unfortunately papain has no action against lipids, oils, cosmetics, or minerals. The enzyme cleaner has a larger molecular size than the lens itself and penetrates only slightly below the surface of a low-water-content hydrogel contact lens. It will, however, build up within a lens of high water content and may leave residual enzymatic activity within the lens matrix, which may be toxic to the cornea.

Other available enzyme cleaners such as Optizyme by Alcon contain not only a proteinase compound but also a lipase and a mucinase. This enzyme, optizyme, is a large molecule called pancreatatin. Pancreatatin contains protease plus lipase and amylase to remove lipids and mucin as well. The large molecule resists penetration into the matrix of high-water-content lenses. Therefore, low- or high-water contact lenses may be soaked for up to 12 hours without pancreatatin penetrating into the lens matrix.

A number of companies' products are now available for special weekly cleaning (see Table 12-5).

COMMENT. Papain is retained in the superficial pores of HEMA lenses and may cause adverse reactions such as burning, stinging, photophobia, redness, and superficial punctate keratitis. Thorough rinsing of enzyme cleaner is important. It is also useful to clean the lens between forefinger and thumb with a surfactant and rinse thoroughly.

Method of use of Hydrocare tablets. The lens is placed with the cleaning tablet and distilled water in a vial. The vial is shaken until the tablet is dissolved. The lens should be left in the vial for a minimum of 2 hours, or it may be left overnight. The lens is then removed, rinsed, and disinfected by the recommended procedure. The lens should remain in the disinfectant solution for a minimum of 8 hours.

We have found that this method of cleaning is the most effective and practical and that it adds considerably to the preservation of the clarity and comfort of a lens. It should be used once weekly by those patients who use thermal disinfection or lay down protein regularly. This can be reduced to only twice monthly for those using a chemical disinfecting system.

We have found that with higher-water-content lenses (more than 60%), the lens should not be left in the enzyme solution for two hours. Thirty minutes should be adequate. The higher the water content, the more retention in the lens.

COMMENT. The use of prepared saline is no longer acceptable. Tap water is too frequently contaminated, and clinically it has been shown to be a source of infection and corneal ulceration. Even deionizers of tap water for purification are not effective unless the prepared saline is made fresh.

Ultrasound

An effective way of cleaning a soft lens is by the use of ultrasound, especially biphasic ultrasound. An ultrasound bath in which the lens is placed in a cleaning solution, such as any of the surfactants, enzyme cleaners, or hydrogen peroxide, will aid in cleaning a very soiled lens. In addition to the ultrasound waves, heat is generated and the combination of heat and ultrasound reinforces the cleaning action of the com-

Table 12-5 ■ Special cleaning products

Product name	Active	Lens type	Company
Opti-Zyme	Pancreatin	H/GP/C	Alcon
Enzymatic Cleaner	Papain	H/GP	Allergan
Ultrazyme	Subtilisin	H	
Protein Remover	Surfactants	H/GP	Barnes-Hind
ReNu	Subtilisin	H	Bausch & Lomb

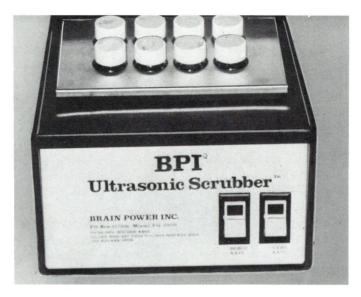

Fig 12-7 ■ Ultrasound unit for in-office cleaning of soft and rigid contact lenses. This unit provides ultrasound in two directions.

pound (Fig. 12-7). As a final action, one can place the lenses in the ultrasound bath in a vial filled with preserved or unit dosage saline solution. Ultrasound units are presently becoming available for home use.

COMMENT. Ultrasound may effectively clean the lens; however, protein may recur more rapidly after an ultrasound bath. If this occurs, replacing the lens is the best recourse.

The disposable-lens concept discussed in Chapter 33 has changed the whole concept of care. It has minimized the amount of care accessories that are required to maintain clean lenses.

DISINFECTION OF SOFT LENSES

Sterilization implies the complete death of all bacteria, fungi, and spores; *disinfection* refers to either physical or chemical procedures that kill common pathogenic organisms but may permit some nonpathogenic organisms to survive. Lens care involves disinfection, which is adequate for soft lenses.

Disinfection of lenses is important to prevent the growth of common organisms that may be present in the environment and cause serious eye trouble. Examples are *Staphylococcus aureus*, *Pseudomonas aeruginosa*, *Candida albicans*, and *Herpes simplex* virus. Disinfection procedures are aimed at removing the presence

of the organisms. Hands and contaminated cosmetics may both represent potential sources of a high number of these organisms. Normally, the conjunctiva and conjunctival cul-de-sac have nonpathogenic normal flora, but this may be significantly altered by the presence of new bacteria not related to soft lens wear. These may in turn contaminate the surface of soft lenses. Disinfection is practical and clinically effective, if proper hygiene and care are used. Soft lenses are usually supplied in a sterile state from the manufacturer. Most lenses with water content below 50% can withstand temperatures of up to 260° F (127° C); therefore the packaged lens can be autoclaved before shipping. Once the vial is opened, however, the lens is no longer sterile and both the practitioner and the patient must maintain a high level of cleanliness and must follow proper disinfection procedures between usage.

There are basically three methods of disinfection that are available commercially for soft lenses:
1. Thermal disinfection
2. Chemical disinfection, and
3. Oxidative procedures, which require the prior use of a cleaning agent and should be followed by thorough rinsing. Ideally, thermal disinfection should be accompanied by regular use of an enzyme cleaner.

Thermal disinfection

Boiling thermal method (100° C). With the boiling thermal method, practitioners have the option of prescribing preserved saline or non-preserved saline solution. Sterile disposable units of preservative-free buffered salt solutions are also available along with canisters.

The pharmaceutically prepared saline solution considerably reduces the effect of contaminants in the distilled water and the errors of users who put the salt tablet in tap water. In the latter situation, there is a fundamental misconception that clear water is pure and free of chemicals and metals, which may in turn have a deleterious effect on the lens.

COMMENT. Salt tablets for home use are no longer recommended because of the problem of water contamination, which may cause serious eye infections. Even pharmaceutically prepared saline solutions are not recommended. Distilled water may be free of metals and chemicals but may still harbor bacteria.

Commercially prepared saline is available without preservatives.

Heat method. These steps are followed in the heat method of disinfection of soft lenses:
1. Lenses are cleaned in the palm of the hand with a surface-acting cleaning agent.
2. Lenses are rinsed well with a saline solution.
3. Lenses are placed in the lens container, which is filled with saline solution.
4. The container is placed in the heating unit.
5. The unit is turned on; it will heat up and cool down in approximately 45 to 60 minutes and shut off automatically. The time cycle will vary from one manufacturer to another. Lenses are now ready for use.

There are four main advantages to boiling:
1. Many consider it to be more effective for disinfection.
2. It is unquestionably cheaper in the long run.
3. About 30% of persons develop adverse reactions to chemicals.
4. The thermal method achieves disinfection in a shorter period of time than chemical disinfection, which requires 4 to 6 hours.

Boiling is used chiefly for soft lenses that have a water content below 60%. Laboratory tests have shown that repeated boiling and cooling of the lens over hundreds of hours has a minimal deleterious effect on the plastic itself. However, degradation of the plastic does occur with repeated exposures to temperatures above the normal boiling point of water. This may cause slow degradation of the plastic and may lead to loss of the original parameters, such as base curve, with a change in the fitting characteristic of the lens. This may be more noticeable with one lens material than with another. Many high-water-content and higher-oxygen-permeable lenses are adversely affected by repeated heating. Extended wear soft lenses of high water content should not be disinfected with the autoclave or heating method.

The patient should use preserved commercially prepared saline. The lens material and the wearability factor may be affected if the patient substitutes salt tablets and tap or spring water, which often contain undesirable impurities, especially unwanted minerals. In addition, the wrong amount of water or the wrong number of salt tablets may result in a lens that is uncomfortable to wear. Commercial preparations are the best.

Another problem with the thermal disinfection system is the coagulation of protein on the lens surface and the baking on of this protein with repeated heating. This results in lack of clarity, mass increase, and an increase in the adherence of immunoglobulin A. This last result may be responsible for giant papillary conjunctivitis because of its allergenic activity. There also may be a resultant change in parameters and fitting characteristics.

Dry heat method (80° C). The new miniature dry heat units that are available do not require water to be added to the unit and subject the lens, in its carrying case, to a minimum temperature of 80° C for 10 to 20 minutes. This time-temperature cycle has been demonstrated to be effective in accomplishing disinfection of the lens. It has been demonstrated that a variety of bacteria, mold spores, yeast, acanthamoeba, and the Herpes simplex virus are all killed in these units (Fig. 12-8).

The miniaturization of these thermal units has made them handy for travel. They are now available in small, cordless, and plug-in models.

Chemical disinfection. A number of care systems is available for the care and maintenance of hydrophilic soft contact lenses. These solutions disinfect, clean, and make the lens comfortable for wear. The antimicrobial agents (preservatives) maintain the sterility of the solution in the bottle and also inhibit organisms on the lens from proliferating. These preservatives

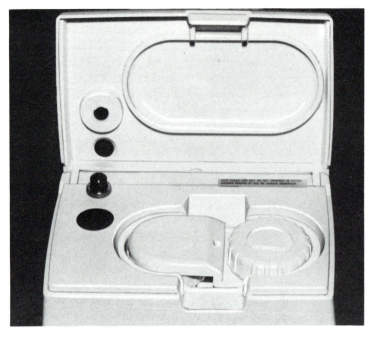

Fig 12-8 ■ Thermal disinfection unit for soft contact lenses. Dry-heat method.

must also not be toxic or cause hypersensitivity.

Chemical solutions containing combinations of chlorhexidine, thimerosal, and EDTA have been shown to be effective in killing organisms. A number of companies have introduced into the Canadian, European, and Asian markets soft-lens disinfecting agents that have shown adequate clinical effectiveness. Individual agents such as sorbic acid and hydrogen peroxide have shown effective antimicrobial properties.

One major problem in developing adequate soft-lens accessory products is the binding of preservatives by the soft lenses. Preservatives like chlorobutanol, benzalkonium chloride, phenylmercuric acetate, phenylethyl alcohol, methylparaben, and benzyl alcohol may concentrate in the lenses and cause corneal changes. Thus one cannot use conventional rigid-lens solutions on soft lenses. Benzalkonium chloride notoriously binds with the soft lens material and can cause severe corneal damage.

Chemicals commonly used for soft-lens disinfection are shown in Table 12-6.

For each manufacturer the percentage of each chemical may vary.

The more common systems for disinfection will be reviewed.

Chlorhexidine-thimerosal system (such as Flexsol and Normol). Flexsol, which was the first

approved chemical for disinfection, is formulated with EDTA, thimerosal, chlorhexidine, and borate buffers along with normal saline. It is permitted to remain in contact with the lens overnight and is then carefully rinsed off with saline solution before the lens is inserted in the eye.

The following are the steps in disinfection:
1. Remove the lens from the eye.
2. Place the lens in the palm of the hand.
3. Pour a few drops of a surfactant cleaner on the lens and rub the lens gently for 20 to 30 seconds.
4. Rinse the lens with saline solution.
5. Place the lens in the container and add disinfecting solution, such as Flexsol, until the lens is well immersed.
6. Store the lens for a minimum of 4 hours before insertion.

On inserting the lens:
1. Remove the lens from the case.
2. Rinse the lens well with saline solution.
3. Insert the lens in the eye.
4. Empty the case and rinse with warm tap water; air-dry the case.

COMMENT. Rinsing the contact lens after using this solution is most important. Chlorhexidine or thimerosal is mildly irritating to the cornea if any remains in the lens or on the lens surface.

Table 12-6 ■ Chemicals used for soft lens disinfection

Chemicals	Example
Thimerosal	Preserved saline
Chlorhexidine	MiraSoak, Flexcare
Chlorhexidine-thimerosal	Combiflex, Flexsol, Barnes-Hind Storage Solution, Hydrosoak
Polyquad®	Optisoft; Opticlean
Thimerosal–sorbic acid products	Permasol
Alkytriethanol ammonium chloride–thimerosal product	Lensept, In a Wink, Oxysept
Hydrogen peroxide	Pliacide, Transoft
Iodine	Soft Tab/Optitab
Dichloroisocyanurate	Sterisoft
Nipastat-thimerosal	
Dymed	Renu
Sorbic acid	Neutralizing solutions, sorbisal, etc.
Chlorine	Chlorox

Fresh disinfection solution must be used daily. Flexcare was introduced as different from Flexsol because the absence of the adsorbable polymer permits the solution to be used as a rinsing solution as well as a disinfecting solution.

Chlorhexidine is rarely used today. Thimerosol is both an irritant and a cause of allergic reactions and has been abandoned by most manufacturers. Most solutions intended for sensitive eyes are made without thimerosal.

Quaternary ammonium solutions. Hydrocare or Allergan Cleaning and Disinfecting Solution and B&L Soaking Solution are used as cleaner and storage solutions. Their main germicide is alkytriethanol ammonium chloride combined with some surfactant agents and buffering solutions. This is a quaternary ammonium compound that binds with surface-acting molecules of the solution and becomes large enough that it does not penetrate into the soft-lens matrix. In this way the solution does not become eluted from the lens while in the eye and produce chemical insult to the cornea.

The reason why quaternary ammonium solutions have fallen into disrepute is because they have an adverse reaction rate of approximately 30%. These adverse reactions include corneal edema, conjunctival hyperemia, and allergic reactions.

Sorbic acid, hydrogen peroxide, and chlorine have been added to the armamentarium of soft-lens disinfectants. The steps in disinfection are similar to the chlorhexidine-thimerosal routine.

COMMENT. Although the lenses can be worn directly after removal from this quaternary ammonium germicide solution, Morgan has pointed out that 15% of persons will develop small intra-epithelial microcystic changes in the corneal epithelium after prolonged use. This is eliminated if the solution is thoroughly rinsed off with preserved saline before use.

We have performed clinical and comparative studies with this solution for over 1 year and have found greater comfort, fewer protein deposits on the lenses, and fewer discontinuances with this disinfectant than with a chlorhexidine-based solution.

We also found that some patients who were unsuccessful with a thimerosol and chlorhexidine system such as Flexsol were successful with a quaternary ammonium system, and vice versa.

Because chemical systems are portable and easy to use, they are a definite convenience for patients when traveling.

Hydrogen peroxide (Table 12-7). This system acts as a cleaning agent and as a good disinfectant for all soft lenses. The excellent performance of 3% hydrogen peroxide is marred only by the fact that patients may fail to neutralize the hydrogen peroxide adequately which may result in chemical burn of the cornea. Ongoing product developments will eventually resolve and simplify care management with hydrogen peroxide. The hydrogen peroxide is similar in all cases but the neutralization differs with each company.

The lens is gently rubbed with a surfactant cleaner and then placed in a specially designed lens container. The container is then filled to a line with 3% hydrogen peroxide and soaked for 10 minutes. It is then transferred to the second

Table 12-7 ■ 3% Hydrogen peroxide disinfectant and cleaner

Manufacturer	Solution
Allergan	Lens Plus, Oxysept Disinfection System
Bausch & Lomb	Quicksept
Barnes-Hind	Concept
Charter	Hydrogen Peroxide System
Ciba Vision	Aosept Disinfection and Neutralization-Storage Solutions
	AODisc Catalyst Solution
	Lens-Sept Disinfection Solution
	Lens-Sept Neutralizing Solution
Wesley-Jessen	Mirasept Disinfection System
Ross Laboratories	Murine PureSept Disinfecting Solution

container, containing preserved normal saline or unit-dosage nonpreserved saline solution and a catalyst (solution or tablet) that breaks down any peroxide into free oxygen and water. The lens is allowed to remain overnight, or for 4 hours or more. It is then shaken and rinsed once again in fresh saline for 3 minutes, after which it is ready to be worn.

Hydrogen peroxide 3% has the ability to penetrate the entire matrix of the soft contact lens in 30 seconds. The D values for hydrogen peroxide are very effective against most organisms. It kills many organisms quickly, including the AIDS virus after 10 minutes. With acanthamoeba, hydrogen peroxide is only effective in 4 hours while heat is preferred as it kills acanthamoeba in 10 minutes.

In clinical experience the lenses containing polyvinylpyrrolidone may become discolored and yellow in time. The use of hydrogen peroxide has a whitening or bleaching effect on the lens.

COMMENT. Hydrogen peroxide is easily decomposed. Light accelerates this decomposition, and hence hydrogen peroxide should be kept away from direct light. The Septicon disc has been practical and effective in neutralizing the hydrogen peroxide and preventing ocular irritation and corneal damage. The present system is somewhat cumbersome for the patient. However, a newly evolved version of this system promises a simple one-step automatic procedure.

About 25 to 50 parts per million of hydrogen peroxide may remain after storage overnight. If any adverse effects are experienced by some patients, one may eliminate these effects by spilling out the saline solution, filling the case with fresh saline, and letting this stand for 5 to 10 minutes before inserting the lenses.

Hydrogen peroxide forms free hydrogel radicals that react against the cell wall of bacteria. The free radical forms water and oxygen, which is neutralized. A platinum disc, a neutralizing solution or tablet, catalyzes the reaction by which hydrogen peroxide is neutralized. The hydrogen peroxide is quite unstable in the presence of a metal, especially platinum.

Although 25 to 50 parts per million of hydrogen peroxide may remain *in situ* in the lens matrix with normal saline neutralization, by using osmotic neutralizers that contain sodium thiosulphite, one can eliminate retention of hydrogen peroxide. These large molecules do not penetrate the lens material but act to draw out hydrogen peroxide by osmosis.

Symed, manufactured by Bausch & Lomb, is both a preservative and a disinfectant. It has minimal toxicity compared to other disinfecting agents. The polymer is positively charged and thus able to cause cell death of micro-organisms. It is also one of the best sensitizing agents. Its kill rate is effective against most organisms.

COMMENT. The basic regimen to be emphasized to patients is that every day they should
1. clean their lenses to prevent build-up of film and debris
2. disinfect to destroy bacteria that gather on lenses
3. neutralize with a rinsing solution to turn the disinfecting solution into a harmless solution
4. use an enzyme or cleaning solution to remove protein once a week

Useful hints on disinfection and cleaning

1. All remarks previously made and those made by the manufacturer are made on the basis of an intact soft lens. If a lens has a slight crack or a roughened edge, bacteria or fungi may penetrate the lens substance and may not be adequately disinfected by some of the techniques of disinfection.
2. Whatever system of disinfection the patient has been instructed in, he or she should continue with that system rather than switch to newer or different systems unless indi-

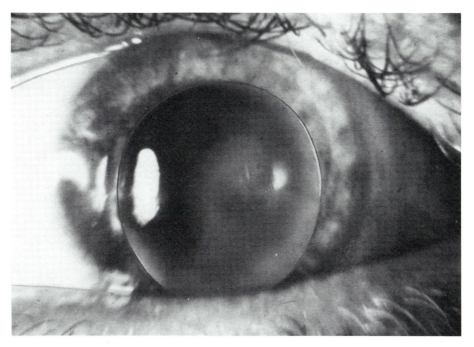

Fig 12-9 ■ Protein deposit on a contact lens. It is considered moderate-to-advanced when seen grossly with the slitlamp.

cated. Some of the different chemicals may react with each other or accumulate and cause irritative problems to the cornea.

3. If a patient is using one chemical system and switches to another, it is important that the lenses be purged in fresh distilled water three or four times to leach out the previous chemical. The lenses should then be disinfected. Alternately, the lenses may be soaked or even shaken for 15 minutes in saline with three or four changes of saline to dilute the chemical. This osmotically removes the chemical. Lenses are then placed in the new disinfecting solution.

4. If protein deposits on the surface of a soft lens are not removed, they lead to reduced visual acuity, interference with oxygenation to the cornea, giant papillary conjunctivitis, and binding of preservatives to the lens. Bound preservatives may produce a burning sensation (Fig. 12-9).

5. Adverse ocular response to disinfecting agents may occur and is manifested by (1) red and itchy eyes, (2) a burning sensation, and (3) diffuse corneal stippling. One may correct this by switching to an oxidizing-agent disinfecting system and to preservative-free saline or an osmotic neutralizing solution.

6. To be effective, the disinfecting solution must be changed daily in the lens-storage case.

7. The friction of rubbing the finger on the lens against the palm with surfactant cleaners tends to shorten the life of soft lenses by causing scratches, particularly if the skin of the fingers or palm is rough.

8. Nonpreserved unit doses of pharmaceutically prepared saline is preferred over salt tablets mixed with distilled water. Chemical impurities have been found in the distilled water and may vary from area to area. Distilled water has been shown to contain 20 times the amount of impurities than triply distilled and deionized water.

9. If an enzyme tablet has turned brown, it has lost its effectiveness and should not be used (Fig. 12-10).

10. Lens cases should periodically be scrubbed clean. Contaminated lens cases play a significant role in infective keratitis. One study has shown that 43% of soft-contact-lens wearers were using contaminated lens cases. Lens cases should be air-dried daily

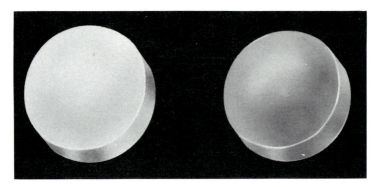

Fig 12-10 ■ The enzyme tablet on the right has become discolored because of oxidation and has lost its effectiveness.

and subjected to boiling water at least once a week.

11. Once a lens container is unsealed, spare lenses or lenses not used regularly should be disinfected at least once a week, either thermally or by a change of the disinfecting solution. We have seen both bacterial and fungal contamination of these lenses when this disinfection procedure is not followed.

12. Studies we have undertaken with Opti-Clean (Polyclens; Alcon, Fort Worth, Texas) surfactant cleaner show that it can remove protein, lipids, and inorganic matter without the use of enzyme tablets in at least 80% of patients.

13. Strong oxidizing agents should be used only infrequently or not at all with HEMA lenses because they degrade the plastic.

14. Patients with dry eyes as suggested by an abnormal Schirmer test or a very thin tear meniscus or a poor BUT (tear film breakup time) often develop deposits more frequently.

15. When a soft lens has heavy white calcium deposits and is professionally cleaned, the lens is more likely to develop deposits much sooner with each succeeding use.

16. In some persons the lens may become coated in a few weeks, whereas in others it may take a year before any significant deposits develop.

17. There are some problems associated with patient preparation of salt tablets: the possibility of contamination, the use of water that does not conform to distilled or purified standards, the use of the wrong type of salt tablets, and patient error in mixing.

18. Kleist has shown that there is an increase in inorganic and organic deposits on lenses that use the thermal disinfection system as compared to those lenses that are chemically disinfected.

19. Cleaning can be effected by swirling the lens in a lens-cleaning solution (Fig. 12-11).

20. Most of today's systems work well if there is sufficient contact time. However, acanthamoeba is very resistant, and special caution should be taken to follow the manufacturer's cleaning instructions faithfully.

Rinsing solutions

A large variety of rinsing solutions are available (Tables 12-8 and 12-9) in aerosol or canister form, which preserves their sterility over a longer period. These solutions may be used to rinse some debris from the lens after cleaning. They are also used to rinse the lens after disinfection

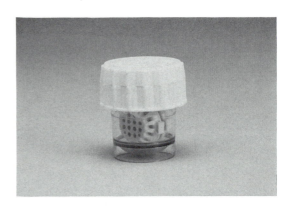

Fig 12-11 ■ Hydromat II—the lens is held in place by a plastic basket and is swirled in order to clean.

Table 12-8 ■ Saline solutions—non-aerosol

Product name	Preservative	Buffer	Company
Boil-n-Soak	Thimerosal	Borate	Alcon
Opti-Soft (OptiPure)	Polyquad	Borate	
Hydrocare	Thimerosal	Borate	Allergan
Lensrins	Thimerosal	Phosphate	
Lens Plus	Thimerosal	Borate	
SoftMate	Thimerosal	Borate	Barnes-Hind
SoftMate ps	Potassium Sorbate	Borate	
SoftMate	Nonpreserved	Borate	
Sensitive Eyes	Sorbic Acid	Borate	Bausch & Lomb
ReNu	Dymed	Borate	
Hypo-Clear	Nonpreserved	Borate	
Murine	Sorbic Acid	Borate	Ross Laboratories
Murine	Nonpreserved	Borate	
Unisol	Nonpreserved	Borate	Wesley-Jensen
Sterile Saline	None	Borate	Blairex
CIBA Vision Saline	None	Borate	CIBA
SOFSAL	None	Borate	Strieter Laboratories

Table 12-9 ■ Saline solutions—aerosols

Product name	Preservative	Buffer	Company
Opti-Pure	None	None	Alcon
LensPlus	None	Borate	Allergan
SoftMate	None	Borate	Barnes-Hind
Hypo-Clear	None	Borate	Bausch & Lomb
CIBA Vision	None	Borate	CIBA Vision
Murine	None	Borate	Ross

by chemicals to reduce the degree of adverse reactions to these chemicals. A toxic reaction may result initially in tiny microcysts of the epithelium, which may break down and lead to find punctate corneal staining.

A list of rinsing solutions may be divided into unpreserved and preserved saline as well as distilled water. Unpreserved saline rinsing solutions may be saline freshly made from salt tablets or individual unit doses or saline or multi-dose aerosol saline.

Preserved saline solutions contain either thimerosal alone in a concentration of 0.001% or potassium sorbate or sorbic acid 0.1% or combinations of either of these preservatives with EDTA (0.1% or 0.01%) or sodium borate 0.22%.

Josephson and Caffrey found that 14% of their patients presented with an adverse ocular response to saline preserved with thimerosal or sorbic acid. Changing to the use of nonpreserved saline solution eliminated this reaction. Symptoms included stinging, burning, itching, and blurry vision. Signs include punctate keratitis, edema, staining, chemosis, hyperemia, infiltrates, and a granular appearance to the bulbar conjunctiva.

COMMENT. The incidence of ocular toxicity, hypersensitivity, and corneal precipitates attributable to solutions is far greater than the frequency of ocular infection. The iatrogenic effect of antibacterial devices is considerable. We rarely see contact lens–induced infections, but inflammatory side effects of antibacterial solutions are common.

Lubricating/rewetting and rehydrating solutions
(such as Adapettes, Clerz II, Comfort, and Opti-tears; see Table 12-10)

Minor degrees of ocular discomfort result from prolonged exposure to environmental conditions such as tobacco, smoke, smog, pollution,

Table 12-10 ■ Re-wetting drops/lubricants

Manufacturer	Solution	Active neutralizer
Alcon	Adapettes for Sensitive Eyes	Sorbic acid
	Opti-Tears	Polyquad
Allergan	Lens Fresh	Sorbic acid
	Lens Plus Re-Wetting Drops	Nonpreservative-saline
	Lens-Wet	Thimerosol
Barnes-Hind	Soft Mate p.s. Comfort Drops	Potassium sorbate
	Soft-Mate Lens Drops	Potassium sorbate
Bausch & Lomb	Lens Lubricant	Thimerosol
	Sensitive Eye Drops	Sorbic acid
	ReNu	Sorbic acid
Blairex	Lens Lubricant	Nonpreservative-saline
Ciba Vision	Ciba Vision Lens Drops	Sorbic acid
CooperVision	Clerz II	Sorbic acid
Ross Laboratories	Murine Lubricating and Re-Wetting Drops	Sorbic acid
Strieter Laboratories	Sofwet	Sorbic acid

and dust. In addition, areas of low humidity will dry out soft hydrogel lens producing discomfort. Those persons exposed to heaters or air conditioners, either in a car or in their work environment, may have dehydration of the soft lenses.

COMMENT. Dehydration of a lens makes it uncomfortable and reduces the clarity of vision. The anterior surface of the lens becomes irregular and spheric instead of regular.

Inadequate tear production is another cause for lenses to dry, requiring special eye drops. There are also persons who are heavy mucus secretors, and the mechanical cleaning of their lenses by a lubricating solution would be helpful. The use of sterile fluid to rehydrate the lens while it is being worn can be helpful in providing comfort and clarity of vision. Fluids today that are manufactured primarily for this purpose also contain a detergent that helps clean the lenses by loosening and dispersing any mucous and inorganic accumulations on the lens' surface.

COMMENT. For those who have symptoms of fluctuating vision or discomfort caused by dryness, it is helpful to add a lubricating drop two or three times daily to their routines.

Ultrathin lenses are more subject to drying because of their thin substance. Persons wearing these lenses often benefit from the use of lubricating drops.

Persons wearing extended-wear lenses may be helped with lubricating drops that contain a cleaning agent in addition to the rewetting agent.

ROLE OF PRESERVATIVES

Preservatives provide protection against chance contamination. Preservatives frequently used are thimerosal, sorbic acid, potassium sorbate, EDTA, and chlorhexidine. Chlorhexidine binds to the lens, and the protein in the tears binds to the chlorhexidine. Laboratory data contrasted with clinical experience frequently provide conflicting results in the efficacy of any one preservative. Many preservatives in rigid lens solutions cannot be used in soft lens solutions because of penetration into the lens resulting in toxic reactions to the eye. However, the same preservatives when used in therapeutic eye drops such as pilocarpine are permissible because of the total lower concentrations.

The agent in soft lenses that is most likely to induce hypersensitivity is mercurial thimerosal, a preservative. In some countries thimerosal has been omitted from the solutions to eliminate the red eye and irritability syndrome that develops in those persons sensitive to thimerosal.

Toxic reactions

With the concentrations of disinfectants for rigid and soft contact lenses required to kill micro-organisms, the cornea and conjunctiva may become irritated. With the use of soft lenses, the preservatives present in the solution may be absorbed into the matrix and later released onto the cornea and conjunctiva. A HEMA lens with a water content of 55% may absorb its equivalent in thimerosal. Reactions to solutions have been reported to occur in 3% to 50% of contact-lens wearers.

While reactions can occur with thimerosal, chlorhexidene, and hydrogen peroxide, studies have shown that thimerosal is the most highly sensitizing agent, causing reactions in 8% to 15% of contact-lens wearers. In the cornea, thimerosal toxicity manifests itself by peripheral infiltrates or punctate keratitis combined with ciliary injection. These reactions subside quickly when the preservative is discontinued.

A mixture of sorbic acid and dymed has been introduced as a substitute to thimerosal. While it is not completely innocuous, it causes less reaction than thimerosal. Sorbates also do not bind to a lens as does chlorhexidine. Solutions preserved with sorbic acid polyquad or dymed have a low incidence of corneal and conjunctival sensitivity.

COMMENT. Josephson and Caffery, in a study of 10 different types of drops used on a population of soft-lens wearers with symptoms of dryness (some of which were supplied with preserved and other with preservative-free saline) found that there was no statistically significant difference in the effectiveness of one solution as compared to another. The only statistically significant difference was between the preservative-free drops and the preserved drops in that patients preferred the preservative-free drops.

SELECTING THE CORRECT CARE SYSTEM

The initial step in selecting the correct care system is to decide on the method of disinfection. One has to decide between the thermal or chemical method. If the lens is not compatible with heat, one must make a decision from among the list of available chemical solutions. Those who have any allergic tendencies should be placed on an unpreserved saline storage system. Those who have abnormal tear chemical patterns or who are more likely to be deposit-formers should be placed on a chemical disinfection system to reduce the tendency for deposit formation.

COMMENT. Any allergic tendency, such as a history of hay fever or allergies to drugs or cosmetics, should be a warning to use preservative-free disinfecting and soaking/rinsing solutions.

We arbitrarily consider some individuals as requiring conventional cleaning routines and others as requiring maximum cleaning routines. Maximum cleaning routines are for those who use the thermal method and those who are rapid deposit-formers. They should use the strongest surfactant cleaner available. Supplementary enzyme cleaning on a weekly basis should be observed. Patients with incomplete blinking may have increased deposit tendencies and may require maximum cleaning routines.

One should be aware that some products made by different manufacturers are identical in chemical composition.

Manufacturers today are constantly researching new and better cleaning agents for soft contact lenses. At the time of this writing, no firm recommendation can be offered because technologic changes are proliferating so rapidly in this area that anything written today becomes obsolete tomorrow.

In addition to the selection of the individual system and the individual specific pharmaceutical vehicle, one should consider the cost factors. The thermal systems cost more initially, but in the years of use may reduce the cost of maintenance. However, the replacement lens cost is increased with the thermal method, which offsets the cost savings of avoiding chemicals. Some patients' lifestyle may be more suited to chemical disinfection or perhaps to conversion to the minimal-care routine of extended-wear lenses. Product availability in some local geographic areas and in some parts of the world may predetermine the care system selected.

SWITCHING FROM ONE SYSTEM TO ANOTHER

The novice fitter can easily become confused with the large variety of care systems that are available for the choices that he may have. Added to the confusion of the fitter is the dilemma of the patient who enters his local drug store and views the special bargains that may entice him to deviate from the solution he is using and to try a new brand. In addition, color-coding of care systems for rigid lenses, gas-permeable lenses, soft lenses, and silicone lenses has not reached the sophisticated level that now identifies red-topped bottles as mydriatric solutions and green-topped bottles as miotic solutions.

The responsibility of the fitter is not only to be acquainted with as many care systems as possible, but also to understand two important aspects: (1) when he should change from one type of system to another and (2) which types can be mixed and still be compatible.

Josephson and Caffrey have outlined one system of care selection (Fig. 12-12). Essentially their view is in agreement with ours in that a history of lens wear and problem analysis is critical to determine when and how to change to another type of care system.

Our method is to divide new patients into two groups: those with previous problems related to allergic reactions and those with no history of difficulty. For the first group, a thermal system usually with unpreserved saline is recommended. For the second group, any one of the disinfectants is recommended combined with a surfactant cleaner and, usually, the enzyme cleaner as well. If an adverse reaction develops, as in red eyes or irritation, one may reduce enzyme-active agents, switch enzymes, switch to another nonthimerosal type of disinfectant, or just switch to the thermal system with unpreserved saline.

The most innocuous system to use for persons who are highly allergic is to clean the lenses with a nonthimerosal surfactant and to soak the lenses at night in fresh unpreserved saline.

Thermal disinfection is slightly more effective if antimicrobial effects are desired. The average life of a lens cleaned by cold disinfection methods is approximately 50% longer than of those cleaned by using heat. Deposits build up with increasing frequency in the case of heat disinfection because the heat tends to denature protein and proteinaceous debris.

The use of vibrating standing waves to clean contact lenses. Vibrating standing waves consist of multilamellar clusters of solution molecules maintained in a highly turbulent state by the application of strong vertically-directed vibrational energy. The waves are automatically generated in the Hydra-Mat II cleaning and storage device when it is used in a Soft Mate automated cleaning unit.

After placing the lenses in the lens baskets and filling the chamber to the line with a cleaning solution, the patient closes the Hydra-Mat and places it in the automatic cleaning unit. Touching the switch immediately generates a continuous strong vertically-directed virbration or energy. This energy produces vibrating standing waves of cleaning molecules that flow through the openings in the lens' baskets as well as up and around the lenses, creating a fountain-like scrubbing action.

The kinetic energy transfers upwards molecular layer by layer; it expends itself and is re-

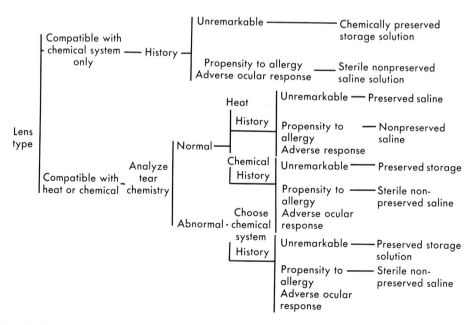

Fig 12-12 ■ Selection of care system. (From Josephson J and Caffrey B: Selecting an appropriate hydrogel lens care system, Am J Optom Physiol Opt 52(3):227-233, March 1981.)

Table 12-11 ■ Products for use with soft contact lenses

Proprietary name	Manufacturer	Preservative	Other ingredients	Sizes
Cleaning products				
Soflens Enzymatic Cleaner Tablets	Allergan Pharmaceuticals Inc.	None	Papain, stabilizers	12s, 24s, 48s
Bausch & Lomb Daily Cleaner	Bausch & Lomb Inc.	Thimerosal 0.004%	Edetate disodium, sodium phosphate, sodium chloride, tyloxapol, hydroxyethylcellulose, polyvinyl alcohol	45 ml
Pliagel	CooperVision Pharmaceuticals Inc.	Sorbic acid 0.1%	Edetate trisodium, Poloxamer 407, sodium chloride, potassium chloride	25 ml
Opticalean II	Alcon	Polyquad	0.001	EDTA Polyuric cleaning beads
12 ml 20 ml				
Opticlean (Poly-clean)	Alcon	Thimerosol 0.004	EDTA Polyuric cleaning beads	12 m 20 m
Preflex	Alcon	Thimerosal 0.004%	Edetate disodium, sodium phosphate, sodium chloride, tyloxapol, hydroxyethylcellulose, polyvinyl alcohol	30 ml
Soft Mate	Barnes-Hind Pharmaceuticals Inc.	Thimerosal 0.004%	Edetate disodium, sodium chloride, tyloxapol, hydroxyethylcellulose	30 ml
Barnes-Hind Weekly Cleaner	Barnes-Hind Pharmaceuticals Inc.	None	Detergents	
Miraflow	CooperVision Pharmaceuticals Inc.	None	Poloxamer 407, amphoteric detergent, isopropyl alcohol	25 ml
Mireup Contact Lens Cleaner	Ross Laboratories	Sorbisol		
Hydroclean	Contactosol Ltd.	Thimerosal 0.001%	Detergents	
Softcon Lens Cleaner	Softcon	Thimerosal 0.001%	Detergents	
Ren-)-Gel	CooperVision Pharmaceuticals Inc.	None	Acidic and basic inorganic poroxy compounds	
Monoclens	Medical Optics Center	None		
Lipofin	Alcon	None	Sodium perborate	
Clean-O-Gel	Alcon	None	Enzymes	
LC 65	Allergan Pharmaceuticals Inc.			
Thermal disinfecting and rinsing products				
Allergan Saline Solution	Allergan Pharmaceuticals Inc.	Thimerosal 0.001%	A sequestering agent, boric acid, sodium borate, edetate disodium	8 oz
Bausch & Lomb Preserved Saline Solution	Bausch & Lomb Inc.	Thimerosal 0.001%	Boric acid, sodium borate, sodium chloride, edetate disodium	8 oz
Bausch & Lomb Saline Solution	Bausch & Lomb Inc.	None	Sodium chloride	14 × 10 ml

Continued

Table 12-11 ■ Products for use with soft contact lenses—cont'd

Proprietary name	Manufacturer	Preservative	Other ingredients	Sizes
Blairex Salt Tablets	Blairex Laboratories Inc.	None	Sodium chloride	135 mg
Durocare	Blairex	Thimerosal		
BoilnSoak	Alcon	Sorbic acid	Boric acid, sodium borate, sodium chloride, edetate disodium	8 oz, 12 oz
Lensrins	Allergan Pharmaceuticals Inc.	Thimerosal 0.001%	Sodium phosphate, sodium chloride, edetate disodium	8 oz
Salette	Medical Optics Center	None	Sodium chloride and buffer	10 ml
Buffered Salt Tablets	Barnes-Hind Pharmaceuticals Inc.	None	Sodium chloride, sodium bicarbonate, edetate disodium	
Pliasol	CooperVision Pharmaceuticals Inc.	Sorbic acid 0.1%	Sodium chloride, edetate disodium, sodium borate, boric acid	4, 8 oz
Soft Therm	Barnes-Hind Pharmaceutical Inc.	Thimerosal 0.001%	Boric acid, sodium borate, sodium chloride, edetate disodium	8 oz
Mirasol	CooperVision Pharmaceuticals Inc.	Sorbic acid 0.1% Thimerosal 0.001%	Poloxamer 407, edetate disodium, boric acid, sodium borate, sodium chloride, potassium chloride	
Unisol	CooperVision Pharmaceuticals Inc.	None	Sodium chloride, boric acid, sodium borate	25 × 15 ml
Opti-Pure	Alcon	None	Sodium chloride	8 oz, 12 oz
Alcon Saline Solution	Alcon	Sorbic acid	Boric buffer system Sodium chloride	

Chemical disinfecting solutions

Proprietary name	Manufacturer	Preservative	Other ingredients	Sizes
Allergan Cleaning and Disinfecting Solution (Hydrocare Disinfecting Solution)	Allergan Pharmaceuticals Inc.	Thimerosal 0.002% Tris (2-hydroxy-ethyl) tallow ammonium chloride 0.013%	Sodium bicarbonate, sodium phosphate, propyleneglycol, polysorbate 80, soluble polyHEMA	8 oz
Bausch & Lomb Disinfecting Solution	Bausch & Lomb Inc.	Thimerosal 0.001% Chlorhexidine 0.005%	Sodium chloride, sodium borate, boric acid, edetate disodium	8 oz
Normol	Alcon	Thimerosal 0.001% Chlorhexidine 0.005%	Sodium chloride, sodium borate, boric acid, edetate disodium	8 oz
Optitears	Alcon			
Optisoft	Alcon	Polyquad .001%	EDTA	8 oz/12 oz
Flexsol	Alcon	Thimerosal 0.001% Chlorhexidine 0.005%	Edetate sodium, polyoxyethylene, polyvinylpyrrolidone, sodium chloride, boric acid, sodium borate	6 oz
Flexcare	Alcon	Thimerosal 0.001% Chlorhexidine 0.005%	Sodium chloride, sodium borate, boric acid, edetate disodium	12 oz
Soft Mate	Barnes-Hind Pharmaceuticals Inc.	Thimerosal 0.001% Chlorhexidine 0.005%	Edetate disodium, conditioning and buffering agents	8 oz
MiraSoak	CooperVision Pharmaceuticals Inc.	Thimerosal 0.001% Chlorhexidine 0.005%	Sodium chloride, boric acid, sodium borate, edetate disodium, Poloxamer 407	4 oz

Table 12-11 ■ Products for use with soft contact lenses—cont'd

Proprietary name	Manufacturer	Preservative	Other ingredients	Sizes
Pliacide	CooperVision Pharmaceuticals Inc.	Iodine 0.1%	Stabilizing agents	5 ml
nutra-Flow	CooperVision Pharmaceuticals Inc.	Sorbic acid 0.1%	Sodium chloride, potassium chloride, edetate disodium, sodium borate	4 oz
Lensept	Am Optical Hydrogen Peroxide			4 oz
Aosept	Am Optical	3%		
Hydrosoak	Contactosol Ltd.	Thimerosal 0.001% Chlorhexidine 0.001%	Salts and buffers	
Sterisoft	Medical Optics Center	Thimerosal 0.001% Chlorhexidine 0.001%	Sodium chloride, edetate disodium	
Lubricating/rewetting eye drops				
Adapettes	ALcon/BP	Thimerosal 0.004%	Povidone, polyoxyethylene, edetate disodium, sodium chloride, and buffering agents	15 ml
Bausch & Lomb	Bausch & Lomb Inc.	Thimerosal 0.004%	Povidone, polyoxyethylene, edetate disodium, sodium chloride, and buffering agents	15 ml
Clerz	CooperVision Pharmaceuticals Inc.	Sorbic acid 0.1%	Hydroxyethylcellulose, Poloxamer 407, edetate disodium, sodium chloride, potassium chloride, sodium borate	25 ml
Comfort Drops	Barnes-Hind Pharmaceuticals Inc.	Thimerosal 0.004%	Tyloxapol, sodium chloride, edetate disodium, borate buffer	
Murine	Ross	Sorbic acid	Sodium chloride buffer agents	
ReNu	Bausch & Lomb Inc.	Sorbic acid		4 oz

generated by continuous operation of the automatic cleaning unit.

The efficiency of the vibrating standing wave has been tested clinically. The following observations have been made at the conclusions of clinical studies. The automated method equaled the digital method in removing protein deposits. The automated method was superior to the digital method in removing lipid deposits. The patient preferred the automatic method because it was easier to use. The use of a vibrating standing wave has been found to be safe and effective and minimizes the handling of lenses; it also encourages patient compliance because of its ease and automaticity. Most of this work was conducted by Murray J. Sibley, PhD. Disinfection should always be performed last, after surfactant cleaning or enzyme cleaning and just before placing the lens in the eye. The reader is referred to Chapter 36 for a more detailed analysis of problems with care systems.

CONCLUSION

New and better products are fast appearing on the market. Table 12-11 indicates some of the products available at this time. This is a multimillion dollar industry as more and more people turn to contact lenses. This era of increasing contact lens wear has been brought about not only by the explosion of new developments in soft and rigid contact lens that make lenses more comfortable and more reliable for visual performance than before, but also by a wider variety of effective care products. New-product development in care systems not only allows lenses to be cleaned and disinfected better, but also tends to simplify the care of contact lenses. The next advance may be an *in vivo* type of drop that cleans a lens perfectly while one is wearing it, and a disinfecting system that works quickly and leaves no sensitizing or toxic products in or on the contact lenses.

13 ▪ *TINTED SOFT CONTACT LENSES*

Recently there has been an increasing use of tinted contact lenses. The manufacturing technology is, however, relatively new. Before modern technology, vegetable dyes, oxidized epinephrine compounds, and biologic stains were used to color contact lenses. However, these pigments were not permanent. The technology has been improved significantly to the point where the dye is impregnated beneath the surface of the lens. Because of this, the newer contact lenses are color-fast; the pigment does not leach out of the lens into the cornea, tear film, or storage solutions.

In recent years, tinting has been accomplished by vat dyes, acid reactive dyes, and diazo dyes. These dyes remain stable; however, hydrogen peroxide- and chlorine-based disinfectants may bleach these dyes.

With opaque lenses, Titmus Eurocon imprints an iris image on a dome of clear HEMA. Wesley-Jessen uses the same process but prints a dot-matrix pattern on the front surface of the lenses. Meshel and Presley have devised a laser method for opacifying a HEMA matrix.

HOW TO FIT

The technique for fitting a tinted contact lens is basically the same as for any soft lens. A trial soft lens should be fitted and the results of
1. base curve
2. diameter and
3. power (if useful vision) is present.
In addition, one should decide on a suitable tint. A number of guides are available to hold over the patient's eye to get the proper enhancement (Fig. 13-1), which is a combination of the existing color of the iris plus the superimposed tint.

The size of the pupil should be assessed in normal room light and a lens of the appropriate size should be ordered.

Contact lenses are tinted for a variety of reasons:
1. Cosmetic Use—Tinted contact lenses can enhance and even change the color of one's eyes.
2. Therapeutic Use—Tinting can improve the appearance of some eyes and even the visual function of abnormal eyes.
3. Handling Tints—To afford the patient with better visualization of the lens.
4. Data Printing—Data, such as lens' specifications, can be imprinted on a lens.

1. *Cosmetic Use*
   a) Color enhancement
   Color enhancement has been most successful in making light eyes more brilliantly blue, green, or hazel. The allure of eyes has been written about by poets and authors since the beginning of time; a tinted lens placed on the eye makes it look richer and more saturated with color. This is because light travels through the lens twice and the second passage results in reflected light bouncing back to the observer from the iris of the contact lens' wearer. A retrospective study that we had undertaken in patients who had been fitted with tinted lenses showed that 60% preferred aqua, 20% preferred green, 15% preferred blue, and 5% opted for other tints.
   b) Color alteration
   Another use of contact lenses is to completely alter the color of the eyes; lenses are most often used to make brown eyes appear blue. Wesley Jessen, CooperVision, Ciba Vision and the Narcissus Foundation all manufacture good lenses

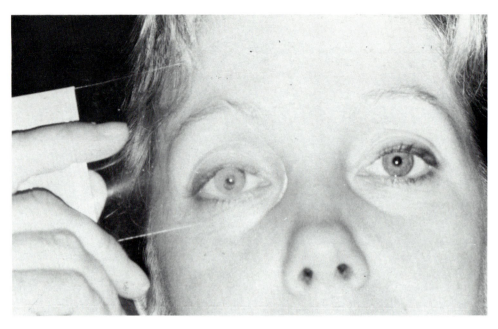

Fig 13-1 ■ Hand-held guide to determine suitable tint to enhance the color of the eye.

that alter eye color. The size of the patient's clear optic zone and the effect of ambient light can have a major influence on the result because color-altering lenses can cause unwanted "tunnel vision." Pupil size is another very important variable. The portion of the lens covering the iris must be totally opaque in order to completely mask the natural brown color of the eyes. Color-altering lenses also play an important role in the movie industry. It is necessary for historical figures such as Churchill, Napoleon, etc. to be portrayed with their natural eye color, but often the actor chosen to play the part has eyes of a different color. To satisfy movie buffs who insist on historical accuracy, actors often have to wear colored contact lenses.

Contact lenses have been used in the movies since 1939. They have been most effectively used in horror movies such as *The Exorcist*. Red glowing lenses were used on the gargoyles in the 1984 movie *Ghostbusters*; reptile eyes were crafted for the commander in *Star Trek*. Even Michael Jackson wore contacts for his animal change in the video "Thriller." White contact lenses were used on Hulk in the television series "The Incredible Hulk." Using contact lenses to

create the illusion of blindness is an old trick that has been used in a number of movies. Audrey Hepburn wore blind eye contacts in the 1967 movie *Wait Until Dark*. Silver mirrored contact lenses were used by Yul Brynner in *West World* in 1973. Elvis Presley's eyes went from blue to brown in the 1960 movie *Flaming Star*. In the 1968 movie *Planet of the Apes*, all the blue-eyed actors became brown-eyed thanks to the use of contact lenses.

Tinted lenses can function as sunglasses for joggers, tennis players, and others who spend a great deal of time outdoors. Ultraviolet blockers are currently available as well.

COMMENT. Some iris colors can be easily changed. A grey iris can be altered to look like any other color; darker or brown irises, however, are more difficult to tint and special opaque lenses are required. The lens diameter must be sufficiently large that none of the natural iris is exposed at the limbus.

2. Therapeutic Use
   a) Covering unsightly corneal scars: Unsightly corneal scars that are not suitable for corneal transplant surgery (usually because of heavy vascularization or patient age) may be masked with a colored lens that has a central black pupil (Figs. 13-2 and 13-3).

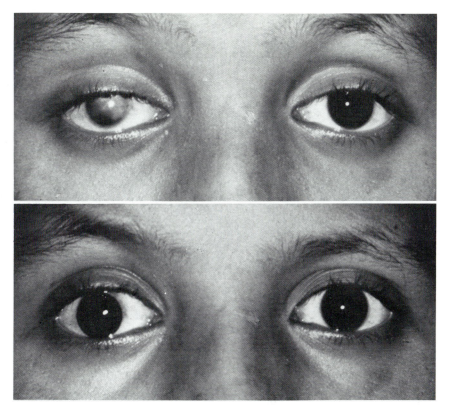

Fig 13-2 ■ Scarred cornea covered by tinted cosmetic contact lens (courtesy Western Technologies, Inc, Phoenix, Ariz).

b) Eyes disfigured by an occluded pupil, large colobomas of the iris, iridoplegia, or defects caused by trauma may be masked by a tinted contact lens.

c) Cataracts and blind eyes that are inoperable may be disguised by a black-out pupil lens on the cornea.

d) Heterochromia can be minimized by fitting a darker brown lens on the lighter iris to make the eyes a matching pair.

e) Diplopia may occur in people who have neurologic disorders, diabetes, etc., that cannot be corrected by surgery. These individuals may have better cosmesis from an occluder lens than a frosted spectacle lens. Occluder lenses may also be of value in strabismus patients who have had unsuccessful surgery.

f) Shrunken unsightly eyes: Patients with endophthalmitis that results in shrunken eyes and collapsed eyelids can be made to look better by soft colored lenses that provide a clear scleral ring, a colored matching iris, and a central black pupil.

These lenses must be large in size (Fig. 13-4).

g) Occluder lens: A fully shaded or opaque lens may be used as an occluder lens in a child who has amblyopia.

h) Aniridia: Darkened lenses with colored or neutral-density tints may be used to protect an albino or a patient with aniridia from the intensity of light.

i) For photophobic patients: Some individuals are extremely photophobic; tinted lenses can reduce photophobia considerably. We have treated two National Hockey League players who have had eye injuries that resulted in permanent widely-dilated pupils and photophobia for which they required tinted lenses. In one case, a star forward with the Chicago Blackhawks had an eye injury that resulted in a dilated pupil and extreme hypersensitivity to even 1/64% pilocarpine. This caused an induced myopia of −6.00 diopters and the forward was unable to play hockey. To counter the effects of the

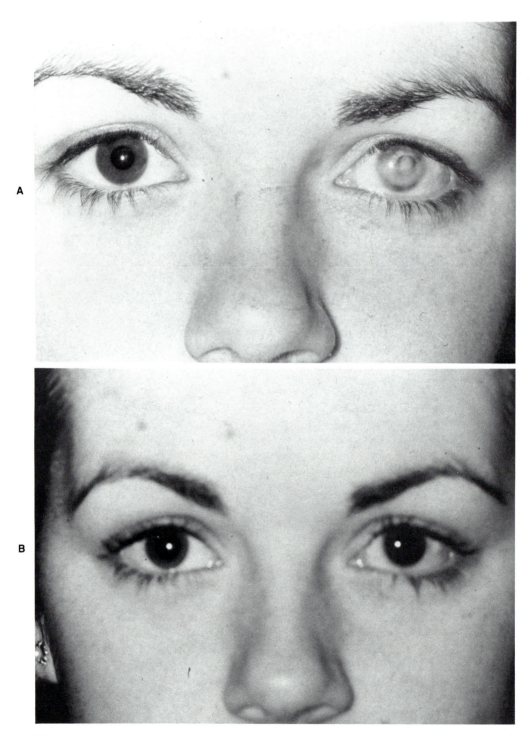

Fig 13-3 ■ **A,** Unsightly corneal scar after failed corneal transplant. **B,** Tinted iris. Print lens used to improve cosmesis.

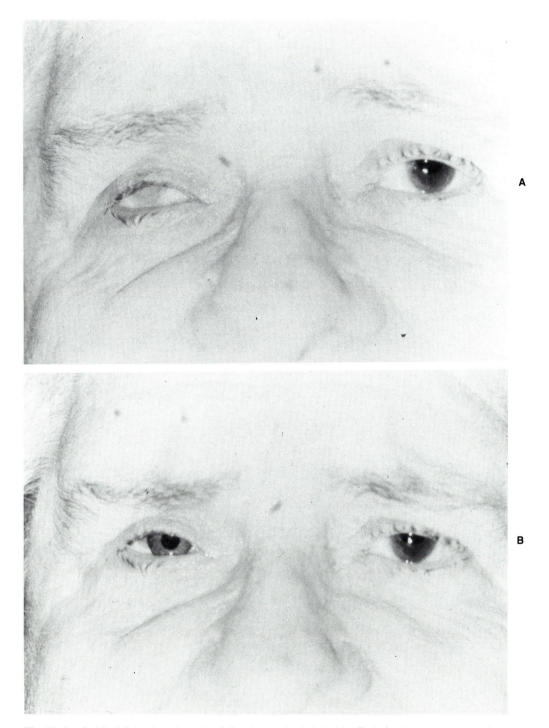

Fig 13-4 ■ A, Unsightly shrunken eye following endophthalmitis. **B,** Left shrunken eye masked by a soft lens with matching iris and pupil.

extreme glare reflecting from the surface of the ice, he was provided with a very dark contact lens and was able to continue playing the game.

3. Handling Tints

Light-handling tints in regular soft or rigid lenses may be helpful when one is looking for lenses or inserting and removing lenses. Deeply tinted lenses should not be used for regular wear because they reduce contrast sensitivity and decrease visual acuity especially when driving at dusk or reading menus in dimly lit restaurants. Light-handling tints are preferred.

DATA INFORMATION TINTING

Meshel and Gregory have developed a method for tinting information onto the periphery of a lens. Such information as the manufacturer's logo, the base curves and power of the lens, or information necessary for identifying the base of a prism ballast toric lens may be put on the lens. Also, a tiny 'L' or 'R' may be put on a soft lens so the wearer can distinguish the right from the left lens.

COMMENT. Although the market for specially tinted lenses is not great and the cost of the lenses is high, they can be extremely useful for patients. The Narcissus Foundation in San Francisco has been a pioneer in developing a process in which the color does not leach out from the lens. What is required for ordering a lens is a brief clinical history, three good-quality, close-up slides of both eyes, K readings of both eyes, the pupil size of the good eye in average room light, and the corneal diameter of both eyes. A trial fitting provides valuable information regarding base curve, diameter, and power, if useful vision is obtained.

14 ▪ *PROBLEMS ASSOCIATED WITH SOFT LENSES*

- ▪ *Patient-related problems*
- ▪ *Problems related to ocular response*
- ▪ *Lens-related problems*
- ▪ *Helpful hints on problem solving*

When a patient has been wearing soft lenses comfortably for a while but then returns with abnormal symptoms, the problems presented must be carefully analyzed and corrected. Because contact lenses now represent a significant proportion of an eye care practice, even practitioners who do not fit contact lenses must be aware of the problems associated with contact lenses so that they may provide a proper examination and evaluation of their patients and thus be able to make a professional diagnosis of the underlying problem. Only then will practitioners be able to construct a treatment plan to remedy the situation.

We have arbitrarily divided the encountered soft lens problems according to their main sources, recognizing that areas of overlap of causation do occur. We shall consider the problems caused by soft lenses in four categories: those related to the patient, to the eye itself, to the contact lens, and to the care systems involved.

PATIENT-RELATED PROBLEMS

Selection of patients for soft lens is by far the most valuable single act that will result in a happy and successful wearer of soft contact lenses. Selecting poor candidates, such as a highly nervous person, a patient with high degrees of astigmatism, or someone who works in a dusty and dirty environment will only result in troublesome visual problems. One should try to avoid, if possible, the following types of patients: those who practice poor personal hygiene, those who are unable to comprehend instructions for the use and care of soft lenses, those who seem to be addicted to alcohol, those who are severely disabled, and those who suffer from diseases of the eye.

Beware of the "challenge" patient. This is the person who has seen four other fitters and tried twelve pairs of contact lenses. Unless you have some special insight into the problem that previously has not been recognized, you are apt to become another unsuccessful contact lens fitter. There are patients who travel from fitter to fitter, professing a high degree of motivation to wear lenses that is basically neurotic.

In evaluating patients one should consider the following specific ocular factors that influence success.

Corneas

Corneas that are flat require a large-diameter lens to maintain stability and centration. Orientals as a group have smaller corneal diameters than Caucasians do, and so a 13.5 mm lens may be optimum for Oriental eyes whereas a 14.5 mm lens may be optimum for Caucasian eyes.

Large-diameter corneas require large lenses to cover the cornea.

Any cornea with deep vertical striae is a result of hypoxia. The lens should be replaced by a thinner lens or one with a higher water content.

Lid abnormalities

Lid abnormalities and size of the eye should be taken into account in selecting the correct diameter for the lens. When faced with a clinical problem, keep in mind that small palpebral fissures require small-diameter lenses. Lid tension may influence one in selecting a small-diameter lens.

Large eyes or eyes with lax or depressed lower

lids that exhibit "scleral show" in which a rim of sclera is exposed below the limbus, may lead to dehydration of the lower portion of the contact lens and subsequent edge lift and ejection of the lens by the lower eyelid. If there is scleral show above or below the cornea or both, then a larger lens is required. A thyroid investigation may also be prudent if such a clinical finding is present. If the patient is involved in body-contact sports such as hockey or football, a larger diameter lens should be selected.

Astigmatic eyes

Astigmatic eyes may require special toric lenses (see Chapter 30). Without these special lenses or rigid lenses, the conventional soft lenses in an eye with astigmatism may result in fluctuating and blurred vision.

It is estimated that at least one third of patients have enough toricity to require correction. In lower spherical powers even ¾ of a diopter of astigmatism may require a toric fit. Failure to deal with this problem causes visual blurring with soft lenses and is a major cause of lens dropout.

Lens discoloration

Lens discoloration may be produced after the patient has used over-the-counter proprietary decongestant drops procured at the local drug store. Such drops contain epinephrine-like compounds. Epinephrine has a tendency to yellow a soft contact lens when used over a prolonged time. Also, nicotine from a smoker's fingers may be transferred to soft contact lenses.

Environmental factors

Environmental factors play a considerable role in the quality of vision with a contact lens. In a dry atmosphere or in an atmosphere in which the wearer is near an air conditioner or behind the heater-blower of a car, the front surface of a soft lens may become dehydrated and rippled, which may result in blurred vision. This is more exaggerated with thin and ultrathin lenses, which lose their small reserve of water faster than standard lenses do. The blurring may be reported as fluctuating or variable rather than steady because each blink restores the surface smoothness of the contact lens and restores clarity of vision. It has been reported that hydrogel lenses can become contaminated by chemical vapors from the environment.

Smoking and soft lenses. Smoking causes:
1. Discoloration of the lens
2. Conjunctival hyperemia—the lens appears tight
3. Increased rate of deposit formation; smokers require more replacement lenses
4. Variable vision—this may be caused by mild corneal edema, dehydration of the lens, and deposit formation.
5. Increased tearing, which in turn can cause decentration of the lens and blurred vision.

Expect poorer results from smokers. Let the patient know about yet another drawback to smoking. Also, the unfortunate person who has to contend with second-hand smoke suffers a similar fate. Smoke-filled rooms present a hostile environment to the contact-lens wearer.

Aphakia

In aphakia, the rupture of the wound is a potential threat, caused by the stress of insertion and removal of a contact lens. Thus wearing daily-wear lenses should be postponed until the wound has healed. Extended-wear lenses are a safer alternative because the tensile strength of a wound is acquired over a long period from the time of surgery.

PROBLEMS RELATED TO OCULAR RESPONSE
Epithelial corneal edema

Epithelial corneal edema results from hypoxia of the cornea. Unlike rigid contact lenses in which the epithelial edema is confined to the central portion of the cornea, soft-lens-induced edema of the epithelial layer of the cornea is diffuse across the entire cornea, thus no charge occurs in the radii.

Edema can be detected clinically with the slit-lamp by maximum retroillumination. Edema is often an indication that the lens is too tight and that a looser lens is required, one with either a flatter base curve or a smaller diameter. The pachymeter can be used to determine an increase in corneal thickness resulting from corneal edema; it can detect even 1% of edema.

COMMENT. If you do not own a pachymeter, performing the following simple tests will be adequate:
1. Placido's disc. The reflection may be irregular and distorted.
2. Retinoscopy. The central reflex will be fractured and irregular.

3. K readings. The mires may quickly become distorted.
4. Retro-illumination. A gray central area appears.

Corneas of patients who have worn soft lenses for 12 hours or more will often show a 6% to 8% increase in thickness as a measure of an adverse effect. Edema at this level may be difficult to detect on slit-lamp examination. Slit-lamp findings are best appreciated through retro-illumination of a gray central disk in relief. For the most part, patients can tolerate this well with no early or late complications. If the resulting edema is so great that slit-lamp edema is detectable, the patient should be instructed to remove his lenses for 2 hours after 8 hours of lens' wear in the early stages of adaptation. If this persists, he should be switched to thin or high-water-content lenses that are more oxygen permeable.

In patients living at altitudes over 8000 feet above sea level, mild oxygen deprivation of the cornea may occur with soft lenses if they are worn for too long a period.

Vertical striae in cornea

Sarver was the first to observe vertical striae appearing in the posterior portion of the corneas of soft-lens wearers. The striae may be seen with the slit-lamp with direct focal illumination. They are indicative of relatively severe corneal edema. They are probably a slight wrinkling in Descemet's membrane brought on by some corneal anoxia.

Folds in Descemet's membrane

Folds in Descemet's membrane have been noted after prolonged wear of a soft lens. In particular, they arise in patients who sleep overnight with their soft lenses on, and are caused by severe corneal anoxia.

Small epithelial microcysts of the cornea may develop (Fig. 14-1). They may result from hypoxia of the cornea caused by the germicide or the preservative used in disinfection. There are thought to be unknown areas of desquamated cells. Less than 15 to 20 microcysts are a normal variant. If more microcysts occur, they may render the cornea susceptible to infection. Fine stippling and punctate keratitis may follow from this and require management.

Compression

An indentation near the area of the limbus is an indication that the lens is too tight. Depending on the size of the lens, it may occur at the peripheral cornea, limbus, or sclera. When it occurs at the limbus or sclera, it is often noted

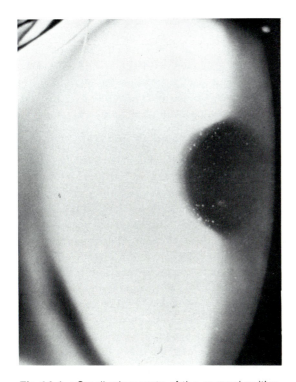

Fig 14-1 ■ Small microcysts of the corneal epithelium as seen by retro-illumination.

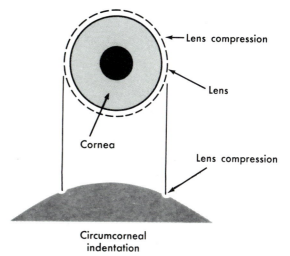

Circumcorneal indentation

Fig 14-2 ■ Circumcorneal indentation. The tight lens compresses the peripheral limbal tissues.

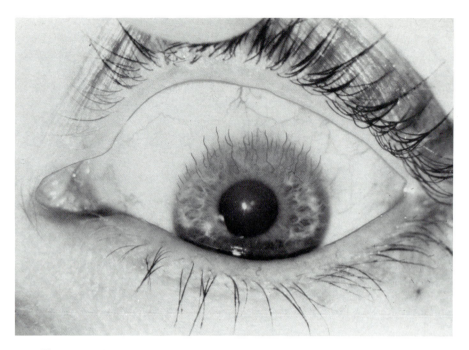

Fig 14-3 ■ Vascularization superiorly from a poor-fitting soft hydrogel lens.

by a blanching of the blood vessels followed later by an indentation (Fig. 14-2).

Vascularization at limbus

Limbic vascularization may be indicative of corneal hypoxia. It also could be caused by an adverse reaction to a tight fit. Fitting a looser lens or one that transmits more oxygen, reducing the total wearing time, or even discontinuing the lens may be required (Fig. 14-3).

Epithelial edema, limbal compression, and vascularization are symptoms that necessitate a change in the lens to a looser lens fit or to a more gas-permeable soft lens, either ultrathin or of a high water content.

If true vascularization occurs (1% to 2% of patients), one of the following remedies can be tried:
1. Switch to a gas-permeable lens
2. Switch to a thinner or more permeable soft lens
3. Switch to an extended-wear lens to be worn on a daily basis
4. Discontinue lens wear.

Photophobia

Sensitivity to light may be the result of a poorly fitting flat lens that irritates the cornea by friction. It also may be caused by a dirty lens, the chemicals used in sterilization, or the lack of proper isotonicity of prepared or preserved saline solution.

Excess tearing

Tearing may be a result of a poorly fitting, a dirty, or a damaged soft lens. It also may be caused by a foreign body under the lens or, in some cases, by an adverse reaction to the elements in the solution care system.

Induced myopia and astigmatism

Wearing conventional standard-thickness soft lenses for a prolonged period greater than 12 hours per day has been shown to produce changes in keratometric readings of the cornea. In some instances there has been an increase in steepness of the cornea; in other instances there has been the development of significant irregular astigmatic error that required several months to subside. For some patients there has developed a permanent form of acquired keratoconus, resulting from chronic oxygen starvation to the cornea. Many of these problems have been remedied with the use of thin and ultrathin lenses or high-water-content soft contact lenses, which permit better oxygenation of the cornea, even for marginal corneas.

Superior limbic keratitis (SLK) is common in

myopic soft-lens wearers and particularly those who wear lenses on an extended-wear basis. No true cause has been found, but SLK may be caused by the mechanical action of the contact lens against the superior tarsus. Symptoms of burning mutation and mucous discharge are present. These may be fine papillary response of the tarsal conjunctiva and even a fine pannus may develop. Removal of the lens usually solves the problem.

Epithelial and subepithelial infiltrates

Small dot-like nummular lesions from infiltrates occur often in the periphery with soft contact lenses and result in localized redness. Some believe that they are caused by chronic hypoxia. The majority of corneal cells lie in the peripheral ring of the cornea, and hence cellular reaction is more vulnerable here. Some observers such as Falasca believe that these subepithelial infiltrates are antigen-antibody reactions brought about by something adhering to the contact lens. The treatment may require steroid drops combined with antibiotics for 2 or 3 days to clear up the reaction, or cessation of lens' wear for a month. Either new lenses or maximum cleaning of the existing lenses is required. If the condition recurs, one may switch to more gas-permeable lenses such as ultrathin lenses, along with a maximum cleaning regimen.

Josephson and Caffrey reported on epithelial and subepithelial infiltrates in contact-lens wearers. Without treatment, infiltrates induced by contact-lens wear had an average recovery time of 2½ months after the lens was discontinued, whereas virus-induced infiltrates took an average of 5½ months to disappear.

I (RS) reported on the separation of toxic infiltrates from bacterial infiltrates; the latter are accompanied by pain.

Staining

Although 2% fluorescein should not be used with a soft lens, it may be important that on reexamination the soft lens be removed and the eye stained with fluorescein. The lens should not be reinserted for 1 hour after fluorescein has been used. If the eye is flushed, the lens may be reinserted after 20 minutes.

High molecular weight fluorescein is available and can be used with low and medium water content lenses. Usually, however, defects in the epithelium can be detected without fluorescein by someone trained to use the slitlamp.

An area of staining in the periphery of the cornea is often indicative of a dry area or an irritated epithelial area from the edge of the lens that occurs because the lens does not center well (Fig. 14-4, *A*). A new lens with better centering properties should be provided. This may involve substitution of a larger diameter lens or a change in the base curve to permit better centering. A peripheral staining area may also be caused by poor edge design, and a new lens may be required.

Arcuate staining in a spotty fashion in the periphery may be a result of poor blending at the junctions of a lathe-cut soft lens (Fig. 14-4, *B*).

Decentration of a lens (Fig. 14-4, *C*) may cause chafing at the edges of the cornea.

Scattered stippled staining of the cornea is often a result of a dirty lens or a lens that builds up particles of protein material and creates anoxia of the cornea (Fig. 14-4, *D*). This lens should be carefully cleaned or replaced.

Generalized stippling of the cornea, often diffuse over the whole cornea, is indicative of environmental toxicity, such as chemicals, oils, or grease. It is most commonly caused by preservatives in contact lens' solutions. It may be remedied if one changes the chemical solution used for disinfection or if one changes to the boiling method of disinfecting the lens with preservative-free saline or to the hydrogen peroxide system with preservatives for saline (see Chapters 12 and 37). Occasionally, it may represent an infectious element and should be treated accordingly.

John Morgan has pointed out small microcystic dot formation in the corneal epithelium that precedes stippling. He found this as a result of germicide toxicity to the cornea, but it may occur with any toxic influence on the cornea.

Foreign-body stains are similar in nature to those seen with persons wearing hard lenses who have linear or curved staining areas on the cornea (Fig. 14-4, *F*).

Inferior staining at the 6 o'clock position of the cornea usually indicates trauma arising from an improper removal technique (Fig. 14-4, *E*). To avoid this, one should keep one's fingernails short.

Staining of the cornea is a cause of concern since these stains represent possible portals for bacterial entry. Even though the patient is comfortable and not complaining, the problem must be solved and, if specific remedies fail, the lens should be changed.

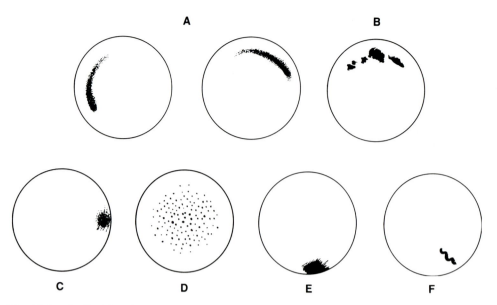

Fig 14-4 ■ **A,** Peripheral arcuate staining caused by decentered, small lenses. **B,** Arcuate staining as a result of poor blend at the junctions of a lathe-cut soft lens. **C,** Chafing at the edge of the cornea because of decentration of a soft lens. **D,** Generalized stippling of the cornea caused by environmental contamination or protein buildup on the lens. **E,** Inferior staining of the cornea resulting from trauma on removal of the lens. **F,** Foreign body stain occurring when a small foreign body finds its way under a soft lens.

Dr. Ira Udell has pointed out that corneal staining may represent dendrites similar to those that the herpes simplex virus produces on the cornea (Fig. 14-5). These so-called pseudodendrites must not be confused with dendritic ulcers of herpes.

COMMENT. Corneal erosion with soft lenses also occurs with the following:
1. Decentration of the lens.
2. Lid gap especially if the lens' edges are bulky and thick.

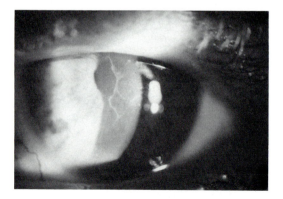

Fig 14-5 ■ Pseudodentrites of the cornea produced by a soft lens. (Courtesy Ira J. Udell, MD.)

3. Truncated lenses, especially if the truncation has not been beveled.
4. Contact lenses too small in diameter to fully cover the lens with blinking.

Allergy versus toxicity

With the widespread use of chemical preservatives associated with soft contact lenses, it is important to differentiate allergy from toxicity (Table 14-1). *Allergy* represents a reaction of the body to a large molecule, usually protein, lipoproteins, and occasionally, polysaccharides. These are referred to as *antigens*. There then results a complex series of events in which the body reacts to the foreign substance and produces an *antibody* resulting in an *antigen-antibody reaction*. A *toxic reaction* is a reaction that a person will show to some applied substance, whether it is a chemical or just a protein molecule. This reaction is a direct insult to the cell. A *toxic idiosyncrasy* is a specialized form of toxicity that happens to just a few persons. The history becomes important. With *toxicity* there is usually a cumulative progressive irritation with the use of any chemical with time. With *allergy*, such as to thimerosal, the history is one in which the patient suddenly develops a red

Table 14-1 ■ Differentiation from an allergic response and a toxic response to a solution used for soft lenses

Allergy	Toxicity
Conjunctival response equal to or greater than corneal response	Corneal response equal to or greater than conjunctival response
Chemosis	Punctate keratitis
Giant follicles	Microcysts

Table 14-2 ■ Signs and symptoms of allergy

Symptoms	Signs
Itching	Chemosis
Burning	Limbal injection
Blurred vision	Conjunctival redness
	Mucous discharge
	Tearing

eye and no longer is comfortable with contacts, or the eyes become hyperemic even with reduced amounts of the agent in question. In our experience differentiation of allergy from toxicity may be noted not only by the medical history, but also by the target that is involved. With allergy, the conjunctiva participates more with conjunctival chemosis and giant follicles. With toxicity the cornea participates more with corneal epithelial punctate changes, beginning with small microcysts to epithelial erosions. When faced with red eyes and suspicion of allergy, one should use Table 14-2 as a guide.

LENS-RELATED PROBLEMS
Tear resistance

Splitting of the lenses has not been a major problem with the newer materials available. However, one must use proper instruction in regard to lens handling to avoid damaging lenses. Needless to say delicacy is required in the handling of the material; fingernails must be kept short. The higher the water content or the thinner the lenses, the more fragile they are. Today's models, however, are within acceptable guidelines for wear and tear. When looking with a slit-lamp, it is often the edges that are first to show nicks, which gradually enlarge into a split (Fig. 14-6).

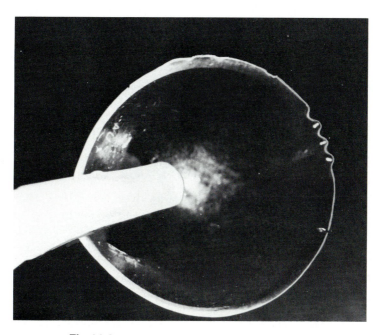

Fig 14-6 ■ Nicking at the edges of a soft lens.

COMMENT. A split lens should be replaced regardless of whether it causes discomfort or irritation. Once the seal of the lens is broken, the lens itself can permit bacteria to enter the plastic.

Hazy or variable vision

If vision is poor, the easiest way to determine if this is a result of a loose lens is to manually manipulate the lens with the eyelid on the patient's eye so that it is objectively centered. If vision clears, chances are the lens is loose and has been gradually slipping off center. If, on the other hand, vision is not improved, some factor other than a loose lens is the cause of poor vision. In that case this procedure should be followed:
1. Examine the patient with the slitlamp.
2. Re-evaluate the fit—the lens may have changed its parameter over time and become tighter or looser, either of which will affect vision.
3. Check that the lens is not inverted.
4. Check the power of the lenses to be sure that the lenses have not been switched between the right and left eye.
5. Check for deposits on the lens.
6. Check protein buildup and the clarity of the lenses.

The most common cause of deterioration in vision with soft lenses is caused by deposit buildup. These deposits are protein, lipids, and inorganic matter. The need for prophylactic cleaning must be re-emphasized to the patient. Lenses often can be restored to normal clarity, but if not, lens replacement is necessary.

COMMENT. When in doubt, replace the lens and do not change the parameters.

Vision may deteriorate because of drying of the lens (Fig. 14-7). Such environmental conditions as dry rooms or dry climates (e.g., Arizona) with low humidity may cause drying of the lens with reduction in visual acuity. Patients who read a great deal, particularly when tired, will have a reduced blink reflex, which in turn will result in drying of the lens. In addition, physical and mental fatigue decrease tear formation; consequently patients will experience irritation with their lenses at the end of a busy day.

Patients should be warned against driving with air-conditioned or heated air blowing in their eyes, since this will dehydrate the lens and cause visual blurring during driving. The blink reflex is also reduced during driving. When a

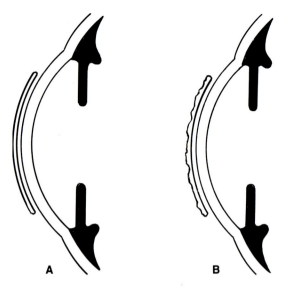

Fig 14-7 ■ A, Normal contact lens. **B,** Dehydrated soft contact lens after exposure to a dry environment, causing blurring of vision.

lens dehydrates, a rippling effect occurs on the front surface and causes blurring.

Occasionally we have found that selecting a lens identical to the one the patient is wearing will significantly improve vision. The initial poor vision is probably caused by defective optics in the first lens.

Cellular debris under a lens may occur if the lens becomes too tight. When viewed with a slitlamp, the lens shows inadequate clearing centrally after each blink, and the patient notes blurring of vision. One may see trapped cellular debris. The remedy is to make the lens flatter for better tear exchange and removal of waste products. Some extended-wear lenses exhibit this trapped-debris phenomenon. This is cleared by either scleral swish or removal for cleaning.

Lens-power changes

In myopia, there may be a steepening of the lens with time, resulting in an increase in minus power. This occurs because a plus tear film becomes present in the central portion of the cornea, which no longer touches centrally, resulting in a pseudomyopia and more minus power required to correct vision (Fig. 14-8, A). The important factor here is that when one is overrefracting a myope who is wearing soft contact lenses and one finds an increase minus power, this may be pseudomyopia and not true myopic

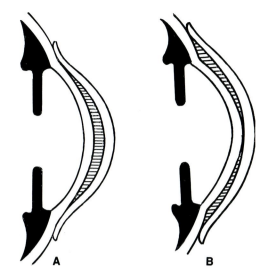

Fig. 14-8 ■ **A,** Plus tear film created by a tight lens behaves as a plus lens requiring more minus power in order for the patient to see. **B,** Minus tear film. In aphakia or high hyperopia, thick plus lenses may fall away from the periphery and thereby form a minus-lens tear film and thus require more plus to correct vision.

change. If the lens has changed in fit, simply replacing the lens with the same-power lens with a correct fit will usually correct the problem.

In aphakia, the opposite holds true. The thicker aphakic lens with aging or with dehydration may become more rigid and stand away from the peripheral cornea and permit tears to fill the interface between lens and cornea. This creates a minus tear layer so that an increase in plus power is required (Fig. 14-8, *B*).

Optic zone

The larger the diameter of soft lenses, the larger the optic zone that permits improved vision. In aphakia a small optic zone can be a real problem because when the manufacturers attempt to reduce thickness a smaller optic zone results. This problem is more prevalent in the higher plus powers and results in fluctuating blurred vision. Some manufacturers hold the optic zone as a constant regardless of power increases.

Edges

Each manufacturer of soft lenses designs edges that are specific for that company. It is a compromise to design an edge that is very thin and well rounded and one that will provide optimum comfort and tear exchange, and yet be sufficiently durable to withstand the wear and tear of handling. If one manufacturer's products do not result in sufficient patient comfort, one should try another manufacturer's lens, which may provide comfort because of better edge design for that patient.

Thin and ultrathin lenses

Thin and ultrathin lenses, though showing increasing popularity, are more prone to damage by poor handlers. They are also more time consuming for the average person to insert; thus one should assess the individual's personality, hygiene, work habits and motivation to determine whether he is a suitable candidate for thin and ultrathin lenses. Certainly the person who gets up in a hurry and rushes off to work early in the morning may find handling these thin lenses frustrating.

We have found that thin lenses wrinkle more easily on the eye causing blurring of vision (Fig. 14-9). They should be fitted tighter than conventional lenses with only minimal movement to overcome this effect and provide stable vision. Generally we initially fit conventional soft lenses 3 to 4.5 D flatter than K, whereas we fit the thinner lenses only 2 to 3.5 D flatter than K. The tighter thin-lens fitting is possible because of the greater oxygen transmission of the lenses.

If a patient reports initial discomfort with an ultrathin lens on the eye, it is likely that either a particle of debris is on the back surface of the lens or the lens is inside out. An everted or inside-out ultrathin lens generally does not affect vision the way an everted standard-thickness lens does, but it will cause greater lens awareness because of the anterior bevel.

Falling out of lens

If lenses continue to fall out, the reason may be that the lens diameter chosen is too small in relation to the palpebral fissure. This may also occur if the lens fits too flatly resulting in edge stand-off, with the lid catching on the everted lid during blinking action. Inadequate tear production may cause drying of the edges and ejection of the lens by the lower eyelid. The accumulation of excess surface deposits may reduce lens hydration and cause dehydration of the lens.

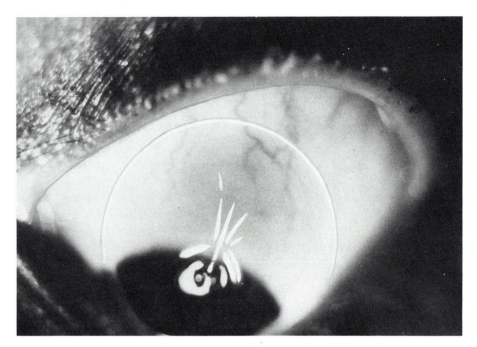

Fig 14-9 ■ Wrinkling of an ultrathin lens demonstrated on looking up when it is on the cornea. This effect results in a degradation of visual acuity. (Courtesy Lester Yanoff, American Optical Corp., Southbridge, Mass.)

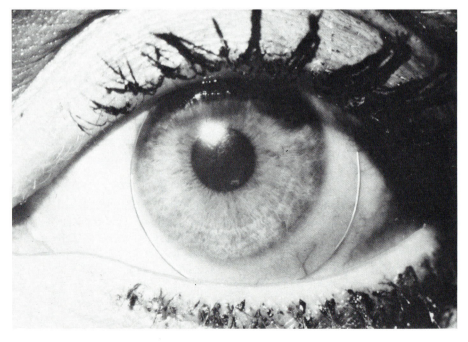

Fig 14-10 ■ Soft lens decentered inferonasally because of a flat lens. Mascara eventually may contribute to clouding, particle discomfort, and decentration.

Care-related problems

Deposits. Deposits are found more frequently in the aphakic patient. Electron-microscopy has shown these spots to be compatible with derivatives of the tear film such as denatured lysozyme, albumin, gamma globulin, and lipids. Often calcium is present. These spots act to irritate the eye and make the lens uncomfortable to wear and may contribute to poor fitting with decentration (Fig. 14-10). If the spots increase in size and number, vision will be affected and a replacement lens will be required. Lens-cleaning procedures should be reviewed with the patient. If deposits continue to recur, the patient should be switched to rigid lenses.

Clinically the deposits may be seen with the slitlamp while the patient is wearing the lens. However, early deposit formation cannot clearly be seen unless the lens is removed, permitted to partially dehydrate, and viewed through the slitlamp or a magnifying lens against a dark background.

COMMENT. Heavy deposit formation can be seen after 3 weeks of wear. If this occurs, switch to a gas-permeable lens.

Thimerosal sensitivity. Thimerosal is sodium ethylmercurithiosalicylate, a compound of organic mercury and thiosalicylic acid. Thimerosal has a broad range of antibacterial activity. A 0.01% solution inhibits the growth of *Pseudomonas aeruginosa*, *Escherichia coli*, and *Staphylococcus aureus*. Clinically it is often used in 0.01% or 0.001% concentrations.

Thimerosal has been the chief component responsible for delayed hypersensitivity of the eye. Patients have had patch tests along with intradermal tests to prove their sensitivity to thimerosal. Typical ocular symptoms are redness, foreign-body sensation, and lacrimation. Ocular examination reveals conjunctival hyperemia, conjunctival folliculitis, and corneal epithelial opacities or punctate keratopathy. Studies have reported about 6% to 8% sensitivity to thimerosal.

Fungus growth. Fungi will occasionally seed on a soft lens and burrow deep into the plastic (Fig. 14-11). Fungi should be clinically recognized and differentiated from protein buildup on a soft lens.

Fungus growth develops on lenses that have not been used for some time and have been stored in unpreserved saline solution. It is important that lenses be continually disinfected both by the practitioner for the inventory or diagnostic set and by patients who wear their soft lenses only occasionally. The problem of fungus growth on stored lenses is one of the major obstacles to the patient requiring a spare pair of

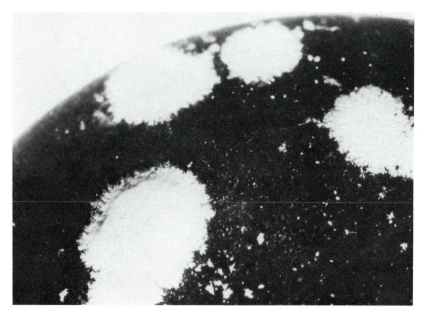

Fig 14-11 ■ Fungus colonies identified as *Penicillium* growing on a hydrophilic lens in a patient wearing a soft lens. (Courtesy Dr. John F. Morgan, Kingston, Ont.)

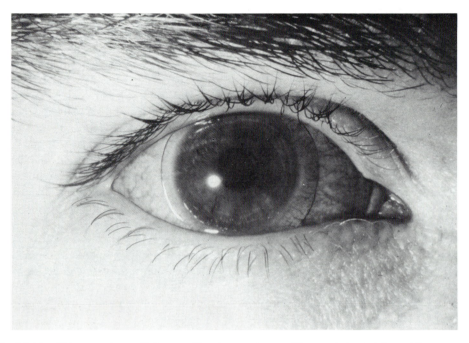

Fig 14-12 ■ Thimerosol sensitivity resulting in a red eye with punctate staining of the cornea.

lenses. Unfortunately the solutions in which the spare lenses are kept are not changed frequently and boiling is neglected.

Infection. There have been several cases of contamination of soft lenses or their containers. Bacteria have been shown to enter fissures in the plastic, whereas fungus has been reported to invade the intact soft lens. However, despite these reports of lens or lens-container contamination, there have been few reports of widespread clinical infection of either the cornea or conjunctiva. We have found only one case of serious inflammatory condition of the cornea as a result of soft-lens wear in a series of a few thousand daily soft lens wearers.

COMMENT. Our low incidence of infection may not be typical. We are compulsive about teaching our patients hygiene, lens care, and proper storage techniques. Also we have a hot line for any problems.

Red eye in contact lens wearers. The most frequent cause of red eyes in contact lens wearers is allergy to thimerosal, an organic mercurial found as a preservative in many soft lens solutions (Fig. 14-12). Thimerosal causes allergy in 4% to 8% of patients. Although red eye is a major problem in clinical practice, there is a variety of possible causes other than thimerosal sensitivity

Table 14-3 ■ Causes of red eye in soft contact lens wearers

Allergy	to thimerosol
	to solutions
	to environment
Infection	bacterial
	viral
	chlamydial
Toxicity	to retained enzyme
	to finger debris
	to cleaning agents poorly rinsed
Tears	quality
	quantity
Tight lens syndrome	
Glued-on lens syndrome	
Incomplete blinking	
Lens thickness	too thick
	too thin (dehydration effect)
Lens changes	deposits
	change in fit
Abrasion	foreign body
	fingernail
	from decentration
Lids	in-turned lashes
	blepharitis
	scleral show and dehydration
Anterior membrane dystrophies	
Lens inside out	

that should be considered. Fortunately, most of the newer solutions do not contain any thimerosal (Table 14-3).

Giant papillary hypertrophy of tarsal conjunctiva (cobblestone conjunctivitis). Spring first drew our attention to this entity and Allansmith and her co-workers have shown that although giant cobblestones appear in 0.5% of normal individuals, they occur in 10% of rigid lens wearers and in 50% of soft contact lens wearers who wear contact lenses for any length of time. It also occurs in persons wearing ocular prostheses. There appears to be some direct relationship to individual sensitivity, to the duration the person is wearing the contact lenses, and to the type of care routine followed. The larger-diameter soft lenses appear to cause an increased incidence of cobblestone conjunctivitis as compared to the smaller-diameter soft lenses.

When this sensitivity occurs, there is often an associated redness, itchiness, and shorter wearing time of the lenses though in many cases it is asymptomatic until the advanced stages. It is important to evert the eyelid under slit-lamp examination to detect early stages of this condition. When the eyelid is everted, a typical vernal type of papillary hypertrophy of the conjunctiva can be seen (Fig. 14-13). Occasionally a large papillary hypertrophy of the conjunctiva may be seen.

The cause of giant papillary conjunctivitis appears to be a combination of allergy (antigen-antibody) reaction and foreign-body mechanical irritation. Fluorescein should be instilled. If the top of the papule stains, this staining indicates the presence of acute inflammation, and steps should be taken either to clean the lenses more completely, switch to new and smaller diameter lenses or those made of a different material, or discontinue lens wear.

HELPFUL HINTS ON PROBLEM SOLVING

1. Impaired reading may occur with soft lens wearers for the following reasons: (a) because of lid-induced flexion of the soft lens when the eyes are rotated downward (this may be improved by instructing the patient to hold the reading material in a higher position), (b) after prolonged reading because

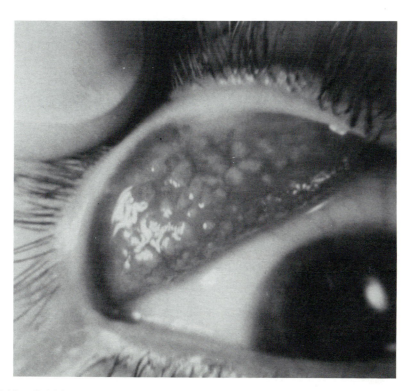

Fig. 14-13 ■ Cobblestone conjunctivitis with papillary hypertrophy of the tarsal conjunctiva seen in a patient who has worn soft lenses for 2 years with chemical disinfection.

of fatigue and the lack of blinking, which leads to excessive drying of the front surface of the lens, or (c) an optic zone that is too small.

2. Discomfort may result from deposit accumulation. This may be overcome by the routine use of an enzyme-cleaning tablet and attention to more careful surfactant cleaning.

3. If peripheral erosions or fine peripheral staining occurs with a soft lens, it may be the result of a decentering of the lens or poor edge finishing.

4. Induced astigmatism and steepening of the K measurement is occasionally found with soft lens wearers who wear their lenses for prolonged times. This is particularly exaggerated if the fit is inadequate. An improvement in fit and a reduction in total daily wearing may be required. A 12-hour wearing time would appear to be optimal for conventional soft lenses. A switch to ultrathin lenses may be required for better corneal performance.

5. A burning sensation along with conjunctival redness may be the result of chemical contamination. This may be transferred from the patient's hands or be caused by the germicide used in asepsis. Occasionally a viral keratoconjunctivitis may cause this, and scattered small gray intra-epithelial non-staining corneal infiltrates may be seen on slit-lamp examination. One must be aware of possible environmental toxic fumes that can produce these symptoms.

6. In those patients who have naturally dry eyes or poor tear formation and are being fitted with soft hydrophilic lenses, a soft lens of low water content should be selected to reduce water demand by the soft lens.

7. Epithelial edema in soft lens wearers is more common with lenses with low water content because they may behave like hard PMMA lenses. A switch to ultrathin or higher water content lenses may be required.

8. Some patients wearing soft lenses, either lathe-cut or spin-cast, develop an increase in myopia with steepening of K readings, or astigmatism. The patient should discontinue wearing lenses for a short while or should switch to a flatter lens or an ultrathin lens.

9. Small bubbles of oxygen or debris trapped under the lens and seen on the slitlamp may be indicative of a steep lens, resulting in a poor exchange of tears under the lens.

10. When lenses fit well at first and then become very loose and decentered, the process may be caused by a loss of shape retention ("memory") of the plastic with time.

11. Repeated blurring of vision resulting from drying of the soft lens, either from environmental factors or from the staring effect caused by fatigue after prolonged reading, may be minimized by the use of Comfort eye drops. This solution hydrates, wets, and cleans the soft lens while the patient is wearing the lens. Other hydrating drops, such as artificial tears, may also be helpful.

12. Farris has pointed out that in some eye conditions, particularly in the elderly, the tears may become hypertonic and result in corneal irritation from a contact lens. There is

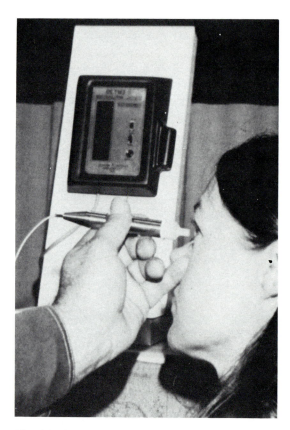

Fig 14-14 ■ Applanation tonometry may be performed over a soft lens without fluorescein or anesthesia by use of the Electro Medical Technology digital applanation tonometer.

value in diluting the salt concentration in the eyes of some persons by the use of Hypotears, a hypotonic tear substitute. This may be used along with soft contact lenses.

13. Sometimes well-fitted lenses may fall out when patients are subjected to low humidity conditions, as in climates similar to that of Arizona or when driving a car with heated or air-conditioned air blowing directly onto their eyes. The lens dries out, the edge everts, and the edge of the eyelid expresses the lens from the eye.

14. There is no indication that soft lenses cause glaucoma, but one should be aware that glaucoma can occur in soft contact lens wearers. One can slide the lens temporally onto the sclera and perform applanation tonometry without fluorescein using the white light of the slitlamp. Alternatively one can use an electronic applanation tonometer (Fig. 14-14) or the Shiøtz tonometer, without fluorescein, after the lens is removed or shifted.

COMMENT. Applanation readings are even more precise without the lens present. For the patient with glaucoma, the lens should be removed. Also there is no indication that soft lenses cause glaucoma.

15. In patients with a high incidence of lens deposits, one should reassess the care system and be sure there is compliance. A new system may be required. One should also reassess the fit because loose lenses tend to reduce any cleansing action by the tarsal conjunctiva.

16. Professional cleaning in the office, aided by an ultrasound unit, may be helpful in increasing the longevity of the soft lens. Ultrasound helps in increasing the action of many chemical agents on the lens and in increasing the speed of the cleaning process.

COMMENT. Although ultrasound can yield an almost-new soft lens, the rate of recurrent deposit formation is faster as compared to that of a new lens. Replacement of lenses is probably the best mode.

17. Thin and ultrathin lenses may be fitted tighter and with less movement than standard lenses. Fitting these lenses in this way minimizes wrinkling of the lens that may result in fluctuating vision.

18. Ultrathin lenses have an exaggerated dehydration effect in dry environments and may produce symptoms of poor vision. With these lenses you are often exchanging corneal problems with patient problems.

19. Avoid ultrathin lens for patients who are poor handlers.

20. A deficient tear state may be present in the elderly, the aphakic or the arthritic. This may result in chronic irritation, red eyes, recurrent infection, and corneal ulcers. Liberal use of artificial tears combined with a reduced schedule of contact lens wear can help in correcting the problem.

21. The aphakic eye is particularly reduced in corneal sensation, and a wearer may have a lens problem or a foreign body under the lens and not recognize it sufficiently early. The low sensitivity of aphakic corneas may mask dangerous symptoms.

22. The aphakic eye that is dry and has excessive mineral concentrations may cause excessive deposit buildup. This may be minimized by daily rinsing of the lens in the eye either by a stream of saline or balance salt solution in the eye or with saline solution in an eyecup as an eyewash. If the lens is to be removed daily, you might as well switch to a gas-permeable lens.

15 ■ *HISTORY OF CONTACT LENSES*

The development of contact lenses is an old story dating back to 1508. The first insight into the concept of covering the optical defects of a cornea with a device is credited by most people to Leonardo da Vinci. Da Vinci made glass water cups that were placed on the eye. He also invented a contact lens with a funnel on one side for water to be poured in.

The first corneal lens was described by René Descartes. In a treatise called *Ways of Perfecting Vision*, Descartes published his findings in 1636. He also used the water principle to neutralize the front surface of the cornea. In the seventeenth century the concept of the cornea as an instrument of vision was already known. Descartes also made from glass a crude elongated corneal contact lens.

In 1801, Thomas Young appreciated the change caused by placing a water-filled lens on his eye. He was aware of the change in power (in his case he became presbyopic) within the eye and knew how to fix it. He noted: "The addition of another lens . . . restores my eye to its natural state."

Sir John F.W. Herschel in 1823 had great insights into irregular astigmatism. He wrote: "Should any very bad cases of irregular corneas be found . . . vision could be improved . . . by taking an actual mould of the cornea and employing some transparent medium."

The scientific design of a contact lens was really evolved by A. Eugene Fick. His lenses had refractive power and were actually tried. He worked on rabbits to obtain correct molds made of glass for the eye. Then from a cadaver's eye he did the same thing to correct problems such as irregular astigmatism. His intention was to replace the scarred cornea with a regular surface made of glass. His first lens consisted of a thin sphere of glass of about an 8 mm radius of curvature. He also experimented with a scleral lens without much success. All his lenses were made with glass, which is about twice the weight of plastic lenses.

E. Kalt, using techniques similar to Fick's, in 1888 made a glass lens to treat keratoconus with the idea of apical touch and flattening of the cornea. Kalt actually saw considerable clinical visual improvement in some of the cases upon which his lens was tried.

From the beginning of the twentieth century to 1948, only scleral lenses made of glass were made. Some of these lens were blown, whereas others were ground and polished. These lenses were mostly applied to eyes with keratoconus, and the wearing time was limited to only a few hours during the day.

The development of plastic was a major breakthrough. In 1947 when Kevin Tuohy began making contact lenses out of plastic rather than glass, a new era of contact lenses were ushered in. The initial lenses caused corneal edema after hours of wear because their diameters were very large, ranging from 10.8 to 12.5 mm. In reality these were scleral lenses.

The next landmark in the history of the hard or rigid lens occurred in Germany in 1952. Wilhelm Söhnges began to use a smaller-diameter, strictly corneal lens that was less than half the mass and weight of the Tuohy lens. After this achievement the contact lens finally emerged from being a research tool of limited use to become a real substitute for glasses as a commercial practical device.

The technology of rigid lenses is still evolving. There are changes in design characteristics and materials. Gas-permeable rigid lenses have crowded out the PMMA hard lenses, and lenses once more are becoming larger in size.

The search for better, more comfortable, safer lenses still persists. New materials of value to the contact-lens fitter are being explored. By the early 1980s, the Scheone acrylates dominated the gas-permeable lens market. More recently, fluorosilon acrylate materials have developed widespread acceptance in providing more oxygen. Through the work of William Isaacson of the 3M Corporaton, the fluorocarbon material entered into the world of the contact lens fitter.

Surgery for the correction of common refractive errors is now a reality. Other solutions to present issues of refractive problems may not be in the form of optical devices but rather through genetic engineering.

16 ▪ SYSTEMS FOR LENS ORDERING

- *Systems based on corneal topography*
- *Systems based on types of lenses*
- *General rules for custom-designed lenses: Parameters to consider*
- *Trial set and inventory method*
- *Difficult cases to fit*

This chapter deals primarily with PMMA lenses, which are fast becoming extinct. However, the basic principles of fitting are fundamental to all rigid lenses and should be understood. This chapter should be considered an outline of basic fitting principles and as an historical reference.

The fitting of gas-permeable lenses, particularly those made of the more popular silicone acrylates and the fluorocarbon silicone acrylates, will be discussed in more detail in Chapters 26 and 27.

Many different philosophies of rigid-lens fitting have been developed over the years. Fitters who believe that the thickness of the lens is of prime importance fit the majority of their patients with microthin lenses. Others believe that the diameter of the lens is the key to good fitting technique. There are fitters who primarily fit large lenses and those who prefer small lenses. Some, who reject thickness and diameter as the ultimate factors, keep both constant and fit their patients largely by altering the primary base curve of the lens. The measurement of the corneal topography is believed by others to be the basis of fit of a lens. A number of devices are available for these measurements. Many fitters believe that trial lenses should be used because of the often repeated statement that the best device for fitting a contact lens is a contact lens. If this is true, perhaps an inventory of lenses is a little better.

There is no doubt that the neophyte lens-fitter is confused by the claims and counterclaims of many who teach lens philosophy. Obviously there is not one but a number of answers, all of which seem to work. In fact, almost any fitting technique can work, since the relative success or failure of a particular method depends largely on the skill and experience of the practitioner. Which to choose? That is the question.

We have used all the systems, and our conclusion is that no system works all the time for everybody. One needs a steady, intelligent, and reliable approach plus alternatives if the customary method fails.

The success of good fitters depends not on how well they fit lenses but on how they deal with any resulting problem.

Special reference has to be made to gas-permeable lenses. Although rigid-lens techniques are applicable to gas-permeable lenses, the approach is different because of the unique facility of this lens. One can take advantage of large-diameter lenses and their improved stability and centration without worrying about hypoxia of the corneal epithelium. Also the fitting of a high-riding lens, satisfactory for gas-permeable lenses, is not consistent with rigid PMMA lens' objectives. Although PMMA lens trial sets are satisfactory for gas-permeable lenses, the diameter of the lenses must be appropriate and the fitting criteria taken into account. What is desirable for PMMA lens fitting is not satisfactory for gas-permeable lenses. The amount of movement of a gas-permeable lens need not be as great as that of a PMMA lens, which entirely depends on tear exchange for oxygenation. Although gas-permeable lenses belong to the general family of rigid lenses, their application, objectives, and complications are quite different. In this chapter, we will try to generalize, but bear in mind that PMMA lenses are fast becoming extinct, giving way to the safer gas-permeable lenses.

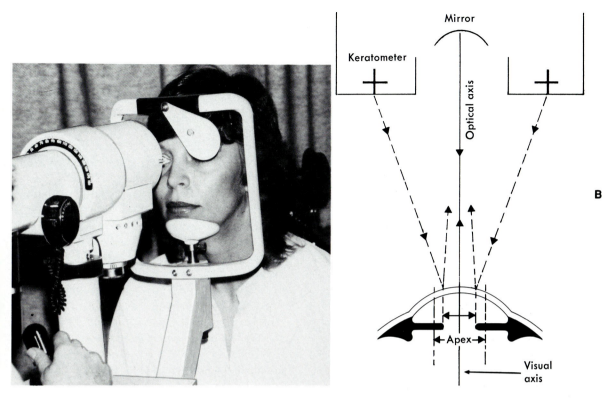

Fig 16-1 ■ **A,** Taking a K reading. **B,** The principle of the keratometer. The visual axis is aligned along the optic axis of the instrument so that the central front surface of the cornea reflects the mires of the keratometer. (**A** from Stein HA and Slatt BJ: The ophthalmic assistant, ed 4, St Louis, 1983, The CV Mosby Co.)

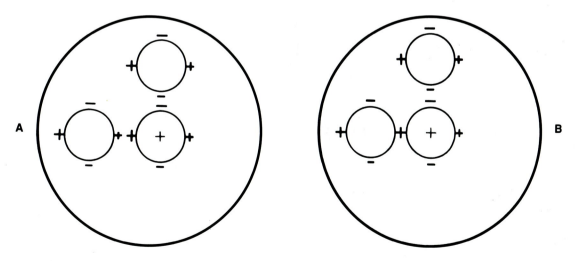

Fig 16-2 ■ Keratometer mires. **A,** Alignment of the mires for axis. **B,** Apposition of the plus-sign mire to measure one meridian of corneal curvature. (From Stein HA and Slatt BJ: The ophthalmic assistant, ed 4, St Louis, 1983, The CV Mosby Co.)

SYSTEMS BASED ON CORNEAL TOPOGRAPHY
Keratometer method

The keratometer method is probably the most commonly used method and is simple to perform. K, the measurement that parallels the steepest zone of the flattest primary meridian, is measured (Figs. 16-1 and 16-2). The steepest zone relates to the apex of the cornea, which is steeper than the peripheral portion.

Method. K readings are taken. The spectacle prescription is recorded in minus cylinder form and the cylinder reading is dropped. If the lens is fitted on K, the power is not changed. If the lens is fitted steeper than K, the plus power of the lens is decreased 0.25 D for each 0.25 D steeper fit. The added steepness causes the lens

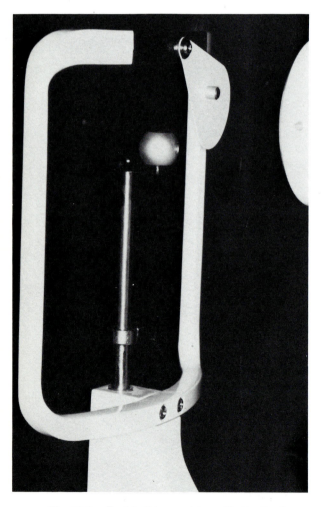

Fig 16-3 ■ Test ball is used to calibrate the keratometer for a given radius of curvature.

to vault the cornea centrally and creates a tear lens of plus power. This is the reason that a slight reduction in the required power is made to compensate. Minus power is increased 0.25 D for each 0.25 D of steeper fit.

The keratometer is designed to measure a spheric surface, with the cornea acting as a front-surface convex mirror (Fig. 16-3). However, frequently the cornea is aspheric and is steeper inferiorly and temporally (Fig. 16-4). The keratometer measures a limited circular area of the cornea, 2 to 4 mm apart, and if one mire is on the steeper side, the result given will be an average. The keratometer reflects only a small segment of the cornea (Fig. 16-5). Each instrument makes an assumption as to the index of refraction of the cornea. The Bausch & Lomb keratometer is calculated for an index of refraction of 1.3375 mm, whereas others are set for 1.332 to 1.336 mm.

The method that we use begins with the base curve, the central posterior curve (CPC). For the PMMA lenses we make the lens about 0.25 to 0.5D steeper than the flattest corneal meridian. If the K readings are 44.00 × 45.00 at an angle of 90 degrees, one chooses a base curve 43.25 or 43.50 D. We recommend an intermediate curve radius 1.0 mm flatter than the base curve. For the peripheral curve we use a standard curve radius 12.25 mm in combination with a width of 0.4 mm. If loosening is required, one can reduce the overall size of the lens and also alter the intermediate and peripheral curves.

The new gas-permeable lenses allow larger diameter lenses in the 8.8 to 9.8 mm range. Larger lenses are used if the cornea is flat and smaller lenses are used if the cornea is steep.

COMMENT. Since this method depends on one measurement, it would be reassuring if that measurement were precise. Unfortunately it is not, and even if it were it would be inadequate.

Despite the fact that keratometry works in a majority of cases, it is probably the least desirable method of lens fitting. The laboratory has the awesome responsibility of determining the peripheral curves, the design of the edge, the diameter of the lens, the thickness of the lens, and the size of the optic zone. This method also precludes any assessment of lid adherence, centration of the lens, and the effect of power on the fit. Its simplicity is its only attractive feature.

GUIDE FOR LENS' DESIGN SYSTEM

System	Comment	Rating
Keratometer	Strictly for beginners; a one-measurement system with faults in the single measurement	*
Topogometer	Attempts to define the topography of the cornea by outlining the corneal cap; rather inflexible; works well, possibly because most of the lenses come out small and thin	**
Nomogram	The number game in disguise; still a one-measurement system; works better than keratometry; good for the novice	**
Corneal mapping	Like the topogometer method except that it adds a permanent photographic record from the corneal scope. Not available to everyone.	**
Microthin lens	A very thin lens must be a small-diameter lens; too limited as a first-choice lens; good for rigid-lens problems or dropouts	**
Custom	No particular philosophy attached to this method; takes into account palpebral fissure size, corneal diameter, pupil size, and corneal topography, which are measured; from this information fitter determines lens size, size of optic zone, type of edge, and thickness; not for beginners	***
Diagnostic lens	Probably the best approach to lens-fitting; provides a dynamic overview of the lens-cornea relationship; requires few modifications for a custom-fit lens that can be universally applied; problems such as effect of power additions to the lens and exact base curves can be immediately determined; trial set does not require a major financial commitment and can easily be replaced if lenses become obsolete	****
Inventory	Its simplicity is its greatest asset; not economic for the occasional fitter, good for the large-volume practice; the system works like a fast-food restaurant outlet—the lens waits for the patient to arrive	***

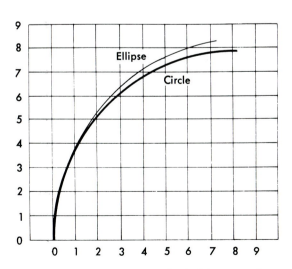

Fig 16-4 ■ The cornea is aspheric; it is not a sphere or a true ellipse. The rate of flattening in its periphery is not symmetric. The keratometer is a limited instrument, designed only for spheric surfaces.

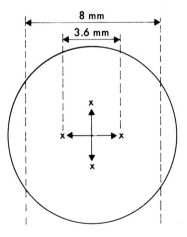

Fig 16-5 ■ The chord diameter (3.6 mm) of the corneal cap spans the linear distance between two points of the cornea. The chord diameter of the corneal cap is usually between 4 and 5 mm, whereas the radius of the corneal cap (8 mm), which measures the curvature of the cornea, is frequently between 6 and 8 mm. The keratometer, which measures a chord area of 3 to 3.6 mm, reflects only a small segment of the cornea.

Topogometer method

The topogometer is an attachment to the keratometer that contains a movable light source so that the visual axis can be decentered from the optical axis of the instrument (Figs. 16-6 and 16-7). One takes K readings across the surface of the cornea by changing the angle of the fixation light. The fixation light is quite handy because it steadies fixation in eyes with poor acuity. Flattening of the cornea is indicated by a change in the radius of curvature.

The topogometer may also be used to scan the corneal cap to detect a steeper zone away from the visual axis. If allowances are not made for such a variation in corneal contour, a lens will fit flat. The topogometer method assists in measuring the size of the corneal cap.

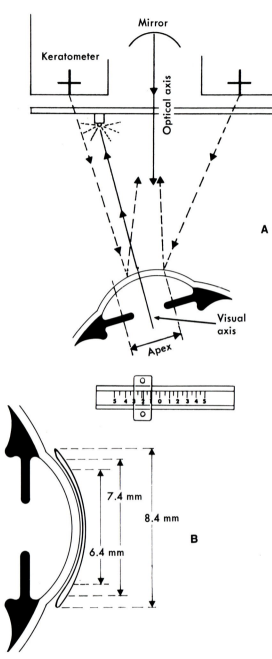

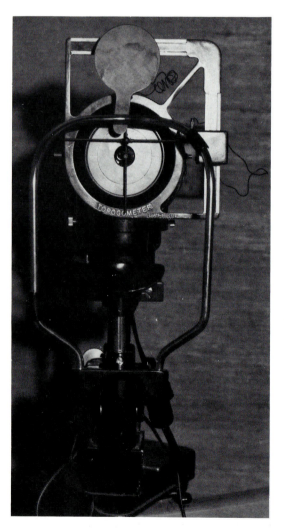

Fig 16-6 ■ The topogometer.

Fig 16-7 ■ A, The topogometer. The visual axis is displaced by the fixation light of the topogometer. The mires are now reflected from a paracentral arc of the cornea. A change in the radius of curvature as the eye is decentered indicates the limits of the corneal cap. **B,** The final diameter of a lens as determined by the formula LD + 2 where LD indicates the longest apical diameter and 2 refers to a 2 mm greater lens size than the longest apical diameter. In this case the longest apical diameter is 6.4 mm; thus the total lens diameter is 8.4 mm.

This approach to keratometery is quite helpful for patients with poor vision, aphakia and keratoconus, where the change of radius of curvature from the apex of the corneal cap to the periphery is great. For ordinary lens patients this method is certainly superior to the K reading method because the optic zone of the lens can at least be ordered so that it coincides with the radius of curvature of the corneal cap.

This technique is also quite popular because most corneas have an optic zone between 5.8 and 6.2 mm, which results in thin, small, steep lenses that have many attractive features. These are discussed more fully in the section on microthin lenses (see below).

This approach to lens fitting is also arbitrary. Once the horizontal and vertical meridians of the corneal cap are plotted, a lens is chosen with a diameter 2 mm greater than the corneal cap diameter. One millimeter is added for stability and movements, and 1 mm is added for proper edge design and secondary curves. The formula is commonly abbreviated to read the LD + 2 method (Fig. 16-8).

Photokeratoscopy with the corneoscope

The photokeratoscope or corneoscope also depends on the cornea acting as a convex mirror to produce a virtual image. Its advantage is that its image reflects the curvature of a larger corneal area than does the keratometer (Fig. 16-9).

The better photokeratoscopes have aspheric targets with an aperture at the center. Behind the aperture a Polaroid camera is mounted to photograph the corneal image for a permanent record.

The annular radius of curvature is derived from assessment of the separation of the target rings in the corneal photograph. In fact the precise margin of the ring may be difficult to identify because of blurring from the film grain. Variability may also be introduced from differences in the photosensitive material on the film. The photokeratoscope does not have any greater accuracy than the keratometer. However it measures more of the cornea, providing information on the periphery as well as the central corneal cap.

The major disadvantage of the system is the expense, which is marginally justified. It is really a variant of an approach to fitting lenses based on a more accurate assessment of corneal topography. No allowance is made for the weight of the lens, the effect of lid lift, the correct lens diameter, or the centration of the lens. These factors can only be judged by a diagnostic lens. On the plus side the photokeratoscope is extremely versatile, being applicable for very flat corneas less than 40.00 D to very steep corneas greater than 50.00 D.

SYSTEMS BASED ON TYPES OF LENSES
Microthin lenses

The core of this fitting system is that the lenses must be thin and lightweight so that they are less likely to mold the cornea and mechanically abrade it. These lenses are small in diameter, usually between 7.8 and 8.6 mm. A reduction in diameter is an inevitable consequence with thin lenses (Fig. 16-10). In fact it is difficult to make a large, thin lens. The center thickness is between 0.08 and 0.12 mm. The peripheral curves are relatively steep with a width of 0.3 to 0.6 mm. The steep narrow edge along with other features in the design of the lens allows the lens to center properly (Fig. 16-11). Also the thin edge does not jar the upper lid, and so blinking is likely to be comfortable and regular in frequency. The thinness of the lens causes some flexure with blinking, which helps tear ex-

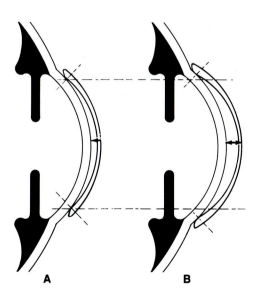

Fig 16-8 ■ **A,** The power of the lens is influenced by the apical vault. **B,** As the vaulting of the cornea is increased, the plus power of the tear film is increased.

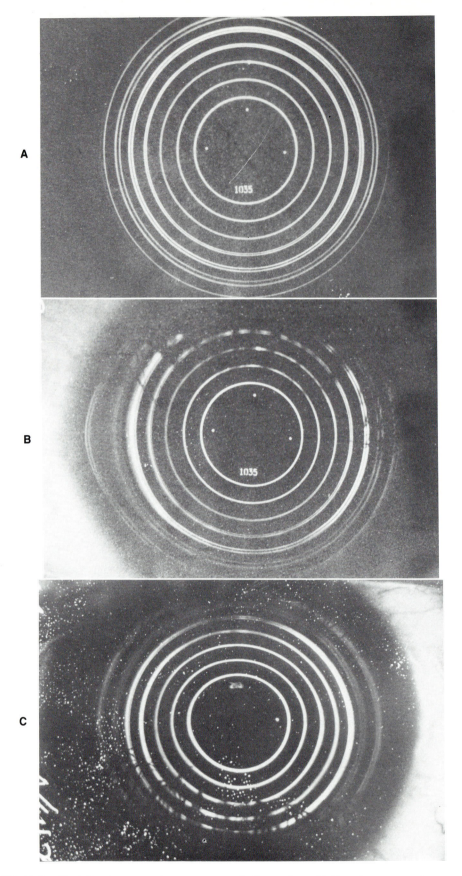

Fig 16-9 ■ Photokeratoscope of corneoscope. **A,** Test sphere. **B,** Regular cornea. **C,** Astigmatic eye (approximately 4.00 D).

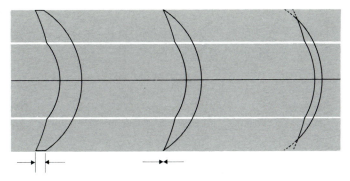

Fig 16-10 ■ Diameter reductions. As the thickness of a lens is reduced, the edge of the lens becomes thinner. Finally, as further reductions in thickness occur, the edge disappears so that a small-diameter, thin lens results.

change by creating a tear pump. The excellent tear exchange with the lightness of the lens usually results in minimal corneal edema after a day's wear, and, as a result, spectacle blur is frequently no more than 15 minutes in duration.

Bending or flexure of this lens may result in the introduction of some astigmatism with the rule to the cornea, and so it is ideally suited for corneas that have astigmatism against the rule.

Eye movement is free from lid irritation when microthin lenses are worn because the lens is usually smaller than the palpebral fissures. These lenses bend slightly on nonspheric corneas because of the capillary forces involved,

creating better alignment between the lens and the cornea. For many fitters this is the lens of choice.

A light, thin lens may be a good solution to some conventional rigid lens problems. For instance, these thin lenses are more comfortable than conventional lenses and can be used as an alternative to soft lenses in cases of rigid-lens' dropouts (Fig. 16-12). In those cases in which significant astigmatism is present they may be the best alternative. In situations where a lens rides low a microthin lens offers less gravitational pull and more lift from the upper lid. At times a large, high-riding lens problem may be solved with small, microthin lenses that may center better. Because of their thinness and small diameter they are useful in those wearers who have a limited wearing time resulting from the presence of corneal edema. Those patients who have induced corneal astigmatism caused by the molding effect of large lenses may be helped with a microthin lens. They cannot see with spectacles, and the time lag in waiting for their corneas to assume their natural shape may

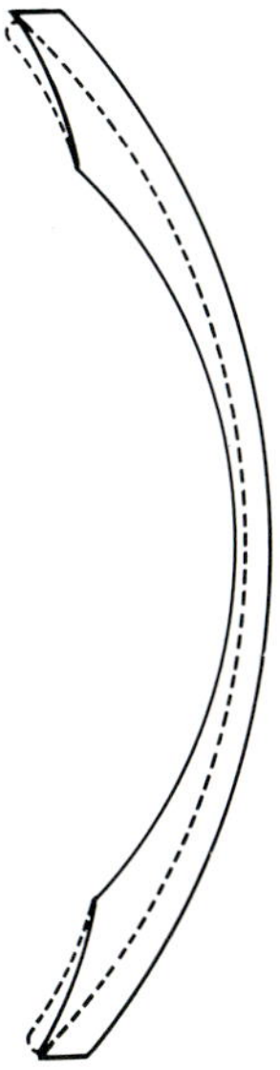

Fig 16-11 ■ The peripheral curves are made steep to allow the lens to center properly. This thin, steep edge provides minimal obstruction to the lid, which adds to the comfort of the lens.

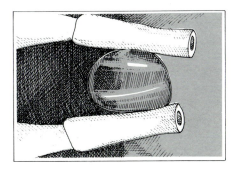

Fig 16-12 ■ Microthin lens, though a rigid lens made of polymethylmethacrylate, is flexible.

Table 16-1 ■ Diameter selection*

Palpebral fissure	Horizontal corneal diameter				
	12.5	12.0	11.5	11.0	10.5
Large	9.2	9.0	8.8	8.6	8.4
Normal	9.0	8.8	8.6	8.4	8.2
Small	8.8	8.4	8.2	8.0	7.8
Very small	8.2 or smaller	8.0 or smaller	7.8 or smaller	7.6 or smaller	7.4 or smaller

*Initial lens diameter in mm.

Table 16-2 ■ Base-curve selection*

Lens diameter (mm)	9.0	8.8	8.6	8.4	8.2	8.0	7.8	7.6	7.4	7.2	7.0
Optic zone diameter (mm)	7.8	7.6	7.4	7.2	7.0	7.0	7.0	6.8	6.8	6.6	6.6
Peripheral curve width (mm)	0.4	0.4	0.4	0.4	0.4	0.4	0.3	0.3	0.2	0.2	0.1
Peripheral curve radius (mm)	Should be flatter than base curve by:										
Minus lenses	1.5	1.5	1.5	1.5	1.5	1.5	2.0	2.0	2.5	2.5	3.0
Plus lenses	1.0	1.0	1.0	1.0	1.0	1.0	1.5	1.5	2.0	2.0	2.5
Blend curve width (mm)	0.2	0.2	0.2	0.2	0.2	0.1	0.1	0.1	0.1	0.1	0.1
Blend curve radius (mm)	Should be flatter than base curve by:										
All lenses	0.7	0.7	0.7	0.7	0.7	0.7	1.0	0.1	1.0	1.0	1.0
Fit steeper than K by (D)	0.12	0.25	0.37	0.50	0.62	0.62	0.75	0.87	0.87	1.0	1.0
	plus 25% of the corneal cylinder (difference between K readings)										

*Minus lenses from −6.00 to −8.00 D should be fitted 0.12 steeper than shown; beyond −8.00 D they should be fitted 0.25 D steeper.

be intolerable. The soft lens is a poor substitute in such cases, since it does little to correct the induced astigmatic error.

How to fit. The following steps are used to fit microthin lenses:

1. Fit either with K readings as a base or by the diagnostic trial lens procedure. The base curve is usually fitted slightly steeper than K by 0.25 to 0.50 D (Table 16-1). Fit the least steep lens that provides satisfactory lens position and lens movement. The diameter and optic zone vary with the base curve and are selected from tables (Table 16-2). The general rules still apply. A flat cornea (42.00 D or less) requires a larger lens (8.6 mm), whereas a steep cornea (45.00 D) requires a smaller lens (8.0 mm).

2. Normally the fit should have slight apical clearance; 1 mm lens movement with blinking is optimal. Minimal lag in ocular rotation is desirable. Central touch can be tolerated because of the thinness of the lens (Fig. 16-13).

3. The fluorescein pattern appears uniform under the lens. Because of the steep peripheral curves a narrower-than-normal band of fluorescein is found at the periphery (Fig. 16-14).

4. With astigmatism from 1.00 to 2.00 D, fit 0.50 D steeper than K. For astigmatism between 2.00 and 3.00 D, fit one third the value of K. These lenses are superior to toric base curve lenses in correcting astigmatism less than 4.00 D.

The microthin lenses seem too good to be true. They have the comfort and rapid adaptability of a soft lens and the optic properties of a rigid lens. There are, however, disadvantages.

DISADVANTAGES. Microthin lenses have the following disadvantages:

1. Microthin lenses frequently cannot be used with some lenses that are likely to be high-riding, as in severe myopia. Their extreme thinness can carry the lens higher.

2. They are especially hard to remove. That nice, thin edge makes it difficult for the upper

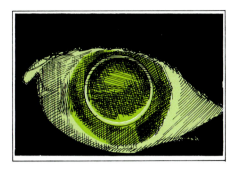

Fig 16-13 ■ Microthin lens fitted on K. The fluorescein pattern shows some central touch and pooling at the periphery of the lens because of the steep peripheral curves.

lid to dislodge the lens. Also the tightness of the fit makes removal awkward.

3. They do not center well in certain patients with high astigmatic corrections.
4. They are difficult lenses to modify in the office because of their size and flexibility. These lenses cannot be held in place with a suction cup. If they are modified, they must be stabilized using a holder with a wax mounting.
5. They warp easily.
6. The base curve may not be stable.
7. Patients with large pupils complain of flare.
8. Because of their thinness, it is easier to damage and break these lenses during handling.

BASE-CURVE SELECTION. The smaller the lens diameter, the more corneal cylinder present, and the smaller the optic zone, the steeper the base curve should be.

LENS THICKNESS (TABLE 16-3). The key to proper performance of ultrathin lenses lies in making them extremely thin. Small lenses of conventional thickness tend to stay down because of their excess weight in relation to their small size. A conventional lens fitted steeper than K will have poor tear exchange, whereas an ultrathin lens tends to flex with each blink. This pumping action provides movement of tears under the lens.

COMMENT. Microthin lenses are particularly useful as starter lenses in patients with small palpebral fissures, tight upper lids, or corneas steeper than 46.00 D. They also provide an alternative to soft lenses for rigid lens dropouts. Microthin lenses are useful for residual astigmatism against the rule, since they flex in the opposite meridian.

Some authors attempt to identify flexible lenses as a separate entity. We believe that all rigid lenses can be made flexible or semiflexible, depending not only on their thickness but also on their material composition. We consider flexible lenses as a subtype of rigid lenses.

The comfort of the lens is largely related to its relatively steep peripheral curves and thin edges, which provide only a minimal obstruction to the lid margin. The comfort is not a function of its size. Even a hydrophilic lens that is reduced in size so that the lid makes contact with its edge will be uncomfortable.

Large lenses with wide peripheral curves

Unless a fitter is committed by tradition to a given lens diameter, there should be some rationale for arriving at a given lens diameter.

Generally a flat cornea is a large cornea and requires a large lens, whereas if a cornea is small, less than 11 mm, or steep, greater than 44.00 D, a small-diameter lens should be considered.

A 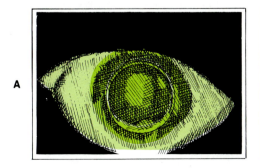 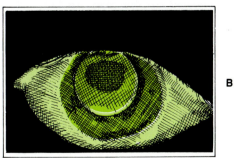 B

Fig 16-14 ■ **A,** Microthin lens fitted steeper than K. The ring of fluorescein around the lens is indicative of the very steep fit. **B,** Microthin lens fitted flatter than K. Large area of apical touch with pooling of fluorescein elsewhere is typical of a flat lens-cornea relationship.

Table 16-3 ■ Recommended thicknesses for minus and plus power lenses

Lens Powers (D)	Diameter (mm)				
	9.0	8.5	8.0	7.5	7.0
			Minus power		
Plano to −0.62	0.18	0.17	0.16	0.15	0.14
−0.75 to −1.37	0.17	0.16	0.15	0.14	0.13
−1.50 to −2.12	0.16	0.15	0.14	0.13	0.12
−2.25 to −2.87	0.15	0.14	0.13	0.12	0.11
−3.00 to −3.62	0.14	0.13	0.12	0.11	0.10
−3.75 to −4.37	0.13	0.12	0.11	0.10	0.10
−4.50 to −5.12	0.12	0.11	0.10	0.10	0.10
−5.25 to −5.87	0.11	0.10	0.10	0.10	0.10
−6.00 & over	0.10	0.10	0.10	0.10	0.10
			Plus power		
+0.12 to +0.75	0.20	0.18	0.17	0.16	0.15
+0.87 to +1.50	0.22	0.20	0.19	0.18	0.16
+1.62 to +2.25	0.24	0.22	0.21	0.20	0.18
+2.37 to +3.00	0.26	0.24	0.23	0.21	0.20
+3.12 to +3.75	0.28	0.26	0.25	0.23	0.22
+3.87 to +4.50	0.30	0.28	0.27	0.25	0.24
+4.62 to +5.25	0.32	0.30	0.29	0.27	0.25

Table supplied with permission of Dr. Stanley Gordon, Rochester, N.Y.

The range of diameters considered is between 8.3 and 9 mm.

Generally a large palpebral aperture, 10 mm or greater, requires a larger lens, whereas a small palpebral aperture, 10 mm or less, should have a smaller lens. Despite these general rules, however, there are fitters who prefer primarily the large-diameter lens as their lens of choice.

Design. These lenses are between 9 and 10 mm in diameter. They have an intermediate curve that is 1 mm flatter than the base curve and a peripheral curve that is 1 mm flatter than the intermediate curve. The optic zone is large, varying from a high normal size of 7 mm to a generous size of 8 mm. This large size would of course eliminate the annoying flare of small lenses. The diameter of the optic zone is usually 1.5 mm less than the corneal diameter.

If fitted properly, these lenses are very comfortable. The large size enables the edge of the lens to remain under the upper lid during blinking.

The wide peripheral curves hold a large reservoir of tear fluid that cushions the lens and assists in tear exchange.

Advantages. This is a good lens for a high-riding lens. The extra weight adds gravitational force to bring it down especially with single-cut plus lenses. This feature is not so relevant with minus lenses. Spheric lenses can be used for corneal astigmatism up to a range of 3.00 to 4.00

D. The lenses are stable, center well, and are easy to handle. They are more comfortable than a smaller lens of similar edge design.

Disadvantages. A large lens has its place in overcoming many fitting problems but as a lens of first choice it has too many drawbacks. There is greater corneal molding because of its bulk. If a lens is reduced from 10 to 8 mm, the entire area of the lens is reduced by 36%. Molding of a cornea can induce serious astigmatic errors of the cornea of 5.00 to 6.00 D in magnitude, which in some cases can be permanent.

This is a difficult lens to handle with small palpebral fissures.

The large lens is poor for steep and for small corneas.

The peripheral curves are complex but must be fashioned precisely. If they do not become contoured to the cornea, the lenses will become very loose.

COMMENT. The disadvantages of a large PMMA lens have been counteracted with gas-permeable material. The positive features still stand.

GENERAL RULES FOR CUSTOM-DESIGNED LENSES: PARAMETERS TO CONSIDER
Primary base curve

Slight apical clearance over the cornea is desirable for many rigid materials. Up to 3.00 D

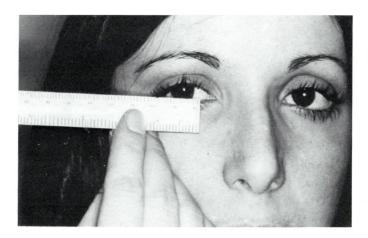

Fig 16-15 ■ Measuring the pupillary and corneal diameter with a ruler. (From Stein HA and Slatt BJ: The ophthalmic assistant, ed 3, St Louis, 1976, The CV Mosby Co.)

of astigmatism can be corrected with a spherical lens. As the degree of astigmatism increases, the base curve must be made steeper. The following is a general guide showing the relationship between the amount of corneal astigmatism and the lens base curve.

Cornea	Base curve
To 0.50 D astigmatism	0.25 D steeper than K reading
0.50 to 2.00 D of astigmatism	0.50 D steeper than K reading
2.00 to 3.00 D of astigmatism	0.50 to 0.75 D steeper than K reading
More than 3.00 D of astigmatism	Bitoric or inside toric lens

The primary base curve may be ordered in diopters or millimeters radius of curvature.

Corneal diameter

The corneal diameter is obtained when one measures the visible iris diameter with a ruler. The most accurate way is to use calipers to determine the limbus-to-limbus diameter after a topical anesthetic is placed on the cornea. Although the cornea is slightly larger, for clinical purposes this amount can be ignored. The diameter of the cornea in the horizontal meridian usually ranges between 10.5 and 12 mm (Fig. 16-15).

Lens diameter

The lens diameter may be determined in various ways. With the microthin lenses the lens diameter must be small, usually less than 8.5 mm.

Lenses over 4.00 D power usually need a diameter of 8.5 mm or more to avoid a high-riding lens. The greater the minus power, the larger the lens.

If the topogometer is used, the lens will be 2 mm larger than the corneal cap, which varies from 5.8 to 6.2 mm. One may calculate the lens diameter in relation to the pupillary size by adding 4 mm to the pupillary diameter.

Generally, large, flat corneas require a large lens, that is, a corneal diameter greater than 11.5 mm and flatter than 44.00 D. Conversely a small, steep cornea, for example, less than 11.5 mm and steeper than 44.00 D, requires a small lens. Without going to extremes the acceptable range of minus-powered lens diameters is between 8 and 9 mm. A large palpebral aperture accommodates a large lens, whereas a small fissure demands a small lens.

Another aid to determining lens diameter is to flash a light into the other eye blurred with a plus lens. This maneuver creates a consensually smaller pupil in the other eye. If the vision is improved by the small pupil, a larger lens is needed.

Increasing the lens diameter with concomitant increase in optic zone without altering the base curve has the same effect as making the lens tighter. It increases apical vaulting. Conversely, reducing the lens size serves to decrease the apical vaulting effect. A change in the clearance of the cornea can affect the shape of the tear film layer and consequently can also affect the power of the lens (Figs. 16-16 and 16-19). Smaller lenses can be fitted steeper than larger

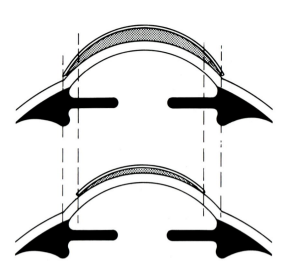

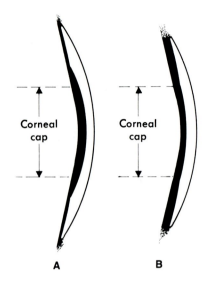

Fig 16-16 ■ As the diameter of the lens is increased, the lens becomes steeper, the apical clearance of the cornea becomes greater, and the shape of the tear film becomes more convex in shape, which adds plus power. Both lenses have the same radius of curvature.

Fig 16-17 ■ Optic zone. Two identical lenses placed on corneas with the same K readings. **A,** The size of the optic zone is too large for the corneal cap, and the lens vaults the cornea. The net effect is the same as if the lens was made too steep. **B,** The size of the optic zone is compatible with the size of the corneal cap, and the lens is comfortable. If the optic zone is too small, flare is frequently experienced.

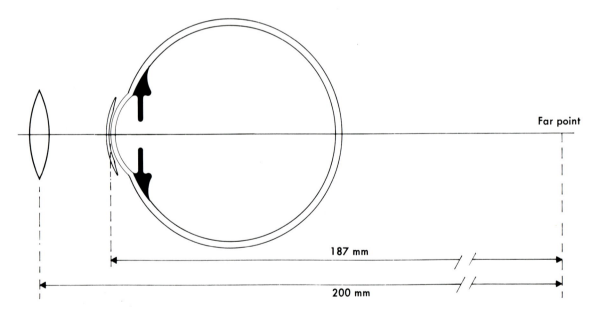

Fig 16-18 ■ Vertex power. The far point of a plus lens is reduced with the shift from a spectacle lens to a contact lens. To achieve the same power, added plus power must be incorporated into the contact lens as follows: 5.00 D hyperopia—in front of the cornea by 13 mm—far point = 200 mm. Far-point distance of contact lens = 187 mm. Power of contact lens = $\frac{1000}{187}$ = +5.34 mm.

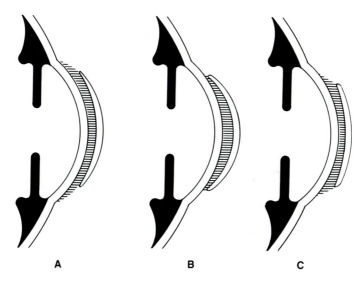

A   B   C

Fig 16-19 ■ Tear power. **A,** Plano power of tear film when the lens is fitted parallel to K. **B,** Plus power of the tear film when the lens is fitted steeper than K. The tear film is convex. Extra minus is required in the final power of the lens. **C,** Minus power of the tear film when the lens is fitted flatter than K. The tear film is concave in shape. Extra plus is required in the final power of the lens. The tear film has an optic density of 1.336, whereas polymethylmethacrylate has an optic density of 1.488.

lenses. A lens of 7.5 to 8.5 mm diameter can be fitted 1.50 to 2.50 D steeper than K, whereas a 9.5 to 10 mm diameter lens should be fitted on K or perhaps 0.25 D steeper. The greater the gas-permeability, the flatter the lens should be. We make our lens at least 0.50 to 1.00 D flatter than we would for a PMMA lens.

Optic zone diameter

The optic zone diameter varies with the pupillary size, the lens diameter, and the palpebral fissure size.

If the optic zone is too small for the size of the pupil, the person will experience flare in dim illumination when the pupillary aperture increases. This person is annoyed by the streaming of lights and may also be subject to fluctuation in visual acuity because at times the pupil is partially covered by the peripheral curve of the lens. Flare occurs as a result of the flatter peripheral curve, creating a prismatic deflection of light passing through it.

For large pupils (5 to 7 mm), that is, for persons with blue eyes, myopia, or anxiety, the size of the optic zone should be increased 0.5 mm. For small pupils (less than 4 mm) for example, for persons who have brown eyes or who are middle aged, the optic zone can be reduced by 0.5 mm.

The optic zone usually varies with the size of the lens. In large, flat eyes with K readings of 42.00 D or under, the optic zone should be larger.

Lens diameter (mm)	Optic zone
9 or greater	1.5 mm less than lens diameter
8.2 to 8.8	1 to 1.3 mm less than lens diameter
8	1 mm less than lens diameter

When in doubt about the correct size of the optic zone diameter, a lens that is larger rather than smaller should be selected. The optic zone of a lens can be made smaller by modification of the lens but cannot be made larger unless a new lens is made.

The lens diameter and consequently the optic zone vary directly with the palpebral fissure size. A small palpebral fissure requires a smaller-diameter lens and hence a smaller optic zone. Decreasing the optic zone (base curve) radius of a lens has the effect of making the fit tighter, whereas decreasing the optic zone diameter or increasing the optic zone radius (making it flatter) will loosen the rigid lens. A decrease in optic zone diameter is the same as an increase in the width of the intermediate curve. Reduction of the size of the optic zone is done in 0.1 or 0.2 mm steps.

The size of optic zone should bear a close relationship to the size of the corneal cap (Fig. 16-17), which can be determined by either the topogometer method or by the corneoscope.

Sometimes the optic zone seems too small because the person experiences halos or fringes around lights. Flare can frequently indicate a flat fit if the lens moves excessively, displacing a peripheral portion of the lens onto the pupillary area.

COMMENT. The factors affecting the size of the optic zone are frequently ignored and its size determined arbitrarily from a nomogram or indirectly from corneal diameter measurements. It is surprising how well a system without any scientific rationale really works. Few practitioners actually measure the size of the corneal cap or concern themselves with the dimensions of the optic zone of a lens.

Thickness of lens

The thickness of a lens varies directly with the power and the lens diameter.

The greater the plus power, the greater the central thickness must be. An aphakic lens is frequently 0.35 to 0.4 mm thick, whereas a myopic lens of -4.00 D is often no thicker than 0.13 to 0.15 mm. If a lens is reduced to less than 0.10 mm, bending or flexure of the lens may become extreme and result in variable vision. A plano lens should have a central thickness of 0.15 mm. For every 2.00 D of minus power 0.01 mm should be subtracted from 0.15 mm. For every 1.00 D of plus power 0.025 mm should be added. The minimum thickness should be 0.10 mm.

The comfort of a lens depends not on its thickness but rather on the edge treatment. A thick lens, however, is likely to ride low and mold the cornea and is less capable of producing tear exchange because of the absence of flex.

If a lens is relatively thin, it will have a tendency to fit tightly, whereas a thick lens may tend to fit loosely and move excessively.

Peripheral curves

The width and the curvature usually vary with the size of the lens, its thickness, and the base curve. For any specified lens diameter the width of the peripheral curve determines the size of the optic zone. A lens can be made looser by either widening the peripheral curves or by flattening them. The choice of which modification to make is often determined by the optic zone

requirements: if the patient has a large pupil and the optic zone is already reasonably small, it might be wiser in this instance to flatten the peripheral curve rather than reduce the optic zone.

Most practitioners rely upon the laboratory to specify the radius of curvatures of the peripheral curves. But any trial set used should have the same peripheral curve as the lenses ordered. A typical posterior peripheral curve is 0.3 mm wide with a 12.25 mm radius. The intermediate peripheral curve is frequently 0.3 mm wide with a 9.0 mm radius.

The peripheral curves are always flatter than the base curve to comply with the flatter peripheral corneal contours.

Blending curves

Blending curves are used to remove the sharp junction of the peripheral and secondary curves and are also used at the secondary base curve junction. Blends can be light, medium, or heavy.

The No. 1 blend is that blend placed between the secondary and base curves. It is 0.5 mm longer in radius of curvature than the base curve.

The No. 3 blend is between the secondary and posterior curves, and its radius is halfway between the radius of the secondary and posterior curves.

Edges

The edges should be smooth, free of sharp areas, and contoured to slip under the eyelids during blinking. On thick edges of high myopic lenses -5.00 D or more, a bevel is added on the anterior surface to contour the lens edge. The lens edge should be contoured posteriorly, since an anterior lens design, though good for tear exchange, causes lid irritation and displacement of the lens.

COMMENT. Any lens over 5.00 D should have its edges beveled. The myopic lens should have that prism base effect trimmed similar in shape to a plus lens, whereas a high-plus lens requires a myopic profile to aid in comfort and lens lift.

Power calculation

The refraction must be expressed in minus cylinder. The cylinder is then dropped, and the sphere is retained as the refractive power. For example,

Spectacle lens power	Contact lens power
-3.00 D -2.00 D $\times$ 180	-3.00 D

If the spectacle lens power is greater than ± 4.00 D an adjustment for vertex distance is required to make the accurate contact lens power. For myopia, less minus power is required in the contact lens form as compared to the spectacle prescription. For example, a spectacle lens power of -5.00 D with 15 mm vertex power would result in a contact lens power of -4.65 D.

For hyperopia more effective power is needed in the contact lens form. For example, a spectacle lens power of $+5.00$ D with 15 mm vertex distance would result in a contact lens power of $+5.41$ D (Fig. 16-18). A vertex table should be consulted.

If the contact lens is not fitted on K, a further modification of power must be made. When the base curve is steeper than the flattest central corneal curve (flattest K reading), a tear lens of plus power is formed (Fig. 16-19). To correct for this the contact lens should be made with less plus or more minus power.

For every 0.25 D that the base curve is steeper than the corneal curve, -0.25 D should be added to the contact lens. For each 0.25 D that the base curve is flatter than the corneal K reading, 0.25 D should be added to the power of the contact lens.

If a trial lens is used, the computation of power is relatively simple, since the spectacle over-refraction is merely added to the power of the contact lens.

A power change of ± 0.50 D can be made on an original contact lens by surface grinding.

Tint

The tint of a lens is used to assist the patient in finding a dropped lens or in retrieving a lens displaced on the sclera. Tinted lenses are not a substitute for sunglasses, regardless of the density of the tint. The cosmetic aspects are really slight because the diameter of most lenses is substantially smaller than the size of the visible iris. At times the color of a pale blue, gray, or green iris can be enriched with an appropriately tinted lens. Even a change of color, for example, from brown to blue, can now be done.

A light blue tint is the most practical. Light blue transmits more light under scotopic and photopic conditions than does any other tint (Fig. 16-20). Activities such as night driving are much safer and more enjoyable for a lens patient with a light blue tint. Blue lenses are easy to locate when dropped on the floor.

One practical advantage to making all the lenses one color is that lost lenses can be replaced more easily from an office that maintains a supply of lenses.

COMMENT. The choice of tint of a lens should be the prerogative of the fitter, not the patient. The tint should be selected on the basis of maximum retinal sensitivity under photopic and scotopic conditions. Green and brown solid pigments used in the plastic have been generally avoided because they were unstable in the plastic. However, this problem has been rectified in recent years, and pigments used for these colors are now virtually as stable as for other colors.

Good fit

A good fit is one in which the lens is centered and moves well and the underlying cornea is free of edematous changes.

The following are sample typical lens specifications for the laboratory and fitting information.

Ideally the geometric center of the lens should coincide with the line of fixation. However, a minus lens often rides 1 or 2 mm higher, whereas a plus lens may ride slightly lower. A lens should not touch the limbus (Fig. 16-21), a situation that commonly occurs during the act of reading. With reading the eyes are lowered and the lenses may be pushed up by the lower lid. If this occurs, the diameter of the lens should be reduced. However reducing the diameter may make the lens looser, and so a steeper base curve may be required.

The lens should be stable when the patient looks straight ahead and should move with blinking, first downward with lid closure and then up as the lid elevates. When the lids are fully open, the lens gently drops. At times the bottom of the lens rotates nasally with blinking. If the upper lid is held, a normal lens will drop 1 to 2 mm in smooth motion, whereas a loose lens will take a rapid fall, often to the lower lid.

With version movements a lens will lag 1 or 2 mm in all directions. If the lens decenters more than this, it is too loose and will be uncomfortable.

During the adaptation period the contact-

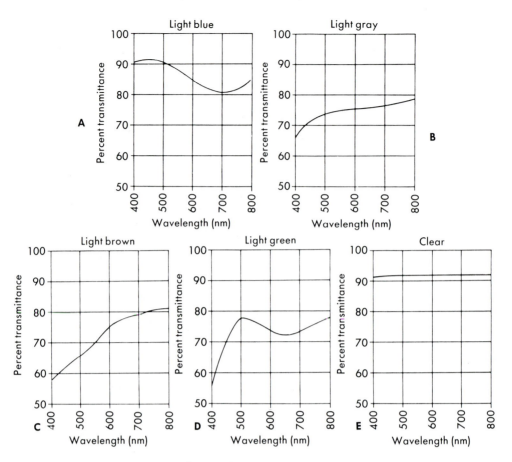

Fig 16-20 ■ Light transmittance. **A,** Light blue tint has the greatest light transmittance in the 500 nm area (91%) and the lowest in the 700 nm area (80%). The wavelength of maximum retinal sensitivity for the scotopic eye is between 500 and 510 nm and, for the photopic eye, around 550 nm. **B,** Light gray tint has less than 80% light transmittance anywhere on the spectrum. **C,** Light brown tint has only 65% transmittance in the 500 nm area. **D,** Light green tint has a maximum light transmittance of 75% in the 500 nm area. **E,** Clear lenses show slightly greater light transmittance than do blue-tinted lenses in the area of greatest retinal sensitivity. (Courtesy American Optical Corp, Southbridge, Mass.)

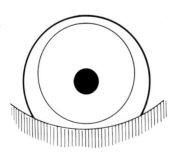

Fig 16-21 ■ Normal position of the lens lies 1 to 2 mm above the edge of the lower eyelid. (From Stein HA and Slatt BJ: The ophthalmic assistant, ed 4, St Louis, 1983, The CV Mosby Co.)

cornea relationship may change because of corneal edema. Some steepening in the area of 0.50 D is common. However, if it exceeds 1.00 D, there is need to re-evaluate the fit.

The integrity of the cornea is best documented by slitlamp examination. The presence of central corneal clouding indicates that hypoxic changes are taking place either because of inadequacy of the tear pump or direct mechanical compression of the cornea.

TRIAL SET AND INVENTORY METHOD (Fig. 16-22)

A trial set system of fitting basically uses a lens as an instrument to detect a proper fit. A

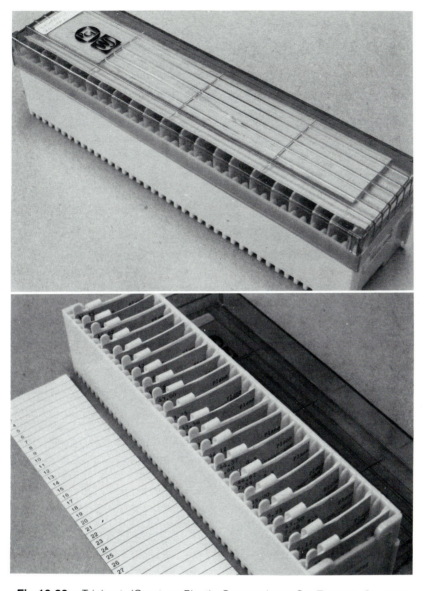

Fig 16-22 ■ Trial set. (Courtesy Plastic Contact Lens Co, Toronto, Canada.)

diagnostic lens will replace the front surface optics of a cornea and therefore can be used to determine major and minor irregularities in the contour of the cornea. The procedure is not just trial and error. By observing the fitting characteristics of each lens one can judge the changes to give the best final fit. Many fitters deplore the connotations of the term *trial lens* and prefer the term *control lens* or *diagnostic lens*.

Trial sets usually contain a small number of fitting lenses with a maximum of about 20. These sets can be stored either wet or dry. If wet storage is used, the solutions should be changed daily. An inventory system operates on a similar principle, but the precise lens can be tried and fitted at the time of examination. An inventory of lenses is basically a large trial set, and so both methods will be considered together.

Since any system is more or less dependent on the skill and experience of the fitter, the beauty of the inventory system is its absolute simplicity. It requires minimal sophistication in lens-fitting because only one parameter is altered at a time and the changes can be made instantly. The base curve can be altered while the diameter is held constant, or the diameter can be varied while the base curve remains constant.

Set

In the past, most PMMA fitting sets contained 400 to 600 lenses with a power range between −1.00 and −7.00 D in 0.25 D steps. The base curve range is between 41.00 and 46.00 D in 0.25 D increments. The diameter choice, between 8.2 and 8.6 mm, was very limited. The tints in the sets were restricted to a choice of blue or gray. Today, inventory systems incorporate rigid gas-permeable material.

Fitting

The base curves are established by conventional keratometry. The diameter of the lens is selected by general principles, that is, small-diameter lenses are chosen for a small cornea with a base curve over 44.00 D.

A lens is selected that is the same as or slightly steeper than the K reading and placed on the eye. After the initial reaction to the lens has subsided, the fitter can assess the final visual acuity, the centration, the fluorescein pattern, and the movement of the lens without delay. If the lens is too loose, a steeper base curve is selected. The desired position of the lens is usually concentric with the limbus for PMMA lenses and slightly superior for high DK rigid lenses. The movement should be 1.0 to 1.5 m upward followed by slow refraction to a near central position. Fluorescein can help determine the quality of a fit. If the lens is too tight, fluorescein will pool centrally to beneath the peripheral curve. If the lens is too flat, there will be a central touch with a pool of fluorescein centrally. If the visual acuity is not up to par, an over-refraction is done and the power is adjusted.

There is nothing else to alter. Thickness, edge, peripheral curves, and optic zones are standardized.

Practical benefits

Seventy percent of rigid lens' candidates can be fitted with a standard set of lenses. Modifications are unnecessary because the lens is simply replaced instead of modified. These lenses are usually of high quality because of the rigid specifications that lend themselves to quality mass production. A custom-designed lens requires more expertise; therefore it is more subject to error.

A fitting set eliminates an enormous amount of paperwork. No longer are ordering, notifying patients of arrival of lenses, sending major adjustments out, and ordering and billing for replacement lenses necessary. When a lens is used, reordering is done by a simple return of the lens case to the laboratory for replacement.

The cost of an inventory lens is less than that of a custom lens.

Patients can be refitted with a temporary lens without a period of being deprived of their lenses. This aspect of an inventory is very important for patients with high refractive errors who simply cannot function with a spectacle correction.

Finally, a patient may be trial-fitted with lenses that are precise for his or her eyes without anyone making a financial commitment to those lenses. Some fitters would regard this point as a drawback, considering a financial commitment to a set of lenses an aid to motivation.

Drawbacks

The blessing of cheaper lenses is offset by the cost of an expensive inventory. Unless there is a reasonable turnover of lenses the inventory can become a "white elephant." Also the set can become obsolete because of new developments. Imagine owning a large inventory of scleral lenses or several hundred of the prototype soft lenses. The present generation of rigid lenses is now being eclipsed by newer, oxygen-permeable lenses.

Custom-designed lenses are still required for special cases such as patients wth high refractive errors, residual astigmatism, keratoconus, and presbyopia, as well as those who require a toric fit.

COMMENT. For the busy practitioner an inventory of lenses can certainly streamline a practice. It is an efficient, fast system that reduces paperwork and the fitter's dependency on the laboratory. The lenses are of high quality and can be applied to a majority of conventional cases. For the occasional fitter a diagnostic set of lenses makes more sense.

The drawback of inventory lies in having to make a commitment to use that inventory. One in effect marries a given laboratory. The link to a laboratory may be attractive in a stable environment, but consider the recent technologic changes. There are new generations of plastics such as silicone, elastomers and polymers, newly fabricated cellulose acetate butyrate (CAB), and various mixtures of plastics that combine PMMA, CAB, silicone, and fluorocarbon.

The designs of lenses are changing. Large-diameter lens are in because of comfort, stability, and centration. New aspheric designs are also making their presence felt. Soft lenses have been changed. They have become hydrated and thinned to unbelievable levels to make them more oxygen-permeable. These are now commercially available as toric lenses, bifocal lenses, and as extended-wear lenses.

There is now a disposable lens.

Do you really want to commit yourself to a large number of lenses that cannot be turned over rapidly? Unless your practice is a high-volume one, it is better to use a trial set or diagnostic fitting set rather than to maintain an inventory.

DIFFICULT CASES TO FIT
Spheric corneas

A rigid lens fitted to a spheric cornea may tend to slide off the cornea or create tight symptoms. An element of corneal toricity is desirable so that the lens is centered. In such cases it is advisable to make the diameter 1 mm larger than normal or large enough so that the lens slips under the upper lid.

Exophthalmic eye

A soft lens is preferable because it offers protection to the cornea and stability of position and does not offend the blinking lid with a hard edge.

Flat corneas (41.00 D or less)

Large, flat corneas provide a poor base for the lens to rest on. The lens tends to slide off, become decentered, or even pop out of the eye. A large-diameter lens is indicated here.

High refractive errors

They cause thick centers or thick edges, depending on whether the refractive error is high hyperopia or high myopia. Thicker lenses are heavier, harder to center, and more likely to cause corneal hypopia and compression.

COMMENT. Most of the difficulties with rigid PMMA lenses relate to corneal edema, lens centration, and lens stability on the moving eye. A gas-permeable lens of large diameter usually will remedy most of these complications. That is why PMMA lenses are becoming obsolete. Updated materials include silicone acrylates and fluorocarbon silicone acrylates. Please refer to Chapters 26 and 27 for details on fitting lenses made of these materials.

17 ▪ INSERTION AND REMOVAL TECHNIQUES

- ▪ Insertion by practitioner
- ▪ Removal by practitioner
- ▪ Insertion by patient
- ▪ Removal by patient
- ▪ Recentering a displaced lens
- ▪ Factors affecting wearing schedule

Basically the novice lens–wearer worries more about the handling of a lens than any other consideration. It seems implausible that a large foreign body can sit comfortably on the naked eye. Normally when anything is brought before an eye, the head recoils, the eye looks away, and the lids close. Because these natural reactions must be suppressed when a lens is brought to the cornea, the patient is suspicious and fearful. There is the nagging fear that the determination and discipline will not be there and that the entire exercise will be a failure. There is also the worry that an unnatural marriage is taking place and that as a result a great deal of suffering will ensue.

The fitter must be gentle and reassuring at all times. The patient should be told what to expect so as to avoid the shock of any unpleasant feelings. The lens should be placed upon the cornea by the fitter initially. A smooth performance can only increase the confidence of an apprehensive patient. In a short time repressed fears are eliminated, for a lens can be tolerated by the cornea, which under usual circumstances will violently reject a cinder or any other tiny foreign body. The insertion and removal techniques are the same for the PMMA lenses and gas-permeable lenses. However, there are a few differences to bear in mind.

The *silicone acrylates* are quite fragile and will split at the edges if handled roughly.

Microthin PMMA lenses are usually fit on K or on the tight side of K. These lenses are more difficult to eject from the eyes with conventional techniques. It may be necessary to add a drop of artificial tears to loosen the lenses.

CAB (cellulose acetate butyrate) lenses may warp with time. The dimensional stability of these lenses is not so good as that of PMMA. They have to be handled with greater care.

Silicone lenses, now primarily used for pediatric aphakes, can become very tight and difficult to remove, that is, produce the sucked-on lens syndrome. Parents should be forewarned and taught emergency techniques for lens removal—eyecup, or dunking the head in a basin of water.

Aphakic lenses are difficult to remove. The manual dexterity of an elderly person may not be sufficient to remove a lens consistently. Also the lids may be lax, and so indirect techniques using the lids are hard to apply. It is important to teach a spouse, relative, or friend to remove the lens should the aphakic elderly person become unable to do so and become agitated in the process.

Children's lenses. Children should be taught to insert and remove their lenses as soon as possible. Dependency in lens handling is not advisable.

Lenses that pop out. If the lens pops out spontaneously or springs forth with a small flick of the lid, it is too loose or too thick at the edges. *Removal should be controlled.* The lenses should not be ejected onto a sink or floor. They may become contaminated or scratched.

Before the end of a lesson in insertion and removal, the patient should have a set of written or typed instructions regarding what to do if lenses cannot be removed. A few instructions may defuse a potential emergency. For example, a small pamphlet, outlining emergency procedures is helpful.

"What to do if you cannot get your lens out of your eye"

1. Add a few drops of tears, saline solution, Comfort drops, or anything that will loosen the lens from the eye.
2. Use an eyecup to wash out the lens.
3. Place the head in a basin of water with the drain closed and blink forcefully once or twice.
4. Add a touch of honey to your finger and once or twice touch it to the lens. This is useful for any rigid lens.
5. Have a friend or relative use a small rubber suction cup to remove the lens. If you have this rubber lens remover, do not apply it yourself.
6. Do not be afraid if the lens is on the white of the eye. It can stay on the white coat (the sclera) without being lost behind the eye or causing ocular damage.
7. Do not work excessively to get the lens out. You may cause a corneal abrasion or ulcer. If the techniques to remove the lens fail after one or two passes, call the doctor, the technician, or the emergency department of the hospital.
8. Do not sleep with the lens on unless you have been told to do so.
9. Do not put any medication in the eye except the fluids to loosen the lens.
10. Do not panic. There is little likelihood you will do permanent damage to your eye no matter what happens.

INSERTION BY PRACTITIONER

(Fig. 17-1)

Insertion by the practitioner should be done first to help patients dispel their fears. If this is done smoothly, patients not only experience a sense of relief and accomplishment but also develop more confidence in the ability of the fitter.

1. Have the person look down and cast his or her gaze away from the approaching lens.
2. Retract the upper lid, place the lens above or beside the cornea, and shift it centrally.
3. Let the lens remain in the eye for about 20 minutes. It is important to forewarn the person that the eye may feel irritated, be sensitive to light, and tear after the lens has been inserted. You may reduce some of this early unpleasant foreign-body sensation by asking the patient to keep his or her head up and gaze downward. It is the impact of the upper lid with the margin of the lens that leads to much of the irritation.

Some authorities will use a topical anesthetic when a trial lens is first employed to reduce reflex tearing. It enables a better assessment of the lens-cornea relationship, since a pool of tears can distort the secondary refraction over the lens and interfere with the normal movement of the lens. The major fault of this approach is that it accustoms the patient to a false sense of comfort.

If topical anesthetics are used, they should be used only once, preferably under special circumstances, as with children, excessively nervous people, or people who tear excessively upon attempted insertion of a lens.

Helpful hints on insertion

1. The fitter should attempt to place the lens on the eye of a novice patient without

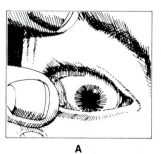 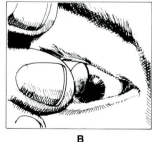 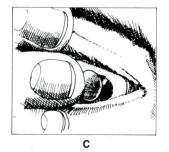

A	B	C

Fig 17-1 ■ Insertion by the fitter. **A,** The lens is placed on the index finger. **B,** The approach is to the side or above avoiding the line of fixation. The upper lid is retracted up and laterally. **C,** Once the lens is applied, the upper lid is used to center the lens.

blocking the line of sight. This avoids the menace of the blink reflex.

2. The apprehensive patient should be asked to open his or her mouth during initial lens insertion. Forced closure of the lids is very difficult to do with the mouth open.

3. The patient should be given something to look at. Controlled fixation invariably makes insertion easy. Both eyes should be kept open.

4. Retraction of the upper lid should be gentle. A forceful maneuver invites a strong lid-closure response.

REMOVAL BY PRACTITIONER

(Fig. 17-2)

Removal of the lens is easier for the practitioner, and the following method should be used:

1. Squeeze the lens off by the thumbs of each hand by applying pressure on the upper or lower lids, respectively.

2. Alternatively, apply the fingers of one hand to the outer canthal region, resting on the upper and lower lids. The patient's eyes should be kept wide open so that the lid

margin can engage the lens. A voluntary blink coupled with a lateral jerk of the lids to increase the lid tension is usually sufficient to dislodge the lens.

INSERTION BY PATIENT

(Fig. 17-3)

There are two natural motions that the novice must overcome—a desire to look away and a desire to close the eyes as the lens is brought near. One can control the blink response by placing the free hand near the margin of the lid and retracting it. The position of the eye can be controlled by fixation. A mirror is most helpful so that the patient can watch his or her own eye.

1. Depress the lower lid with the middle finger while the index finger carrying the lens is gently applied to the cornea.

2. Slowly release the lids to avoid accidental ejection of the lens. Release the lower lid first and then the upper.

Alternate approaches

1. Retract the lids with the index finger retracting the upper lid and the middle fin-

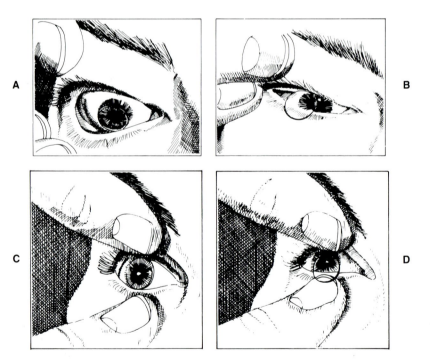

Fig 17-2 ■ Two methods of removal by the fitter: (1) **A,** The lids are held wide apart and pulled laterally. **B,** The lid margin catches the upper and lower edges of the lens and displaces it. A scissors movement by the lids ejects the lens. (2) **C,** The thumbs of both hands are placed on the upper and lower lids, respectively. **D,** The lids are brought together, squeezing the lens off the eye.

ger depressing the lower lid. Carry the lens on the index finger of the other hand.

2. For the nervous patient the lens-carrying finger is the middle one. It is supported by the fourth finger, upon which it rests as the lens is carried toward the cornea.

Helpful hints on insertion

1. Most lenses are lost or damaged in the first few months because of clumsy handling techniques. The novice should be extra-careful with the lenses during this period. Drains should be closed before the lenses

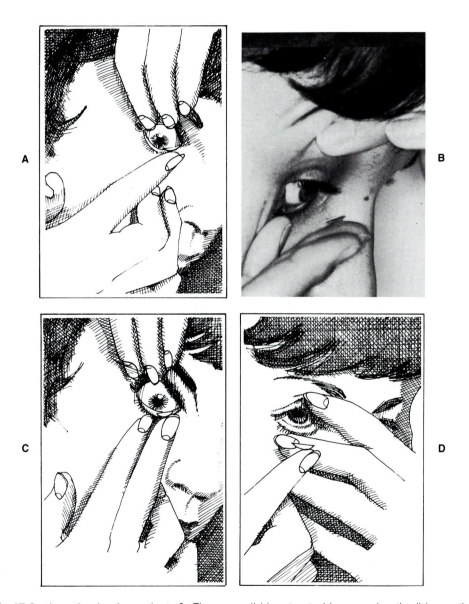

Fig 17-3 ■ Insertion by the patient. **A,** The upper lid is retracted by grasping the lid near the margin and retracting it. The left hand is used to elevate the right upper lid. The patient's gaze is directed downward, and the lens is carried to the eye by the index finger of the right hand. **B,** Incorrect method—the upper lid should be grasped near the lid margin, and the lens should rest on the tip of the finger. **C,** For the unsteady or tremulous patient, the middle finger carrying the lens rests on the index finger. **D,** The lids are separated by the index finger retracting the upper lid and the middle finger depressing the lower lid. The index finger of the free hand brings the lens to the eye. *cont'd*

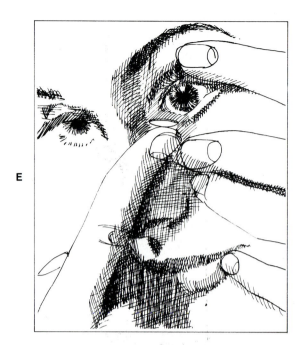

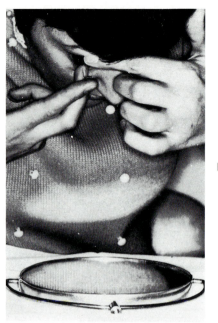

Fig 17-3, cont'd ■ **E,** The lids are separated laterally between the index and middle fingers while the hand opposite the eye carries the lens. **F,** Use of a mirror for insertion of a lens.

are rinsed with water. A good lens case should have a rinsing chamber so that the risk of accidental loss can be eliminated. A dropped lens should not be grasped directly between the thumb and forefinger; instead the finger should be moistened and the lens lifted. Insertion and removal should initially be done over a desk covered by a white towel so that the lens is easy to find if it falls and so that it can be cushioned on impact.

2. Suction-cup devices may be used by an assistant in dealing with children or the elderly. They should not be given to a new lens patient. If the lens happens to be decentered upon removal, a suction cup may take off the corneal epithelium.

3. The patient should be told to be gentle and that the lens will adhere to the eye if brought close enough. Some patients will try to ram the lens on the cornea and will abrade it.

REMOVAL BY PATIENT

(Fig. 17-4)

Removal of the lens may cause more apprehension than insertion does. Failure to insert a lens results in frustration. Failure to remove a lens creates a problem that can result in panic.

Fear that the lens cannot be removed makes the exercise more difficult, and a vicious cycle can result. Furthermore, with the use of microthin lenses, removal of a lens is even more difficult without a thick edge for the lid to dislodge.

The simplest method is the following:

1. Look downward, open the lids wide so that the edge of the lid will engage the edge of the lens, draw the lid tight by a lateral pull of the index finger, and blink. The lid should dislodge the lens.

2. Cup the other hand under the eye to catch the lens.

Alternate approaches

One-handed method. Draw the upper lid up and out with the thumb while the same hand is cupped under the eye to catch the lens.

Scissors technique. Hold the upper lid by the index finger and the lower by the middle finger, apply lateral traction to the lids, and squeeze the lens off by a scissors motion.

RECENTERING A DISPLACED LENS

(Figs. 17-5 and 17-6)

The displaced lens must first be located. A lens that is decentered inferiorly, temporally, or nasally is usually easily seen. If the lens if dis-

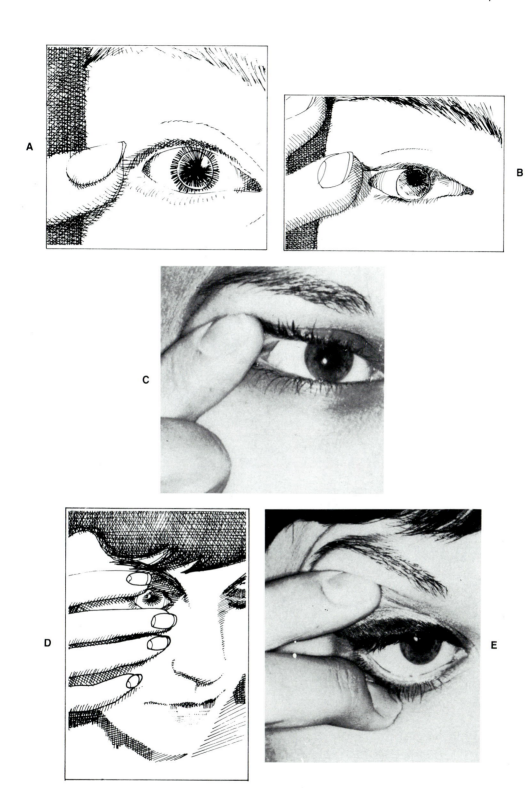

Fig 17-4 ■ Removal by the patient. **A** through **C,** The index finger tugs at the lateral canthus in an outward and upward direction. If the lids are held widely open, the edge of the lid margin should engage the lens and dislodge it. **D** and **E,** The open-handed scissors method. The lids are opened widely and the index and middle fingers are applied to the upper and lower lids to squeeze the lens off the eye.

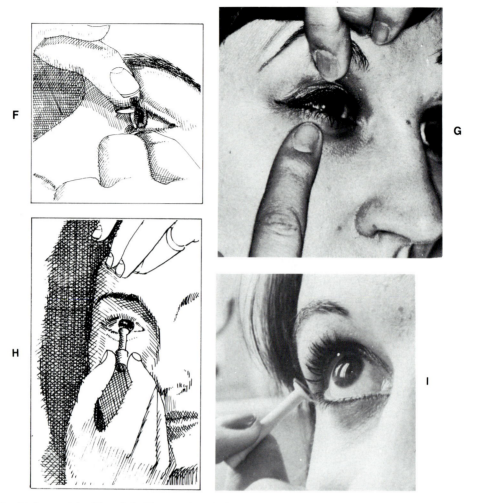

Fig 17-4, cont'd ■ **F** and **G,** The two-handed scissors method. **H** and **I,** The use of a suction cup is best delegated to an assistant to avoid inadvertent application of the cup to the cornea.

placed upward, assistance is often needed to find the lens in the superior cul-de-sac. The eye must be rotated downward and the lid retracted; under good illumination the lens can easily be located.

The following approaches may be successfully used to replace the lens onto the surface of the cornea:

1. Manipulate the lens by the fingers through the closed lid until it is centered.
2. Move the eyes in a direction opposite to the position of the lens. The lens is centered by manipulation and held there; then the eye is rotated centrally, sliding under the held lens.
3. Push the lens into position by using the upper and lower lid margins. This method applies only to superiorly and inferiorly displaced lenses.
4. Pinion the lens by the index fingers of both hands and rotate the eye slowly and deliberately toward the lens until it moves under it.

Lost lenses

There have been reports of lost lenses found in the upper fornix and even embedded in the conjunctival tissue above the tarsus. A complete search includes eversion of the lids. At times the lost lens may become glued to its mate.

Helpful hints on recentering

1. The patient should manipulate the lens gently through the lids. If too much pres-

sure is applied, the lens becomes more adherent to the conjunctiva and is almost impossible to dislodge. If such a contingency occurs, the patient is best advised to use a suction cup or to put some eye drops into the eye to relieve the suction effect of the lens upon the eye.

2. The lens must climb the limbal ridge to mount the cornea. If pushing movements are forceful, the edge of the lens can get caught on the limbus and cause corneal abrasions and irritation to the eye.
3. At times a practitioner will have difficulty in finding the lens. The most common hid-

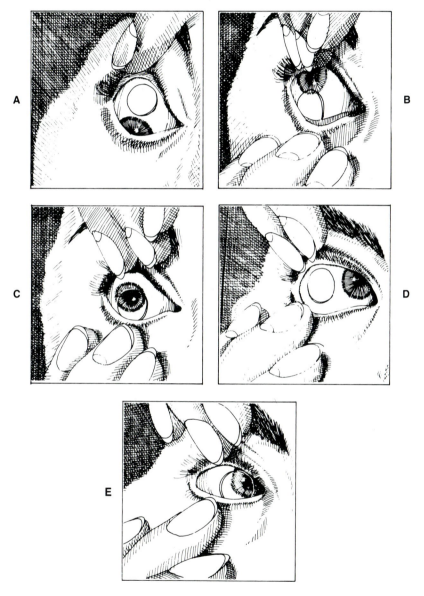

Fig 17-5 ■ Recentering a lens. **A,** The lens is displaced upward. The chin is raised and the eye is lowered while the edge of the upper lid is used to engage the lens and push it down. **B,** The lens is displaced downward. The eye is raised and the lower lid is depressed with the index finger. **C,** Through the lid, the lens is pushed up by an upward movement of the finger. At the same time, the eye is lowered. **D,** The lens is displaced laterally. The eye is moved medially while the index and middle fingers of each hand push the lens centrally. **E,** With the fingers exerting pressure through the lid, the eye is then rotated under the lens.

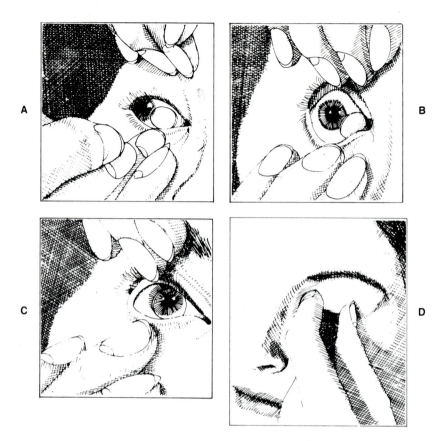

Fig 17-6 ■ The lens is displaced medially. The eye is rotated laterally. **A,** While the fingers are used to secure the lens, the lids are opened and the eye is rotated medially, **B. C,** The eye rotates under the fixed lens. **D,** The lens can frequently be palpated through the closed lid and moved centrally. While it is held there, the eye is rotated under it.

ing place is the superior cul-de-sac. In this case the upper lid should be everted. Fluorescein stain will accent the presence of a lost lens.

FACTORS AFFECTING WEARING SCHEDULE

The rapid adaptation of the presence of a rigid lens depends on several factors:

1. Gas permeability. A gas-permeable lens will benefit the cornea because it reduces the shock of sudden corneal hypoxia. Also the lens has a large diameter and is slightly high-riding. In ideal cases, the upper edge of the lens will be under the upper lid, a position thus eliminating lid impact, which is a major source of discomfort.

2. Edge treatment. If the edges are beveled on their anterior aspect especially for re-

fractive errors greater than 4 diopters, an accelerated schedule may be tolerated, that is, a myopic contour on the periphery of an aphakic lens.

3. Good tear presence, which means a good aqueous tear flow, an intact mucin layer, and an anterior sebaceous film to prevent dehydration. Dry eyes or corneas with a short tear-film breakup time require a longer period of adaptation and shorten the tolerance to full-time wear.

4. A normal blink response. If the patient blinks infrequently or incompletely without lenses, he or she will suffer a long time with the introduction of any kind of lens. The lens will drop to a low position and generally behave as though the lens fit were tight.

5. Favorable anatomic lid position. If the upper lids are retracted above the superior

limbus, or if the lower lids are high, skirting the lower limbus, then lens displacement by the lids will be inevitable and the discomfort factor greater.

6. Tight lids as found with many Oriental lid configurations with strong lid adherence may make a good fit intolerable. The lens will be excessively raised by the action of the lids.

7. Large heavy lenses. Large heavy lenses are more likely to cause corneal edema and lid irritation. If the lenses are not permeable to oxygen, one must proceed very slowly. These lenses tend to ride low, do not rise adequately with a blink, and cause excessive 3 and 9 o'clock staining.

8. An excessive response to a lens. Some patients, especially fair-skinned people, immediately tear, develop puffy lids, and complain of pronounced photophobia. These persons are usually identified in the process of a trial fitting. These individuals may become very apprehensive and show many compensatory reactions to the negative reception of the lens. To reduce lens movement and lid sensation, the person may tilt his head backwards. He may not move his eyes for fear of losing a lens; his eyes are literally frozen with fear. This discomfort may be accentuated when he looks up, a position that makes the lens drop low and strike the lower lid. The patient reacts by squinting the lids close together because of fear of any vertical lens motion. Such patients suffer too much with any rigid lenses and frequently are better off with soft lenses.

9. Corneal edema. Signs of clinical corneal edema in the initial fitting lenses would indicate a slower schedule. Corneal edema may be manifest with the slitlamp through direct or indirect illumination or retro-illumination. It may become apparent through staining of the cornea with fluorescein, which may show central corneal epithelial stippling. A change in K readings, a change in pachometry, or an alteration of the quality of Placido's disc may indicate excessive corneal edema. If clinical corneal edema is clinically evident, the initial wearing schedule must be slowed.

10. The size of the refractive error may be important. With high hyperopes such as aphakic persons, the lenses are three times thicker in the center than that of a myope's lens.

A thick lens may negate the permeability features of lenses, drop low because of gravity, fail to ride up with blinking, and be more prone to cause corneal edema through hypoxia or compression.

The secret to large heavy lenses of high refractive errors is the treatment of the edges. If the edges are not thinned out, they will be bulky, engage the upper lid with blinking, and create considerable discomfort.

A high myope has his own problems except that the added thickness to the lens is at the edges. These lenses are frequently high riding, uncomfortable because of thickened edges, and more prone to cause peripheral corneal erosions. The wearing schedule should be simple and easy to remember. One schedule is to have persons wear their lenses 1 hour every morning, afternoon, and evening on the first day. On each subsequent day 1 hour is added to the schedule three times a day, so that by the third day the lenses are being worn 9 hours a day. The patient is seen on the fourth day after the lenses have been worn 8 hours. By the fifth day the breaks in lens wear can be obliterated. The lenses are first worn through the lunch break and then finally through the afternoon to the evening, so that by the seventh day the lenses are worn full time.

The wearing schedule is highly variable and should fit into the office pattern of the practitioner. One conservative approach is as follows:

Contact lens wearing schedule

First and second day	2 hours in, 1 hour out
Third and fourth day	3 hours in, 2 hours out
Fifth and sixth day	4 hours in, 2 hours out
Seventh and eighth day	5 hours in, 2 hours out
and so on	

Patients are reassessed at the end of 2 weeks for reinforcement sessions on handling of the lenses, office modifications if there are signs of poor fit, and appraisal of the corneal epithelium. Changes in the cornea should not be tolerated. These include staining of the cornea, corneal edema as viewed through retro-illumination or specular reflection, changes in the K readings of 0.60 D or greater, or 0.50 D of spectacle blur.

The wearing schedule must be adjusted to the person's needs. If all systems are favorable, the patient may adapt in a week to the presence of a rigid lens. If there are clinical problems, a month may elapse before full-time wear is established.

COMMENT. With gas-permeable lenses, liberty can be taken in accelerating the adaptation cycle. Frequently we can "adapt" an eye in 4 or 5 days.

Some people can adapt to a rigid lens in a day. However, these people are impossible to define, and so it is risky to use this type of speedy schedule. For those fitters who wish to attempt this kind of fast fit, it is prudent to keep the patient in the office for the first day and check for corneal edema on the first, fourth, and eighth hour of wear. If there is no corneal edema, full-time wear can be attempted.

Basically we advocate a slower schedule because it reduces the chances of sudden hypoxic symptoms. In the beginning it is not wise to accentuate your patient's fears and anxieties about wearing lenses.

Patients who miss 2 or more days of wearing time should revert to their original wearing schedule. If only 1 day is missed, rest periods of 1 hour each at noon and at 6:00 PM are helpful to avoid an overwear reaction. One rest period can be gradually eliminated after 2 days, and the other can be eliminated in 4 days.

When returning home, the patient should be instructed not to persevere with unsuccessful insertions or removals if the eye becomes red and painful. After the initial visit the patient should be seen in 1, 2, and 4 weeks.

COMMENT. Young teenagers frequently have to be restrained when they first obtain lenses. They are anxious to demonstrate their new lenses and frequently will overwear them while attending a party or social function.

Some fitters advocate continuous wear of lenses during sleep. This is possible with gas-permeable lenses of high DK, especially for short naps. The subject of continuous wear of lenses is discussed in detail in Chapter 33.

Liberties, such as short naps, can easily be taken with gas-permeable lenses. If the patient is not careful and wears gas-permeable lenses too fast and too long, corneal edema may occur, but not with the acute painful episode that characterizes PMMA overwear or more precisely acute hypoxic reaction.

18 ▪ *OFFICE MODIFICATION OF RIGID LENSES*

- Polishing compounds
- Blending transition or junction zones
- Reducing optic-zone diameter
- Reducing overall lens diameter
- Flattening intermediate curves
- Adding minus power
- Adding plus power
- Removing scratches
- Polishing and refinishing lens edges
- Adjusting peripheral curves
- Flattening the base curve
- Identifying the lens
- Fenestrating the lens

Some practitioners' disillusionment with soft lenses combined with the advent of new and better rigid lens materials has given cause for the "dusting off" of many a modification unit. Certainly oxygen-permeable materials and improved lens designs give sophistication in fitting, which lessens the need for modifications. However, they may be necessary in some cases, and when this is so, faster and better service can be given to the patient by having modification equipment available in the office.

An added advantage of in-office alteration is that the patient's wearing schedule is not disrupted. Rigid lenses should be worn for a consistent number of hours daily, and if such minor adjustments cannot be done in the office, the wearing schedule will be seriously affected. The patient may be willing to put up with such disruptions initially, but any repetitions that prolong this may culminate in a dissatisfied patient and some irritation with the fitter.

There are many types of modification units available, ranging from the sophisticated and rather expensive to the simple and moderately priced. The simplest unit is recommended for the average lens office; if necessary more elaborate equipment can be added as the need arises (Fig. 18-1).

The following is a list of in-office adjustments that can be made to rigid and rigid gas-permeable lenses.

1. Blending transition or junction zones
2. Reducing optic-zone diameter
3. Reducing overall lens diameter
4. Flattening intermediate curves
5. Adding minus power
6. Adding plus power
7. Removing scratches
8. Polishing and refinishing lens edges
9. Adjusting peripheral curves
10. Identifying the lens
11. Fenestrating the lens
12. Flattening the base curve

All the adjustments that can be made to a lens will have the effect of loosening the fit or increasing tear flow between the lens and cornea. Any adjustments to tighten the fit of a lens necessitate the fabrication of a new lens.

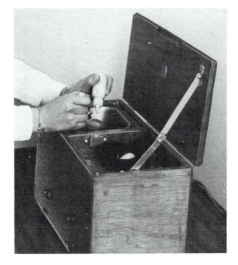

Fig 18-1 ▪ Modification unit for rigid lenses.

POLISHING COMPOUNDS

Most polishing compounds used in lens modification are abrasive agents such as Silvo or Xpal mixed with oil or water. When one is working with gas-permeable materials, a fine compound such as Xpal is the most desirable. It may be mixed with an equal quantity of conventional RGP cleaning solution. Silvo is coarser and lends itself to more scratching of the gas-permeable lenses. There are several commercially available polishing solutions for gas-permeable lenses. BPI of Miami, Florida, and Polymer Technology Corporation of Wilmington, Massachusetts, are two companies that market these solutions. They are already mixed to the proper consistency and are preferred by us especially to polish lenses that are made of the more sensitive fluoro-silicone acrylates.

BLENDING TRANSITION OR JUNCTION ZONES

The junction zones between the central, intermediate, and peripheral posterior curves can be examined with an instrument called a *profile analyzer*. The blends may also be evaluated by observing the reflection of a fluorescent tube on the posterior surface of the lens. If the reflection toward the edge of the lens is a soft "J"-shaped curve, the blending is adequate. If the reflection shows more of a sharp "V" shape, the blending

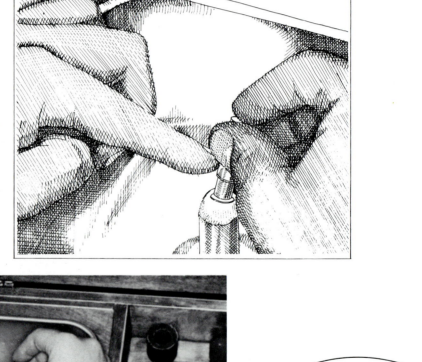

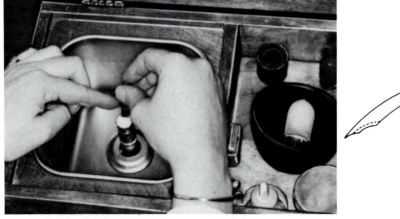

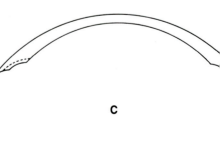

Fig 18-2 ■ A and **B,** Blending junction zones. **C,** Blending transition zones to eliminate sharpness of junction zones.

is poor and the junctions are sharp. If these junction zones are not smooth, they can interfere with the tear exchange under the lens, thus causing "tightlens" symptoms. If the junction zones are extremely sharp, they may cause irritation in the same manner as a sharp lens edge (Fig. 18-2).

To blend the transition zones of a lens, a radius tool is used, the radius of curvature of which is halfway between either the central posterior curve (CPC) and the intermediate posterior curve (IPC), or the intermediate posterior curve and the peripheral posterior curve (PPC). The radius tool should be covered with a felt-surfaced polishing tape. This tape is usually 0.2 mm thick, and its thickness must be taken into consideration when the alteration is made. For example,

CPC	42.00 D or 8.04 mm
IPC	38.00 D or 8.88 mm
Halfway radius	40.00 D or 8.44 mm
Less allowance for tape	0.20 mm
Thus select tool	= 8.24 mm

Since tools are standardized and come in increments of 0.2 mm, ranging from 7.6 to 10.0 mm, an 8.2 mm tool should be used. The unit also has 11.0 and 12.0 mm tools.

Either the lens is held by a suction cup (convex side against the holder, concave side against the tool), or it is mounted with double-sided adhesive tape on a small lens block. The lens block is supported against the rotating radius tool by a pencil or other pointed object inserted into a hole on the top of the lens block. This enables the lens to spin freely while the radius tool rotates. A polishing compound is used in blending to prevent scraching of the lens surface.

Blending a lens takes only a few minutes. Practice enables the fitter to estimate how long it will take to smooth out these transition zones.

COMMENT. Sometimes blending can make a fit tighter by bringing the lens closer to the cornea.

Fig. 18-3 illustrates the pattern of a fluorescent tubelight on the posterior surface of a lens. It is a fast way to evaluate blending.

REDUCING OPTIC-ZONE DIAMETER

If blending a lens does not alleviate the problems of tight fit, the next modification would be to reduce the optic-zone diameter. The optic zone determines the stability of the lens, and the size and curvature of this zone determine how loose or tight the fit will be. This modification is similar to that of blending a lens. A tool is selected that has a radius of curvature halfway between that of the central posterior curve and the intermediate or peripheral posterior curve and the intermediate or peripheral posterior

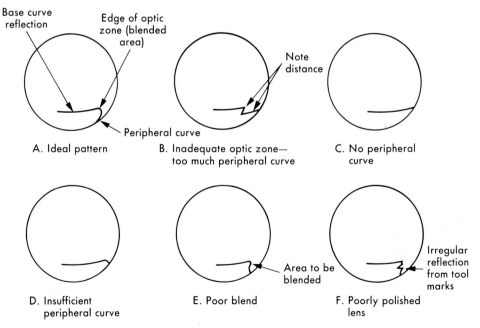

A. Ideal pattern

B. Inadequate optic zone—too much peripheral curve

C. No peripheral curve

D. Insufficient peripheral curve

E. Poor blend

F. Poorly polished lens

Fig 18-3 ■ Verification of blending transition zones with fluorescent tubelighting.

curve, allowing 0.2 mm for the thickness of the tape. The length of time of polishing will determine how much the optic zone needs to be reduced.

Another method of reducing the optic zone is to increase the width of the intermediate or peripheral curve. One does this by using a diamond-impregnated tool of the same radius as was used in the original grinding of the intermediate and peripheral zones with grinding maintained for a longer period. This type of tool should be soaked in water before use and should be kept moistened while the lens is being modified, to avoid burn spots on the lens. Polishing compounds should not be used with this type of tool. After the diamond-impregnated tool is used, the surface of the lens will be quite rough, and so it must be polished with a regular tool covered with velveteen, using a polishing compound.

REDUCING OVERALL LENS DIAMETER

The trend in fitting gas-permeable lenses is to use larger diameters than those with PMMA, as has been the practice. It is therefore important that a fitter be knowledgeable in the reduction of lens diameter. If blending, reduction of the optic zone, or flattening of the intermediate and peripheral curves does not solve the problem of a tight lens, reduction of the diameter may solve the problem. Again, with experience in lens-fitting this may be the first modification done if the diameter of the lens appears too large. A good rule of thumb to follow in the reduction of diameter is: reducing the overall diameter of a lens by 0.1 mm is the equivalent of blending the peripheral curves 0.2 mm. The diameter may be assessed on a V-groove diameter gauge (Fig. 18-4). There are several techniques available for reducing the diameter of a lens.

Razor-blade technique

The lens is centered and mounted on a spindle with double-sided adhesive tape, and the blade is contoured around the lens edge as the lens rotates. Accurate centering of the lens is of the utmost importance (Fig. 18-5). The blade must be kept wet or moist; otherwise the friction it creates will cause the lens to crack. After this the lens edge must be polished. Adjustments to the peripheral curves may then become necessary. Variations of this technique involve the use of files or other grinding material (Fig. 18-6).

Conic-stone technique

In this technique a diamond-impregnated 60- or 70-degree hollow stone is used. The lens is held with its convex side against the suction cup

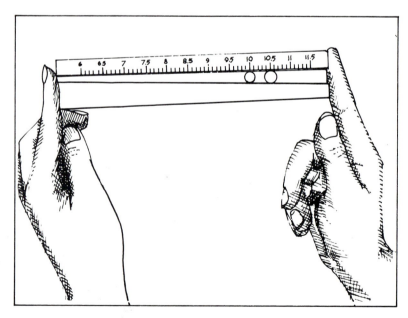

Fig 18-4 ■ Diameter gauge. The lens is inserted at the widest opening and allowed to slide to its position of rest.

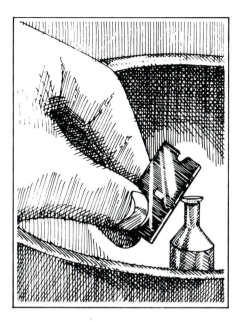

Fig 18-5 ■ Reducing diameter with razor blade.

and gently rocked in the hollow tool (Fig. 18-7). Care must be taken to keep the tool wet during this procedure. Once the diameter of a lens is reduced, the peripheral and intermediate curves have to be reapplied and blended and the edge of the lens refinished. Therefore the diameter should be reduced to approximately 0.1 mm larger than the finished diameter. For example, a lens with a diameter of 9.5 mm that needs to be reduced to 9.0 mm should initially be reduced to 9.1 mm; the edge refinishing and polishing will yield a lens of 9.0 mm diameter.

COMMENT. Most laboratories work on a diameter tolerance of 0.1 mm.

FLATTENING INTERMEDIATE CURVES

The intermediate curve of a lens can be flattened when one blends the lens with a felt-covered tool of a flatter radius than the intermediate curve of the lens.

ADDING MINUS POWER

Up to −1.00 D can be added to a lens by use of a velveteen- or sponge-covered drum tool (Fig. 18-8). The lens is held on a suction cup (concave side against the holder) away from the center of rotation of the drum tool. The lens is rotated a full 360 degrees against the rotation of the drum for one or two turns. The drum tool must be kept wet with polish during this procedure.

Another method of adding minus power is to use a velveteen cloth, which is placed on a thin foam backing. A 4- or 5-inch diameter circle of polish is put on the cloth. The lens is held against the cloth with the index finger, and the lens is rotated around the circle with the lens being

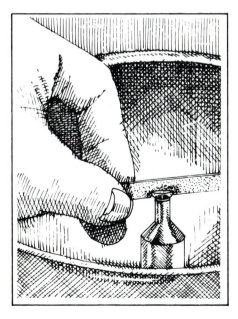

Fig 18-6 ■ Reducing diameter with emery board.

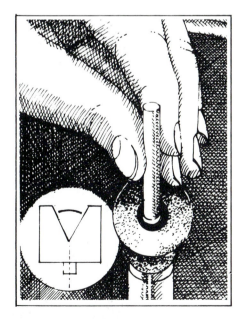

Fig 18-7 ■ Reducing diameter with conic stone.

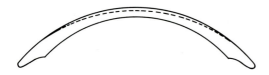

Fig 18-8 ■ Adding minus power.

kept free of any wobble. It should be rotated clockwise for three rotations and counterclockwise for three rotations, after which the power is inspected. Care must be taken not to use excessive pressure because this will cause distortion in the optic figure.

ADDING PLUS POWER

Up to +1.00 D can be added to a lens. The procedure for adding plus power is similar to that for adding minus power, but the lens should be held slightly off the center of rotation of the drum tool and rotated so that the lens thickness is reduced more at the edge than at the center; thus the anterior curve is steepened.

REMOVING SCRATCHES

Scratches on the anterior surface of a lens will interfere with the wetting characteristics of the lens. In this age of gas-permeable rigid lenses, this can be an extensive problem. As a result of the "softness" of some of the gas-permeable materials and the difficulty in wetting them, the lenses may require regular polishing. The accumulation of mucus, oils, and fat lipids in the scratches causes poor wetting of the lens and thus foggy vision. In addition, there can be discomfort from the rough lens surface.

To remove scratches from the anterior surface of a lens, place the lens on a suction cup, concave side against the holder, apply the front surface of the lens against a rotating felt-covered drum tool and gently buff and polish the front surface (Fig. 18-9).

To remove scratches from the posterior surface of a lens, a steep tool such as one with a 6.9 mm radius is used. The tool should be covered with a narrow strip of molefoam, approximately 1⅛ inches wide and 2 to 2½ inches long. The tool is wet with polish, and the concave side of the lens is placed on the tool using a suction cup while the tool spins. Scratches on the inside of a lens cannot easily be removed without causing changes in the curvature of the lens, which often necessitates replacement of the lens.

POLISHING AND REFINISHING LENS EDGES

There are several methods available to the fitter for polishing and refinishing lens edges, including the rag-wheel, felt-disc, and Con-Lish methods. Of these three, the one most often used is the felt-disc method because of its simplicity.

Rag-wheel method

The rag wheel is mounted on the spindle and the lens is held on a spinner. A suction cup or brass rod may be used, but one must take care to avoid burn spots by turning the tool by hand. Liberal use of a polishing compound is also recommended to reduce the incidence of surface burn caused by friction. The lens should be held against the rag wheel in three positions for equal time: (1) 45 degrees above horizontal, (2) horizontal, and (3) 45 degrees below horizontal.

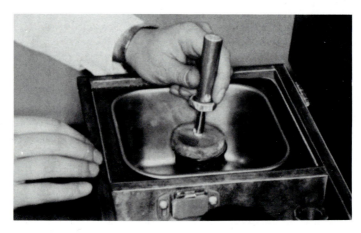

Fig 18-9 ■ Polishing lens on velveteen with Silvo polish to remove scratches.

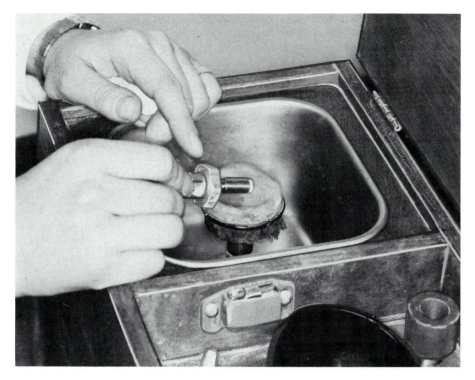

Fig 18-10 ■ Use of a felt disc in polishing edges of rigid lens.

Felt-disc method

A small, round disc covered with moleskin or velveteen is used in this method. The lens is fixed to a spinner with double-sided tape, and a polishing compound is used. The spinner is held at a 45-degree angle against the disc, midway between the center of rotation and the circumference of the disc. The lens should be gently pressed while the angle is being simultaneously reduced to 10 degrees. This process is used for both sides of the lens and is an excellent method for in-office adjustments (Figs. 18-10 and 18-11).

Con-Lish method

Five separate tools are used in this method. Four tools have concave cones of different degrees—40, 60, 90, and 140—and the fifth tool is a flat tool. All the tools are lined with velveteen or moleskin, and the lens is held with double-sided adhesive tape on a rod or by a suction cup. The procedure is as follows:

1. Place lens convex side down on 60-degree tool for 10 seconds at 110 rpm.
2. Place lens convex side down on 40-degree tool for 5 seconds at 110 rpm.

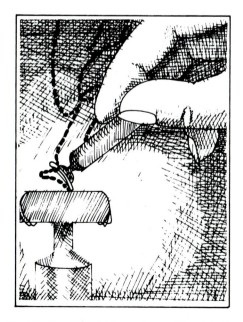

Fig 18-11 ■ Refinishing edges with a felt disc.

3. Place lens concave side down on flat tool for 20 seconds at 110 rpm.
4. Place lens concave side down on 140-degree tool for 15 seconds at 110 rpm.
5. Place lens concave side down on 90-degree tool for 10 seconds at 110 rpm.
6. Place lens concave side down on 60-degree tool for 5 seconds at 110 rpm.
7. Place lens concave side down on 40-degree tool for 2 seconds at 110 rpm.

The advantage of this method is that it standardizes the shape of the lens edge and is therefore good for duplication. Another advantage is that it produces an edge with the outside shaped away from the eyelid and the inside shaped away from the cornea. This method is good for lenses with relatively thick edges.

ADJUSTING PERIPHERAL CURVES

Peripheral curves can be flattened, widened, or blended. The basic technique for flattening or widening the peripheral curves is to use a diamond-impregnated tool of the appropriate radius. The diamond tool should be soaked in water before use and kept wet during use. Silvo polish or other polishing compounds should not be used with such tools. The lens is held with a suction cup with its concave surface against the tool away from the center of rotation. The lens is rotated in a direction counter to the rotation of the tool. Once the desired peripheral curve is achieved, the lens should be polished with a felt-covered radius tool soaked with polishing solution.

FLATTENING THE BASE CURVE

Although infrequently done, flattening of the base curve of a lens can be done. The base curve of most rigid lenses can be flattened by about 0.50 diopter or 0.10 mm. The lens is with its convex side against the suction cup, and the concave side is placed against a tape-covered tool of the same radius of curvature as the lens. The lens is held directly on the center of the tool. Polishing solution should be added every 5 seconds to avoid burning and blurring of the optic figure. The base curve should be rechecked on the optic spherometer (Radiuscope) after every three of these 5-second applications on the tool.

The principle of this procedure is that the outer edge of the tool is rotating faster than the center and so a greater amount of material will be taken off at the periphery of the tool than at the center, resulting in a flatter lens. This is *not* recommended for fluorosilicone acrylate materials.

IDENTIFYING THE LENS

If one requests it, most laboratories will put an identification mark such as a red dot, on the right lens, but again this can be done very simply by the fitter if the need arises. A toothpick shaved to produce a fine point or a similar thin-pointed object is dipped in lens identification ink, which is available from most lens manufacturers. After the toothpick is dipped into the ink, the tip should be touched to a piece of paper to remove any excess ink. The peripheral, convex surface of the lens should then be touched with the tip of the toothpick, After several minutes the lens should be rubbed with the fingers over the spot to remove any excess ink, and the lens should then be allowed to dry completely for 10 to 15 minutes before use.

Unfortunately ink or nail polish will wear off the lens with time. A small hole can be burred into the front surface of the lens with a dental burr or a small hand-held drill after which the hole is filled with nail polish. This type of identification never wears off; even though the nail polish may rub off, the red mark becomes a white dot because of the hole in the lens. This method is very good for office use. A small, inexpensive instrument may be purchased to burr the hole into the lens.

More elaborate instruments are available to mark "R" or any other letter on the lens.

FENESTRATING THE LENS

Putting a hole in a lens is not a way of allowing more oxygen to get to the cornea. Only 1 mm around the hole benefits from an added oxygen supply. Bascially fenestration has the effect of loosening the fit of a lens. Holes can be made on the center of a lens or at the outer periphery. Although this cannot be done with the modification unit, a small fenestration instrument can be purchased if necessary (Fig. 18-12). The fenestration unit contains drill bits, mounting arbor, dental wax to hold the lens in position, and a countersinking bit for removing burrs from the posterior surface of the lens. A fine oil is used to prepare the drill for cutting into the plastic lens without causing the heat to be absorbed by the lens itself. Fenestrating a lens affects the tear lens dynamics. The holes provide oxygen only in the area under the lens near the holes.

COMMENT. Although all the previously mentioned adjustments to lenses are possible, the ones most commonly done are blending transition zones, adding minus power, removing sur-

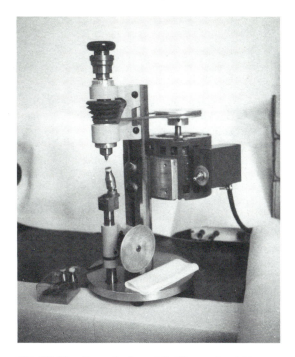

Fig 18-12 ■ Fenestration drill. There should be no visible cracks dispersing from the drill hole area because of stress caused by the drilling operation.

face scratches, and dotting or redotting lenses for identification.

Hands-on practice

The only way to become proficient in the art of lens modification is with practice. One must obtain a modification unit and work with contact lenses. If possible, go to a nearby RGP laboratory for some instruction. It is to the laboratory's advantage that the fitter be able to solve many of the minor lens modification problems in the office. Most laboratories will be more than happy to supply you with reject lenses with which to practice.

Surface-cracking. Surface-cracking has occurred with some of the RGP plastics. Surface-cracking has been reported by Grohe, Norman & Caroline as a result of a number of factors. See the outline that follows.

A. Mechanical pressure
   — Manufacturing process
   — Modification/polishing
   — Handling/flexing
B. Physical factors
   — Heat accumulation
   — Rapid temperature change

— Alkaline pH
— Ultraviolet radiation
— Dehydration/evaporation
— Polymer composition
C. Organic fluids
   — Alcohol
   — Some solvents
   — Some surfactants

If cracking does occur, micro-organisms can enter the fissure, be retained, and eventually produce corneal ulceration. Overpolishing can induce irreversible cracking. Microcracks may occur that may not be identified with standard low-power magnification.

In addition, overpolishing of high-DK material can result in scorching of the material because of heat buildup.

It is recommended that copious amounts of the manufacturer's recommended polishing solution be used in a continuous delivery to minimize heat buildup. Much slower spindle speeds may be required to decrease friction. Alternatively, hand-polishing, using lighter digital pressure, may be the best method.

All modifications outlined in this chapter may be applied to any rigid lens that has not been surface treated in some manner. Some helpful hints are as follows:

1. Use a fine polishing compound for all modifications to PMMA, CAB, and PMMA-silicone materials. When this is done, the same tools and pads may be used for adjusting any lens. Although the modification may take longer with the harder materials, it is not necessary for a total cleanup of the equipment after each adjustment.

2. Apply light pressure for short periods before checking the result. It is very easy to overadjust a lens.

3. Constantly add polishing solvent to avoid friction buildup, which will distort the lens.

Knowledge and expertise in making any of these adjustments increases the confidence of the fitter, which in turn is communicated to the patient.

Since many people lose at least one lens per year, it is advisable that each patient have a spare set of rigid lenses. This eliminates the problem of losing wearing time and the possible resulting overwear reaction that may occur if the patient tries to resume the same wearing schedule.

19 ▪ *LENS SOLUTIONS FOR CLEANING AND DISINFECTING RIGID LENSES*

- ▪ *What is wetting?*
- ▪ *Wet or dry storage*
- ▪ *Combination solution*
- ▪ *Cleaning the lens*
- ▪ *Lens cases*
- ▪ *Gas-permeable lens care*
- ▪ *Patient responsibility*

WHAT IS WETTING?

A drop of liquid on a solid may behave in one of two ways: it may aggregate in droplets because of *cohesion*—the attraction of molecules in the liquid for each other—or it may spread over the surface of the solid because of *adhesion*—the attraction of molecules in the liquid to the molecules in the solid.

The relative values between the forces of adhesion and cohesion are expressed as the angle of contact—θ (theta) (Fig. 19-1). For water and glass, θ is 0 degrees, which is complete wetting of the solid by the liquid. Mercury on glass

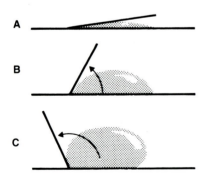

Fig 19-1 ▪ The smaller the angle of contact (θ), the greater the spreading of a liquid over a solid. A rigid lens is hydrophobic and has a 60-degree angle of contact with water. **A,** Low-wetting angle; **B,** wetting angle of polymethylmethacrylate rigid lens; **C,** large wetting angle with droplet of mercury.

has a θ value grater than 90 degrees; it does not spread but gathers into spheric droplets. A hydrophilic solid has a contact angle of 0 degrees, since a liquid will spread over its surface. Polymethylmethacrylate is relatively hydrophobic; its contact angle with water is 60 degrees.

Wetting solution

A wetting solution serves to improve the wettability of the lens. This allows the tear film to uniformly spread over the surface of the lens rather than break up into droplets (Fig. 19-2). It also coats the lens and helps to prevent oils and debris from being transferred from the finger to the lens (Fig. 19-3). During insertion it helps the lens adhere to the finger.

Tears will also wet polymethylmethacrylate, provided that the lens that is inserted into the eye is perfectly clean. There is a time lag, however, and the patient may experience discomfort until the tears coat the lens.

Saliva has been used by some patients as a wetting agent. Natural saliva is an excellent wetting agent because it contains a conjugated polysaccharide similar to that of the precorneal tear film. However, *Pseudomonas aeruginosa* is found as an indigenous oral flora in the saliva of 6.6% of the population. Besides this microbe, yeasts, fungi, protozoa, gram-positive and gram-negative cocci, and rods make up part of the host oral flora of saliva. Urine on the other hand is usually sterile. Neither is advocated, though the latter is the cleaner of the two.

Wetting solutions are composed of the following:

1. A preservative—benzalkonium chloride (BAK) or thimerosal
2. A wetting agent—polyvinyl alcohol, poly-N-vinylpyrrolidone (PVP), or ethylenediaminetetraacetic acid (EDTA).

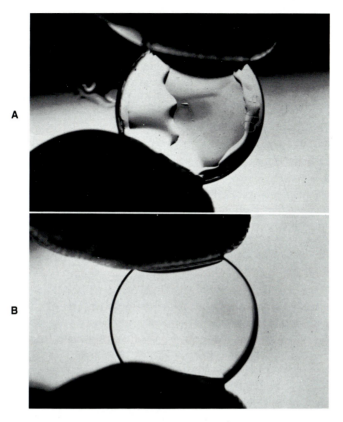

Fig 19-2 ■ **A,** Improperly cleaned and wetted lens. **B,** Lens properly wetted. (From Camp RN, Moore CD, and Soper JW: Handling of the lens—insertion, removal, cleaning, and storage. In Girard LJ, editor: Corneal contact lenses, St Louis, 1970, The CV Mosby Co.)

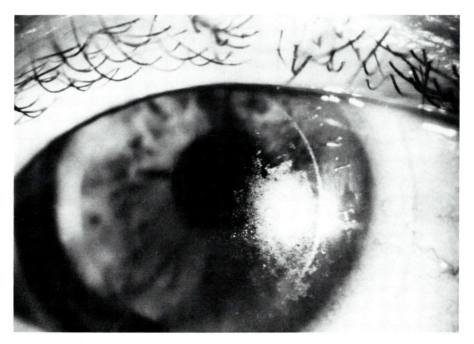

Fig 19-3 ■ Poor wetting of the surface of a Silsoft lens after it had been lost from the eye for 24 hours.

3. A buffering system—the pH of the solution should be compatible with that of the precorneal film, 7.3 to 7.8
4. Methylcellulose—viscosity and cushioning effects
5. Sodium chloride—control of tonicity

Commercial solutions vary as to the concentrations of ingredients, buffering systems, and the substitution of act-alike compounds. No household product can be used as an effective substitute.

Improved wetting of a rigid lens has been aided by incorporating cross-linking agents that have an affinity for water and are part of the polymethylmethacrylate molecule. This new material, commercially sold under different trade names, is considered to be stable and easily fabricated and has a very low degree of water absorption. Improving surface wettability aids comfort and reduces lens awareness. Lenses of this material have a reduced surface friction and resist the accumulation of mucus and other debris on their surface. One drawback is that, over time, these lenses lose some of their wetting properties. The clinical significance of the slightly reduced wetting angles and the manufacturer's claims is controversial.

COMMENT. Some concerns have been expressed that preservatives diminish the wettability of solutions. However, Dziabo and others have shown that preservatives have little effect on altering the wettability of RGP lens solutions.

Storage solution

A storage solution primarily functions to eliminate or reduce to tolerable levels pathogens contaminating the surface of the lens. It also serves to clean the lens and keep it wet. Wetting of the lens should follow soaking to render the lens more hydrophilic (more wettable). Characteristics of some brands are shown in Table 19-1.

Soaking solutions should be changed daily after use. Some of the solutions evaporate, whereas in others activation of the preservative occurs by debris introduced into the solution by the lens or the patient's finger. The cost of a daily change of soaking solution is not great (approximately 10¢ per day), which is certainly within the means of any lens wearer.

The active disinfection ingredient in a soaking solution is the preservative. The common preservatives are benzalkonium chloride, chlorobutanol, and organic mercurials.

Benzalkonium chloride. Benzalkonium chloride is a quaternary ammonium compound. It is an effective germicide but in high concentrations (0.03% 1:2000) can cause superficial punctate keratitis, whereas in weak solutions it is not strong enough to provide a germicidal effect. Presently, concentrations of 1.75, 0.0133% solutions are used. Benzalkonium chloride is the best and most effective preservative against *Pseudomonas*. Benzalkonium chloride can reduce surface wettability over time on certain silicone acrylates. It has been reported that BAK, which is positively charged, will bind and

Table 19-1 ■ Gas-permeable wetting & soaking storage solutions: some comparative systems

	Barnes-Hind GP Wetting & Soaking	Allergen Wet-N-Soak	Boston Conditioning Solution*
Approved for these lenses	Polycon, Paraperm, Boston, Optacryl, and all other silicone/acrylates	Paraperm, Fluoroperm, Polycon	Boston, Boston Equalens, Paraperm, Polycon, and all other silicone/acrylates
Wetting agents	0.5% PVA	2.5% PVA	0.5% PVA
Viscosity	20 cs; moderate	35 cs; high	23 cs; moderate to high
Solids' content	1.9%	2.5%	2.5%
Preservatives	Chlorhexidine gluconate 0.005%, EDTA 0.02%	Benzalkonium chloride 0.004%, EDTA 0.05%	Chlorhexidine gluconate 0.006% EDTA 0.05
Tonicity	Isotonic	Isotonic	Hypertonic
pH	7.1	7.0	7.0

*Similar to Bausch & Lomb Wetting & Soaking

concentrate on negatively charged silicone-based lens material and that, over time, this binding will render the surface hydrophobic. This may lead to an unstable tear film, corneal dry spots, and superficial punctate keratitis.

Chlorobutanol. Chlorobutanol is a relatively slow bactericide and fungicide that possesses synergistic activity when combined with benzalkonium chloride. It is volatile, and conceivably its concentration can fall below useful levels. In recent years, some manufacturers have removed it from their products or have reduced its concentration by 50%. Bacteria can attach itself to chlorobutanol.

Organic mercurials. Organic mercurials are largely bacteriostatic in activity and are not as effective as other preservatives against gram-negative organisms, especially *Pseudomonas*. However, in high enough concentrations and when used with other agents, they can be an effective disinfectant. Thimerosal is the most commonly used mercurial. It can be irritating and sensitizing after repeated instillations and is now being eliminated from most contact lens' solutions.

WET OR DRY STORAGE

Dry storage was the most favored in the days of PMMA lenses. Its advocates claimed that *Pseudomonas* had been cultured from soaking solutions and that a dry lens minimized the replication of bacteria.

However, with the new silicone acrylates and fluorocarbon silicone acrylates, the fitting with lenses that have been "conditioned" by a conditioning and storage solution has become crucial. These conditioned lenses are more comfortable to insert and to wear. Also, a rigid lens tends to flatten with hydration so that when the lens is stored dry it is constantly changing and only becomes stable after 24 to 48 hours of hydration.

Ordinary tap water is sometimes used by patients for storage. This should be discouraged because the halogen component of tap water can be irritating and sensitizing to the tissues. Also, tap water creates a hypotonic layer of water on the surface of the lens, which can be irritating when the lens is inserted.

COMMENT. We highly recommend wet storage for the rigid gas-permeable lens because it renders it more comfortable and results in greater accuracy and reliability in fitting. This is also our recommendation for our trial-fitting sets.

COMBINATION SOLUTION

A combination solution is one with chemicals that permit cleaning, soaking, and wetting or just soaking and wetting. The major advantages of a combination solution are improved patient compliance, convenience, and some economy. The chemicals perform adequately together, but certainly not as well as when the individual solutions are used separately. For instance, the preservative is usually benzalkonium chloride with ethylenediaminetetraacetic acid (EDTA) as a synergist. This preservative inhibits wetting so that a lens stored in a combined solution may cause discomfort upon insertion. In some combined solutions the preservative phenylmercuric nitrate 1:25,000 has been shown to be relatively ineffective against *Pseudomonas*. Thimerosal as a preservative has the same disadvantage. At the present time there is no all-purpose solution that is not a compromise.

CLEANING THE LENS

If a lens becomes smudged with dried mucus, oil, nail polish, nicotine, or a nonsoluble cosmetic (Fig. 19-4), it can be cleaned by the patient with a cleaner. Comparisons of cleaners are outlined in Tables 19-2 and 19-3. Some household cleaners, such as shampoo, may be used on PMMA lenses. However, some detergents of this type may be harmful to the softer gas-permeable materials or, if not properly rinsed off, may act as an ocular irritant.

Basic methods of cleaning

Basic methods of cleaning rigid lenses include friction rubbing, hydraulic cleaning, ultrasonic cleaning, and spray cleaning.

Friction rubbing. This is the application of a cleaning solution to the surface of the lens, followed by rubbing the lens between the thumb and forefinger or forefinger and palm. This is the least efficient method and over a period of time can lead to warping or scratching of the lens because finger roughness is quite common.

Hydraulic cleaning. In this method the lens is placed in a container that permits back-and-forth pumping action. Frequently, this is accomplished by manual agitation of the entire unit. This is an excellent method.

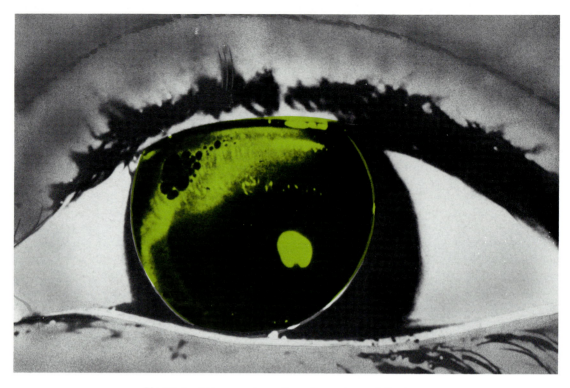

Fig 19-4 ■ Mascara deposit on the surface of the lens.

Table 19-2 ■ Representative gas-permeable cleaners

	Barnes-Hind GP Daily Cleaner	Allergan Easy Clean/GP	Boston Cleaner*
Approved for these lenses	Polycon, Paraperm, Boston, Optacryl, and all other silicone/acrylates	All silicone/acrylates	Boston, Boston Equalens, Paraperm, Polycon, and all other silicone/acrylates
Cleaning methods	Hydrodynamic cleaning with Hydra Mat II or digital Highly concentrated cleaning agents	Manual	Manual—contains insoluble, abrasive particles
Preservatives	Potassium sorbate 0.13% EDTA 2.0%	None	None

*Similar formula to Bausch & Lomb Concentrated Cleaner

Table 19-3 ■ Intensive cleaners for gas-permeable lenses

	Barnes-Hind GP Protein Remover	Allergan ProFree/GP
Approved for these lenses	Polycon, Paraperm, Boston, Optacryl, and all other silicone/acrylates	Polycon
Cleaning methods	Hydrodynamic cleaning with Hydra Mat II; patented combination of 3 surfactants	Papain Enzymatic Cleaner
Preservatives	Potassium sorbate 0.13%; EDTA 0.1%	EDTA

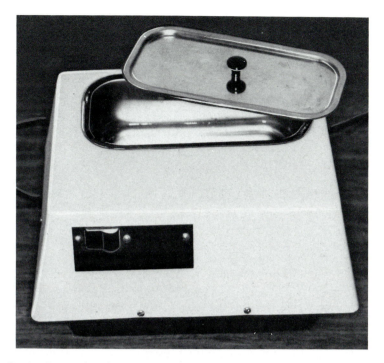

Fig 19-5 ■ Sonic cleaner for cleaning lenses. This device is excellent but too expensive for home use.

Ultrasonic cleaning. In ultrasonic cleaning the lens is placed in a cleaning solution through which ultrasonic waves are passed. Ultrasonic cleaning is efficient and excellent for the practitioner but too expensive for home use (Fig. 19-5).

Spray cleaning. The lens is placed in a perforated storage and cleaning kit (e.g., Swisher, Alcon/BP), which is then placed under running water.

We have had the opportunity of reporting on a double-blind study using the Barnes-Hind cleaner and the Boston cleaner on rigid gaspermeable lenses. Both cleaners were essentially effective in improving comfort; the Barnes-Hind solution significantly reduced corneal staining. Since this study, both cleaners have been improved and are now equally effective.

Routines used by lens solution manufacturers

Barnes-Hind Pharmaceuticals, Inc. Lenses are cleaned by friction cleaning or hydraulic cleaning with the Hydra-Mat II. With hydraulic cleaning a liquid cleaner is added to tap or distilled water and the lenses are put in a container that permits back-and-forth pumping action.

The lenses are placed in a soaking container (Hydra-Kit) that is filled with soaking solution (Soquette [benzalkonium chloride 0.01%, chlorobutanol, EDTA]). The lenses are removed in the morning and wetting solution is added. The storage unit (Aqua Cell/Mate) has inner and outer containers. The inner houses the lenses, and the outer contains tap water plus a cleaning agent. Manual agitation of the unit cleans the lenses.

Alcon. The lenses are soaked in Contique, which is really three solutions—wetting, soaking, and cleaning—in one. The lenses are stored in a simple flip-top case that allows safe rinsing of the lens in a separate storage compartment.

Allergan Pharmaceuticals, Inc. The lenses are placed in a receptable that fits into a storage case. The container is filled with a combination cleaning and soaking solution (Wet-N-Soak). This solution has a cleaning agent and preservatives that include phenylmercuric nitrate 1:25,000. The lenses should remain in the solution for 4 hours; the solution should never be reused. Before removal of the lenses, the unit is shaken five or six times. The lenses are rinsed and a wetting solution is applied to them before insertion. The wetting solution contains a wetting agent (polyvinyl alcohol with methylcellulose) and preservatives (EDTA and benzalkonium chloride 1:25,000). A weekly cleaner, ProFree/GP, is formulated to remove protein. The tablets are dissolved in distilled water for 2 hours; the lenses are rinsed and disinfected.

LC 65 is a daily contact lens cleaner and safely removes the accumulation of undesirable film and deposit on all rigid and soft lenses.

Bausch & Lomb concentrated cleaner is rubbed on both sides of the lens for 20 seconds and then the lens is placed in Bausch & Lomb wetting and soaking solution. This contains chlorhexidine 0.006% polyvinyl alcohol and hydroxyethyl cellulose. The lens should be soaked for at least 4 hours or overnight. The solution binds to the lens surface and enhances its wettability.

Clean the lens with Boston cleaner using the manual method. The solution will have some soft abrasive action on the lens. Then place the lens in Boston conditioner solution for 4 hours. This will wet and disinfect the lens. The solution contains PVA (polyvinyl alcohol) 5%, HEC (hydroxyethyl cellulose), EDTA 0.05%, and chlorhexidine gluconate 0.006%.

The manufacturers of the Boston cleaner also make rewetting drops called Boston Reconditioning Drops that contain chlorhexidine 0.006% and EDTA 0.05%, which when instilled in the eye, rewet and lubricate the lens, prolong wearing time, and remove debris.

COMMENT. Each approach to cleaning and storage has its drawbacks, but each leaves the lens reasonably free of deposits. The greatest contamination comes from dirty lens cases, dirty fingers that carry the lens to the eye, and to some extent, from the eye itself, which harbors some pathogens on its surface. Wetting the lens with saliva will also negate any chemical decontamination attempts. The most important factor in lens cleanliness is still good patient hygiene.

If a patient does get an infection, it is important to do cultures and sensitivities of the lens case used and of the conjunctiva as well.

LENS CASES (Figs. 19-6 and 19-7)

The design of the case is less important than the material of which it is made. The lens-holding basket or compartment should be of a softer plastic than the contact lens so that the incidence of surface scratching is lessened. The patient should also be well instructed not to slide the lens out of the case compartment. This will reduce scratching and the need for frequent lens polishing or replacement. The design of the case should be such as to allow a finger to be touched to the concave side of the lens, which will then

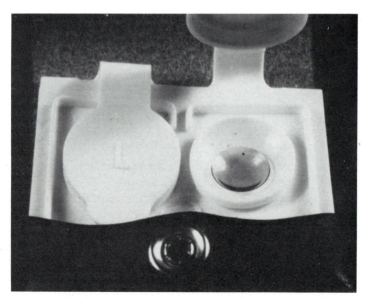

Fig 19-6 ■ Snap-top case is compact, inexpensive, and requires very little solution. The lens is easily exposed to contamination, it frequently is not immersed in soaking solution, and with time this case leaks. This case has limited use and is best for use as a mailing unit.

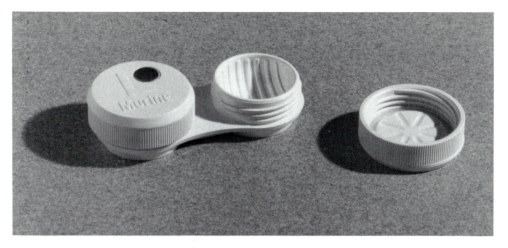

Fig. 19-7 ■ Nonstub wells with threaded caps. Lens case may be used for hard, soft, or extended-wear lenses for heat or chemical disinfection or storage.

stick to the finger when the finger is withdrawn.

A proper lens case can prevent a number of problems. Ideally the lens case should fulfill the following requirements:

1. It should have a removable basket that will allow the lens to be rinsed without loss
2. It should be stored loosely; patients tend to crack or bend lenses upon removal if they are fixed in a snap-on device
3. It should allow total immersion of the lens if it is going to be stored wet
4. It should be easy to clean; the snap-top variety is probably the easiest to contaminate
5. It should be made of plastic and should not contain any sponge rubber that can concentrate the chemicals of the soaking solution
6. It should be distinguished from mailing cases; the compartments of mailing cases are too shallow for germicidal solutions.

GAS-PERMEABLE LENS CARE

Rigid gas-permeable lenses encompass a range of lens materials and material combinations broader than that of either soft or traditional rigid PMMA lenses. The care of a gas-permeable lens is simpler than that of a soft lens because cleaning is not so critical for the survival of the lens. Also, heat sterilization is not used. Caring for a gas-permeable lens is a little more complicated than for a PMMA lens because deposits may form on the lens and should be removed.

Common gas-permeable materials in use today are silicone-PMMA combinations, the fluorocarbon (Advent™) lens and the fluorocarbon silicone acrylate lenses. Although the development of the gas-permeable material has been of great benefit to both fitter and patient, these lenses have at the same time been accompanied by some characteristics not previously encountered.

Wetting and soaking

Most gas-permeable lenses tend to be somewhat hydrophobic. This is especially so in the case of silicone-PMMA materials and the fluorocarbon silicone acrylate lenses such as the Boston, Paraperm, and Polycon lenses. It is the silicone component that makes wetting more difficult. As in the case of any contact lens, poor wetting leads to patient complants of blurred vision and discomfort. It is of importance that a compatible wetting agent be used with the gas-permeable lenses. Soaking in the same solution when the lenses are being stored is also recommended.

Most patients have the best wetting from wetting-soaking solutions that use EDTA as the primary agent. Polyvinyl alcohol, commonly used in rigid lens wetting solutions, does not seem to provide as good results as other agents. Some manufacturers, in an effort to obtain approval to market their lenses faster in the USA, did so in conjunction with soft lens care systems. This method, however, is not acceptable from a practical standpoint, and soaking the lenses in a soft lens storage solution does little more than keep them moist. There is little or no surface treatment or increased wettability achieved by these solutions.

Cleaning

The hydrophobic aspect of the gas-permeable lenses combined with their oxygen permeability can create a smearing such as that seen on a PMMA lens. However the coating is more of the proteinaceous and lipid type, which we would expect to see on a soft lens. The deposit, which is creamy to white in color, interferes with the comfort and clarity of the lens. One can best appreciate the presence of the deposit by looking at the lens under the slitlamp after the lens has been rinsed and dried.

Because of the nature of the deposits, most soft lens surfactant cleaners do an adequate job of removal. In some 5% to 10% of patients wearing gas-permeable lenses, it is necessary to supplement daily cleaning with weekly enzymatic cleaning to keep protein deposits in check.

Giant papillary conjunctivitis may occur from the protein deposits. It is usually found under the upper lid and has a cobblestone-like appearance. Each papilla usually has a blood vessel in the center in contrast to a follicle, which is virus induced and has a blood vessel on its surface. Also, virus-induced disorders frequently have a swollen pre-auricular node.

The tarsal side of the conjunctiva becomes heaped into large papules and produces even more protein, and so the circle of events goes faster. If the inflammation is giant papillary conjunctivitis, which can occur with hard or soft lenses, the reaction is usually seen on the center of the tarsus. With pure allergic reactions, the elevations are usually more at the edge of the tarsal plate.

Approximately 5% of rigid lens wearers eventually get giant papillary conjunctivitis, whereas it can occur in some form in 20% of soft lens users. Oddly enough, its frequency is less with extended wear lenses. People with this problem benefit from the weekly soft lens enzyme cleaners currently available. After one uses these proteolytic enzymes, the lenses should be rinsed with nonpreserved saline solution and conditioned with wetting solution before being inserted into the eyes. Enzyme tablets are most useful for rigid lenses and should be used at least once or twice a week to reduce deposition.

Tap water should not be used as a rinse for lenses. Tap water in many cities may be contaminated with bacteria, including *Pseudomonas*. This is also true of distilled water taken off the pharmacist's shelf. In one survey we conducted on drugstore-purchased distilled water, some 50% of the samples were contaminated. The best rinse is physiologic saline solution. It is not contaminated when purchased and is not hypotonic like water. Contamination increases once the bottle of saline has been opened and left for any time because of the lack of preservative.

COMMENT. Giant papillary conjunctivitis ensures a continuous supply of protein debris to the surface of the lens. Vigorous cleaning of the lens and the local application of steroids to shrink the papillas may not be sufficient to stop the reaction permanently. Frequently the patient needs a new lens or a different type of lens. At times the patient has to resort to glasses for a while because a permenent solution does not seem to exist.

Cleaning devices

Some manufacturers advocate that patients clean their gas-permeable lenses with a velveteen cloth soaked in cleaner. This approach is not recommended because it may result in a distorted optic figure or unwanted lens adjustments by the patient.

Patients who are extremely rough in handling their lenses may use a cleaning device such as the Hydra-Mat II (Barnes-Hind Pharmaceuticals, Inc., Sunnyvale, Calif.) in which the lenses are rinsed in a dilute solution of cleaner. This type of cleaning, though not as effective as careful digital cleaning, may be best for the less careful individual. There are also a number of concentrated laboratory cleaners available to remove lipids, vaseline, body oil, etc., from the lens.

Gas-permeable solutions for the Boston lens

The Boston Lens has its own wetting and soaking solution, which has a hydrophilic component that binds to the surface of the contact lens, thereby enhancing its surface wettability. Other solutions are not recommended because of their ineffectiveness in wetting the surface of the Boston Lens. The Boston Lens conditioning solution is, however recommended for all RGP materials.

Polymer Technology Corporation has introduced a new conditioning solution under the label "Boston Advance" conditioning solution for rigid gas-permeable leanses. The Boston Advance solution contains polyaminopropylguanide (PAPB) as a preservative. It has been shown to be effective against *Acanthamoeba*, the AIDS virus, and *Serratia marcescens*. It has shown promise in its ability to combat the biofilm that maintains the *Serratia* contaminant. This may reduce lens intolerance through contamination.

The wetting component of the Boston Advance solution has been tripled while its viscosity has been reduced. This increased initial comfort upon insertion of the lens encourages more rinsing of the lens with the conditioning solution.

The Boston Lens also has its own special cleaner, which is recommended. This cleaner contains emulsifying agents in addition to a friction-causing component.

If cleaning is required on the part of the practioner prior to lens-dispensing or subsequent to lens wear, Polymer Technology provides a laboratory-type surfactant. The method of application the company advances is as follows. To clean the outside lens surface, attach a rigid suction lens holder to the concave surface and rub the outer surface in a circular motion over a taut piece of velveteen that has been saturated with the Boston Lens Practitioner Cleaner. To clean the inside surface, apply the lens holder to the outside surface of the lens. While rotating the lens, rub the velveteen, soaked in the appropriate solution, over the inside surface.

Care should be taken to instruct patients to exercise proper handling during cleaning. The lens should be cleaned by rubbing it in the palm of the hand with a finger. Rubbing between the thumb and forefinger tends to flex and stress the lens. Proper handling will reduce lens fatigue and damage.

Preservatives—a necessary troublemaker

Preservatives keep the solutions free of contamination while in storage and use. A solution without a preservative becomes contaminated within 48 hours. *Pseudomonas*, which thrives in a wet environment, is the most serious pathogen. Preservatives also reduce surface contamination, especially by fungi, and act as a defense mechanism against the sloppy patient who will not change nonpreserved solutions regularly.

Commonly used preservatives in gas-permeable lens solutions are the following:

Benzalkonium chloride (BKC)—It acts by a surface action on microbial organisms and can cause damage to the cornea. Primarily used as a preservative for rigid lenses and for regular topical eye medication. It is not used for soft lenses because it is absorbed into the lens itself to the cornea. The absorption can reach toxic levels. It acts by a surface action on microbial organisms.

Chlorhexidine—used for soft lenses; has a tendency to bind protein to the lens.

Thimerosal (TH)—a mercurial that competes with the respiratory mechanism of microbial organisms by releasing mercury. It can be toxic to the tissues or act as a sensitizing agent.

Ethylenediaminetetraacetic acid (EDTA)—deprives the organism of essential metal ions and disrupts the bacterial wall. EDTA is frequently found in soft lens solutions but is also present in some gas-permeable solutions. It tends to bind protein to the lens. If the concentration of the solution is reduced from 0.50 to 0.25, the binding effect is considerably reduced.

Chlorobutanol (CB)—It is rarely used because of its volatility, and so it can become excessively concentrated in solution and reach toxic levels.

Some gas-permeable lens cleaners have preservatives that are especially troublesome, causing either toxic or allergic reactions. A toxic reaction is one that is harmful to tissues at the usual normal levels of concentration. It is caused by a direct insult to cells in its metabolism. With toxic material, there is usually a patient history of progressive intolerance to the material used. An allergy is a reaction to an antigen, and the allergic inflammation is attributable to a specific antigen-antibody reaction. In the eye, the conjunctiva is the target organ of an allergy, whereas the cornea is the target organ in toxicity.

Chlorhexidine, though not directly toxic to the eye, binds proteins, fats, and mucus to the lens and renders it hydrophobic. The altered lens becomes an irritant to the eye and the eye becomes red. Most preservatives in full concentration are toxic to tissues. However, in many cases toxicity is not a problem because the preservatives of ocular solutions are immediately diluted by tears.

Whereas chlorhexidine causes toxicity, thimerosal, a mercury-based preservative, is likely to cause an allergy. With an allergy, the patient is asymptomatic for a long time and suddenly develops redness in an eye because of contact with the allergen. The typical history is that a patient uses this agent for 6 months or longer with no side effects and then suddenly develops an allergic inflammatory reaction. The eye simply becomes red and irritable with no change in the power or fitting characteristics of the lens. Although most preservatives can cause toxicity and allergic reactions, they are a necessary evil because they are needed to keep solutions free of contamination while the solutions are in the storage case.

The following presumptive adverse reactions to preservatives have been reported: papillary conjunctivitis and superficial punctate keratitis (BKC, TH, CB); follicular keratoconjunctivitis (TH); allergic contact dermaconjunctivitis (TH and CB). BKC (Zephiran) is probably the most potentially irritating preservative of those in common use. By itself, BKC 0.01% solution can cause severe loss of microvilli, disruption of plasma membrane, degeneration of superficial epithelial cells, and retardation of healing. This level of concentration of benzylkonium is most commonly used in ophthalmic drugs, including over-the-counter preparations.

There may be no clinical difference between an allergy, toxicity, and infection, except for the difference in history and the cytologic appearance, which would show a higher degree of eosinophils in the case of a patient who has an allergic response.

COMMENT. The weekly cleaners seem to be more toxic to the corneal conjunctival surface than the daily surfactant cleaners. When solution reaction is suspected, do an office cleaning, reassess the lens, and omit the use of the weekly soft lens cleaners first. Diagnosis of a toxic effect is nearly always presumptive but can be proved by eliminating or substituting a nontoxic preparation. Also, it is important to reassess the lenses once the offending solution is removed and the eyes have returned to normal (usually with the help of topical steroids). It is possible that the eyes may have become red because of tight-fitting lenses.

LENS CASES

With the increasing softness of RGP lenses, a proper lens case is important. If a smooth-walled case is selected and the patient places the lens concave side down in the case, the lens may warp or even invert upon removal from the case and may be inserted incorrectly in the eye.

PATIENT RESPONSIBILITY

Patients must be taught lens hygiene, proper insertion and removal techniques, and must be given an appropriate lens-wearing schedule. They should be advised to have their lenses periodically inspected for damage, scratching, or chipping. The steps involved in hard lens hygiene include the following:

1. Hand washing. This should be done preferably with a mild, non-ionic soap.
2. Lens cleaning. Both sides of the lenses should be cleaned by rubbing them with a hard lens cleaner. After this cleaning the lens should be rinsed with sterile saline solution.
3. A more thorough cleaning with an enzyme cleaner should be performed at least once a week with rigid gas-permeable lenses.
4. Wetting solutions. Wetting solution may be applied just prior to placing the lens on the cornea. These drops can be used to rewet the surface of the gas-permeable lens; the drops aid in preventing protein and mucous build-up on the lens surface.
5. Storage solution. Lenses should be stored overnight in a storage case filled with soaking solution meant for rigid lenses. This solution should have a disinfectant to prevent bacterial contamination of the lens.

20 ▪ ADAPTIVE SYMPTOMS TO RIGID LENSES

- *Edges*
- *Excessive movement*
- *Lid impact*
- *Excessive lens awareness*
- *Flare*
- *Optic-zone size*
- *Decentration*
- *Photophobia*
- *Tearing*
- *Difficulty with reading*

There is no doubt that the symptoms initially labeled as adaptive were really limitations of the design and material of PMMA lenses. An adaptive symptom is usually manifested in the first few weeks of contact lens wear. Yet a patient can adjust to a soft lens within a few minutes. So the duration and severity of these turbulent initial lens reactions are not attributable to the rejection of the device but to the nature of the device itself.

Many early reactions to PMMA were hypoxic in nature. When the corneal thickness is measured on an eye in which a PMMA lens has been applied, with a -4.00 diopter model being used, the thickness can increase by 10% or more. Yet, when silicone is used, the increase in thickness of the cornea of the unadaptive eye is 4% or less, which is a comfortable margin of safety.

Sudden shock to the cornea causes corneal edema and its symptoms of flare, sensitivity to light, tearing, inability to tolerate the lens, and the defense mechanisms of the lids, including abnormal blinking reactions. With time, corneal hypothesia occurs, and these reactions may be reduced. Also, if staring abates, proper tear exchange can reduce corneal edema to a tolerable 1% to 2%.

At times, the reactions of an early new rigid-lens wearer are simply the normal responses to a bad or tolerable fit. For example, a small thin interpalpebral lens may be acceptable if the lens moves minimally. The reduced mass and thinness of the edges enable the lid to traverse the border of the lens without impact. The same fitting technique with a large-diameter lens would be intolerable, and clouding of the cornea would invariably result. Not only would there be corneal edema, but there would be blink inhibition to avoid contact with the heavy and thick edges.

Ideally, a rigid lens should become tolerable in a few days. Today, there are modifications in design and oxygen permeability that permit faster physical and physiologic adaptation to the application of a lens.

In addition, patient selection is important. The fitting of a rigid lens on a high school student enjoying a summer vacation is a matter different from the application of a lens on an advanced student studying for a doctorate. If an eye is engaged in reading, the blinking rate is altered and may go down to as much as 75%. So the novice lens wearer may be faced with evaporation of tear film on the surface of the lens with resultant deposit formation, symptoms of a tight fit because of a lack of lens movement, and symptoms from a hypoxic cornea. The oxygen permeability of some widely used rigid lenses varies with the mode of measurement (Table 20-1), but it is apparent that PMMA has no permeability whatsoever.

Adaptation time

The adaptation time to any rigid lens may be reduced significantly if gas-permeable lenses are used. Keep in mind that the permeability of any lens is a function of its thickness. In a $+6.00$ diopter lens the transmissibility at the center of

Table 20-1 ■ High-DK fluoropolymer rigid gas-permeable contact lenses

Trade name	Manufacturer	Material	DK
Advent	Allergan/3M	Fluroforon A	100
Fluoperm 30	Paragon	Fluorosiloxane acrylate	30
Fluoperm 60	Paragon	Fluorosiloxane acrylate	60
Fluoperm 92	Paragon	Fluorosiloxane acrylate	92
Boston equalens	Polymer	Fluorosiloxane acrylate	71
Boston equacurve	Polymer	Fluorosiloxane acrylate	71
Fluorex	GT Laboratories	Flusilicon A	70
Quantum I	B & L	Fluorosilicone acrylate	92
Quantum II	B & L	Fluorosilicone acrylate	210
Boston EXPFS	Polymer	Fluorosilicone acrylate	203

the lens with a thickness of 0.3 to 0.4 mm may be virtually zero, with good transmissibility being enjoyed in the same kind of lens −4.00 diopters and 0.1 mm thick. Adaptability is then a function of oxygen transmissibility of a lens, and that transmissibility in turn is governed by the thickness of the lens.

Today an individual can usually tolerate the higher DK rigid lenses for almost an entire day initially. We, however, are still recommending a first-day wearing schedule of four hours, and an increase of one to two hours daily. This minimizes early and adaptive symptoms. Initially, displeasure and discomfort is a recognized feature of learning to cope with rigid lenses. The major causes of such reactions appear to be as follows:
1. Poorly contoured or thick edges
2. Excessive movement
3. Lid pressure or impact
4. A lens that is stored dry
5. A lens that causes mechanical abrasion of the cornea.

EDGES

There is the possibility that the laboratory's quality control may be poor and must be checked by the practitioner with the optic spherometer (Radiuscope) and profile analyzer for evidence of careless manufacturing. However, the edge of the carrier of the peripheral flange may not be refined. For example, any aphakic lens should have a minus carrier to avoid the weight of the lens combined with the lid pushing a thick lens excessively low, instead of carrying the lens to its desirable upward position with each blink. High minus lenses should have a plus carrier to permit the contact lens to center lower. Poor edges will make the process of adaptation much longer, if the patient is ever able to adapt.

EXCESSIVE MOVEMENT

Older PMMA lenses needed movement because tear exchange was the only vehicle for oxygen exchange. This movement of the lens caused lid impact and discomfort because the lens rode over a wider surface of the cornea. Ideally, the lens is fitted high under the upper lid so that there is less lid impact, and the degree of comfort and the period of adaptation are therefore decreased.

Another design feature is that these lenses can be made 9 mm or greater so that they have greater stability. One drawback of the larger lens, however, is the problem of thick lens edges, which if not refined cause a lid gap and 3 to 9 o'clock staining. Lid gap occurs when there is a gap between the edge of the lens and the cornea sufficient to cause drying of the cornea at this site and subsequent desiccation.

Flexure is another serious problem with the higher DK lenses. The larger the diameter and the softer the lens, the more the lens drapes on the cornea to induce a change in power as well as a glued-on syndrome. This will be discussed more fully later. Suffice to say that the lens needs to be made thicker to stabilize it on the cornea and reduce flexure.

LID IMPACT

Lid impact is more likely to occur when the lenses are small, movement is excessive, and the lenses are decentered inferiorly on the cornea as opposed to lenses covered superiorly by the margin of the lid.

A soft lens, if made small enough to be an interpalpebral lens, creates considerable interaction with the lid margin and is quite uncomfortable. So the initial discomfort of a lens can be decreased considerably by changes in its design. The lid should not engage the upper edge of the lens.

EXCESSIVE LENS AWARENESS

Lens awareness is caused by the conscious presence of a foreign body on the eye. However, like a new filling in a tooth, the feeling of "something there" should recede. Frequently patients who are very aware of their lenses and are anxious about their presence will demonstrate their fear in other ways, such as not blinking, moving their eyes, especially upward, or tilting their

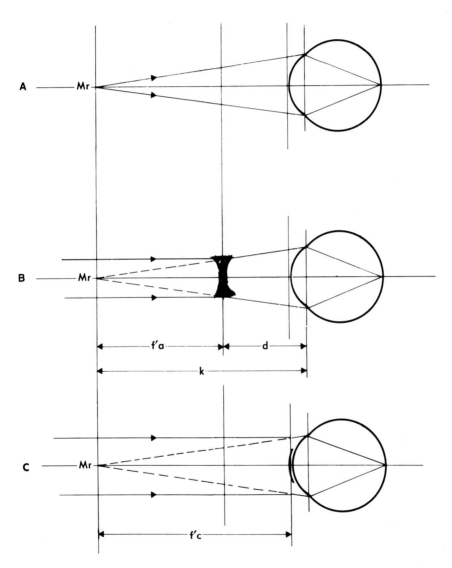

Fig 20-1 ■ **A,** Rays of light in the myopic eye in the uncorrected state diverge from a far point in front of the eye (Mr) and are focused on the retina, **B** and **C.** The focal length of the correcting spectacle lens (f′a) is less than the focal length of the correcting contact lens (f′c). Thus in myopia a weaker contact lens is needed as compared to a spectacle lens. It should also be noted that rays of light diverge after leaving a spectacle lens with the result that more accommodative effort is needed as compared to the accommodative demands of an eye corrected with contact lenses. A person with myopia who wears spectacle lenses and is developing presbyopia may find reading glasses a necessity when the switch is made to contact lenses.

head backward in an effort to reduce lens movement.

If the fit is good and the quality control of the lens is satisfactory, the use of a tear substitute or comfort drops may be sufficient to decrease the awareness of the lens.

FLARE

Seeing lights with a sunburst quality, especially at night, is a common initial symptom. There are two major reasons for flare, and they are related to the size of the optic zone and decentration of the lens (Fig. 20-1).

OPTIC-ZONE SIZE

At times the optic zone may be adequate for the light-adapted eye but insufficient for the dark-adapted eye, in which the pupil dilates. Light streams in through the optic zone and around it because the optic zone is too small for the dilated pupil. Because of the movement of the lens, some flare may be acceptable, but it can be reduced when the optic zone and the lens diameter are enlarged.

A simple test to measure the adequacy of the optic zone is to have a patient simply observe in a dark room the quality of the square white blank image of your projector. If there is a great deal of streaming of lights, the lenses should be changed.

DECENTRATION

A decentered lens may be one that is off center and partially covering the pupil or a lens that is too flat and moving excessively. In both instances the remedy is either a larger or steeper lens. Obviously, if the optic zone is moving or not centered, flare will be excessive.

Initially some patients are extremely sensitive to light from oncoming cars when driving at night. If there are no faults in the fitting or lens movements, with time the flare decreases in intensity and usually is acceptable.

PHOTOPHOBIA

The pronounced sensitivity to light gradually recedes after the lenses have been worn 1 or 2 weeks, but in many cases it persists in a low-grade form. Some patients require sunglasses to go out on a cloudy day, whereas others are unable to work because of intolerance to fluorescent light. This is a more common symptom in blue-eyed individuals. If this does not abate after 2 or 3 weeks, it ceases to be an acceptable complaint and probably is indicative of persistent corneal edema.

The causes listed in Table 20-2 may be active in the production of photophobia.

Most of the time photophobia is the response to low-grade corneal edema. The solution is frequently a gas-permeable lens. Many people have photophobia when outdoors; it persists and requires the presence of deeply tinted sunglasses.

When photophobia occurs indoors, it is pathologic, especially if it persists. Such patients are really ocular invalids if they have to wear their sunglasses at night or indoors. Besides ruining contrast and resolution, the acuity that occurs with night driving is unacceptable.

How to cope with unacceptable photophobia:
1. Perform quality control on the lenses.
2. Consider higher-DK gas-permeable lenses.
3. Check fit—if the lenses are too mobile, try a slightly steeper fit.
4. Make sure the optic zone of the lens is sufficient for the size of the pupil.
5. Tint the lens. If it is to be done, choose gray

Table 20-2 ■ Causes of photophobia

Cause	Observe	Treatment
Corneal edema	Change in K readings or appearance of mires; pachometer change	If the lens fits, switch to a high-DK gas-permeable lens
3 and 9 o'clock staining	Dry spots on cornea Deficiency of tears Lid gap because of thick edges	Tear film assessment and treatment; modify lens edges
Large lens	Type of refractive toric cornea Blend and adequacy of peripheral curves	Use refined edges with good peripheral lens profiles May require switch to smaller lens Modification of lens required

because it causes the least distortion of the color spectrum.

6. Use an ultraviolet filter in a lens—it may reduce photophobia.

TEARING

Tearing usually stops after the patient becomes adjusted to the lenses. Sometimes the pooling of tears under and on the lens can create irritating reflections, and the patient complains of glare. A teardrop may dislodge the lens and create discomfort and variable vision because of the lens sliding around so much.

Dealing with tearing involves looking into several causes:

Inspect the edges—thick edges are uncomfortable and cause tearing.

Check the lids. Lid impact can cause frothing because of the excessive liberation of sebaceous material. In addition, the lens develops a greasy film over its surface.

Inspect the periphery of the lens—even a new lens may have a poor edge profile.

Check the lens with a profile analyzer.

Look for signs of corneal edema that persists.

Change the fit, or change to a higher-DK gas-permeable lens.

DIFFICULTY WITH READING

More accommodation and convergence is required when a moderate-to-high myope exchanges his glasses for contact lenses (Fig. 20-1). There is an increase in accommodative demand and a loss of base in prism. With a young person these changes can be quickly overcome, but in a person close to 40 or older with depleted accommodative reserves, reading becomes a chore.

Added to these difficulties is the change in blink rate, which is often 75% less in a person doing concentrated work, and further problems may occur. The lens is not moved, and so tear exchange is poor. The eye may feel dry or gritty. Also evaporation occurs on the lens surface and the visual acuity may become blurred. Dry spots may appear on the cornea just under the lens, and symptoms of burning may result. These normal conversion symptoms can be ameliorated but not eliminated.

1. Do not prescribe rigid lenses for students in the intense part of their year of study.
2. Warn patients over the age of 35 about the possibility of a reading handicap.

Table 20-3 ■ Alterations in blink patterns

Blink pattern	Treatment
Lid retraction	A large lens, preferably gas-permeable with the upper edge of the lens harbored under the upper lids
Lid flutter	Blinking exercises Good edges Normally tolerated lens movement
Incomplete blink	Blinking exercises and not voluntary forced lid closures
Infrequent blinking	Reschedule fitting if the patient needs his eyes for extensive reading or driving

3. Use of supplementary drops during periods of retarded blinking as in driving, studying, and typing, is helpful.
4. Consider higher-DK gas-permeable lenses if the blink rate is normally infrequent or if the blink rate is retarded by the demands of the patient's occupation or hobbies.

Alterations in blink patterns may ensue. Changes in the blink rate, excursion, and style may occur if the rigid lens is perceived as something foreign, to be avoided by the lids at all costs. The types of alterations that may be expected are shown in Table 20-3.

Although a high myope may be adversely affected by contact lenses as he becomes presbyopic, the hyperope gains significantly. He or she may be able to read for several more years by switching to contact lenses.

Precautions

There are several precautions that can be taken in order to minimize adaptive reactions to rigid lenses:

1. Although one generally avoids fitting lenses to a patient who has recently become pregnant or has gone off or on birth control pills, gas-permeable lenses are tolerated despite hormonal changes.
2. Avoid fitting rigid lenses on patients who are in emotional distress.
3. Rigid lenses should be avoided in dry dusty working conditions, in arid places like Arizona, and in polluted environments such as hair-dressing shops.

4. Do not prescribe rigid lenses to any myopic person who is edging into the presbyopic range because the lens may deplete his accommodative reserve (Fig. 20-2).
5. Do not use rigid lenses on patients who have lid deformities, such as ptosis, retraction of lids, or active blepharitis.

Ideally, there should not be any reaction to rigid lenses when they are first applied or worn on an intermittent basis (though they should not be worn in this way). Adaptive symptoms are attributable to a combination of irritation by the lens and corneal hypoxia, both of which can and should be minimized. Today the introductory period of rigid lens wear is relatively smooth for the patient and is usually acceptable.

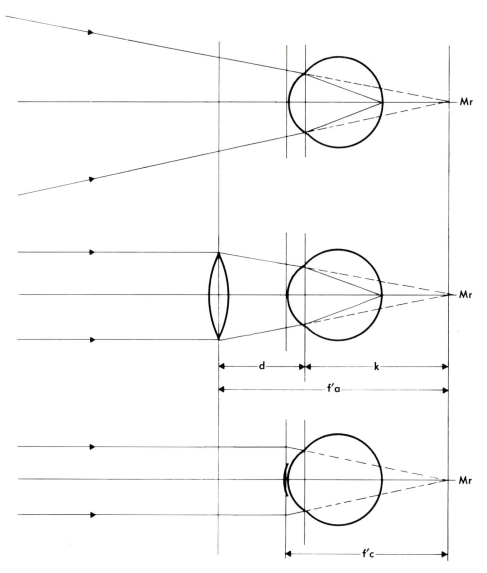

Fig 20-2 ■ Rays of light in the hyperopic eye that are uncorrected and converging toward the far point, which is behind the eye (Mr). The focal length of the spectacle lens (f'a) is greater than the corresponding focal length (f'c) of the contact lens. Thus in hyperopia a stronger contact lens is needed as compared to a spectacle lens. By the same token the hyperopic eye requires less accommodative effort when corrected with contact lenses. For the person with hyperopia who wears spectacle lenses and is developing presbyopia, this means that with contact lenses, reading glasses may not be required or may at least be postponed for a few years.

21 ▪ *FITTING PROBLEMS AND THEIR SOLUTIONS*

- *Symptoms of an inadequate fit*
- *Checking the old lenses—a must!*
- *Fitting problems related to the cornea*
- *Role of blinking in fitting problems*
- *Use and limitations of fluorescein in assessing fitting problems*

With the use of gas-permeable lenses, the problems have changed. The lenses are larger, override the superior limbus, create lid gap if the edges are not beveled, and create extensive 3 and 9 o'clock staining with greater frequency and severity than PMMA lenses do. However, corneal edema is not a serious problem with gas-permeable lenses. Acute corneal hypoxia (the so-called overwear syndrome) has been virtually eliminated (at least we have rarely seen a case). For this advantage alone these lenses have merit.

The various problems, from massive corneal edema with vertical striae on Descemet's membrane to epithelial microcysts, have been effectively checked with the gas-permeable lens. But some of the PMMA complications were the result of chronic hypoxic changes in the cornea plus the added effect of molding, which produced an irregular corneal surface or a severe toric distortion in corneal shape. We have been dealing with gas-permeable lenses over 10 years and permanent changes in the cornea contours have not been observed.

Also, fitting problems of a PMMA lens and lower DK gas-permeable lenses, may be remedied with a higher-DK gas-permeable lens. This is seen in any ill-fit PMMA lens that causes corneal hypoxia. In refitting the patient with corneal edema and distortion, one may use a gas-permeable lens right away without waiting for K readings to stabilize or the corneal surface to gain total regularity. This advantage represents considerable progress because these patients were unable to wear this PMMA lens or see clearly with spectacles and became visual cripples. The waiting period was often days. But commonly it was months before the corneas stabilized to prelens K readings. Because PMMA is still not a historic curio, we shall have to concern ourselves with its problems.

SYMPTOMS OF AN INADEQUATE FIT
Flare or streaming of lights

Frequently this is caused by a lens with a small optic zone that can be overshadowed by a large pupil. The typical story is that the person cannot stand driving at night because of the streaming that is perceived around lights. When the pupil is dilated under dim illumination, there is a prismatic displacement of light coming in from the periphery of the lens. The same effect can occur from a lens that is decentered. In such a case the optic zone is displaced, and the pupil will not be fully covered. Flare may be induced in aphakic patients who have had a sector iridectomy and are fitted with a lenticular lens fitted over a widely exposed coloboma. Corneal edema from any cause can create the same symptom. With the sensation of flare the zone of streaming of lights is always opposite in direction to the displacement of the lens. If the lens rides low the fringe of light will be above.

The detection of flare is quite simple. In the darkened examining room have the person look at the square right of a visual acuity chart and report any distortions. If the flare is uniform, the optic zone of the lens is too small and it must be enlarged. If streaming occurs in only one direction attention must be directed toward centering the lens (Fig. 21-1). If the pupil is too large for the optic zone of the lens, constriction

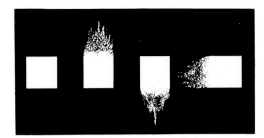

Fig 21-1 ■ Flare: The zone of streaming is always opposite to the displacement of the lens. Such a lens requires recentering. Uniform flare indicates that the optic zone of the lens is too small.

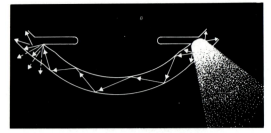

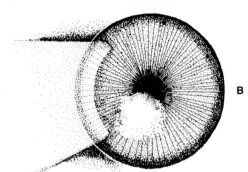

Fig 21-2 ■ **A,** Corneal edema can be detected grossly when the beam of the slitlamp is angled 45 to 60 degrees at the limbus. **B,** Specular reflection. The internal reflection of light through the cornea makes the central edema stand out as a gray haze. The cornea is employed as a fiberoptic channel.

of the pupils by the application of light to one eye will abolish the flare. Flare around lights is rarely encountered at near range because of the synkinetic near reactions, which include pupillary constriction.

Large-diameter gas-permeable lens should be considered in anyone with large or widely dilated pupils. This group usually consists of young, blue-eyed, and myopic people. Their pupils are 4 mm or greater and enlarge to 5 or 6 mm in dim illumination. The pupillary aperture is still smaller than the optic zone of a PMMA lens, but not when one considers the movement of that lens with blinking.

Gas-permeable lenses are effective because of the following:
1. The optic zone is normally large.
2. The movement of the large lens is less than that of a PMMA lens.
3. The lens is more likely to stay centered, especially with blinking.

Blurred vision

The most obvious cause of blurred vision is "incorrect power" of the lens and is simply handled by refracting over the lenses. If the manifest refraction brings the vision to normal by adding equal power to each eye but of the opposite sign, the lenses were probably switched.

At times the hazy vision may be caused by a "grease smudge or coated lens." This becomes obvious the moment the retinoscope is used. An irregular reflex always ensues from the optically disordered front surface of lenses stained with a greasy deposit.

The most worrisome cause of hazy vision is "corneal edema." Corneal edema always means a poorly fitting lens. When the edema is severe

enough to create epithelial erosions that pick up fluorescein stain, it indicates severely decompensated corneal epithelium. For more subtle changes the slitlamp is used to best advantage.

Heavy edema accumulations in the cornea usually represent epithelial and stromal involvement. One can easily detect it by angling a broad slitlamp beam 45 to 60 degrees at the limbus (Fig. 21-2, *B*). By oscillating the beam, the specular reflection of light traveling throughout the cornea will make the central area of edema stand out in relief as a central, gray haze (Fig. 21-2, *A*). This device uses the cornea as a fiberoptic channel. Fine corneal edema and epithelial bedewing can also be demonstrated and are seen as a stippling of the epithelium. They are best seen in the shadow of retro-illumination (Fig. 21-3).

The best antidote to corneal edema is a gas-permeable lens. This becomes most important with lenses with high refractive errors and thick centers (plus lenses), or thick edges (minus lenses), which are prone to cause corneal edema.

If a DK gas-permeable lens is used, the following points must be checked:

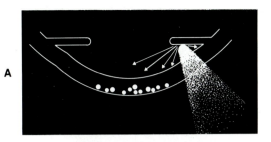

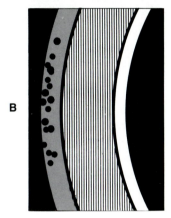

Fig 21-3 ■ **A,** Fine corneal edema. This is best appreciated through retroillumination. **B,** The corneal epithelium has a stippled appearance.

1. Is the lens warped? Check the lens on the Radiuscope.
2. Is the lens centered? Displacement can occur with blinking or eye movement. When this occurs, the lens, which normally rests on the central spheric portion of the cornea, is shifted to the flatter more ellipsoid section. The fit is then imperfect and molding of the cornea is a common complication.
3. Is the lens tight? Remember that small thin lenses are designed to be a little tight. A different lens may be needed.
4. Any change greater than 0.50 D in comparison with the amount found before a contact-lens fitting is considered significant. Usually the K readings are steeper and may be blurred.

Burning

If burning occurs soon after the lenses have been inserted, it probably means that the lens is dirty or that the wetting agent used is irritating the eye. However, if the burning occurs after several hours of wear, it invariably suggests a poorly fitted lens or faulty blinking patterns.

Burning is the symptom of equivalent of corneal edema and is a complaint to which one must pay attention.

Spectacle blur

This is such a common finding after wearing rigid lenses that it has been accepted as being a normal sequela of lens removal. However, many authorities now believe that spectacle blur in excess of 0.50 D is symptomatic of a marginal fit. The thicker the lens, the greater will be the severity and duration of blur. Also, the larger the lens diameter, the more prominent spectacle blur is. It may be caused by corneal molding induced by the presence of a massive lens—certainly a microthin lens is less likely to cause spectacle blur of any consequence. The usual duration is variable. It may be present for only a few minutes to half an hour, or it may persist for hours after the lenses have been removed.

Excessive spectacle blur of the type that lasts hours is usually caused by excessive corneal edema created by the presence of a poorly fitting lens (Fig. 21-4). Such a patient should be seen at the end of the day and examined for corneal edema, changes in the K readings, alterations in the refraction (the tendency is invariably toward being more myopic). Spectacle blur of this intensity should not be accepted as a minor deviation of a normal lens event.

The tear exchange must be improved and appropriate alterations in the lens made depending on whether the lens is too flat, tight, and so on. Persistent flattening of the cornea by a poorly fitted lens can induce permanent changes in the corneal curvature. For those fitters whose sole interest is safely fitting corneal lenses, this sequela should be regarded as a grave complication. The nuisance value of spectacle blur to the patient is one of the major drawbacks to rigid lens wear.

Corneal edema causes an increase in the radius of curvature of the cornea and produces a refractive change in the direction of myopia. This permits the eye to accept more minus correction.

Spectacle blur from corneal edema can be resolved with the use of a higher-DK gas-permeable lens. In some cases, the relief is dramatic. The wearer can read or watch television within minutes of removing the lenses. This asset is one of the main features of a gas-permeable lens system.

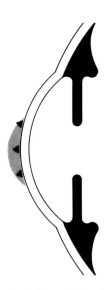

Fig 21-4 ■ Spectacle blur. With a rigid lens corneal edema is confined to the corneal cap, which results in a radical change of the corneal curvature. The location of the edema is central whether the lens is fitted steep or flat. Upon removal of a poorly fitted rigid lens there is often noticeable spectacle blur because of an increase in myopia.

Not all spectacle blur can be eliminated. In the higher grades of refractive errors, the aberration of spectacles in itself causes blurring of vision and discomfort. Nothing can be done about this type of spectacle blur. The person with a −8 D prescription will find the quality of vision poor regardless of the permeability of the lens or its fitting when the switch is made to glasses. That person will suffer chromatic aberration, spheric aberration, restriction of visual fields, image minification with myopic lenses, and parallax because the spectacle lens does not move with the eye. It is helpful to warn patients with large refractive errors of this spectacle-induced disturbance because they may harbor the notion that their prescription is incorrect.

There are solutions to the problem of excessive spectacle blur. To increase the tear exchange, a fitter can do the following:

1. Reduce the diameter of the lens
2. Blend the lenses better
3. Flatten and extend the peripheral curve
4. Switch to a microthin lens

The easiest modification is to flatten the curvature of the peripheral curve.

Blending the junction between the optic zone and peripheral curve is effective, but his method reduces the size of the optic zone. Reducing the optical zone may cause flare if the original lens was selected with the smallest optic zone.

The treatment of spectacle blur is important because it enables the patient to switch more comfortably from one system to the other. For the new patient, it is alarming that the new contact lenses cause impaired visual acuity with spectacles.

COMMENT. The best solution to aggravating spectacle blur is a higher-DK gas-permeable lens and avoidance of PMMA and low-DK lenses.

Mucus formation on lenses

This is a common complaint and has a variety of causes, none of which is too serious. Eyeliner, mascara, and lash thickeners, especially those that are water-insoluble, can cake on the surface of the lens. Although the lens fitter is not supposed to be a beautician, it is helpful to warn female patients to keep their eyeliner behind the lash line, to confine the mascara to the outer half of the eyelashes, and to use water-soluble products. At times a poor edge of the lens can cause lid irritation and hypersecretion from the meibomian glands. Such a lens will appear greasy and coated, as though there is a film over it. Patients will usually complain of some discomfort and a lack of clarity of vision. Frequently they will take their lenses out two or three times a day to try and clean them. With this kind of history the lens periphery is suspect and the junction zones must be checked with the profile analyzer.

At times mucus secretions may be whipped into a froth by the fluttering action of the lids. This froth has the appearance of foamy, translucent bubbles and is seen around the lens edge.

A surface scratch, which consists of a ridge and a gutter (Fig. 21-5), can also irritate the lid. The lid is annoyed by the ridge, which can be eliminated with polishing. Too many gutters, however, require that a new lens be made because they fill up with debris and impair the transparency of the lens. It should be remembered that polymethylmethacrylate is more vulnerable to scratching than even the poorest grades of glass. However it is firmer than gas-permeable lenses are.

Imperfect lens edges account for more problems than any other defect. They can cause corneal abrasions, lid irritation, excessive meibom-

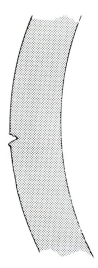

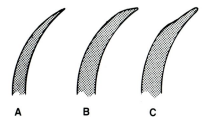

Fig 21-6 ■ Imperfect edges. **A,** Too sharp; **B,** too blunt; **C,** below center with lenticular ridge.

Fig 21-5 ■ A scratch consists of a ridge and a gutter. Only the ridge is removed with polishing.

ian gland secretion and dirty lenses, pronounced photophobia, and decreased lens tolerance (Figs. 21-6 and 21-7). The edges should be tapered so that they glide smoothly under the upper lid. The direction should be slightly posterior to prevent edge stand-off and displacement by the blinking lid. If the edge is too posterior (close to the corneal epithelium), tear exchange will be hampered.

Other complications with hard lenses

Toric or irregular cornea. Large amounts of astigmatism can be induced by a lens that is warped or fits poorly. Sometimes the astigmatism lasts for months and occasionally is permanent. The best treatment is prophylaxis. K readings of the cornea should be checked regularly, and quality control inspections of the contact lens should be done to check for warpage.

Persistent corneal edema. This is probably the most frequent complication and causes persistent redness around the limbus, flare, photophobia, haziness of vision as the day wears on, excessive and intolerable spectacle blur, and corneal erosion.

The presence of corneal edema is a sign of a poorly fitted lens, which must be corrected. Gross edema of the type that produces a gray blot on the apical zone of the cornea usually demands attention. Patients can tolerate corneas with microcystic edema indefinitely. They shorten their wearing time, take one or two

breaks during the day, and glumly accept the murky vision of excessive spectacle blur. The fitter often tries to ignore such cases or treat them marginally. Such patients are told that the corneal edema will get better with time, are given a variety of drops ranging from vasoconstrictors to tear substitutes, or have their lenses fenestrated (the latter frequently works but does not deal directly with the cause). Any corneal edema causing a steepening of the K figures greater than 1.00 D requires reassessment.

Perhaps one of the most common forms of persistent corneal edema is 3 and 9 o'clock staining. These wedge-shaped corneal erosions at the nasal and temporal margins of the cornea may be indicative of a tightly fitted lens, inadequate blinking, or poor tears. It may occur when everything seems to be normal. Treatment is directed against the precise cause and, if no cause is found, consists in the use of tear substitutes. Some fitters ignore the problem because it may not bother the patient or because it may not result in an ulcer.

Extreme complications. Some extreme complications that are frequently discussed because of their serious nature include the following:

PERMANENT LOSS OF VISION. In 1966, Joseph Dixon and others reported loss of vision in 14 eyes from PMMA lenses. Since that time, a number of eyes using soft and rigid lenses have been lost. The main reason has been serious corneal infection by bacteria, fungi, and viruses. The microcysts that result from hypoxia that may result from contact lens wear permit a portal of entry for these organisms to penetrate the cornea and allow a scarring process as well as a full-blown endophthalmitis.

KERATOCONUS. It is controversial whether an ill-fitting rigid lens or a lens with low-frequency

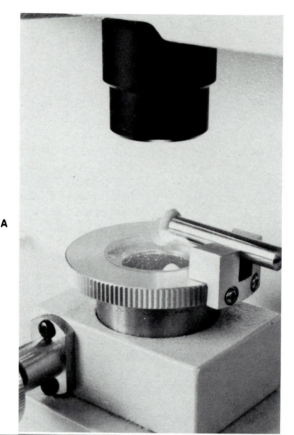

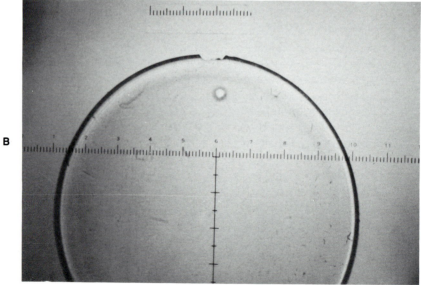

Fig 21-7 ■ **A,** Lens in position for inspection with shadowgraph. **B,** Chipped edge seen through shadowgraph.

low-DK can induce corneal warpage permanently and produce keratoconus. However, we do know that a lens that reduces corneal hypoxia when fitted to a keratoconic patient can aggravate the keratoconus.

ENDOPHTHALMITIS. Although we have never had a patient develop this disease with gas-permeable lenses, it frightens us enough to demand strict hygiene from our patients and never to lose respect for possible serious contamination.

Checking the old lenses—a must!

It is important to check the old lenses. The profile analyzer is perhaps the most important piece of equipment for verification of the blend. Improper edges, though, are the most common cause of lens intolerance. The optic spherometer (Radiuscope) is useful to obtain the radius of curvature of the lens and to check for warpage. Warpage can be detected on the Radiuscope by noting that the line patterns do not come into focus at the same plane. Other parameters should also be checked, including the power, diameter, and thickness of the lens.

The next step is to check the fit of the lenses on the cornea. If the fit of the lens is grossly off, this will be obvious. At times, however, the fit is a little tight or a little loose and the fitter is not positive if anything is really wrong. It is helpful then to assess the patient after the lenses have been worn for several hours. By that time there may be a little more corneal edema, and the situation may be easier to appraise. It is important to keep in mind that the adequacy of a lens-cornea relationship may be related to the movement of the lids. The blinking pattern should be analyzed. The symptoms of a tight lens that shows little movement may be caused by incomplete blinking motions.

Tight lens. A tight lens is a lens that hugs the cornea too tenaciously and shows little movement with blinking. The fluorescein pattern typically shows a dark band around or near the periphery of the lens with pooling in the center. A person wearing such a lens may be comfortable in the morning, but as the day progresses he or she develops hazy vision, burning sensations, and an inability to tolerate the lens during the day. Removing the lens is frequently a struggle because it clings strongly to the cornea.

It is important to distinguish between a tight lens and a steep fit; the two are not always synonymous. A steep fit may be normal, as with microthin lenses, or may cause symptoms of a tight lens because either the peripheral or primary base curve impinges on the cornea.

Some causes of a tight lens include the following:

STEEP BASE CURVE. When the base curve of the lens is much steeper than the corresponding radius of curvature of the corneal cap (Fig. 21-8), such a lens requires replacement with a flatter base curve. Because this solution is expensive and requires a new lens, many fitters prefer to make adjustments to the original lens. The peripheral curves are flattened and widened, and additional blending is often helpful. This technique works if the apical vault is great, since widening of the peripheral curves allows the lens to settle closer to the surface of the cornea (Fig. 21-9).

Reducing the diameter of the lens accomplishes the same thing. Each time a lens is made smaller, one must add new peripheral curves to alleviate some of the stricture of a tight lens.

STEEP PERIPHERAL CURVES. In this case there is minimal apical vault but tear exchange is hampered by steep peripheral curves (Fig. 21-10). The remedy is simple—the peripheral curves must be widened and flattened.

DECENTERED LENS. When a lens is decentered, the optic zone of that lens is usually displaced to a flatter area of the cornea. The infringement of the steeper optic zone to a flatter corneal periphery results in a poor fit because

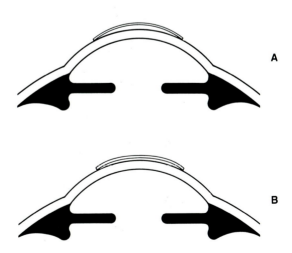

Fig 21-8 ■ A, Tight lens—base curve is too steep. **B,** Peripheral curves flattened—apical vault effect is decreased.

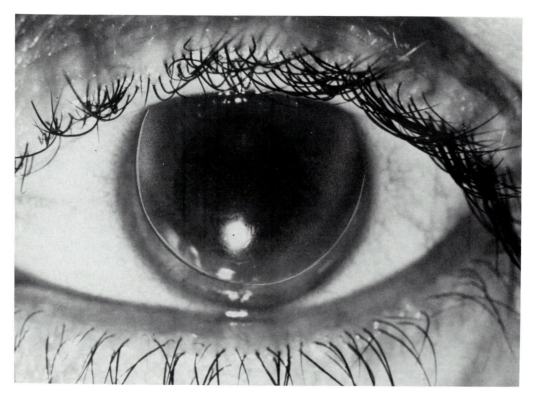

Fig 21-9 ▪ Tight lens with compression of the cornea in the region of the blend.

of the trapping of tears under the center of the lens. A steep zone of the lens displaced to a flat area on the cornea is always noticeable; however, if the infringement is intermittent, the patient may tolerate it.

If a lens is decentered, it will cause the same symptoms that a tight-fitting lens does. However, tight symptoms can also occur when a lens that is too loose has been decentered. This can occur with a lens fitted too flat or displaced by a toric cornea.

Too large a lens. An increase in the diameter of a lens increases the apical vaulting and makes the fit tighter. Reduction in lens diameter is a simple modification.

INFREQUENT AND INADEQUATE BLINKING MOVEMENTS. If blinking is incomplete or infrequent, the normal tear exchange and oxygenation of cornea will not take place. A lens normally moves with the action of a blinking lid. The upper lid pushes the lens down as the lid is lowered and then raises it up several millimeters as the lid is lifted. If the lid does not blink properly, the lens will not move sufficiently and there will

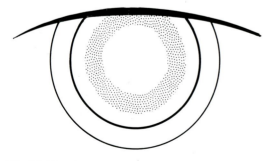

Fig 21-10 ▪ Steep peripheral curve with absence of fluorescein staining in the mid-periphery.

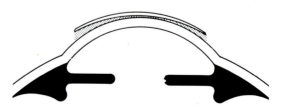

Fig 21-11 ▪ Flat lens. Note concave meniscus of tears, edge stand-off, which allows for easy displacement by the lid, and minimal apical clearance.

be stagnation of tears. Such a lens, showing relatively little movement, will behave like a tight lens and give rise to tight symptoms. Blinking exercises are an even simpler remedy than office modifications of a lens in this situation.

Loose lens. A loose lens does not conform to the cornea because it is either too flat or too small in diameter and, as a result, moves too freely on the cornea.

Such a lens may be tolerated initially, but eventually the excessive movement or the apical corneal compression causes problems. Excessive lens movement leads to flare, intermittent hazy vision, and frustration from a lens frequently decentering or actually popping out of the eye. People with marginally flat lenses lose them with the slightest provocation (Fig. 21-11), including yawning, coughing, laughter, or a swift slap on the back by a well wisher. The weight of the lens bearing down on the corneal cap may cause a burning sensation after prolonged lens wear, or foggy vision and severe spectacle blur after the lenses have been removed (Figs. 21-12 and 21-13).

A lens may be loose because the peripheral and secondary curves are too wide or the optic zone is too wide. A lens made inordinately thick may also fit too loosely on the cornea. The primary base curve may be too flat, in which case a new lens is required.

Smaller diameter lenses can be worn with good movement patterns, but the lenses must be fitted steeper than normal to compensate.

The correction of a flat lens requires a new lens with steeper base curves and peripheral curves.

If the diameter of the lens is too small, it should be increased to improve stability and centration. A larger-diameter lens is more likely to be hidden by the upper lid so that it is less likely to be jarred out of position by the margin of the lid.

The symptoms of corneal edema, which occur with any poorly fitting lens whether flat or steep, are photophobia, burning, hazy vision, and excessive spectacle blur.

For a large-diameter lens of high refractive error that is too loose or too tight, a gas-permeable lens is the best solution. A gas-permeable lens can be fitted tighter because of its permeability. Its larger diameter leads to centration and retardation of lens movement, which checks the faults of a loose lens.

Low-riding lens. A low-riding lens may cause tight symptoms because of the inferior displacement of the optic zone if there is a lack of adequate movement, resulting in tear stagnation (Fig. 21-14). The lens can also irritate the lower lid by mechanically abutting against it with each successive blink. If the lens drops below the limbus at the 6 o'clock position, it can create vascular compression. Such a lens is uncomfortable to wear and is optically undesirable.

The most common cause of low-riding lenses is a thick, heavy, plus lens such as that prescribed for the ordinary aphakic patient (Fig. 21-15). Not only is the lens weighted down by gravity, but also the convex anterior peripheral curve does not give the upper lid a proper edge to lift it. A low lens is frequently a lens that is flat or too small. Low lenses are common with patients with exophthalmos or just very promi-

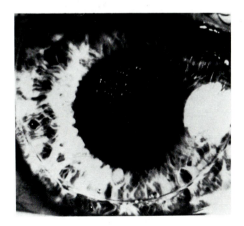

Fig 21-13 ■ Punctate staining of the cornea after flat-fitting lens is removed. (From Stein HA, Slatt BJ, and Stein RM: The ophthalmic assistant, ed 5, St Louis, 1988, The CV Mosby Co.)

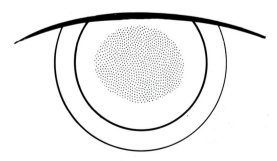

Fig 21-12 ■ Large central touch indicative of a flat lens.

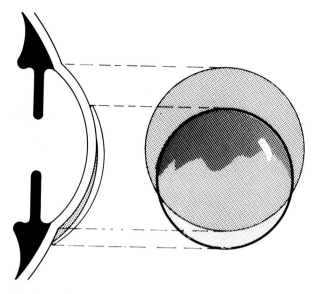

Fig 21-14 ■ Low-riding lens. Note vascular compression in the limbal region, corneal touch at the superior portion of the lens, and a wedge-shaped prism of tears with the base downward.

nent eyes. In such cases the lens diameter must be increased to permit more upper lid traction.

In large, flat, aphakic eyes the lens of choice is a lenticulus with a minus carrier. If the cornea is steeper than 45.00 D, a small-diameter, 7.8 mm, thin lens can be employed. For ordinary high-plus lenses, +3.00 D or greater, a mi-

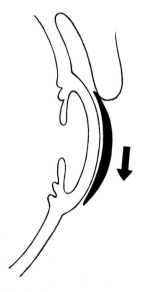

Fig 21-15 ■ A plus lens having a steeper anterior curve will tend to be pushed into a downward position by the upper eyelid. Such lenses tend to ride low.

crothin lens is frequently a satisfactory solution to the problem of a low-riding lens. Stronger powers can be added without making the lens heavy and bulky.

High-riding lens. Like all displaced lenses a high-riding lens suffers from a steep optic zone of a lens resting on a relatively flatter corneal periphery or even a limbal zone.

The most common cause of a high-riding lens is a high-minus lens that has a relatively prominent concave anterior surface. The periphery of the lens, which is similar to an hourglass, presents a ridge that is easily grasped by the upper lid and raised (Fig. 21-16).

Other causes include pronounced astigmatism with the rule and a high lower lid. A flat lens can be displaced upward, and a steep lens with a large optic zone may also ride high. The correction of this problem is not easy. The many solutions are indicative of the complexity of the situation and not of its simplicity.

Reducing the lens diameter seems to be the most direct route. Unfortunately this tactic often aggravates the condition and makes the lens ride even higher. This occurs because the lens is lighter and is more easily pulled up by the traction of the upper lid. Also the upward movement of a lens is basically stopped by the lens riding on a flatter peripheral area of the cornea or sclera. Therefore, if two lenses of different diameters have their uppermost edge riding to the

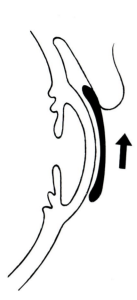

Fig 21-16 ■ The thicker and concave anterior edge of a minus lens permits the upper eyelid to lift the lens and hold it in a superior position. Such lenses tend to ride high.

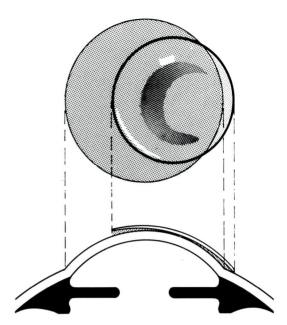

Fig 21-17 ■ A horizontally displaced lens caused by +2.25 D astigmatism against the rule. Note edge stand-off on the corneal side, limbal compression, and flat fit with paracentral corneal touch.

same point, it is apparent that the smaller-diameter lens will show a larger upward decentration than the larger lens will.

Incorporating a prism ballast, which makes the lens heavier, tends to bring it down. If this is combined with reducing the peripheral bevel on the periphery of a myopic lens, grasp of the upper lid is reduced. As a result the gravitational effect of the lens is increased while the lifting power is minimized.

This is a good solution for high-riding minus lenses. A minus edge can be converted to a plus edge, that is, from a concave to a convex surface. This is called a plus-carrier lenticular lens.

If the cause is a pronounced astigmatism with the rule, a bitoric lens may be needed, though frequently a large-diameter spheric lens works as well but without the attendant problems caused by a toric lens.

Patients with high lower lids usually have small palpebral apertures. A small, microthin lens is most helpful for this sort of problem.

It is important to recognize that a high-riding lens is not a single entity. At times trial and error must be used to correct it. For instance, reducing the diameter of the lens can make it better or, paradoxically, worse.

The high-riding lens is not a problem for the gas-permeable lens because it is designed to fit that way. The problem with gas-permeable lenses usually is a central or even low fitting position. When the lenses are low, 3 and 9 o'clock staining is intense and the lenses cause great discomfort. In such cases, the diameter may have to be reduced to allow the lids to lift the lens. Another solution is to fit the lens flatter to promote wider lens excursions so that the lens can be carried upward to the superior limbus.

Horizontally displaced lens. The most common cause of a nasal or temporal displacement of a lens is astigmatism against the rule (Fig. 21-17). If the astigmatism is 2.00 D or less, a spheric lens fitted steeper than K by 1.00 D is often enough to remedy the problem. For added stability and centration a large lens with a large optic zone should be employed.

Since there are no clear-cut numbers as to how much steeper than K is right for an individual patient or how large is large with respect to diameter, the simplest approach is to simply use trial spheric lenses. If a spheric lens will not become centered, a toric one must be employed. Again a gas-permeable lens is probably the best solution.

EDGES—HOW TO ASSESS THEM. The treatment of the edge of the lens becomes more important with the use of gas-permeable lenses. These lenses are made large in diameter, 9.2 mm or greater, as opposed to a small microthin rigid lens, which may be 7.8 mm. Not only is there a 40% increase in the mass of the lens, but also the edges become very thick in the process.

A myopic profile on the anterior surface must be placed on lenses of a high-plus nature of +5 or over, to reduce the increased edge thickness.

Similarly a plus profile must be used to treat a high-minus lens, that is, −5 D or greater, so that again the edges are treated.

If the edges are not dealt with adequately, the following problems may occur:
1. Lid gap, which results in a very thin tear film at the meniscus of the lens edge.
2. Low-riding lens because of the lids pushing the lens down. This is especially true for high-plus lenses such as aphakic lenses.
3. Three and 9 o'clock staining.
4. Formation of dellen.
5. Discomfort because of lid impact. A blinking upper lid can create considerable pain if it engages a thick lens.

The edges should be checked with the profile analyzer and the shadowgraph with the lens being viewed in profile.

In the silicone-PMMA combinations, the edges are often made too thin and they chip and fragment easily.

Good edging is difficult to fabricate because the problem of too little or too much is quite an easy trap to fall into.

SCRATCHES ON THE LENS. In times of frustration in dealing with a complaining patient many fitters will simply clean and polish the lenses and hope for the best. Unfortunately this works only if there is accumulated mucus, grease, or salt crystals on the surface of the lens or actual scratches in the plastic. It is not a remedy for an ill-fitting lens.

If scratches are abundant, the furrow in the plastic will fill up with foreign debris, causing ocular irritation and hazy vision. A deeply scratched lens can be salvaged by removal of the disturbing ridges that line the furrows; however, if the scratches are very deep, removal of the ridges is not enough because the gutters will continue to collect dirt and foreign matter. In this case a new lens is needed.

Polymethylmethacrylate lenses, combined with silicone, are very soft and are more subject to scratching than lenses made of even the poorest grade of glass. Because of this tendency to scratch, patients should be advised to be very careful with their lenses, especially regarding the following:
1. The lens should not be slid across a surface when one is picking it up.
2. Friction cleaning should be done gently, not vigorously, because this can cause scratches or warpage.

WARPAGE OF A LENS. Warpage of a lens should be suspected in any patient who has been comfortably wearing lenses and then develops an intolerance to them. One can detect its presence by checking the lens curvature for cylinder with either an optic spherometer or a keratometer. Frequently the signs of warpage are gross and can be seen when one holds the naked lens with a smooth forceps in front of a good light source. If the plastic is internally fractured, the site of disruption in the lens looks frosted, like a series of crisscrossing translucent lines or a single, linear break. This disruption of the plastic can be appreciated when one holds the lens under an incandescent light.

The most common cause of warpage is rough handling. Frequently an edge is internally cracked as it is pulled out of its container. Excessive pressure in the lens with cleaning can also cause ruptures in the plastic. Other causes include grasping a dropped lens between the thumb and index finger and excessive squinting with the lens in place.

Lenses should be replaced if the warpage is creating residual astigmatism and visual difficulties or symptoms of corneal compression. If the warpage is excessive—greater than 0.50 D—lens replacement should be done to prevent induced corneal molding. Warpage of a lens can mold a cornea to a toric shape permanently.

The other factor that causes induced toricity of the cornea is corneal edema. A soft cornea is more easily molded by a bulky ill-fitting lens.

FENESTRATED LENS. The prime purpose of fenestration in a lens is to make a marginal fit tolerable. It is particularly useful in a tight lens. The apertures serve to diminish the suction-cup effect created by a blinking lid pressing on a lens that is vaulting the cornea. It does not affect materially the presence of corneal edema.

FITTING PROBLEMS RELATED TO THE CORNEA

The cornea should be assessed for corneal edema and its radius of curvatures checked with the keratometer. If there is corneal edema, the fit of the existing lens may be difficult to assess. An edematous cornea will exaggerate or even distort a pre-existing marginally poor fit. For example, if the lens is tight, the edema will be confined to the apical cone of the cornea. When fluorescein is used to evaluate the fit, there will be corneal touch resulting from forward protrusion of the center of the cornea. Such a lens will appear to be fitting flat.

In cases of severe corneal edema the patient should be seen early in the day before the cornea becomes swollen and obsures the normal fitting pattern. The radius of curvature of the cornea should be evaluated in order to determine the presence of induced corneal astigmatism. These figures must be compared to previous K readings to determine the change in corneal curvature.

Corneal edema from an ill-fitting lens can be detected with the following:
1. Slitlamp—using indirect illumination or specular reflection
2. K readings
   a. Change in curvature
   b. Change in the quality of the mires—a muddy pattern with breaks and blurriness
   c. Distortion of the mires
3. Pachometer
4. Retinoscope—an irregular retinoscopy reflex
5. Placido's disc—distortion of the circle on the reflected image of the cornea.

Changes should be picked up when the corneal edema is present—large gray haze in the central area of the cornea, striae of Descemet's membrane, corneal erosions, large swing in the K readings, and pronounced changes in the refractive error to a more myopic correction.

ROLE OF BLINKING IN FITTING PROBLEMS

Patients, expecially PMMA lens wearers, with an unsatisfactory blink response frequently complain of intolerance to their lenses. The symptoms may be subtle or expressed as a total inability to wear their lenses. Some of the more common complaints include the following:
1. Failure to wear the lens for a full day. The patients can't wait to remove the lenses at 5 or 6 o'clock when they reach home.
2. Inability to wear the lenses for reading, studying, or driving.
3. Tight lens features:
   a. Spectacle blur that is excessive
   b. Burning of the eyes
   c. Grittiness of the eyes
   d. Poor vision
   e. Haloes and fringes around lights
   f. Discomfort and intolerance of the lens
   g. Whitish strands on the lenses
4. A tendency to remove the lenses three or four times a day to clear them.
5. Excessive photophobia—tinted lenses are worn indoors and outdoors.
6. Discomfort symptoms—burning, irritation, pain with movement of the eyes, and so on.

Ocular signs of poor blinking

1. Erosions of the cornea inferiorly where the blink motion is arrested.
2. Deposits on the lens that is not polished by the action of the lids. With a rigid lens, a whitish film from deposited protein forms a band on the exposed inferior portion of the lens.
3. Features of a tight lens:
   a. Poor movement
   b. Lenses low and not rising properly with a blink motion
   c. Apical corneal edema
   d. Inferior corneal erosions
   e. 3 and 9 o'clock staining
4. Episcleritis and, at times, formation of dellen.
5. Features of corneal edema:
   a. Change in the quality of the mires of the keratometer
   b. Irregular astigmatism that one best appreciates by noting the distortion of the retinoscopy reflex or alteration of Placido's disc reflection
   c. Slit-lamp findings of corneal edema usually best appreciated through indirect or retro-illumination
   d. Change in pachometry readings, indicating corneal edema and increased corneal thickness
6. Dry spots on the corneal surface.

Purpose of blinking exercises

Blinking exercises, which in reality are a series of voluntary lid-closure movements, assist apprehensive patients who are excessively aware of their lenses. By consciously completing a blink patients soon learn to lose their fear of the lens. Also the lids get the feel of the lens and become accustomed to riding over the edge.

To avoid excessive contraction of the lids, the patient is asked to close the eyes slowly and naturally. The index fingers of both hands are placed just lateral to the outer canthi so that they can feel any excessively forceful contractions. When the eyelids are closed, the patient is asked to pause for a moment. The eyes are then opened naturally, followed by another small pause before the exercise is resumed.

A series of 10 exercise blinks performed 10 times a day is usually adequate to correct faulty blink patterns. Most faulty blink patterns can be corrected with a week of earnest effort.

A change in the blink rate is not the only reason why many persons with myopia find it difficult to read when they first obtain lenses. Myopic spectacles offer the patient a base in prismatic effect, resulting in a decrease in the need to converge. The greater the refractive error, the greater the prismatic deviation of the spectacle lenses. A person with severe myopia who changes to wearing contact lenses frequently feels uncomfortable at first because of the need to converge. There is more accommodative demand from a contact lens compared to a spectacle lens of the same power. Rays of light are diverged by a minus spectacle lens before reaching the cornea, and so more accommodation is required. With contact lenses the convergence of light at the contact lens and the cornea are virtually the same. So a first-time myopic wearer of contact lenses requires more focusing power to read than previously was exerted with spectacle lenses.

If the person experiences hazy vision when reading is first attempted, this may indicate a loss of centration of the lens. When the eyes are lowered in the reading position, the lens may be displaced upward by the margin of the lower lid. This problem can be eliminated when the diameter of the lens is reduced.

Finally, differentiation must be made between those patients who had poor blinking habits before wearing their lenses and those with faulty blinking induced by the wearing of lenses.

Persons in the latter group are those whose poor blinking habits can be easily corrected by blinking exercises.

USE AND LIMITATIONS OF FLUORESCEIN IN ASSESSING FITTING PROBLEMS

The fluorescein pattern offers the clinician additional information regarding the fit of rigid lenses. A positive test is quite helpful in confirming or supporting a diagnosis of a tight or flat lens. However a normal fluorescein pattern is not necessarily evidence of an adequate tear exchange. It is possible that a patient, seen too early in the day and fitted marginally, when first viewed, was shown to have a perfectly acceptable staining pattern. The time of examination may therefore be significant. The fluorescein paper acts as a Shirmer's test No. 1, which promotes reflex tearing in the unanesthetized eye. A flush of tears can certainly change the contact-cornea relationship, especially if the lens was initially slightly tight. There is no standard fluorescein test. What is normal for one lens may be abnormal for another. In view of these drawbacks many authorities regard the presence of corneal edema detected by slit-lamp examination as a better sign of poor tear exchange. It is undoubtedly more reliable, and there are still diagnostic clues provided by this simple, rapid test that cannot be determined in any other way.

A good method to apply fluorescein is to add a drop of anesthetic to the dry, sterile, fluorescein-impregnated paper and touch it to the upper sclera. This minimizes reflex tearing, and there is better control of the amount of fluorescein liberated. A single drop of fluorescein is adequate.

Take care to avoid dripping fluorescein on the patient's clothing because it stains vividly and is extremely difficult to remove.

Fluorescein in solution form is rarely used today because it has been shown to support the growth of *Pseudomonas aeruginosa*.

The following are staining patterns associated with various lens characteristics:

Normal-lens-pattern lens with slight apical vault (Fig. 21-18). There is a slight vault over the apical zone of the cornea with slight central pooling with an absence of stain in the intermediate area. The peripheral portion of the lens should have a pooling of stain, indicating that the edge is not bearing on the cornea. The newer high-

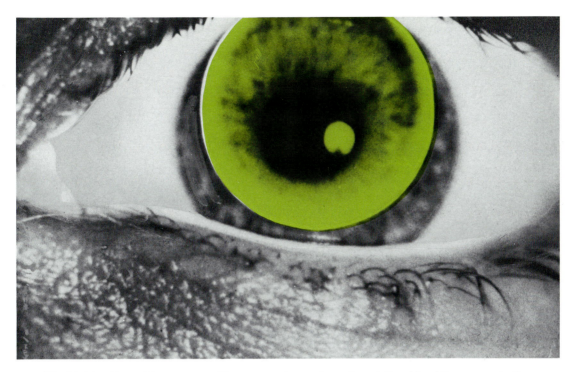

Fig 21-18 ■ Normal lens pattern. The pattern depends on the relationship of the cornea to the diameter, base curve, and material. Fluoronated lenses usually should exhibit more central bearing than silicone acrylates.

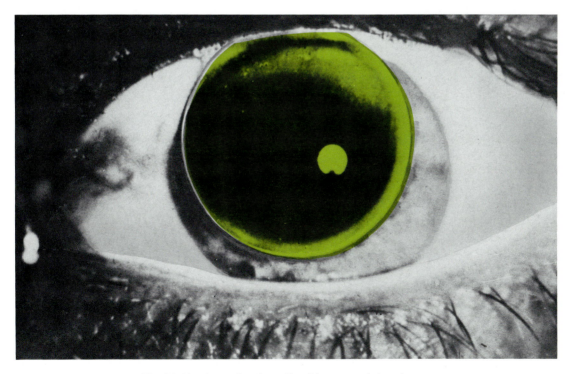

Fig 21-19 ■ Lens fitted too flat. Narrow peripheral zone.

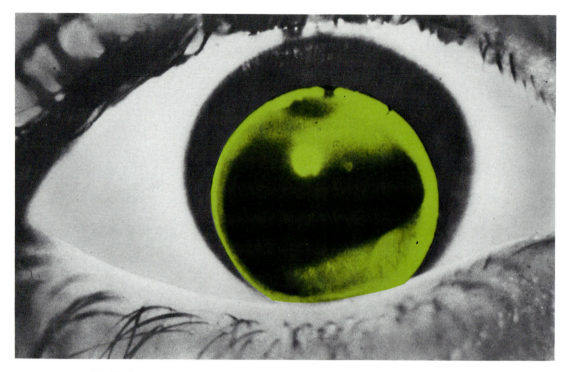

Fig 21-20 ■ Astigmatic fit. A band-shaped area of touch is characteristic.

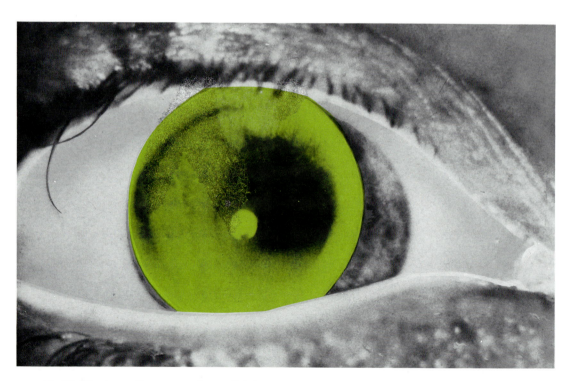

Fig 21-21 ■ Lens diameter too large. This lens is too large for the corneal size. More importantly, it is too large for the size of the palpebral fissures. The lens should not extend from lid to lid.

DK fluoronated silicone acrylates can be fitted flatter and can reveal control central bearing.

Lens fitted too flat (Fig. 21-19). Typically with a flat lens there is apical touch with little fluorescein in the area of contact. The lens may also be decentered, a common finding with a flat lens. In this case the apical zone was too small. A large optic zone steepens a lens, whereas a smaller optic zone flattens it. This error was corrected by increasing the size of the optic zone from 6 to 7.3 mm. No other changes were made. There was apical staining of the cornea after the lens was removed.

Lens fitted too steep. The classic picture of a tight lens is central pooling with an intermediate or peripheral zone of touch. In this case the lens is also decentered. A steep lens does not ensure centration; the centration was corrected by adjustment of the blend.

Astigmatic fit (Fig. 21-20). Characteristically there is a band-shaped area of touch on the flattest meridian. The degree of astigmatism was 6.00 D in this case, which is frequently too much for a spheric lens to vault. Over 3.00 D of astigmatism usually requires a toric lens.

Lens diameter too large (Fig. 21-21). The lens is in contact with both upper and lower lids with the eye in the primary position, and there is some central pooling. A large lens is effectively a steep lens and will present essentially the same fluorescein pattern. Note the frothing superiorly.

Lens diameter too small (Fig. 21-22). This lens is too small in diameter; as a result it is carried too high on the cornea by the action of the lid.

Foreign-body stain (Fig. 21-23). A false eyelash became trapped under the lens and created a typical abrasion.

Decentered lens (Fig. 21-24). The decentered lens overrides the flatter peripheral portion of the cornea and the limbus. This lens was too flat.

Ultrathin lens pattern (Fig. 21-25). The lens is fitted steeper than K, which is acceptable with such a lens. The central pooling indicates a steep fit, which is present and, in this case, desirable.

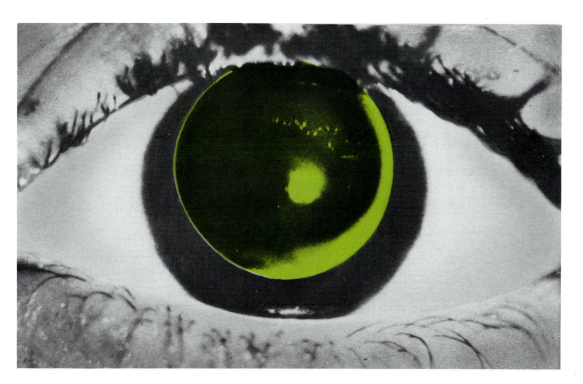

Fig 21-22 ■ Lens diameter too small. This lens showed too much movement. The looseness of the fit was improved by fitting with a larger diameter lens. The patient complained of streaming of lights because the size of the optic zone of the lens was too small to cover the pupil of the eye, which became semidilated in dim illumination.

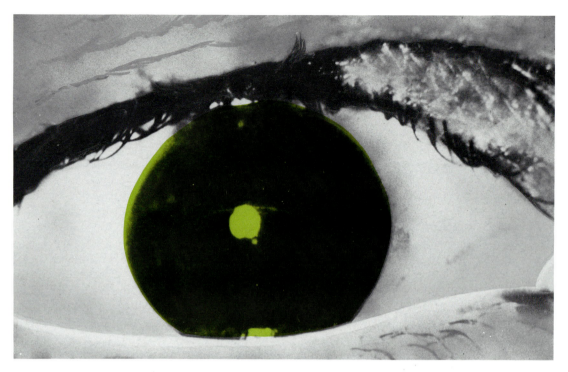

Fig 21-23 ■ Foreign body stain. An arc-like abrasion was caused by a small foreign body.

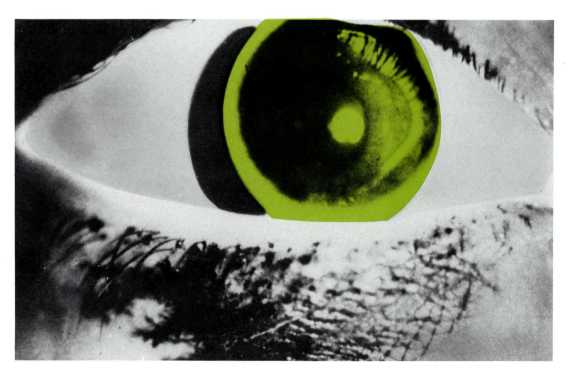

Fig 21-24 ■ Decentered lens. The lens has shifted to a flatter portion of the cornea. The decentered lens then acts as a tight-fitting lens. Flare is also a problem because the optic zone no longer covers the pupil.

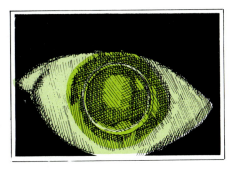

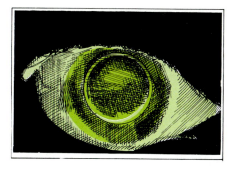

Fig 21-25 ■ Microthin lens fitted steeper than K. The ring of fluorescein around the lens is indicative of a very steep fit.

Fig 21-26 ■ The fluorescein pattern shows some central touch and pooling at the periphery of the lens because of the steep peripheral curves.

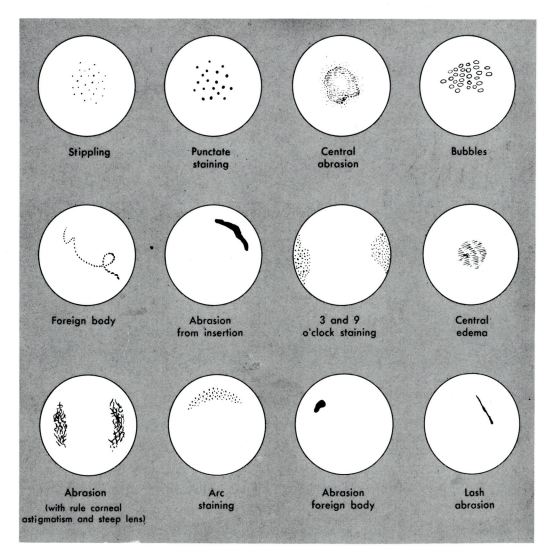

Fig 21-27 ■ Abnormal staining patterns. Notice that stippling, punctate staining, central edema, and central abrasion are largely apical and caused by an ill-fitting polymethylmethacrylate lens. (From Stein HA, Slatt BJ, and Stein RM: The ophthalmic assistant, ed 5, St Louis, 1988, The CV Mosby Co.)

Lens fitted on K (Fig. 21-26). A slight accumulation of fluorescein is present centrally. As will all microthin lenses a definite band of fluorescein is found at the position of the peripheral curve, which normally is fitted steep. This fitting pattern is also acceptable.

Abnormal staining patterns (Fig. 21-27)

Corneal edema from either a steep or flat lens is invariably central in location. It can create stippling, punctate staining, and central corneal hazing, which results from edema in the corneal cap.

Mechanical abrasions from foreign bodies create irregular superficial epithelial scratches. If the lens is fitted too flat, a central abrasion will occur because the area of central clearance becomes converted to central touch, and compression of the cornea occurs. If the blend is too sharp or the peripheral curve too steep, the imprint of this poor fit leads to arcuate staining.

In 3 and 9 o'clock staining, a triangular wedge of corneal staining appears at the margins of the cornea.

There are several causes of the finding of 3 and 9 o'clock staining.

Lid gap. A lid gap occurs largely with large-diameter rigid lenses. It is particularly prone to occur with gas-permeable lenses whose edges have not been reduced in size.

A gap occurs between the margin of the lens and the cornea. The meniscus of tears becomes very thin or absent at this border. It is a lens-induced dry spot.

The degree of staining is intense and often associated with episcleritis and even formation of dellen. It is particularly prone to occur with lenses that are low, that is, not brought up to a high position with a blink.

Low-riding lenses. Poor lid adherence may be a factor in causing a low-riding lens that results in 3 and 9 o'clock staining. If the lens is low, the lens should be made flatter, thinner at the edges, or smaller in diameter.

At times, the lens will rise with a blink and then suddenly drop to a low position. Such a lens requires a little alteration; flattening the blend and peripheral curves will frequently solve the problem.

Poor blinking. The incomplete blinker dehydrates the exposed position of the eye—the 3 and 9 o'clock portion. The lines of protein dehydration across the lens indicates its presence; its treatment is blinking exercises.

Poor tear film. A poor tear film occurs with people with an insufficient tear film to support a large-diameter lens.

With these people, supplementary tears during the day and a bland ointment at night (such as Duratears) may be enough to remedy the problem.

The staining of the cornea is caused by desiccation of the corneal epithelium and not by corneal hypoxia.

22 ▪ COMPLICATIONS OF RIGID LENSES

- Keratoconus—a complication of contact lens wear?
- Corneal edema
- Corneal staining
- Vascularization
- Prolonged lens pressure
- Loss of corneal sensitivity
- Acute corneal crisis (overwear reaction)
- Care-related problems
- High-altitude risks
- Inclusion blennorrhea
- Birth control pill intolerance
- Fitting problems
- Crazing and cracking

There is no doubt that contact lenses can cause complications despite the flippant way they are regarded by the media, some commercial optical shops, and the general public. Contact lens are advertised as a commodity, no different from shoes. It is no wonder that people are lax in their contact lens hygiene. They have no respect for the device.

Most serious ocular complications occur as a result of patient neglect. Failure to clean the cases in which the lens are stored can result in the growth of *pseudomonas aeruginosa*, a virulent organism that can penetrate a small corneal ulcer and cause endophthalmitis. Over 25 years ago, when rigid lens complications were surveyed, 14 eyes become blind in a one-year period and a few required enucleation because of total loss of ocular function and severe pain. This calamity was the result of infection from dirty cases and contaminated lenses. Dirty hands, dirty fingernails, dirty contact-lens cases, dirty habits such as using saliva as a wetting agent, and failure to change soaking solutions on a regular basis are the most common causes of serious ocular infections. Today the number of contact-lens wearers is much higher and so is the incidence of serious damage. Perhaps a warning should be printed on each contact-lens case stating that "contact lenses may be damaging to the eye if a strict hygienic procedure is not carried out."

KERATOCONUS—A COMPLICATION OF CONTACT LENS WEAR?

An area of controversy is whether keratoconus can be caused by a contact lens. Most contact lens fitters do not believe that it is possible. The increased incidence among contact lens wearers is probably attributable to the fact that the early symptoms of keratoconus may be progressive myopia. Both myopia and keratoconus begin in teen-agers. Most corneal edema in rigid-lens wearers is apical in location—on the corneal cap. Keratoconus usually is decentered, inferiorly and nasally, but not in the exact location where corneal edema is detected. Early keratoconus may be accelerated by the wearing of a contact lens, but in our opinion there is insufficient evidence to implicate rigid lenses as a cause of keratoconus.

CORNEAL EDEMA

As higher-oxygen-permeable lenses are introduced to the fitters' armamentarium, many of the conditions described below may become of historical interest. We hope so. However, one must be cognizant of the ill effects of corneal hypoxia that may often be induced by poor fitting with resultant inadequate tear exchange.

Corneal edema is probably the most frequent complication and causes persistent redness around the limbus, flare, photophobia, haziness of vision as the day wears on, excessive and intolerable spectacle blur, and corneal erosion.

The presence of corneal edema is a sign of a poorly fitted rigid lens, which must be corrected. Gross edema of the type that produces a gray blot on the apical zone of the cornea usually demands attention. Patients can tolerate cor-

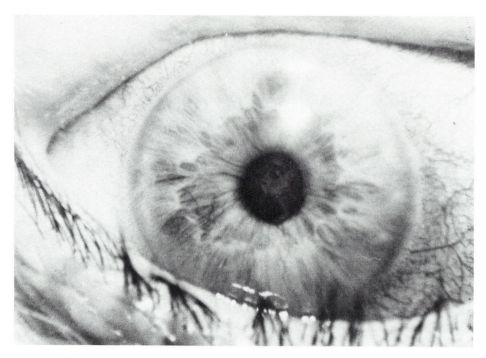

Fig 22-1 ■ Corneal edema centrally causing pain and blurred vision.

neas with microcystic edema indefinitely. They shorten their wearing time, take one or two breaks during the day, and glumly accept the murky vision of excessive spectacle blur. The fitter often tries to ignore such cases or treat them marginally. Such patients are told that the corneal edema will get better with time, are given a variety of drops ranging from vasoconstrictors to tear substitutes, or have their lenses fenestrated (the latter frequently works but does not deal directly with the cause). Any corneal edema causing a steepening of the K figures greater than 1.00 D requires reassessment. Corneal edema can assume a variety of forms and cause a variety of troubles for the contact lens wearer (Fig. 22-1).

CORNEAL STAINING
Stippling

Stippling or small dots in the central position of the cornea may arise from lens defects in which there is inadequate tear exchange. This results in stagnation of tears and anoxia to the cornea, heat retention, and inability to dissipate the end products of metabolism from the cornea. Changing the peripheral curve, blending the junctional zones, thinning and rounding the

edges, or selecting a more appropriate diameter may correct this problem.

Punctate staining

Punctate staining in large areas may occur at the points of contact of either the edge of the lens, one of the curves of the lens, or the edge of the optic zone. It is a result of compression of the lens on the cornea. The lens may be too flat, have a sharp blend (which needs to be extended), have poor edges or edge profile, or be warped.

Arcuate staining

A poor edge that is not well rounded or one that is too sharp like a knife-edge can cause corneal insult of an arcuate nature. The junctional zones must be smooth and gently float over the peripheral cornea, or they may induce an arcuate staining defect. A lens that constantly decenters and positions itself eccentrically may cause arcuate staining.

3 and 9 o'clock staining (Fig. 22-2)

Three and 9 o'clock staining is sometimes referred to as *peripheral corneal staining* or *nasal and temporal staining*. It is usually light punc-

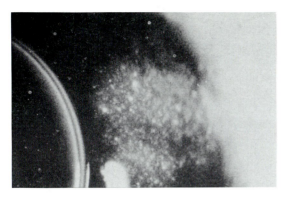

Fig 22-2 ■ 3 to 9 o'clock staining.

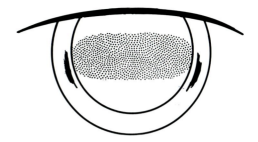

Fig 22-3 ■ With-the-rule astigmatism demonstrating compression at the 3 o'clock and 9 o'clock positions from the edges of the contact lens.

tate staining found at the horizontal margins of the cornea but may coalesce to form a concentrated area of staining. Inadequate tear film, inadequate blinking, lid tension, and the relationship of the lens edge to the cornea are contributing factors. Redness is usually found adjacent to the area.

The presence of staining in the 3 and 9 o'clock positions of the cornea has three major causes:

1. Dehydration effect
2. Thick lens edge with lid gap
3. Expression effect

The dehydration effect on the cornea is one of the major causes. The 3 and 9 o'clock staining may be mild or cause a severe episcleritis or even marginal dellen of the cornea with ulcer formation. Physiologically, the mucoid layer from the goblet cells of the conjunctiva does not cover this area of the corneal epithelial cells and permit adequate wetting. It may lead to stromal thinning. This may occur with lacrimal insufficiency, a problem that has to be addressed. The thick edges of a contact lens permit a gap of the mucoid layer in the area of the edge and result in desiccation.

Mild staining is not significant, but more advanced staining will often reduce the patient's wearing time considerably. The use of blinking exercises and artificial tears can lessen this considerably. Redesigning the lens with thinner edges or making the lens larger to bridge the defect in the case of gas-permeable lens will often help. With gas-permeable lenses this complication is common and is believed to be a complication of lid gap (drying of the tear film at the margin of a thick lens) and a low-riding lens, which impedes tear flow. To remedy this prob-

lem, one may also make the lens smaller with thinner and more polished edges. With gas-permeable lenses, one must thin the edges, that is, use a myopic profile on an aphakic lens, and the lenses must not be permitted to ride low.

Compression effect occurs every time the eyelid sweeps down and compresses the edge of the lens against the cornea. This is much more significant if there is a cylinder present. In with-the-rule astigmatism, this compression occurs in the 3 or 9 o'clock position. In against-the-rule astigmatism, it will occur in the 6 pm position (Fig. 22-3; see Figs. 29-6 and 29-7).

VASCULARIZATION

Vascularization can occur because of a number of factors caused by a poor-fitting rigid lens. There may be chronic decentration of a rigid lens that continually rides on the limbus, creating a vasogenic effect. This is more troublesome with thick lenses. There may be improper venting of the metabolic products of the eye, such as lactic acid with its subsequent buildup behind the lens. Improper venting also leads to thermal buildup with a subsequent vascular response and injection. Vascularization of the cornea is more likely to occur with soft lenses, which produce limbus-to-limbus corneal edema, whereas PMMA and gas-permeable lenses create corneal swelling in the corneal cap away from the limbal vasculature.

PROLONGED LENS PRESSURE

When a lens touches centrally on the cornea in any excessive amount, it causes a flattening effect of the apex, resulting in a reduction of the myopic refractive error. Slight touching with graduated flattening of the curve of the lens and subsequent changes in the eye are the basis of orthokerotologic treatment. With regular lens fitting, flattening of the cornea is not desirable.

If the pressure area is excessive and the touch area becomes more than slight, there may be degradation in Bowman's membrane with resultant scar formation on a permanent basis. Because of this, moderate apical touch should be avoided with standard PMMA lenses. Slight touch may be valid in keratoconus. Soper-designed PMMA lenses with a deep central curvature permit maximal clearance at the apex. Gas-permeable lenses of the Soper design are one step better because if the cone does progress between visits, with prolonged pressure on the apex, the improved oxygenation of the cornea will prevent degradation of epithelium and Bowman's membrane and preserve corneal integrity.

Undue pressure or irregular corneal pressure on a normal healthy cornea may result in a change in corneal architecture in a manner that may result in astigmatism, not only of the regular type but also of the irregular type. Repeated keratometric monitoring is required for assessment of this phenomenon.

LOSS OF CORNEAL SENSITIVITY

The wearing of a rigid PMMA contact lens has been shown to decrease the corneal sensitivity. If a rigid lens is worn for 1 to 2 months, the corneal sensitivity is rapidly regained by overnight removal of the contact lenses. However, if the lenses have been worn for years, it may take several months for the corneas to regain their normal sensitivity. This is probably not a true atrophy of the corneal nerves but an adaptation effect to a constant foreign-body stimulus. It returns when lenses are aborted or a switch is made to a high-DK lens.

Does this decrease in sensation put these patients at risk by eliminating a valuable warning sign of pain? Patients wearing PMMA lenses may have a corneal pathologic condition and not feel it. Included are the finding of 3 and 9 o'clock staining, corneal edema, and induced alteration of corneal topography.

COMMENT. One curious result of placing gas-permeable lenses on an eye with chronic corneal edema is the resumption of corneal sensation. Patients may initially find that the new lenses are more difficult to wear because of an increase in that sensation that may be interpreted as irritation. Patience is vital if the lens fits, otherwise your patient will not view your efforts char-

itably. If you have exchanged old comfortable PMMA lenses for uncomfortable gas-permeable lenses, the patient will believe that the new device is worse than the old. The patient should be forewarned about this contingency.

Endothelial changes

Many reports, particularly with PMMA lenses, have implicated corneal changes after prolonged wearing of contact lens. The main thrust of these reports has shown that when specular microscopy is performed on longterm wearers, the endothelial cells are altered. This alteration occurs in the form of polyhedral cells as well as larger polymegathism of the endothelial cells. There have been no reports of loss of cells or decrease in cell density. The higher-DK gas-permeable lenses have not revealed this pathology but the wearing time is still too short for reliable data.

Does this imply altered function of these cells and could it be a precursor to disaster later on? No one seems to be certain. However, new techniques with microscopes that can identify these cells under high magnification in 3D (an advance over 2D specular microscopy) are beginning to show that there is only a slight swelling on the surface of these cells, but the intercellular substance between cells is intact and that there is probably no loss of function. Edlehauser's studies have shown that the barrier effect of the endothelium remains even on longterm contact lens wearers. The change probably reflects some cell stress but none that is of significant proportion.

ACUTE CORNEAL CRISIS (OVERWEAR REACTION)

An acute corneal crisis is usually related to PMMA lens wear. It is strictly attributable to acute hypoxia of the corneal epithelium. Generally it occurs with a teen-ager who normally wears these lenses all day and then continues to wear them until 3 am. The normal wearing time is exceeded, and the corneal epithelium cannot tolerate the anoxia for such a length of time.

This condition always seems to begin in the early hours of the morning, several hours after the person has taken out his or her lenses the night before. Invariably there is an early morning phone call from a frightened mother that her child is totally blind and in excruciating pain.

A drop of local anesthetic goes a long way in

reducing the patient's discomfort and furthermore in facilitating examination of the cornea. The typical clinical findings are central epithelial erosions, pronounced ciliary injection, swelling of the lids, and constricted pupils.

The cure is dramatic. With bilateral firm patching, an analgesic for pain, a hypnotic to allow the distressed patient to obtain some sleep, and a short-acting cycloplegic to relieve the ciliary spasm, the condition resolves in approximately 24 hours.

After such an occurrence the lens should not be worn for approximately 4 or 5 days until all signs of irritation and corneal edema are gone. A renewed, controlled wearing time is mandatory.

The patient should then be warned about overwearing the lenses. For any casualty of an overwear reaction, a 1-week rest period when renewed wear is established is advisable.

If there is no history of actually overwearing the lens, attention should be directed to reassessment of the fit of the lens. If the lens is slightly steep or flat, it may be tolerated, but not for a full day. This situation is not a true overwear reaction, though from the patient's point of view there is no difference in symptoms.

The best treatment is prophylaxis. The patient should trade these lenses in for oxygen-permeable lenses.

COMMENT. In our hands PMMA lenses have become obsolete and the acute corneal crisis is only of historical interest. However, milder forms of acute corneal crisis do occur and have to be dealt with.

CARE-RELATED PROBLEMS
Scratches and cleaning

Feldman has pointed out that secretions of the meibomian glands will fill in the furrow of a scratched lens and will be difficult to remove because of the raised edge of the furrow. Polishing of these rigid lenses is required to permit adequate cleaning of lipoid material. Lester has suggested that edge buildup of material may be a causative factor in 3 and 9 o'clock staining.

Foreign body under lens

Any person who wears contacts may have a foreign body enter his eye. Because the tear exchange under a hard lens is about 50% to 80% with each blink, it is very easy for a conjunctival foreign body to enter and remain between the lens and cornea. In this position it will usually irritate and frequently scratch the corneal surface.

Of more particular concern is inadequate cleaning of a lens and leaving particulate matter on the inner surface of the contact lens. Not only may this matter act as a physical irritant to the cornea, but also chemicals remaining may cause toxicity to the underlying cornea. Careful washing of one's hands and using recommended care solutions are of utmost importance.

Fingernail scratches

Inadequate insertion technique with long fingernails is a frequent cause of corneal abrasions. This is usually noted by telltale markings on the inferior portion of the cornea. At least 6% of contact lens wearers experience corneal abrasions.

Improper care routines

The gas-permeable rigid lenses of the silicone-PMMA material do not wet well with standard rigid lens solutions. These standard rigid lens solutions will often impair the wetting surface of the newer gas-permeable lenses so that the person wearing these lenses will have blurred vision. One must follow recommended care systems.

Infection

The committee on Contact Lenses of the American Association of Ophthalmology reported in 1966 in the Journal of the American Medical Association on 14 eyes lost or blinded in patients wearing contact lenses from a population of almost 50,000 contact lens wearers. There were 157 other eyes permanently damaged in this series, attesting to the serious problems that can be caused by contact lenses. All the blindness was caused by the result of a serious infectious process, hand-to-eye contamination.

HIGH-ALTITUDE RISKS

People who live in high-altitude locations, such as Denver, Colorado, may experience great difficulty with hard as well as soft contact lenses. In all probability the decreased tolerance is directly related to the decreased oxygen content found in high altitudes. Also the relative humidity at 5000 feet is lower than at sea level. The lowered humidity tends to increase the evaporation rate, and protein and salt deposits tend to crust on the surface of the hard lens. In addition to these problems the rare atmosphere allows more infrared and ultraviolet rays to pass through the lens with more intensity. The infrared rays create more heat and more evaporation. A polymethylmethacrylate lens acts as an insulation that raises the oxygen demands of the corneal epithelium. Coupled with the normal hypoxia of a lens covering the cornea, the added stress may be intolerable. The ultraviolet rays can create corneal epithelial irritation under the PMMA lens.

As one would expect, people who wear lenses in high-altitude locations frequently complain of photophobia, grittiness in the eyes, inability to tolerate their lenses for a full day, and burning sensations. Frequently they display superficial punctate staining of the epithelium, dry patches on the cornea, and 3 and 9 o'clock perilimbal congestion and keratopathy. These symptoms and signs frequently disappear when such a person either visits or moves to a low-altitude environment. Stewardesses frequently have trouble with their lenses while in flight. In the Boeing 747, for example, when flying at 31,000 feet the cabin is pressurized to equal the pressure of about 5000 feet, whereas at 42,000 feet the cabin pressure is equivalent to an altitude of 7000 feet. Thus the atmospheric pressure is not at sea level. In addition, the air-conditioning system dehydrates the cabin, and so there are less tears to carry oxygen.

For permanent high-altitude dwellers who wear lenses, a reduction in wearing time to a range of 8 to 10 hours must be made. Other approaches include the use of multiple fenestrations, small microthin lenses, and the use of artificial tears during the day. Sometimes rigid lenses must be abandoned and, if the indications are present, soft lenses substituted, which usually are satisfactory.

Skiers do not seem to have any problems with their lenses and in fact enjoy them more while skiing. In all probability this comfort is caused by the increased tear production, stimulated by the cold and wind, and the cooler temperatures that prevent heat accumulation under the lenses. The hypoxia of high altitudes is compensated by the hypothermia of a cooler environment.

Gas-permeable lens again are an excellent choice for the high-altitude dweller. Not only is the oxygen permeability better but also the thermal conductivity is enhanced. The temperature of the cornea is not raised by the presence of the lens. Regular PMMA acts as an insulator and consequently raises the oxygen demands of the cornea. With silicone-PMMA lenses, there is heat transfer through the lens and the oxygen needs of the cornea are reduced.

COMMENT. Ski goggles are still required for the protection of the corneas while contact lenses are worn.

INCLUSION BLENNORRHEA

An inclusion blennorrhea is a venereal disease that causes a subclinical infection resulting in follicular conjunctivitis, a few subepithelial infiltrates of the cornea, and a soft, palpable, preauricular node. This condition is tolerable until the patient tries to wear a lens and then suddenly develops symptoms that naturally are blamed on the presence of the lenses. These cases are best treated with sulfonamide drops until the punctate keratopathy and follicles disappear. The duration of the disease can seem to be endless, lasting from 6 weeks to 3 or 4 months, during which time lenses cannot be worn.

BIRTH CONTROL PILL INTOLERANCE

Women who begin wearing lenses and then begin taking birth control pills frequently find that they can no longer tolerate their lenses. Vision becomes hazy, the wearing time is reduced, and the eyes are unusually sensitive to light. Some authorities believe that this results from a change in the tear film, whereas others who witness a haziness of the keratometer mires believe that there is an alteration in the shape or texture of the cornea itself. Women already on birth control pills usually do not suffer such reactions. Intolerance to rigid lenses has also been a problem during the early stages of pregnancy.

FITTING PROBLEMS

Fitting problems will be reviewed under each of the newer materials. The silicone acrylates (Chapter 25) and problems such as flexure are specifically related to the newer and softer material. Methods of fitting have to be altered to provide a thicker lens if flexure occurs.

Bubbles are related to high-riding lenses that tend to vault the area between the corneal apex and the upper limbus. This causes tiny bubbles of froth to be trapped under the lens, resulting in epithelial wrinkling.

CRAZING AND CRACKING

The newer rigid lenses that contain silicone have been reported by a number of observers to show a peculiar surface crazing. This appears as interconnecting cracks on the lens surface. The etiology may be a manufacturing problem that may continue to grow because of dehydration and hydration effects on the lens.

COMMENT. This overview of contact lens problems will be expanded under each material discussed. Fortunately, many of the problems of rigid lenses that we have seen previously are becoming less serious and the fitter is able to concentrate his or her energies on fitting high cylinders, presbyopes, tints and other more interesting aspects of contactology rather than constantly handling serious problems. The more serious defects that affect epithelium and endothelium are reviewed in Part IV, Chapters 36 to 40.

23 ▪ *HOW TO ENSURE YOUR RIGID LENSES ARE WHAT YOU ORDERED*

G. Peter Halberg

- Diameter
- Surface quality and edges
- Base curve
- Power
- Central thickness
- Surface quality
- Blend

If the lens received from the laboratory is faulty or does not conform to the design specifications ordered, the fit of the lens will be poor. No laboratory can mass-produce quality lenses all the time. Fitters must be able to verify the lens not only for their own satisfaction but also to keep the lens laboratory alerted to the fact that its work is being inspected. This helps to raise the standards for everyone concerned. With the advent of gas-permeable rigid lenses, the rigid lens has an important new role and must be critically evaluated.

DIAMETER

The first parameter to be checked is the diameter of the lens. The diameter of rigid lenses can be assessed with a diameter gauge (Fig. 23-1). Care should be exercised not to use any force while inserting the lens into the gauge. The lens should fall into the proper position by its own weight. The lens should check in at at least two meridians for roundness. It should also be dry, as a wet lens will have a water collar at the edge and will appear larger. The tolerance for diameter should be ±0.05 mm. The diameter of rigid lenses can also be assessed with a measuring loupe, which serves the dual purpose of measuring the diameter and the width of the peripheral and optic zones. In addition the hand loupe serves to assess the surface quality of the lens (Fig. 23-2).

SURFACE QUALITY AND EDGES

A more elaborate and precise check of the surface quality and diameter of the lens can be performed with the various projector type of inspection devices available. Typical of these projection devices is the Wesley-Jessen Inspectocon (Figs. 23-3 and 23-4).

COMMENT. It is important to check the edges, since an imperfect edge is probably the greatest source of discomfort from wearing rigid lenses.

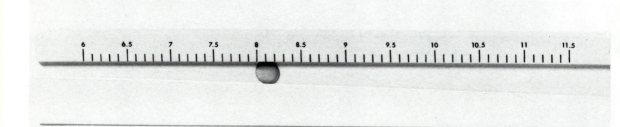

Fig 23-1 ▪ Diameter gauge for rigid lenses.

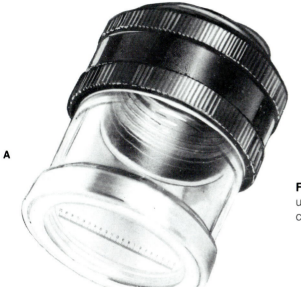

A

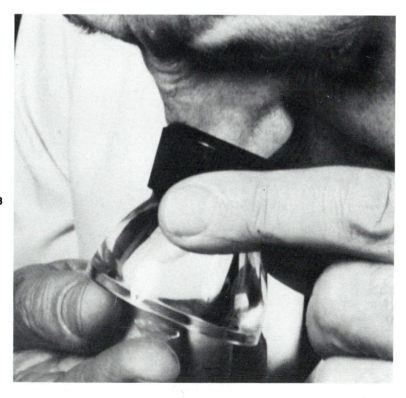

B

Fig 23-2 ■ **A,** Measuring hand magnifier. **B,** The use of a hand magnifier to inspect a rigid or soft contact lens.

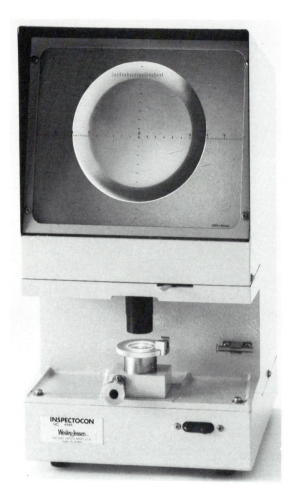

A

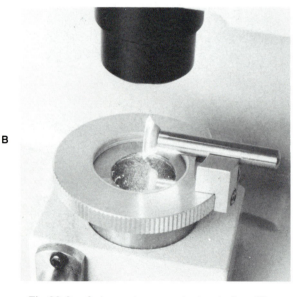

B

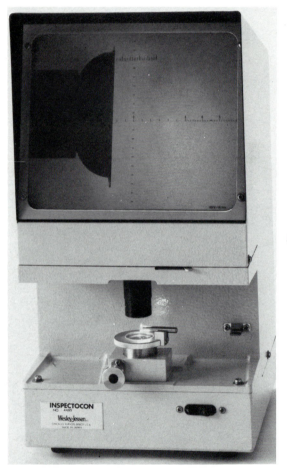

Fig 23-4 ■ **A,** Inspectocon projection device has provision for examination of the lens edge in a profile view.

Fig 23-3 ■ **A,** Inspectocon projector device. (Courtesy Wesley-Jessen, Chicago.) **B,** Close-up of a lens attached to a suction cup for inspection by Inspectocon projector.

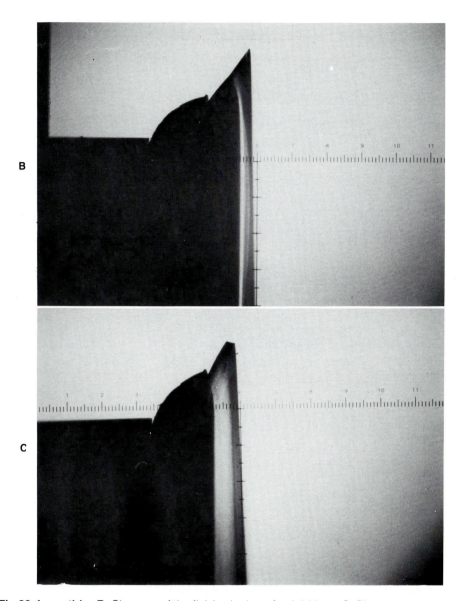

Fig 23-4, cont'd ■ **B,** Close-up of the finished edge of a rigid lens. **C,** Shadowgraph projection of a thick blunted rigid lens edge.

BASE CURVE

The curvature of the lens can be assessed by the Bausch & Lomb keratometer or the CLC Ophthalmometer of the American Optical Corporation (Figs. 23-5 to 23-7). A holder is at- tached to the keratometer that has a receptacle for the lens and a concave test plate. The lens is held in the well of the holder with an adhesive substance such as clay or cream. An excellent type of holder (called Con-Ta-Check) is one that

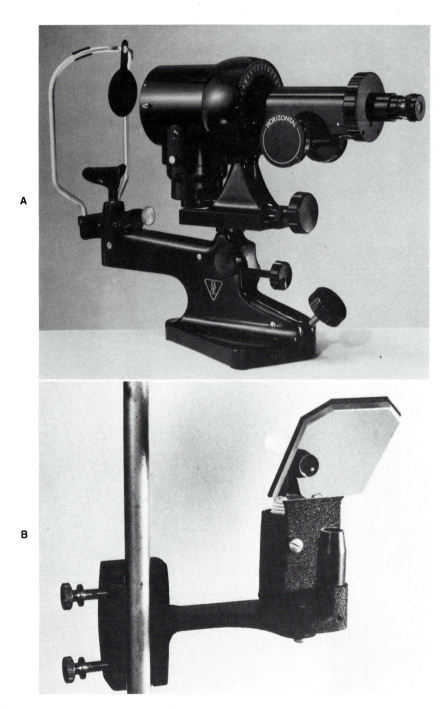

Fig 23-5 ■ **A,** Bausch & Lomb keratometer. **B,** Con-Ta-Check attachment for keratometer. (Courtesy Wesley-Jessen, Chicago.)

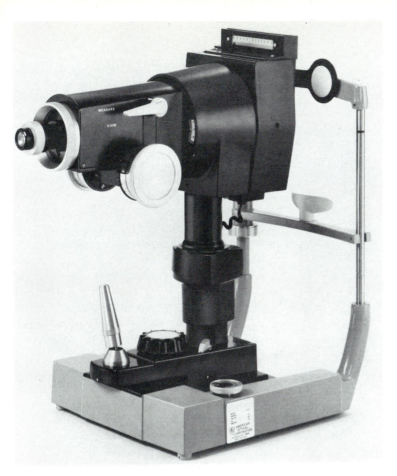

Fig 23-6 ■ CLC Ophthal-mometer. (Courtesy American Optical Corp, South-bridge, Mass.)

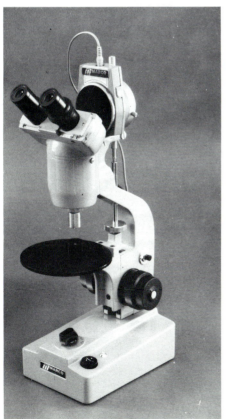

Fig 23-7 ■ Binocular Digital Radiusgauge optic spherometer for measuring the radius of curvature of a contact lens. Note the digital readout. (Courtesy Marco Medical Products, Jacksonville, Fla.)

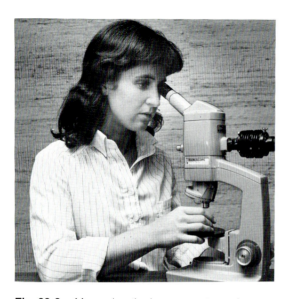

Fig. 23-8 ■ Measuring the base curvature of a contact lens with the optic spherometer (Radiuscope). (From Stein HA Slatt BJ and Stein RM: The ophthalmic assistant, ed 5, St Louis, 1988, The CV Mosby Co.)

allows the lens surface to be placed horizontally while the keratometer remains in its normal position. A front-surface mirror placed at a 45-degree angle to the optic axis of the keratometer reflects light from the mires to the lens. For optic purposes it is the same as if the lens were placed in front of the keratometer. By allowing the lens to lie flat, no adhesive substance is needed; this eliminates annoying distortions. The lens is placed so that its convex surface is in contact with the fluid, which can be glycerin, water, or wetting solution. Because the refractive index of the fluid approximates the index of the lens, the convex surface is neutralized and the posterior lens surface is measured.

More reliable inspection and measuring of the lens curvature can be performed with the Radiuscope (American Optical Corporation), Figs. 23-8 and 23-9.

The Contacto Gauge (Fig. 23-10, *A*) works on the same principle as the optic spherometer (Radiuscope, Fig. 23-8) but is lower in price and has the added advantage of a built-in thickness gauge.

Besides being a part of the routine verification of a lens, evaluation of the base curve is the best

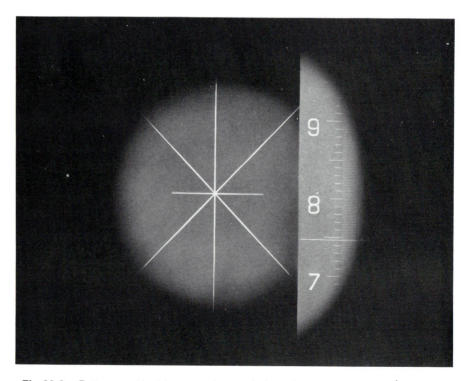

Fig 23-9 ■ Pattern and inside measuring scale in optic spherometer (Radiuscope).

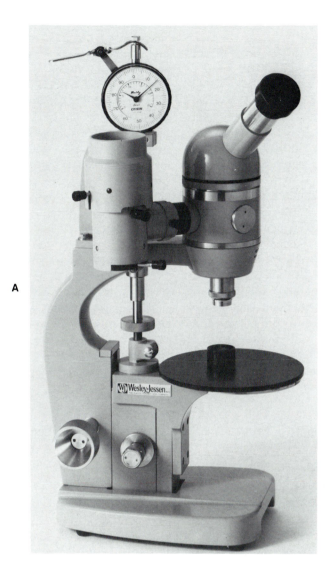

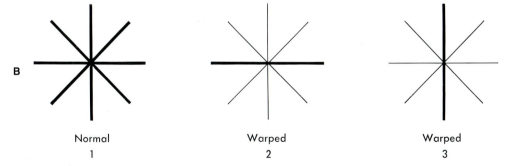

Normal
1

Warped
2

Warped
3

Fig 23-10 ■ **A,** Wesley-Jessen Contacto Gauge with built-in thickness gauge. **B,** Warpage is indicated if the mires are not in focus in all principal meridians as indicated in 2 and 3.

method for determining warpage. Contented lens-wearers who suddenly develop hazy vision, intolerance to their lenses, or astigmatism must be suspected of having a warped lens. The base curve should be accurate to within 0.025 mm of specifications (Fig. 23-10, *B*).

The optic spherometer is specifically designed to measure the optic-zone radius. It is more accurate than the keratometer, is simple to use, and yields rapid results. It is an excellent instrument for determining the base curve or the presence of warpage. Its major disadvantage is its cost.

The technique is straightforward. The concave surface of the lens is used as a concave mirror. The convex surface is neutralized by a drop of glycerin placed under the lens. The image is reflected from the posterior surface of the lens and is viewed on the lens and at the radius of the mirror. The focusing device is adjusted to its lowest position until the bottom image comes into sharp view. This image should be adjusted for zero. The barrel is moved upward until the first image is seen. The radius of curvature is read in hundredths of a millimeter.

POWER

The dioptric power of a rigid lens is determined with the lensometer. Since most lensometers are designed for large, flat posterior curvatures of spectacle lenses, they cannot be completely converted to measure the power of a highly curved, corneal lens. An error in power is introduced that is equal to the sagittal depth at the back of the lens and the plane of the aperture. This error can be reduced with an accessory conic choke, which reduces the aperture size. The convex side faces away from the eyepiece, that is, against the lensometer stop when the power at the front-vertex surface is measured. However, most laboratories measure the back-vertex power; that is, the concave surface is placed away from the examiner and toward the lensometer stop. This is done because refractors, corrected trial lenses, and spectacle lenses are all specified this way. This is the back-vertex or corneal-plane—vertex power of a lens, the most reliable one to use. This difference in approach can yield different results. The practitioner should make sure that he or she and the laboratory are doing the same thing. Plus lenses

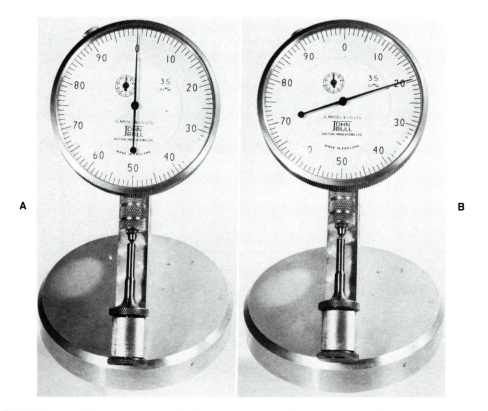

A   B

Fig 23-11 ■ **A,** Before measuring, thickness gauge must be set to zero. **B,** Thickness gauge.

show less plus for front-vertex powers than for back-vertex powers. The lens power should be exact within ±0.25 D of power ordered and less than ±0.12 D of uncalled-for astigmatism.

CENTRAL THICKNESS

A thickness gauge is the most useful device for measuring central thickness. The most reliable measurement is calibrated in tenths of a millimeter, but some lathe-cut machines (Wesley-Jesson) for fabricating lenses are set for thousandths of an inch, and so one must make a conversion, for example, 0.001 inch = 0.02 mm.

The most common instrument used is the dial gauge. The lens is placed convex side down on its base. A spring-plunger tip is released until it touches the lens. The amount by which the plunger is separated from the base indicates the thickness of the lens (Fig. 23-11).

All gauges have arrangements for zero setting. Before measuring, the gauge must be set meticulously to the zero point.

SURFACE QUALITY

Surface quality of the rigid lens can also be assessed by use of attachments for the slitlamp, which then permit detailed inspection in diffuse or slit illumination, or both. If necessary, one can use monochromatic light, switching in the various filters available on the slitlamp. Fig. 23-12 shows a simple device readily available for slit-lamp inspection of lenses. The holder rotates the slitlamp, and the lens is held in place by a standard rubber suction cup.

A more elaborate slit-lamp inspection device is the Zeiss prismatic lens holder, which will fit on the Zeiss photographic slitlamp and with some ingenuity can be easily attached to other slitlamps. We use it on the 900 Haag-Streit slitlamp by inserting the metal rod of the prismatic device into the Hruby lens-holder socket (Fig. 23-13).

BLEND

The transition zones of the rigid lens in our view should be thoroughly blended. Instantaneous assessment of the transition zones can be achieved with the profile analyzer, a product of Gulf Coast Contact Lens, Inc., of New Orleans (Fig. 23-14). This instrument gives an optic projection of the inner (concave) surface of a narrow section of the lens diameter, vividly displaying any defect that may be present in the blending. One look at a poorly finished transition zone in the profile analyzer will make it instantly clear to the fitter why the patient cannot tolerate the otherwise well-fitting lens. In our view this is an essential quality-control instrument in medical lens practice (Fig. 23-15).

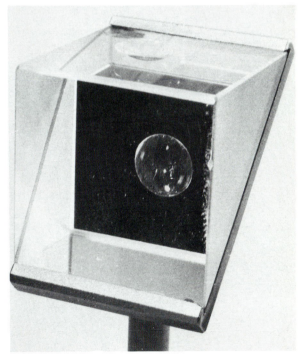

Fig 23-13 ■ Zeiss prismatic lens inspection device for the slitlamp. The lens rests on top and is reflected in the vertical plane for viewing by the slit lamp microscope.

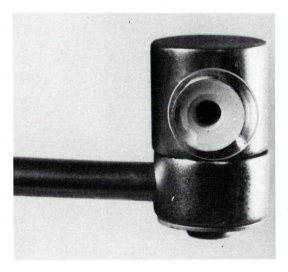

Fig 23-12 ■ Holder for lens in slitlamp inspection.

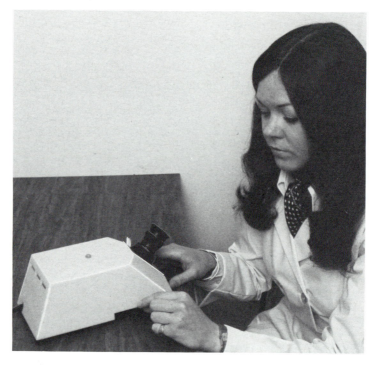

Fig 23-14 ■ Profile analyzer used to evaluate the blend of the peripheral curves of a lens. (From Stein HA, Slatt BJ and Stein RM: The ophthalmic assistant, ed 5, St Louis, 1988, The CV Mosby Co.)

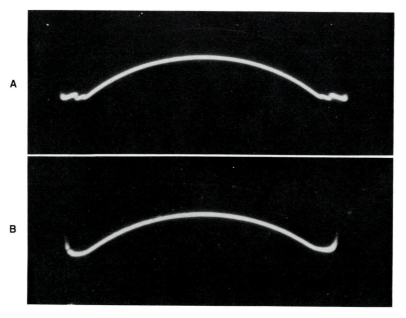

Fig 23-15 ■ **A,** Poorly finished transition zone as determined by the profile analyzer. **B,** Perfect transition zone with ski contour at its periphery.

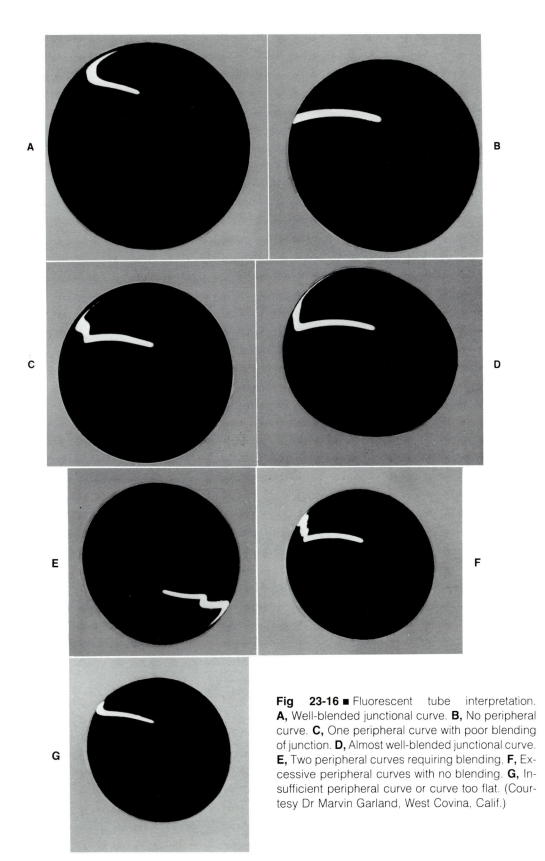

Fig 23-16 ■ Fluorescent tube interpretation. **A,** Well-blended junctional curve. **B,** No peripheral curve. **C,** One peripheral curve with poor blending of junction. **D,** Almost well-blended junctional curve. **E,** Two peripheral curves requiring blending, **F,** Excessive peripheral curves with no blending. **G,** Insufficient peripheral curve or curve too flat. (Courtesy Dr Marvin Garland, West Covina, Calif.)

A sharp junction at the blend is a major source of rigid lens defects, but a faulty edge creates more problems. If a profile analyzer is not available, Honan and Garland have described the following technique to examine the peripheral curves and blend of a rigid contact lens.

The fluorescent tube should be in front of and higher than the examiner. The examiner should position himself so that the bare fluorescent tube is *directly* in front of and parallel to the examiner's shoulder. One should be situated slightly back from the fluorescent tube so that the reflection is thinner and easier to interpret. The lens must be held so that the reflection of the light on the posterior surface of the lens falls on the inferior portion of the lens, approximately 65% to 75% of the distance from the top to the bottom of the lens. The lens must be tilted and positioned slightly to the side so that the reflection is continuous to the edge of the lens. The positioning of the lens under the fluorescent tube is the most difficult part to perform. Wearing a loupe or using a hand magnifier helps one to see details better.

An ideal blend in peripheral curve should show a J-shaped or ski pattern in a nice smooth curve. The J is horizontal and curves inferiorly at the edge (Fig. 23-16, *A*). If there is no pe- ripheral curve present, the reflection of the fluorescent tube continues to the edge in a straight or upward pattern (Fig. 23-16, *B*).

If there are peripheral curves, the area where the reflection starts to curve inferiorly is a junction of the optic zone and peripheral curve. If the peripheral curve is poorly blended, the reflection appears as in Fig. 23-16, *C*. An almost well-blended curve is shown in Fig. 23-16, *D*. If there are two peripheral curves requiring blending, this pattern appears as in Fig. 23-16, *E*. If there are excessive curves, the pattern looks like a Z as shown in Fig. 23-16, *F*. Appropriate blending will convert this pattern to the ideal J or ski pattern. If there is an insufficient peripheral curve or the peripheral curve is too flat, this deficiency is shown in Fig. 23-16, *G*.

COMMENT. Quality control of contact lenses starts with the manufacturing phase. However, the practitioner should have sufficient equipment to determine that the specifications conform to what was requested, the edges are smooth and carefully lathed, and a proper blend is constructed between curves. Without these assurances, one cannot adequately analyze improper fitting and proceed to rectify the problem.

24 ■ *CELLULOSE ACETATE BUTYRATE (CAB) LENSES*

■ *Advantages*
■ *Disadvantages*
■ *Fitting the CAB lens*

This lens may soon be of historical interest, but a short description is presented because at the time of writing, the lens was still in the marketplace.

The gas-permeable cellulose acetate butyrate (CAB) lens is made of a unique plastic (cellulose acetate butyrate, a cellulose derivative) that has the ability to permit oxygen to diffuse into and carbon dioxide to diffuse out of the lens. This gas-permeable plastic, which is made from natural substances, was developed by Eastman Kodak for photographic purposes. Cellulose is derived from wood and cotton, acetic acid from vinegar, and butyric acid from natural gas. Although the plastic has been available since 1938, it was not used as contact lens material until 1974. It was the first of the gas-permeable lenses.

The material's prime attraction appeared to be that it was not flammable. This plastic dissipates heat much better and wets much easier than the plastic of which ordinary hard lenses are made, and thus permits tears to flow better under it. Kodak is still the prime manufacturer of this material.

ADVANTAGES

The CAB has the following advantages over PMMA:
1. Longer wearing time.
2. Reduction of corneal edema, spectacle blur, and overwear syndrome.
3. Elimination of edge glare seen with smaller lenses because lenses can be fitted larger.
4. Permeability to oxygen 40 times greater than that of soft lenses but not so much as the pure silicone lenses or the silicone-PMMA varieties.
5. Larger optic zone; consequently increased visual field and less flare.
6. Better heat conductivity.
7. Very tough and difficult to break.

The CAB lens has a smaller contact angle than the PMMA lens, making it more wettable than the PMMA lens. This advantage is particularly helpful in patients with moderately dry eyes. The surface tension is 35 degrees lower and the wetting angle 18.5 degrees less than those of PMMA. Although the major advantage of this plastic is its permeability to oxygen and carbon dioxide, the newer rigid lenses, including silicone-PMMA combinations and the fluoronated silicone acrylates, are much superior.

DISADVANTAGES

These lenses have the following disadvantages:
1. Visual acuity may be reduced because of poor surface optic patterns.
2. Some lens awareness because of thickness at the center and the edges.
3. Susceptibility to scratches and chips.
4. Center and edge thickness is much greater (approximately one third) when compared to silicone-acrylate lenses.
5. Unavailability of toric lenses and prism ballasts, color, and other special designs.
6. Lack of stability. Lenses frequently change after hydration and occasionally steepen after several weeks. Also the lenses can warp after 1 year of wearing time. Lens warpage, however, is not too much of a problem if the lens is not manufactured too thin.

261

7. Verification of the base curve requires rapid measurement after drying of the soaked lens since the properties of the same lens differ depending on whether it is wet or dry.

The primary disadvantage of CAB is its low module of elasticity or poor shape retention. The material does not retain its contours when flexed or distorted. Clinically, this leads to warpage of the lens from handling during cleaning procedures. The material tends to be distorted by a lathing bit, and during manufacturing the material may require special hardeners to keep it compact. One method to retain hardness is boiling the buttons in silicone oil. Unless excellent quality controls in the fabrication are present, the softness and heat sensitivity of the materials can result in unsatisfactory peripheral curves and edges. Finishing procedures require care. Special compounds must be used in its fabrication. The polishing compounds should be cool or cold and water-based. Ammonia-based compounds like Silvo hydrolyze and the lens material can turn it yellow. Alcohol and petroleum products also cause opacification of this material. The plastic must be bathed at 98° F (39° C) for hours after finishing.

The finished lens is relatively thick in contrast to the thin PMMA or hydrogel lenses. The recommended minimal central thickness is approximately 16 mm. These lenses are fit steeper initially, since the material tends to flatten because of its inherent softness or perhaps its molding to the corneal surface. As with any gas-permeable lens, the permeability feature allows for larger diameters, which in turn allow one to have a larger optic zone than a smaller-sized PMMA lens would have. The large lenses which are about 9 mm in diameter, also afford stability and centration. The steeper base curves are permitted because of the ancillary feature of diffusion of oxygen. There is less movement to a good fit, and hence there is more comfort. In the aphakic lens, the added thickness of the lens makes warpage less of a problem. However, the thicker lenses also significantly reduce oxygen permeability, and such a reduction makes extended wear unsatisfactory or marginal.

COMMENT. The authors feel this lens will soon be of historical interest only, so detailed fitting methods have been omitted from this chapter. Excessive lens flexure may cause unwanted astigmatism with CAB lenses.

The CAB lens is made of a tough, gristle-like material that may have microscopic waves. Verification of the base curve on the optic spherometer may show errors as a result of the very small segment measured. The keratometer, which measures a larger area, will show the true base curve.

FITTING THE CAB LENS

Any size, curvature, or thickness similar to regular rigid lenses can be ordered. A good fit is one that is positioned somewhat high with minimal movement but with complete corneal clearance. One should fit either from a trial set or from K and refractive error measurements. There is a high index of refraction to this plastic; consequently about 0.50 D more plus than the normal refractive power is required.

25 ▪ *SILICONE-ACRYLATE LENSES*

Gas-permeable lenses have added a new dimension to the fitting of rigid lenses. Because of the ability to transmit oxygen, they have significantly reduced the complications of rigid PMMA lenses that are attributed to anoxic changes in the cornea. Also, because of the ability to design larger rigid lenses than before, one can overcome the optic disadvantages of the PMMA lenses. With this technologic improvement to the time-honored PMMA lens, the silicone-acrylate (sometimes referred to as *silozanyl-acrylate*) lenses have replaced PMMA lenses and have heralded the era of the gas-permeability of contact lenses. Other gas-permeable lenses, such as the styrene lens of Wesley-Jessen (Chicago) and the rigid fluorocarbon lenses are challenging the position of preeminence enjoyed so far by silicone-acrylate lenses.

Today there are over 21 million North Americans who wear contact lenses. 5 million people are now wearing RGP lenses whereas in 1982 there were only 2 million who wore rigid lenses.

The search for a highly gas-permeable contact lens material has been pursued since the late 1950s. The use of silicone as a contact-lens material dates to 1958 when Becker of Dow Corning in Pittsburg fabricated a crude contact lens from silicone rubber. Dow Corning donated a great deal of time and money to the development of a pure silicone contact lens, both hard and soft, that provides excellent oxygen permeability. However, eventually this was abandoned except for special custom designs intended for the pediatric aphake. The mixture with PMMA appeared to have become a more acceptable and commercially viable alternative.

Although silicone is highly oxygen-permeable, it is also hydrophilic with a tendency to flexure. Because of this, other monomers are added. These include methyl methacrylate for rigidity and optical performance and to provide dimensional stability and reduce flexure and warpage. Methacrylate and/or hema may be added to improve wettability.

The recent introduction of fluorocarbon and fluorocarbon silicone-acrylate lenses (see Chapter 26) has made possible better wetting properties, increased oxygen performance, and lower deposits. The silicone acrylates alone have a higher surface reactivity because of negative surface charges that attract such protein as denatured lysozyme.

The principal silicone-acrylate lenses are known clinically as Polycon I or II (Sola/Barnes Hind, San Diego, California). Boston lenses I, II, and 4 and the Equalens (Polymer Technology Corporation, Wilmington, Massachusetts) are lenses derived from the gas transmission buttons, giving rise to a number of trade names, and Menicon O_2 (Toyo Contact Lens Company, Tokyo, Japan). In addition, Optocryl 60, Paraperm, and B&L Gas Perm are other entries in the field. These lenses should be differentiated from cellulose acetate butyrate (CAB), basically a wood product that is also gas permeable but thicker and less stable, being subject to warpage. Rigid lenses of 100% silicone are available but are confined to specific areas such as in the treatment of pediatric aphakia.

THE LENS
Material considerations

The essential component of this group of gas-permeable lenses is silicone that has been mixed with PMMA. After oxygen, silicon is the second most abundant element in the earth's crust. From its position below oxygen in the periodic table, one would expect silicon chemical behavior to be similar to that of carbon, but it is not. During the past several decades, there has been a burgeoning synthesis industry so that today thousands of organosilicones are known.

The preparation of silicones starts with the isolation of pure silicon or silicon carbide. For contact-lens usage, most polymers stem from silicon oxide and carbon groups—R_2SiO—and various polymers are added. Organosilicone polymers are polyacrylates and have radicals attached to make the material more functional.

> Methyl groups contribute to flexibility.
> Phenyl groups contribute to stiffness.

Increasing the length of the organic group attached to silicone increases its softness and water repellency. As the ratio of organic groups to silicone decreases, the polymer becomes less fluid, less soluble, and harder to produce (that is, goes from a rubbery to a glassy state).

The oxygen bond of the silicone contributes to high heat resistance, oxidation resistance, and permeability toward gases.

Pure silicone polymers are soft and nonwettable (hydrophobic). In combination with polymethylmethacrylate (PMMA), the hardness and stability of the silicone are enhanced. To ensure sufficient wettability, there is a polymerization of the silicone with additional hydrophilic monomers. When this is done, no surface treatment or special solutions are thus required to attain good surface wettability. Different additives such as dimethacrylate may be used to enhance tensile strength and resistance to deformation.

In the marriage of silicone with PMMA, normally the addition of silicone decreases wettability, stability, and strength. This has been overcome by some manufacturers of silicone-acrylate lenses: the wettability, stability, and strength of the hybrid material has been maintained when the two components are mixed, usually in the ratio of about 65% PMMA and 35% silicone. However, silicone does have an adverse effect on a contact lens. There is an increase of mucus and protein in a high-silicone lens. In addition, flexure becomes a problem with wearing silicone. Other polymers may be added (e.g., ITA conate) to ensure physical stability. Polymer corporation has added ITA conate, which is an attempt to counteract the softeners of the material and to avoid lens flexure.

Table 25-1 reflects the technical comparisons of the numerous available lenses. Silicone polymers fall between PMMA and CAB (cellulose acetate butyrate) in terms of hardness on the Shore D scale.

PMMA	88.5
Silicone-PMMA	84.0
CAB	77.5

In terms of wettability, silicone-based gas-permeable lenses are close to PMMA and CAB—between 23 and 25 degrees. These can be reduced with special bonding.

Fabrication

The fabrication of silicone-based lenses is similar to that of PMMA lenses. However, the silicone polymer is somewhat more sensitive to heat and pressure. Thus the diamond-tipped cutting tool must always be sharp; carbon-tipped tools are not satisfactory. Compressed air cooling of the diamond tip is advisable.

Wax or pitch polishing is strongly recommended, especially for outside surfaces. Pillow pads may be used for base curves. White Nissel wax is ideal for polishing base curves. Conventional non-ammoniated polishes may be used for edge finishing and generating peripheral curves. However, polishing compounds with a particle size less than 0.4 μm should be used for polishing both surfaces. If done properly, the optic quality of these lenses should match that of PMMA.

Aliphatic (saturated) hydrocarbons solvents are best for the removal of wax, pitch, and tape adhesive. Alcohols, esters, ketones, and aromatic hydrocarbons will damage the plastic and should be avoided.

Because these lenses may be less resistant to breakage and more subject to flexure than

Table 25-1 ■ Available specifications of some silicone-acrylate gas-permeable lenses

Rigid oxygen-permeable lenses	Manufacturer	Index	Hardness		Permeability (DK × 10^{-11})	Wetting angle
			Shore D	Rockwell		
		(1.490)	(95H)	(94H)	(0)	(25°P, 46°H, 50°A, 20°)
(Polymethyl-methacrylate for comparison)						
Polycon I	Syntex Ophthalmics	1.479	86	71H	5.0; 5.82 ± 0.9132‡	22°P, 43°H, 56°A, 30.4°R
Polycon II	Syntex Ophthalmics	1.479	N/A	N/A	10.0	50°A, 15°R
Boston Lens I	Polymer Technology	1.471	116 79H	85	116 79H; 10.66 ± 0.7590‡	22°P, 47°H, 29° others
Boston Lens II	Polymer Technology	1.471	N/A	N/A	12.6	24°
CABCurve	Hydrocurve	1.475			4.2†	56°S, 24°B
Modified CAB	Hydrocurve	1.475	76		4.2	20°S, 13.5°B
W/J Airlens	Wessley-Jesson	1.533	86		12.2	54°B
Sil-O₂-Flex	Fused Contacts	1.47	89		7.7 5.2†; 8.2 Hill	25.4°P
Menicon O₂	Toyo Contact Lens	1.481	N/A	N/A	7.5 10.5†; 9.1 others	16° to 23°
Optacryl 60	Capital	N/A	N/A	N/A	12.4	N/A
Persecon	Titmus-Eurocon	N/A	N/A	N/A	N/A	N/A
Oxyflow	Hirst	1.47		31	32.01 22.0†	42.3°H
Alberta (SM38 and XL30)	Calgary Contacts	1.469	88		8.73 ±1.0872§	24.8° to 30°, 30.4°P
Calgary (XL20)	Calgary Contacts	N/A	N/A	98H	4.05° 1.8246§	28°, 46°H
Oxyflex	Cantor & Silver	1.47	N/A	N/A	13.0 7.2 others	23°P

†Morris: RM (rotation of mirror) = 21° to 25°; eye = 35°.
‡Morris, 1981.
§Morris, 1982.
N/A, Not applicable.
A, Advanced; *B*, bubble; *H*, Hirst; *P*, poster; *R*, receded; *S*, sessile drop.

PMMA lenses are, they are frequently made slightly thicker than regular rigid lenses.

The following are common problems in quality control.

Lens warpage. The presence of warpage usually indicates that excessive heat was applied during the blocking or lathing procedures or that excessive force was applied as the lens was removed from the blocking pitch or wax. If this problem persists after you confirm the alignment and sharpness of the diamond tool, reduce the depth and speed of each cut and check the results of increasing the turning speed of the lathes.

Poor surface optic properties. If this problem is present, increase the polishing time using a polishing compound. Also, the alignment or sharpness of the cutting by the diamond tool may be unsatisfactory.

COMMENT. Silicone polymers that are made with PMMA can be made as thin as regular rigid lenses. The only problem with these hybrid lenses is they are slightly more brittle and tend to chip easily at the edges.

Thermal conductivity

PMMA acts as a thermal insulator. Not only does it create corneal hypoxia, but by insulating the cornea it also raises the basal metabolic rate and increases the oxygen demand of the epithelium of the cornea. However, silicones, either in the pure form or mixed with PMMA, are thermal conductors, which take the heat of metabolism away from the corneal surface and thereby decrease oxygen requirements.

Thermal conductivity:	$10,000$ cal/sec/m^2/°C/cm
ASTM test	C 177
CAB	6.4
PMMA	5.0
Silicone	12.6

Optic and surface properties

These silicone polymers transmit most of the light in the range of the visible spectrum, that is, 400 to 750 nm. Commercially available contact lenses have a refractive index in the range of 1.35 to 1.45.

For the investigation of the wettability of polymers, most reports deal with angle measurements. However, these measurements are not absolute because the figures change drastically when lenses are worn. For example, the addition of protein or lipid to the surface of a lens effec-

tively reduces its wettability and permeability. As one might expect, surface coatings reduce vision and comfort.

UNDERSTANDING GAS PERMEABILITY

The permeability of a contact lens is largely related to the following:
1. Permeability of the polymer, or D_1
2. Solubility coefficient or partition coefficient, or K_1
3. Thickness of the lens

Permeability can be enhanced by increasing DK or reducing the thickness of the lens.

The permeability coefficients of contact lens materials to oxygen are usually expressed at a constant relative humidity (water-vapor activity) and at a constant temperature, preferably at 34° C (Table 25-1).

Silicone groups offer high oxygen-permeability, whereas an ordinary PMMA lens has no oxygen permeability. Also, pure silicone polymers are chemically stable and transparent. Unfortunately, in the pure form they are not very wettable. The incorporation of moderate amounts of silicone monomers by copolymerization with PMMA increases the permeability of oxygen through these lenses without losing the dimensional stability of the lens.

True gas-permeable rigid lenses are those that transmit oxygen from one side of the lens to the other side. It should be noted that a cosmetic HEMA lens of 38.6% water content and 0.15 mm center thickness allows no physiologically significant oxygen to reach the cornea. All rigid and most conventional soft lenses present a barrier to oxygen diffusing directly to the cornea. After wearing a nonpermeable test lens, the cornea develops an increased demand for oxygen. With PMMA, for example, with the lens being -4.00 D, the application of such a lens to the cornea can increase its thickness by 10% or greater because of hypoxia.

If a goggle is placed over the eye with different percentages of oxygen until that oxygen degree producing the same corneal demands as the test lens is found, it is said that that value represents the equivalent oxygen performance of the lens. Without proper oxygen, the cornea becomes hypoxic. A silicone lens that is gas permeable creates only a 4% increase in corneal thickness when first applied to the eye.

Edema results if the available oxygen falls below the level of 1.5% to 2.5%. This can be measured with the pachometer as an increase in corneal thickness. Glycogen (glucose-storage level) begins to dissipate if there is less than 5% oxygen available.

The amount of equivalent oxygen in air is 20% with the eyes open. With the eye closed as in sleep and with no lens applied to the eye, the amount of oxygen drops to 7% equivalent of oxygen to the corneal surface. It is therefore desirable that gas-permeable day-wear lenses allow between 7% to 10% oxygen to the cornea. Normally the present-day gas-permeable silicone-acrylate lenses provide about 7% equivalent oxygen performance (EOP). However, with adequate blinking the tears introduce more oxygen, and so the EOP in the blinking state is over 8% (Fig. 25-1). Permeability of one manufacturer's lens from another will vary considerably (Tables 25-2 and 25-3). As technology improves, each

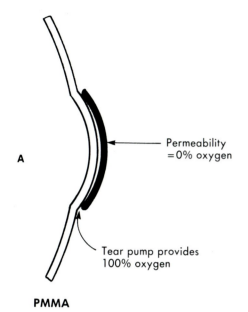

A

PMMA

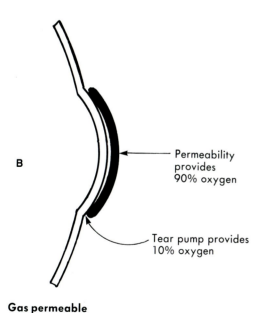

B

Gas permeable

Fig 25-1 ■ **A,** Normally with a polymethylmethacrylate lens, 100% of the oxygen must be provided by tear pump. **B,** With the gas-permeable lens, 90% of the oxygen diffuses through the contact lens, and so only 10% is required through the tear pump.

Table 25-2 ■ Oxygen permeability (DK)

Silicone	Highest permeability
Pure	
Fluorocarbon	
Equalens	
Fluoroperm	
Boston Lens	
Alberta	
Polycon	graded in ml O_2–cm^2/sec ×
CAB	mm Hg at room temperature
HEMA	
PMMA	Lowest permeability

Table 25-3 ■ Relationship between center thickness and equivalent oxygen performance for gas-permeable contact lens materials*

Center thickness (mm)	Equivalent oxygen performance (%)
HEMA (hydroxyethyl methacrylate) (35% water)	
<0.05	6.0-3.0
0.05-0.10	3.0-2.0
0.10-0.20	2.0-1.0
>0.20	<1.0
CAB (cellulose acetate butyrate)	
<0.05	7.5-6.5
0.05-0.10	6.5-3.5
0.10-0.15	3.5-2.0
0.15-0.20	2.0-1.0
>0.20	1.0
Silicone-organic copolymer	
<0.10	12.0-9.0
0.10-0.20	9.0-7.5
>0.20	7.5-6.0
Polycon	
<0.10	10.0-7.8
0.10-0.20	7.8-4.5
>0.20	4.5-2.5
Permalens	
<0.10	19.0-15.0
0.10-0.20	15.0-10.0
>0.20	10.5-8.5

*Modified from Goldberg J: Int Contact Lens Clin 6(6):64, 1979.

manufacturer tries to leapfrog over the other in the production of a better material.

TEAR-LAYER OXYGEN

Oxygen at the corneal site under a gas-permeable contact lens reaches the cornea through tear exchange and by diffusion through the lens itself. Diffusion is controlled by the difference between external and internal oxygen tension. The factors that control the available oxygen supply are quite variable, as in the following:

1. Different eyes may have different oxygen needs. The difference may be in the integrity of the corneal epithelium and the nature of the tear film. For example, a cornea with a previous epithelial nebula from trauma or with dry spots will have oxygen needs different from those of a totally normal corneal epithelium.
2. Time of day in which the oxygen supply is measured is important. With fatigue or reading or any activity in which the blink rate is down, the oxygen supplied through tear exchange will be depressed.
3. The external oxygen tension is a variable that is partially dependent on altitude and weather conditions. Oxygen tension decreases when the altitude is increased. The oxygen pressure at sea level is 155 mm Hg whereas in Mexico City it is only 126 mm Hg; at the top of Mount Everest it is between 20 and 30 mm Hg. Under a contact lens it varies from 0 to 30 mm Hg. An oxygen tension greater than 20 mm Hg is required to supply the cornea's adequate oxygen needs.

COMMENT. Certainly the use of gas-permeable lenses must be appreciated in high-altitude places like Aspen where the oxygen pressure is considerably lower than it is at sea level.

ADVANTAGES OF A GAS-PERMEABLE SILICONE-ACRYLATE LENS
(see box below)

1. *More comfort.* The high-riding lens with minimal movement is a very comfortable lens. It is much more comfortable than a small 8 mm ultrathin intrapalpebral lens.
2. *Rapid adaptation.* The gas-permeable lens can frequently be worn for full-time day wear within a week.
3. *Spectacle blur.* Blur that is largely caused by corneal hypoxia is reduced. It is not eliminated because some spectacle blur is attributable to the aberrations of conventional spectacle lenses and is not related to corneal edema, or induced myopia, or molding of the cornea.
4. *Corneal distortion.* Corneal distortion from an ill-fitting PMMA lens will usually disappear with gas-permeable lenses. The distortion is best appreciated when one notes the irregular mire pattern of the keratometer by observing the irregular reflex from a retinoscopy light or the muddy reflex from the reflection of a Placido disc. Good refractions with stable corneas are frequently found 4 to 12 weeks ater a gas-permeable lens is worn. Of great importance is that an oxygen-starved cornea can be immediately covered with a gas-permeable lens and the repair can occur under the lens. With rigid lenses a period of days or weeks, even months, may be required before K readings and mires are stabilized. During this time, the patient is incapacitated in visual needs.
5. *Larger lens permitting better centration.* Better centration makes the lens more stable and less irritating because of smaller excursion, and a large lens can mask astig-

---

■

ADVANTAGES AND DISADVANTAGES OF SILICONE-ACRYLATE LENSES*

Advantages	Disadvantages
Greater oxygen transmissibility	Softer than PMMA and scratches and chips easily.
Surface tension 40% higher than PMMA.	Poor shape memory. The lens does not spring back when flexed or distorted. A change of shape of the lens is more likely to occur with fabrication or usage.
Increased comfort and wearing time. Larger diameters mean a larger optic zone, which reduces annoying flare.	
Reduced spectacle blur.	Deposit formation occurs.

*From Stein HA, Slatt BJ, and Stein RM: Ophthalmic assistant, ed 3, St. Louis, 1988, The CV Mosby Co.

matism of the cornea of up to 4 diopters.

6. Rigid lenses also permit greater ease and economy in handling hygiene-related problems and, in particular, daily cleaning routines. However, there is a decreased fragility.

7. Newer rigid lenses are inherently safer for extended wear than soft lenses. Although this in part is due to the greater oxygen transmission of the material, it is also a result of a reduced tendency to trap metabolic debris.

8. Giant papillary conjunctivitis (GPC) does occur with rigid lenses but with far less frequency than other soft lenses. Cleaners are also effective on rigid lenses and polishing pads may be used to help prevent build-up.

9. *Greater safety*. The incidence of an acute hypoxic syndrome, better known as an *overwear reaction* is minimal. We have not seen a single case in over 1000 cases fitted. Long-term hypoxic changes, which include corneal molding, corneal hypesthesia, and irregular astigmatism, do not occur as with PMMA lenses.

10. *Less flare and better vision*. There is less flare because the optic zone is usually large enough to accommodate a young, blue pupil dilating in dim illumination. With a lens 9.5 mm in diameter the optic zone is 8.4 mm and is larger than the entire diameter of many PMMA lenses. This reduces glare from lights to provide better vision.

11. *Masking of astigmatism*. Gas-permeable lenses in a spheric form can mask large amounts of astigmatism. The large lens offers stability and centration. Up to 5 diopters of astigmatism can be attempted with a regular lens. With corneal astigmatism of 1.00 D the base curve should be 0.20 to 0.30 flatter than the flattest K. With corneal toricity of 4.00 D or greater, the selected base curve should be on K.
    Rule. As the corneal astigmatism increases, so should the steepness of the base curves and center thickness increase (see Harrison-Stein nomogram).

12. *Sucked-on or glued-on lens syndrome*. Reported with pure silicone lenses greater than 12 mm in diameter, the sucked-on lens syndrome is more likely if the patient has a marginal tear film. It has not been reported with silicone-acrylate lenses but has been noticed with fluorocarbon silicone acrylate lenses.

In this syndrome the lens adherence to the epithelium becomes advanced toward the end of the day when the blink rate is decreasing and the tear film has shown some evaporation, with the visible formation of dry spots. Also, these lenses, which are usually silicone, are fitted a little steep to allow for perfect nonfluctuating acuity.

Clinically what occurs is that the lens movement ceases and the eye suddenly becomes inflamed. There is circumcorneal injection, corneal edema with striae of Descemet's membrane, iritis, and so on. The patient is in severe pain and has pronounced photophobic and extremely blurred vision.

COMMENT. This complication can result in the dividing of the epithelium when the lens is removed. The lens is best removed with an eye cup with saline solution so that pulling off of the entire epithelium is avoided. This type of response is to be anticipated in large fluorocarbon silicone acrylate lenses that are fitted steeper than the flattest corneal meridian. The steep fit can be recognized early because it may cause pressure at the 6 to 12 o'clock meridian, which causes lens buckling at the horizontal meridian. This creates against-the-rule astigmatism.

DISADVANTAGES OF A GAS-PERMEABLE SILICONE-ACRYLATE LENS
(see box on p. 268)

1. *Quality control*. Quality control must be excellent because the large diameter can create edge and peripheral curve problems. Check edges and peripheral curve profile with the profile analyzer. If the edges are thick, as one might find with a high myope, lid impact will be excessive and the lenses uncomfortable. Also, lid gap becomes a problem. The frequency and severity become common and severe. Many patients develop exposure episcleritis and formation of dellen. The edge thickness for a regular myopic lens should be no greater than 0.09 mm.

2. *Increased fragility of lens*. More care is required in the cleaning of these lenses because breakage can occur.

3. *Waxlike deposits*. Because silicone is lipophilic, lipid deposits may form on the lens.

After 12 months of wear, creamy deposits are best identified when the rinsed and dried lenses are examined with the slitlamp. Appropriate cleaners can be used to clean the lens.

4. *Protein deposits*. If protein deposits are excessive, they may not come off manually. The lens is cleaned with a soft-lens cleaner, or some of the specific cleaning agents for gas-permeable lenses. Avoid rigid-lens cleaners because cleaners with polyvinyl alcohol can degrade the wettability of the lens.

For professional cleaning the lens is held with a suction cup, and the outer surface is rubbed in a circular motion with velveteen saturated with the appropriate cleaner. One cleans the inside surface by applying the suction cup to the outside surface and applying the cloth impregnated with cleaning solution gently. This procedure must be stressed because the lens edge may fragment and chip with excessive manual application.

5. *Easily scratched surfaces*. Gas-permeable lenses are softer than PMMA ones and tend to scratch more easily.

COMMENT. It is advisable to select your patients with the softness of the plastic in mind. Teenagers who are rough with their lenses and may be a little careless when handling them are often better off with PMMA lenses, which are hard and resistant to breakage.

6. *Initial transfer irritability*. Patients who are being refitted with gas-permeable lenses for induced toricity, corneal edema, irregular astigmatism, or excessive spectacle blur may on initial exposure be unhappy with the comfort of a gas-permeable lens even if the lens is perfectly fitted.

This paradox occurs because the corneal sensation frequently improves when a gas-permeable lens is worn. The same patient who will tolerate corneal edema, corneal erosions, or infiltrates of the epithelium, may be quite irritable with new lenses that are gas permeable. Usually the *symptoms of increased corneal sensation* last 2 to 4 weeks. Unless the practitioner is aware of this change in corneal sensation, he or she will make endless modifications on a perfectly fitted lens for a patient who seems impossible to satisfy.

PATIENT SELECTION FOR GAS-PERMEABLE SILICONE-ACRYLATE LENSES

As of this writing, silicone acrylate lenses are the most commercially available of all lenses. Higher and higher DK lenses are being manufactured. However, fluorocarbon silicone acrylate lenses are fast surpassing high-DK lenses (See Chapter 26). Consequently, this chapter may eventually become outdated as has the chapter on silicone contact lens that was written for the last edition (see below).

Indications for a gas-permeable lens
Giant papillary conjunctivitis
History of soft-lens damage
Keratoconus or irregular cornea
Corneal astigmatism up to 5 diopters of astigmatism
Epithelial infiltrates with soft lenses
Rotational instability with toric soft lenses
Rigid-lens dropout
    Poor comfort
    Corneal edema
    Flare and glare

Dating back to 1976 when gas-permeable lenses became available to us in limited quantities, we have always selected patients who would benefit the most from the features of gas-permeable lenses. These candidates are as follows:

1. PMMA wearers who develop corneal edema caused by chronic hypoxic changes; also those patients who end up in the emergency room of a hospital because of acute hypoxia or *overwear syndrome*.

2. Patients who have persistent spectacle blur after removing their glasses. This is caused by corneal edema producing an increase in myopia.

3. PMMA rigid-lens wearers who cannot achieve satisfactory wearing time.

4. Patients with high degrees of corneal toricity that may be more simply remedied by a rigid lens than a soft toric lens.

5. Patients who develop flare with standard PMMA lenses. The gas-permeable lenses may be made larger with a larger optic zone.

6. Patients who have developed warped corneas with PMMA lenses. It has been traditional to advise these patients with corneal warpage to discontinue use of their lenses until their eyes are stable; that is, the K readings are normal, mires undistorted, and the refrac-

tions back to baseline findings. Unfortunately such advise may make a visual cripple of the person. The induced astigmatism may last for months. Refitting these people with gas-permeable lenses of the same measurements as that of their rigid contact lenses will in most cases permit the cornea to regain its normal undistorted mires.

7. Patients whose corneas developed vascularization from hypoxia at the limbus.
8. Keratoconus patients with thinning or scarring of the cornea.

COMMENT. Over 97% of our patients fitted with a rigid lens for astigmatism over 1.25% could be fitted with a gas-permeable spheric lens, whereas less than 3% required a toric gas-permeable lens.

The least successful candidate for this lens has the following:

1. A large corneal diameter.
2. Lids that barely cover the upper limbus.
3. Inadequate blink responses—incomplete blink, infrequent blinking, and so on.
4. A low centration despite modifications in the lens.

FITTING GAS-PERMEABLE SILICONE-ACRYLATE LENSES

Obviously there will be differences from one company to the next and from one expert to another according to preferences and clinical experience. We shall attempt to deal with general principles and be specific on occasion to present a broad picture.

Which lens to choose

There is available, even now, a large selection of gas-permeable lenses. One might assume that the higher the permeability of a lens, the more desirable the lens. We did a study on two lenses. At that time only the Boston and Polycon lenses were available. The Boston Lens had a DK value greater than 10, whereas the DK value of the Polycon lens was 5.5. Thus one lens had almost twice as much oxygen permeability as the other. The following considerations were made.

CORNEAL EDEMA. There was no difference in the function of the two creas.

CORNEAL COMPLICATIONS. There were more problems with the Boston lenses. These early lenses had thick edges with all the attendant problems.

DURABILITY. The Polycon lens was better because it was less fragile.

WETTING ANGLE. The Polycon lens had a lower wetting angle.

CARE. They were both about the same.

Today the silicone acrylate lenses have much greater oxygen-permeability but the same comments are probably still valid. The design of the lens is of fundamental importance.

Conclusions. The design characteristics of the lens is as important as its permeability. A lens with good quality control should be chosen over a lens with sloppy manufacturing techniques. Note the following points:

1. The laboratory that can produce reproducible high-quality control lenses.
2. A lens laboratory that customizes a lens if needed.
3. A lens that uses a variety of cleaners so that availability is not a problem.
4. Any lens that will effectively eliminate corneal edema.
5. A thin lens with thin edges that do not break.

Positioning the lenses

The ideal fit for any gas-permeable lens is one in which the lens position is high, even when the lens overlaps the superior limbus (Fig. 25-2). The upper lid should cover a position of the lens during the full cycle of each blink. The purpose of the high-riding lens is to tuck the edge of the lens under the lid to avoid lid impact. This "full-sweep" blink also enhances lens surface wetting. The engagement of the upper lid margin with the edge of the lens is a major cause of discomfort. Even a soft hydrogel lens will be uncomfortable if it is made small and interpalpebral.

At times, the ideal may not be achieved (Fig. 25-3). The position of the upper lid may be too high to cover the upper position of the lens or there may be excessive astigmatism, which because of the corneal topography, resists the upper motion of the lens. In these cases, the central position may be accepted, provided that the patient accepts this type of fit, or modifications can be made. The lens diameter may be reduced to increase the lid lift, or a flatter base curve can be chosen. A central fit on the cornea is adequate, but a low-riding lens is unsatisfactory. When the lens is low, the blink rate is frequently suppressed to a minimum or the blink itself is

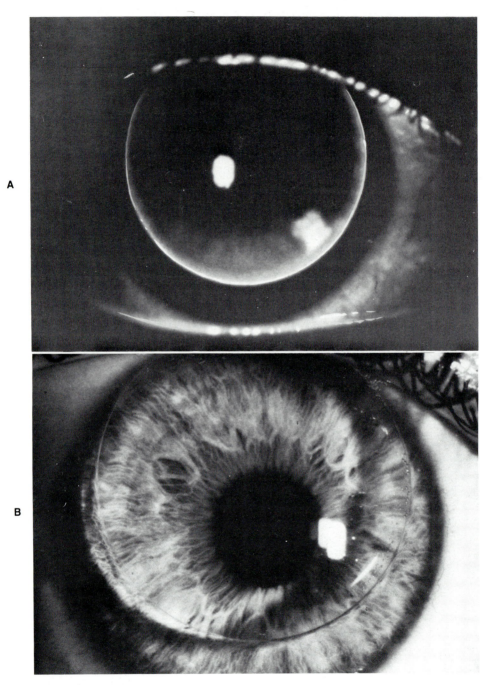

Fig 25-2 ■ A, Large gas-permeable rigid contact lens with upper edge under upper lid. Normal fit. **B,** A moderately large diameter rigid gas-permeable lens, 9.4 mm, which centers high.

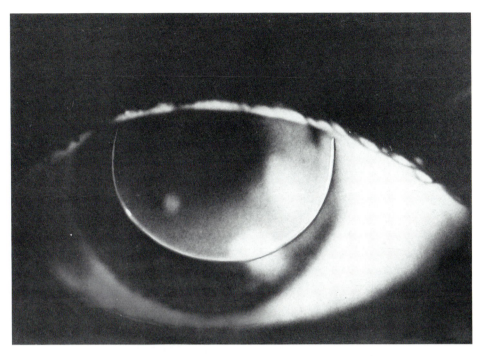

Fig 25-3 ■ A flat-fitting lens riding too high.

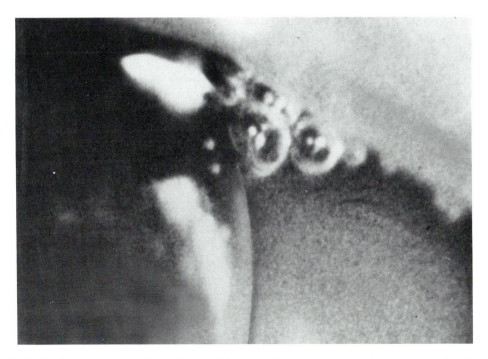

Fig 25-4 ■ The gap at the edge of the eyelid and contact lens may lead to corneal desiccation if the lens is thick.

incomplete. Also, a low lens is frequently a source of lid gap, which causes 3 and 9 o'clock staining of the cornea. The margin of the upper lid slides over the low lens, and it bridges the nasal and temporal cornea between the edge of the lens and limbus. Lid gap is especially common with highly myopic refractive corrective lenses because the edges of the lens are prone to be thicker than usual and the trough between the edge of the lens and the margin of the cornea is likely to be deep (Fig. 25-4). Because these lenses are usually of large diameter, the proper edge treatment is essential (Fig. 25-9). A plus edge or configuration for myopic lenses with power greater than −4.00 D and a minus edge for lenses +4.00 D or greater is appropriate.

COMMENT. Staining patterns with fluorescein are most helpful in evaluating an ideal fit, a steep fit, and a flat fit (Figs. 25-5 to 25-7).

SYSTEMS FOR FITTING
Diagnostic lenses

For trial lenses, some fitters use lenses made of PMMA because they can be stored dry. We tend to use trial sets made of the same material, to be used and left in conditioning solution. It is best to use large-diameter trial lenses. For example, for the Boston lenses, a trial lens of 8.5 mm diameter is chosen. The base curve should be 0.5 to 1.5 steeper than the flattest K. If the lens is high or just overriding the limbus, the lens power is determined by an over-refraction. If the lens rides excessively high, a larger diameter is chosen sufficient to cover the pupil in dim illumination. *As the diameter of the lens increases to 9 mm or greater, the lens base curve should be made flatter*—to the flattest corneal meridian. This rule applies to all gas-permeable lenses.

For those who wish to work with diagnostic sets we have identified the most commonly used lenses in our practice to serve us as a diagnostic set (Table 25-4).

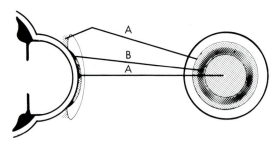

Fig 25-5 ■ Ideal fitting with light peripheral touch.

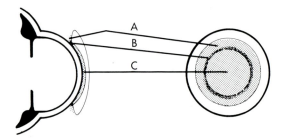

Fig 25-6 ■ Steep fitting spherical lens central pooling of fluroescein with heavy peripheral bearing.

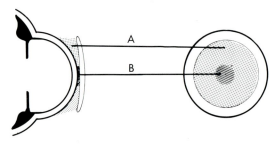

Fig 25-7 ■ Flat fitting spherical lens demonstrating central touch with absence of fluorescein centrally.

Table 25-4 ■ Diagnostic set for gas-permeable lenses

Base curve (D)	Diameter (mm)	Power	Peripheral curve width (mm)
40.00	9.6	−3.00 −6.00	0.6
41.00	9.4		0.6
42.00	9.2		0.5
43.00	9.0		0.5
44.00	8.8		0.5
45.00	8.6		0.4
46.00	8.4		0.4
40.00	9.8	+14.00	0.6
41.00	9.6		0.6
42.00	9.4		0.5
43.00	9.2		0.5
44.00	9.0		0.5
45.00	8.8		0.4
46.00	8.4		0.4

Diagnostic set:
  14 minus lenses
  7 plus lenses

COMMENT. Polycon uses three standard diameters for myopes: 8.0, 9.0, and 9.5 mm. The initial 9.0 mm lens is usually chosen flatter than the flattest K, but the final lens is not chosen in terms of the base curve but from the *positioning of the lens* and *its comfort*. At times, the lens rides high after a blink and then drops. The after-blink position should be maintained in the high-riding position. If it is not, a flatter lens should be chosen.

If the lens rides low, increase the diameter and make the base curve flatter. Ideally the apex of the lens should not slide below the center of the cornea between blinks. Lenticular lenses should have a minus carrier. If the lenticular lens is low, choose the smallest single-cut lens with a base curve steeper than K.

Inventory fitting

There is a belief among some fitters that lens design and manufacturing is of primary importance and that soft lens systems may be applied to the gas-permeable lens. In effect, one manufacturer (Syntex Ophthalmics) believes that three diameters of lenses for myopia, 8.5, 9.0, and 9.5 mm, will satisfy almost all requirements for patients, and they recommend 9.5 and 10.0 lens' diameters for aphakia. If adequate base curves are available, these lenses will simplify fitting.

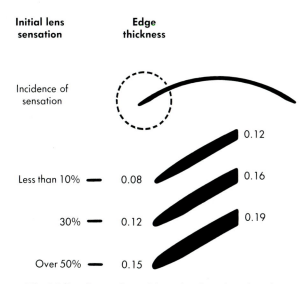

Fig 25-8 ■ Sensation of lens is directly related to edge thickness. Lens edges must be made thin to reduce lens sensation. Over 50% of patients with a lens edge 0.15 mm as noted in the lower lens will complain of sensation because of lens-lid impact.

For myopic patients, the larger 9.5 mm diameter is recommended for levels of high astigmatism and also for flatter corneas.

COMMENT. Inventory fitting by lenses with preselected diameter simplifies fitting because one has fewer variables to deal with. In addition, one can rely on the quality control in providing lenses and controlled edge designs by one manufacturer.

Lid sensation is directly dependent on the edge finishing. It must not be left thick but must be thinned out to minimize lid sensation and the uncomfortable fitting of a lens that lies under the upper lid (Fig. 25-8). A good reliable laboratory is most important.

Polycon, in an effort to maintain as high a permeability as possible, manufactures all minus lenses to a center thickness of 0.08 to 0.1 mm. This may not allow for lens flexure on high astigmatics. Custom lenses of greater enter thickness may be better for these cases because the thicker lens marks the corneal toricity.

Harrison-Stein nomogram method of fitting

The ideal method of fitting silicone-acrylate lenses is from a trial set where the lens is placed on the eye. However, there are a number of low-volume fitters and occasional fitters who do not wish to have and maintain a standard fitting trial set. We have developed, over the past few years, a nomogram that is designed to be a guide for the best possible starting point in lens selection (Table 25-5). With a nomogram, one may order the lens directly by referring to the nomogram for the initial lens factor.

The nomogram takes into account the progressive increase in diameter required for flatter corneas and the decrease in diameter for steeper corneas. The second factor takes into account the increased thickness required for the soft silicone-acrylate lenses to avoid flexure on the cornea. The base curve is selected according to the corneal toricity. If the corneal cylinder is 0.75 D or less, we select the flattest K. If the corneal cylinder is between 1 and 2 D, we add one fourth of the difference of the two Ks to the flattest K reading. If the corneal cylinder is over 2 D, we add one third of the difference to the flattest K.

EXAMPLE. If the flattest curve of the cornea was 42.0 D and the cylinder axis was less than 75°, we would select a lens 9.2 mm in diameter

Table 25-5 ■ Harrison-Stein nomogram: initial lens selection

If corneal cylinder < 0.75:	select flattest K.
1.00 to 2.00 D:	add ¼ of difference of 2 K's to flattest K.
> 2 D:	add ⅓ of the difference of 2 K's to flattest K.
	(All plus prescriptions over +2.00 D should be in lenticular form.)

Base curve (D)	Diameter (mm)		Peripheral curves (mm/D)
	Minus power	Plus power	
40.00 and 40.25	9.6	9.8	0.2/36.00 0.2/31.00 0.2/27.50
40.50 and 40.75	9.5	9.7	
41.00 and 41.25	9.4	9.6	0.2/36.00 0.2/31.00 0.2/27.50
41.50 and 41.75	9.3	9.5	
42.00 and 42.25	9.2	9.4	0.3/32.00 0.2/27.50
42.50 and 42.75	9.1	9.3	
43.00 and 43.25	9.0	9.2	0.3/33.00 0.2/27.50
43.50 and 43.75	8.9	9.1	
44.00 and 44.25	8.8	9.0	0.3/34.00 0.2/29.00
44.50 and 44.75	8.7	8.9	
45.00 and 45.25	8.6	8.8	0.2/36.00 0.2/29.00
45.50 and 45.75	8.5	8.7	
46.00 and 46.25	8.4	8.6	0.2/36.00 0.2/30.00
46.50 and 46.75	8.3	8.5	

and provide the lab with the details of the peripheral curves.

In developing this nomogram, we have reviewed almost 1000 eyes. We found that 75% could be fitted on a first-fit basis using this nomogram and most of the remainder fitted with less than two subsequent lenses.

WEARING SCHEDULE

A simple safe conservative wearing schedule, such as the following example, can be applied to most patients.

Day	Hours
1	4
2	5
3	6
4	7
5	8
6	9
7	10
8	11
9	12

Additional hours may be added until the person is wearing gas-permeable lenses full time. Despite their permeability, we do not now recommend wearing of these lenses on an extended basis overnight.

In many cases an accelerated schedule can be used.

Day	Hours
1	2 hours morning, afternoon, and night
2	same
3	3 hours morning, afternoon, and night
4	same
5	4 hours morning, afternoon, and night
6	same
7	full-time wear

Most adaptation is of a physical nature (lid-lens) rather than physiologic nature (cornea-lens).

CARE OF GAS-PERMEABLE LENSES

Giant papillary conjunctivitis, which is an autoimmune papillitis of the upper tarsal conjunctiva, occurs with gas-permeable lenses but not with the same frequency as with hydrogel lenses. It is important to keep these lenses clean. Daily nonsensitizing cleaners such as Pliagel assist in reducing the incidence of papillary conjunctivitis. After cleaning, a saline solution, preferably one without preservatives, should be used to rinse the lens. At times, reactions can occur to the saline solution and the cleaners. Usually, it is the preservative thimerosal that is the sensitizing agent. In such cases, nonpreserved saline solution made fresh daily or dispensed from an airtight container should be used. Weekly or bimonthly cleaning may be necessary. Soft-lens weekly cleaners can be best used for the more thorough cleaning. How does a patient know the lenses are dirty? After cleaning, the lenses should be clear and transparent. If the lens is exposed to a light source, the dirty deposits will become visible instantly.

Special solutions are required for silicone-acrylate lenses. The wetting and soaking solutions used at least 15 minutes before insertion conditions the lens and improves its wetting angle. They also remove any accumulation of surface deposits.

COMMENT. It has been our experience that wetting agents composed primarily of polyvinyl alcohol do not wet silicone-PMMA lenses as well as EDTA does.

APHAKIC GAS-PERMEABLE LENSES

The large lenticular contact lens is recommended in aphakia. The trial lens should have a large diameter and myopic edge (minus carrier) design. The base curve should show minimal clearance. If the lens rides low, use a double lenticular design. If the lens is not successful, attempt to fit a steeper single-cut lens.

COMMENT. With the thickness required for an aphakic lens, the permeability of the lens at its center is drastically reduced. For example, the Boston Lens with outer lens thickness of 0.1 has a DK value of 10, whereas at a thickness of 0.30 to 0.40, the usual range of an aphakic lens, the DK value drops to 5. CAB at a center thickness of 0.1 has a DK value of 4, whereas at 0.3 to 0.4 mm thickness the DK value drops to less than 2. For extended-wear purposes, the equivalent oxygen performance should be 7% or greater. The lack of permeability to support the oxygen requirements of the cornea during sleep makes the silicone acrylate gas-permeable lens a questionable choice for extended wear. For this reason, a gas-permeable lens is not so useful for the aphakic person. Central permeability is lowered, but it is still higher than that of PMMA, yet PMMA may be chosen because it is sturdier and less likely to fracture peripherally during handling.

If higher peripheral permeability is required, a lenticular lens with a wide flange of plano or plus design may be manufactured.

SPECIAL PROBLEM SOLVING WITH GAS-PERMEABLE SILICONE-ACRYLATE LENSES

Many of the major and disabling complications of PMMA lenses have been eliminated by the use of the new generation of gas-permeable lenses. However, there are still a number of lens-regulated problems of the gas-permeable lenses that need to be addressed. By understanding these problems and solutions, practitioners are able to direct their attention to achieving happiness and success in a lens-wearer.

Three and 9 o'clock staining

There are several causes for 3 and 9 o'clock staining.

Lid gap. A lid gap occurs largely with large-diameter rigid lenses. It is particularly prone to occur with gas-permeable lenses whose edges have not been properly thinned.

A gap occurs between the margin of the lens and the cornea. The meniscus of tears becomes very thin or absent at this border. It creates a lens-induced dry spot. The degree of staining is intense, often associated with episcleritis and formation of dellen. The staining of the cornea is attributable to desiccation of the corneal epithelium and not to corneal hypoxia. It is particularly prone to occur with lenses that ride low, that is, those that are not brought up to a high position with a blink. Poor lid adherence is another cause of a low-riding lens.

The treatment is to make the lens flatter, thinner at the edges or smaller in diameter.

At times, the lens will rise with a blink and then suddenly drop to a low position. Such a lens requires a little alteration; flattening the blend and peripheral curves will frequently solve the problem and permit tear flow.

Poor blinking. The incomplete blinker dehydrates the exposed position of the eye at the 3 and 9 o'clock portions. Lines of protein accumulation caused by dehydration across the lens indicates its presence.

Poor tear film. Some people have an insufficient tear film to support a large-diameter lens. For these people, supplementary tears during the day and a bland ointment (such as Duratears) at night may be enough to remedy the problem.

Corneal compression

On cylindrical corneas with the rule, compression of the lip-lid onto the contact lens may cause erosions at 3 and 9 o'clock at the edge of the lens. Similarly, with against-the-rule corneas, compression and erosion may occur at 6 o'clock.

COMMENT. Three and 9 o'clock staining is more common with large gas-permeable rigid lenses. Despite the intensity of the corneal erosions and episcleritis, patients do not seem to have much pain. Some fitters do not treat it because it may be an asymptomatic condition; this is an error. Breaks in the epithelial integrity should not be tolerated. More often than not, these patients primarily complain of the redness of their eyes.

Lens-flexure problems

The softer silicone component that is added to the silicone-acrylate mixture combined with the thin-designed lenses permits the lens to flex with each blink because of the pressure effect of the eyelid on the lens, which may rock on a toric cornea. This phenomenon results in blurring of vision, along with a residual astigmatism that is not corrected by the tear film.

Against-the-rule corneas create even more lens flexure as the lid sweeps over the lens. Steeper fitting of the lens also will create more opportunity for lens flexures. Smaller lenses may produce even more flexure than the larger-diameter lenses, which have a greater stabilizing force.

These problems of lens flexure are problems that are presenting themselves because the new generation of lenses are being used to correct astigmatism. These problems were apparent with soft HEMA lenses in the early years. Their use for corneal toricity was minimal because one soon learned that the soft HEMA lenses draped entirely over the cornea since they did not have any hard component. These lenses did not significantly correct large measures of corneal astigmatism.

To remedy this problem, one needs to increase the thickness of the lens. This will vary with the degree of corneal cylinder present. As a general rule, one should increase the thickness by 20% to 30% for larger lenses and 40% to 60% for the smaller lenses because the smaller lenses are more subject to flexure.

The lens should also be fitted high under the upper lid because doing so minimizes flexure, which may occur with an interpalpebral lens.

COMMENT. Because of lens flexure with the silicone-acrylate lenses, we use a trial set made from the material to be dispensed. Some fitters, however, believe that this factor can be estimated quite reasonably and that PMMA lenses used in trial sets are preferable because they maximize the durability of the trial set and minimize the care required in conditioning the wetting angle of the lens.

Lens breakage

Gas-permeable lenses, because of their soft component, are liable to breakage. Patients must be taught the same careful care and cleaning routine that one has learned to establish for soft lenses.

Fabrication more difficult

The manufacturer of these lenses does require more sophisticated care or the breakage rate in fabrication can be very high, particularly if they are made thin. A good manufacturing facility is important. This additional manufacturing capability may be reflected in a higher cost than that of PMMA lenses.

More deposit formation and greater drying

The new generation of lenses has a greater propensity to pick up proteins and lipids onto their surface than PMMA lenses have. They are not quite so vulnerable as the soft lenses. The lenses also dry easily between blinks. If one watches the patient carefully with the slit-lamp, one can readily see the evaporation of the tear film and a drying of the lens surface.

A number of good cleaners specifically designed for gas-permeable lenses are available for these lenses. Conditioners are also important to maintain the proper wetting angle of the contact lens.

CLINICAL PEARLS ON THE GAS-PERMEABLE LENS

1. In regard to thickness, not all gas-permeable lenses are the same. The CAB lenses tend to be thicker than the PMMA-silicone lenses. CAB usually has a center thickness of 0.19 mm compared to 0.10 mm for Polycon (silicone-acrylate). However, some of the recently developed CAB lenses (Rynco) are very slim. Edge thickness of CAB is often 0.18 mm, whereas edge treatment of

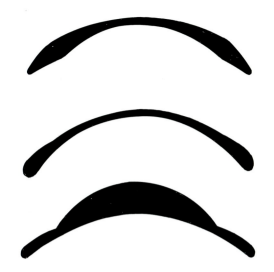

Fig 25-9 ■ For large refractive errors, the edge treatment is essential.

silicone-acrylate can be refined to 0.08 mm. Thinner lenses mean better permeability, but thinner edges also mean greater breakage.

2. Large refractive errors require special attention to lens edges so that irritation is minimized (Fig. 25-9).

COMMENT. For every 1 to 2 D of corneal cylinder we order the lenses 0.04 mm thicker to reduce lens flexure. We think this is an important factor.

3. PMMA-silicone is not a homogeneous mixture when manufactured into buttons. Therefore permeability may vary slightly from one lens (of the same material and manufacturer) to another.

4. PMMA-silicone lenses must be well finished, as with blended edges. Despite their forgiving properties, quality in manufacturing is still all important.

5. The reduction in spectacle blur with a well-fitted gas-permeable lens is impressive. Close to 90% of rigid lens patients sampled were vastly improved when the switch to a gas-permeable lens was made. Of course, the smaller the refractive error, the better the result because the distortions, minification, and aberration of a thick-lensed glass system still cannot compare to the visual accuracy obtained by use of any contact lens.

6. Frequently a lens will ride high just after a blink and then drop. When lens drop occurs, it usually means either a flatter lens is required or the blink is incomplete. If the latter is the case, the patient needs to do blinking exercises.

7. Gas-permeable lenses are best fitted steeper and larger than are comparable PMMA lenses.

8. Signs of corneal disaster under a PMMA lens include the following:
   a. The retinoscopy reflex on the naked cornea is irregular.
   b. There is irregularity from the reflection of a Placido disc.
   c. The mire reflection from the keratometer is distorted.
   d. Corneal edema is present with changes also in the corneal thickness. This change is apparent when one measures the central corneal thickness through the pachometer.
   e. Corneal hypoesthesia occurs.
   f. There is corneal pitting and erosions of the epithelium.
   g. There is a change in the refractive error because of greater astigmatism, greater hyperopia attributable to flattening of the cornea, greater myopia in a mature adult, or suspicion of diabetes.

COMMENT. When one is removing a PMMA lens, if the keratometer mires are distorted, refraction is difficult to refine and visual acuity is reduced. The contact lens should be checked for warpage with the Radiuscope. What should be done? Refit with gas-permeable lenses preferably when the keratometer reading and refraction are stable. If vision is too poor with spectacles, it is permissible to refit immediately with gas-permeable lenses. Our experience tends toward refitting directly with a higher-DK lens.

9. Gas-permeable lenses should be considered in any area where the temperature is generally warm or hot. Lenses such as the gas-permeable lens have a 25% greater thermal conductivity than PMMA lenses do, permitting a greater dissipation of heat. A PMMA lens acts as an insulator, increasing the metabolic activity of the epithelium and increasing the oxygen demand. So, if you live in Arizona or Texas, a gas-permeable lens should be on top of the list.

10. Flexure may result in astigmatism, which is aggravated if the lens is very thin, the fit is

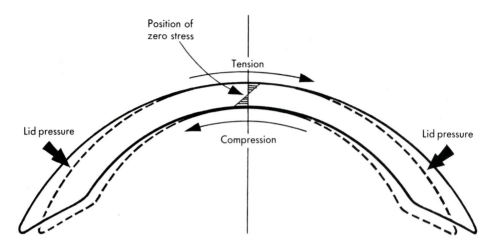

Fig 25-10 ■ Flexure-induced residual astigmatism. This is aggravated by thin lenses, against-the-rule toric corneas, steep fits, interpalpebral designs, hydrogel lenses, and silicone-acrylate lenses.

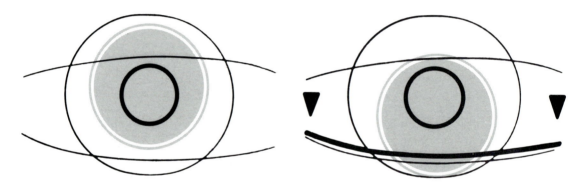

Fig 25-11 ■ Blinking may cause the lens to ride low.

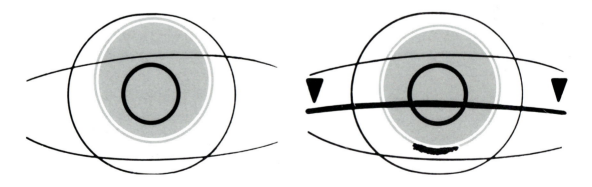

Fig 25-12 ■ Blinking may cause arcuate epithelial defect if edges are thick.

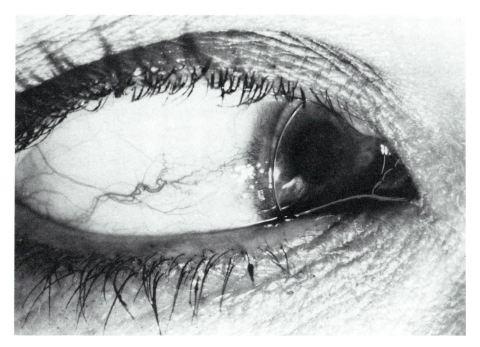

Fig 25-13 ■ Three to 9 o'clock staining and neovascularization caused by edge thickness with drying of the cornea at the edge of the lens.

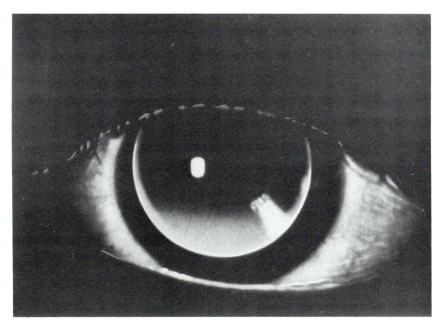

Fig 25-14 ■ A gas-permeable rigid lens fitted on a cornea with 4 diopters of astigmatism. Note the dark horizontal flat band.

steep, or there is against-the-rule astigmatism (Fig. 25-10).

11. The major flaws of these lenses are improper edges. Because these lenses are frequently large in diameter, the edges tend to be thicker. There should be a plus-carrier lenticular lens for high-minus lenses. A minus-carrier lenticular lens should be used for low-minus lenses. A minus-carrier lenticular lens should be used for high-plus lenses. Any projection device will illuminate the edge profile. The integrity of the edge design is easily checked with the profile analyzer or the soft-lens analyzer.

12. Blinking may cause an epithelial defect at the 6 o'clock position (Fig. 25-11). This is particularly true if the edges are thick or the lens is steep. It will also occur if there is against-the-rule astigmatism with the flatter meridian vertically.

13. Blinking may also predispose to the lens riding low (Fig. 25-12). This may also occur if there is a moderate amount of with-the-rule astigmatism with the flatter meridian placed horizontally. It may also occur if the lens is heavy or the edges are thick.

14. Lid gap or a thick lens may result in a gap of mucin tear film at the corneal surface adjacent to the contact lens. This may result in drying of the cornea, corneal erosion, and eventually vascularization (Fig. 25-13). This usually occurs at 3 and 9 o'clock.

Summary of advantages. It would seem that gas-permeable lenses have many more virtues than PMMA lenses do.

They are more comfortable.

They are safer.

They are better for use in warm climates or areas of low oxygen tension because of their thermal conductivity.

They are easier to adapt initially, and the adaptation time is reduced by 50%.

Some of these lenses are more wettable than other types in this classification.

They can hide up to 5 D of corneal astigmatism without going to a toric lens design (Fig. 25-14). They undoubtedly will cause fewer changes in the endothelial cell complex of the cornea in the long run.

They are useful in keratoconus and in postgraft cases with irregular astigmatism and are better tolerated in children.

They give more satisfactory results in cases of piggyback fitting.

They cause less flare, glare, and photophobia because they have a large optic zone, and they relieve hypoxia created by an ill-fitting rigid lens.

They rarely require fenestration.

They are fitted with rigid-lens tril sets. Inventory is not generally required.

Why don't all wearers abandon PMMA and use gas-permeable lenses? They are doing so. PMMA lens sales are dropping 10% to 15% per year. Eventually they will be an anachronism.

One advantage of PMMA lenses is that they are durable and may be useful for teen-agers who are rough with their lenses.

26 ▪ FLUOROCARBON AND FLUOROCARBON SILICONE ACRYLATE LENSES

Harold A. Stein and *Keith Harrison*

- Methods of fitting
- Some fitting features
- Available lenses
- Three and 9 o'clock staining
- Lens modification
- Fluorocarbon lenses and care systems
- Summary

Lenses containing fluorine may be classified according to the material of which they are made, such as fluoralkyl acrylates, fluorosilicones, and perfluoropolyethers. Each of these materials has characteristics of its own. The most popular material is fluorosilicone, which can be easily adapted to many designs. A number of companies manufacture these materials today.

Around 1979, PMMA was crossed with a silicone molecule, making a new copolymer that had superb oxygen transmission as well as other characteristics that rendered it better than existing materials. This material soon became the state of the art in rigid-lens materials and superceded CAB and styrene. Today fluoropolymer, either in its pure form or combined with silicone, is the trail blazer. It should be remembered that there is a variety of silicones available as well as a variety of possible methods of linking, so each manufacturer has its own formulation and uses different varieties of silicones to cross-link materials to form its specific copolymer. The addition of fluorine to the silicone acrylate provides some oxygen-permeability via solubility and not by diffusion of oxygen within the material. Each material ingredient adds to the total performance of the lens (Fig. 26-1).

The only truly pure fluoropolymer lens was developed by 3M, now marketed exclusively by Allergan as the Advent™ lens. This lens derives its oxygen permeability completely from its flu-orine-containing component whereas other fluorinated silicone acrylates derive their oxygen permeability from silicone as well as fluorocarbon. Today it is being suggested that this material should be classified in an entirely new category of material, distinct from all other RGP materials.

Although there are a number of fluorosilicone acrylates available today, the DK of each material varies as do the wetting angles and other physical properties. Reliable laboratories differ in their findings. DK/L values are important because some materials require thicker lenses to minimize flexure. Table 26-1 lists some of the high-DK fluoropolymer and fluoropolymer silicone lenses available today. Manufacturers of RGP lenses have been competing with one another to produce a higher-DK lens. How high is high enough? One important feature is that some of these materials are required to be thicker. Because of this, higher DKs (permeability) are of value in lens design so that the DK/L (transmissibility) where L is the thickness will provide sufficient protection to the cornea even if the lens is manufactured in a thicker dimension (see box on p. 284).

METHOD OF FITTING
Diagnosing lens fit

The first lens selected may be based on either a nomographic selection or from a diagnostic set of lenses. In reality, the method of selection does not matter a great deal as long as the fitter realizes that the initial lens placed on a patient's eye should be considered a "trial" lens whether or not it was selected through the use of a nomogram. The following are important considerations that must be made in order to properly fit rigid gas-permeable lenses.

Trial lenses. For the most accurate results, it

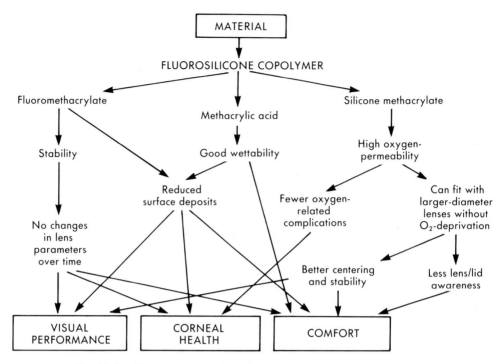

Fig 26-1 ■ Characteristics of the fluorosilicone copolymer materials.

■

ADVANTAGES OF THE HIGHER-DK LENSES

Newer higher-DK lenses offer significant advantages over hydrogel lenses. These advantages are:
1. Increased oxygen-permeability
2. Greater potential for extended-wear performance
3. Venting of debris because of the larger tear layer and because of greater exchange with each blink
4. More durable than hydrogel lenses and thus need to be replaced less often
5. Mask a greater degree of astigmatism without special lenses
6. Easier to insert and remove
7. Economical to maintain
8. Less risk of infection because of the absence of porosity
9. Larger-diameter lens possible. When manufacturing a lens with a larger diameter, a larger optical zone is permitted, which minimizes flare and maximizes vision (Fig. 26-2).
10. More resistant to deposit formation than either hydrogels or silicone acrylate lenses

---

is always recommended that the trial lenses be of the same material and design as the ones that are to be used. Due to slight differences in surface wetting, flexural resistance, and specific gravity, the actual "on eye" performance may vary slightly from one material or laboratory design to another. Therefore, the diagnostic evaluation should also be performed with lenses from the same manufacturer who will be producing the lenses that are to be ordered.

Nomogram. Four years ago we published a nomogram for fitting gas-permeable silicone acrylate lenses (see Chapter 24). We stated then

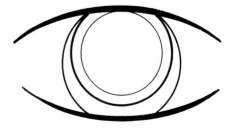

Fig 26-2 ■ Superior fitting of a fluorosilicone acrylate lens. Note the larger optical zone and the larger diameter permitted by the higher-DK material.

Table 26-1 ■ High-DK fluoropolymer rigid gas-permeable contact lenses

Trade name	Manufacturer	Material	DK
Advent	Allergan/3M	Fluroforon A	100
Fluoperm 30	Paragon	Fluorosiloxane acrylate	30
Fluoperm 60	Paragon	Fluorosiloxane acrylate	60
Fluoperm 92	Paragon	Fluorosiloxane acrylate	92
Boston equalens	Polymer	Fluorosiloxane acrylate	71
Boston equacurve	Polymer	Fluorosiloxane acrylate	71
Boston equalens RXD	Polymer	Fluorosiloxane acrylate	45
Fluorex	GT Laboratories	Flusilicon A	70
Quantum I	B & L	Fluorosilicone acrylate	92
Quantum II	B & L	Fluorosilicone acrylate	210
Boston EXPFS	Polymer	Fluorosilicone acrylate	203

that polymethylmethacrylate (PMMA) lenses "are becoming obsolete due to the development of rigid gas permeable lenses." That prediction has now come true: the laboratories that manufacture rigid lenses report that PMMA is rarely chosen for first-fit lenses. Although still relatively new, it appears that current silicone acrylate materials have reached their full potential—to raise the oxygen transmissibility of silicone acrylate any further requires increasing its siloxyl content substantially. But the problems created by raising the siloxyl content are considerable: loss of dimensional stability, loss of effective wetting, and decreased comfort. However, new rigid gas-permeable (RGP) materials, which contain a fluorinated monomer, have overcome the limitations of PMMA and silicone acrylate materials, thus opening the door to safer, more comfortable contact lens wear than was possible with any previous rigid lens materials.

During the past three years, we have worked with lens materials (from Polymer Technology Corporation, Paragon Optical, Bausch & Lomb, and 3M), that contain either a fluorinated monomer or a fluorocarbon. While these fluorinated contact lenses permit greater oxygen transmission, preservation of corneal integrity, and reduction of corneal insult, they also exhibit less flexure resistance. This can cause visual instability and a "glued-on" syndrome if a proper fitting routine is not followed. Historically, fitting routines have had to be changed when contact lens materials changed. Because of their lower resistance to flexure, the new materials require a flatter fitting strategy.

We maintain that the ideal method of contact lens fitting is through the use of diagnostic lenses. However, practitioners who do not maintain a set of trial lenses can benefit from our experience. With that in mind we have developed the first nomogram for the fitting of fluorinated silicone acrylate lenses.

Methods

We conducted an 8-month prospective study to determine the best techniques for fitting the following lenses, all of which are made of fluorine or fluorocarbon-containing materials: Boston Equalens (Polymer Technology Corporation, Wilmington, MA), Paraperm EW II (Fluoroperm, Paragon Optical, Mesa, AZ), Alberta N (Progressive Chemical Research Ltd., Calgary, Alberta, Canada), Fluorofocon A (3M Visioncare, St. Paul, MN), and Quantum (Bausch & Lomb Canada Ltd., Markham, Ontario, Canada). This series of fittings was done on 814 patients (1578 eyes). The group included first-time contact lens wearers, as well as previous wearers of soft, PMMA, and silicone acrylate lenses. Myopia was the most frequent indication for lens fitting, and most patients had less than 1.75 D of astigmatism (Table 26-2).

Table 26-2 ■ Refractive error

Condition	No. of eyes
Myopia	1,125
Hyperopia	216
Early keratoconus	144
Aphakia	93
Corneal cylinder	
0.75 D or less	441
0.87-1.75 D	789
1.87 D or more	348

(From Harrison K and Stein HA: CLAO J 14:3, July 1988.)

Results

As shown in Table 26-3, we achieved success with the first lens selected for 1246 eyes (78% of the sample). Lenses for an additional 173 were acceptable after additional blending or finishing of the edges. Therefore, a total of 1419 of the lenses initially ordered were fit successfully. This represents a 90% first-fit success rate for the nomogram used in these fittings. First-fit success was defined as comfortable wear for at least 10 hours per day achieved with the original lenses within a 45-day period.

Flatter or smaller lenses than those initially fit were required for 41 eyes, whereas steeper or larger lenses were required for 46 eyes. Lenses thicker than the suggested standard were used for 78 eyes to reduce lens flexure.

Larger diameters than those used for silicone acrylate lenses were selected in order to encourage upper lid attachment and proper positioning of the lenses. The wide peripheral curves used and the excellent wetting properties of the fluorinated lenses reduced staining at the 3 and 9 o'clock positions.

Fitting procedure

The nomogram that we tested in these fittings is shown in Table 26-4. This nomogram acknowledges two common guidelines for contact lens selection: (i) The flatter the corneal curvature, the larger the lens required; and the steeper the corneal curvature, the smaller the lens required. (ii) The size of the lens optic in millimeters should relate to the mean corneal curve radius measurement in millimeters—i.e., a cornea with a mean radius of curvature of 7.8 mm (43.00 D) will require an optic approximately 7.8 mm in diameter. The following are guidelines for using the nomogram.

Table 26-3 ■ Results of nomogram fitting (number of eyes)

Number of eyes	1,578
First-fit success	1,246
Required blending or widening of peripheral curves and/or edge finishing (in office)	1,73
Increased lens thickness required	78
Lens too light; refitting with flatter or smaller lens required	41
Lens too loose; refitting with larger or steeper lens required	46

(From Harrison K and Stein HA: CLAO J 14:3, July 1988.)

Base curve selection: When the corneal toricity is 0.75 D or less, the initial base curve selection should be 0.75 D flatter than the flattest K value. When the corneal cylinder measures between 0.87 D and 1.75 D, it is advisable to select a lens base curve 0.25 D flatter than the flattest K. Corneas with a cylinder of 1.87 D or greater should initially be fitted with a lens 0.25 D steeper than K. Thus:

> K reading: 42.00/42.75
> *Initial base curve selected:* 41.25
>
> K reading, 42.00/43.50
> *Initial base curve selected:* 41.75
>
> K reading, 42.00/44.50
> *Initial base curve selected:* 42.25

Diameter and peripheral curve selection: Once the base curve determination has been made, refer to the nomogram. It will indicate the required lens diameter and peripheral curves, providing the laboratory with the information needed to produce the appropriate lens.

Power selection: In order to calculate the correct lens power: 1) refer to the vertex compensation chart, when applicable; and 2) alter the lens power by $+0.25$ D for each 0.25 D that the base curve is flatter than the flattest K reading or -0.25 D for each 0.25 that the base curve is steeper than K.

Thickness selection: When the final lens power has been calculated, apply it to the thickness chart (Table 26-5). As shown on this table, lens power and corneal toricity determine the most appropriate center thickness for the lens. If there is lens flexure on a given toric cornea, we first attempt to correct for the flexure by selecting a lens with a flatter base curve rather than simply increasing the center thickness. It should be noted that an increase in thickness of .03 mm may reduce lens oxygen transmissibility by 15% to 20%.

Other considerations: When applying our nomogram to hyperopic correction, the best results are achieved with lenticular lens designs. This is possible in almost all instances where the prescription calls for correction greater than 2.00 D. Practitioners should also note that the center thickness chart is not applicable to plus-power corrections, since the lens thickness in these cases is dictated by the relationship between the diameter and the correction required. In all cases, lens edges must be well blended to ensure

Table 26-4 ■ Harrison-Stein nomogram for fitting fluoronated silicone acrylate lenses

Initial Lens Selection

If corneal cylinder ≤ 0.75 D	Base curve 0.75 D flatter than the flattest K
If corneal cylinder 1.00-1.75 D	Base curve 0.25 D flatter than the flattest K
If corneal cylinder > 1.75 D	Base curve 0.25 D steeper than the flattest K

Base curve	Diameter* (mm)	Peripheral curve†		
8.44 & 8.39 mm 40.00 & 40.25 D 8.33 & 8.28 mm 40.50 & 40.75	9.8 9.7	.3/9.10 mm .3/37.00 D	.2/10.50 mm .2/32.00 D	.2/11.50 mm .2/29.00 D
8.3 & 8.18 mm 41.00 & 41.25 D 8.13 & 8.18 mm 41.50 & 41.75 D	9.6 9.5	.3/9.10 mm .3/37.00 D	.2/10.50 mm .2/32.00 D	.2/11.50 mm .2/29.00 D
8.04 & 7.99 mm 42.00 & 42.25 D 7.94 & 7.89 mm 42.50 & 42.75 D	9.4 9.3	.2/8.90 mm .2/38.00 D	.2/10.00 mm .2/34.00 D	.2/11.50 mm .2/29.00 D
7.85 & 7.80 mm 43.00 & 43.25 D 7.76 & 7.71 mm 43.50 & 43.75 D	9.2 9.1	.2/8.90 mm .2/38.00 D	.2/10.00 mm .2/34.00 D	.2/11.50 mm .2/29.00 D
7.67 & 7.63 mm 44.00 & 44.25 D 7.58 & n7.54 mm 44.50 & 44.75 D	9.0 8.9	.2/8.70 mm .2/38.75 D	.2/9.50 mm .2/35.50 D	2./11.00 mm .2/30.75 D
7.50 & 7.46 mm 45.00 & 45.25 D 7.42 & 7.38 mm 46.00 & 46.25 D .2/11.00 mm .2/30.75 D	8.8 8.7	.2/8.70 mm	.2/38.75 D	.2/9.50 mm .2/35.50 D
7.34 & 7.30 mm 46.00 & 46.25 D 7.26 & 7.22 mm 46.50 & 46.75 D	8.6 8.5	.2/8.40 mm .2/40.00 D	.2/9.20 mm .2/36.75 D	.2/10.50 mm .2/32.00 D

(From Harrison K and Stein HA: CLAO J 14:3, July, 1988.)
*Diameter specifications apply to both plus and minus power lenses.
†Peripheral curve radii are expressed in both diopters and millimeters for convenience.

Table 26-5 ■ Center thickness chart

Power (D)	Thickness (mm)		
	Cylinder ≤0.75 D	Cylinder 0.87-1.75 D	Cylinder >1.75 D
−0.25	.19	.21	.25
−0.50	.18	.20	.24
−0.75	.18	.20	.24
−1.00	.18	.20	.24
−1.25	.17	.19	.23
−1.50	.17	.19	.23
−1.75	.17	.19	.23
−2.00	.17	.19	.23
−2.25	.17	.19	.23
−2.50	.16	.18	.22
−2.75	.16	.18	.22
−3.00	.15	.17	.21
−3.25	.15	.17	.21
−3.50	.14	.16	.20
−3.75	.14	.16	.20
−4.00	.13	.15	.19
−4.25	.13	.14	.18
−4.50	.11	.13	.17
−4.75	.11	.13	.16
−5.00	.11	.13	.15
−5.25	.11	.13	.15
−5.50	.11	.13	.15
−5.75	.11	.13	.15
−6.00 and over	.11	.13	.15

good venting of tear debris during blinks and to reduce the possibility of mechanical irritation.

COMMENT. This nomogram, like our original nomogram for silicone acrylate lenses, takes into account the need to fit each patient individually. Although we believe that the use of diagnostic lenses is the best approach to fitting, many practitioners believe that they are too busy to work with diagnostic lenses or have an insufficient patient volume to justify large sets of diagnostic lenses. These practitioners have benefited from the use of nomographic lens fitting. The simplified system presented here, which yielded a 90% success rate in the first fitting of fluorinated RGP contact lenses, can be useful to all practitioners as a strating point in the selection of lenses made from this new generation of materials.

SOME FITTING FEATURES
Diameter base curve relationship

The diameter of a cornea will usually vary directly with its radius of curvature. More simply stated, the flatter the cornea, the larger it is

likely to be, just as the steeper the cornea, the smaller it is likely to be. The nomogram that follows shows that for a corneal curvature of 40.00 diopters, the required lens diameter will be approximately 9.8 mm, whereas a corneal radius in the 47.00 diopter range will require a smaller lens, somewhere in the vicinity of 8.5 mm. This principle is applicable except when the cornea is abnormally large and steep or small and flat or when the upper eyelid is positioned too far above the limbus to provide any upper lid attachment. Cases such as these may require either large and steep lenses or small and flat ones. It is in such cases that diagnostic fitting is of the greatest benefit.

Positioning and movement

The lens should always be positioned over the visual axis. Ideally it will sit so that the upper eyelid attaches slightly over the lens edge. This will cause the lens to appear to be approximately ¼ to ½ mm superior when in the primary position. When normal blinking occurs, the lens should move down smoothly with the upper lid, stopping no farther than the lower corneal limbus. When the eye opens after the blink the lens should move upward again with the eyelid, lagging down 1 to 2 mm after the eye is once again fully open.

The absence of any upper lid attachment in cases of a superiorly positioned upper eyelid (i.e., above the corneal limbus) makes it necessary to fit lenses that are slightly smaller and steeper. This digresses from that which would be the case for the same fit where upper lid attachment is a factor in the lens positioning.

We are always concerned when fitting rigid gas-permeable lenses that the vertical lag be enough to allow for good tear pump action with the blink. The movement cannot be excessive to the point where visual stability is compromised. In most cases, an acceptable amount of after-blink lag would be 1 to 2 mm.

Another important factor for optimum lens performance is horizontal movement. A well-fitted rigid gas-permeable lens should move from limbus to limbus when the patient's gaze is directed back and forth laterally. This movement will help sweep the lens edge tear meniscus over the entire horizontal meridian through normal eye movement. The horizontal movement and dragging of the tear meniscus will add to the surface wetting of the cornea and help prevent the onset of 3 and 9 o'clock desiccation.

In evaluating the fluorescein patterns of a fluorosilicone acrylate lens on an eye, we try to achieve:
1. minimal apical clearance or bearing under the optic of the lens as shown by an absence of fluorescein pooling centrally,
2. less bearing in the mid-periphery than we would expect to see with a silicone acrylate lens; ideally, less than 180 degress of mid-periphery bearing, and
3. a wide pool of fluorescein in the periphery of the lens.

Non-attachment fits

When selecting a trial or diagnostic lens for a "non-attachment" fitting, we select a lens base curve that is on or steeper than the flattest K reading. When the corneal cylinder is 0.75 D or less, start with a lens on K, i.e.:

K reading: 42.25/43.00
Base curve selected: 42.25 D or 8.0 mm.

When the corneal cylinder is greater than 0.75 D, the base curve selection will, on the average, be K or half of the difference steeper than the flattest K reading, i.e.:

K reading: 42.00/43.50
Total corneal astigmatism: 1.50 D

Half of the total corneal astigmatism: 0.75 D

Flattest K reading: 42.00

Add ½ T.C.A: 0.75

Base curve: 42.75 D or 7.9 mm.

The total diameter of the lens optic should be as close as possible to the radius of the base curve when expressed in millimeters. Therefore, the diameter of the lens optic in the first example would be 8.0 mm and the diameter of the lens optic in the second example would be 7.9 mm. The peripheral curve width including blending would be 0.5 mm, thus requiring a total lens diameter of 9.0 mm and 8.9 mm respectively. It must once again be stressed that this is the way in which to select a proper diagnostic or initial-fit lens; however, individual evaluation is essential in order to achieve success.

Rx determination

The most accurate prescription is obtained by over-refraction on a diagnostic lens that fits adequately. Vertex distance adjustment tables may be used for nomographic fitting and they must also be taken into account when the over-refraction exceeds 4.00 diopters. For example:

Diagnostic lens Rx: −3.00 D

Over-refraction: −2.50 D

Rx to be ordered: −5.50 D

Diagnostic lens Rx: − 3.00 D

Over-refraction: −8.00 D at a vertex distance of 12 mm

Adjusted vertex Rx: −7.25 D

add diagnostic Rx: −3.00 D

Rx to be ordered: −10.25 D

The result of the over-refraction should always be spherical. If there is refractive astigmatism present it is the result of either residual astigmatism or lens flexure. As previously stated, lens flexure can be corrected via flatter base curve selection and/or increased center thickness. In order to determine if a lens is flexing on a cornea, we take K readings over the lens while it is being worn. The degree of flexure will be indicated by a toric K reading. If there is no flexure present, the K reading over the lens will be spherical.

Toric designs

The development of RGP materials has created a universal interest in the fitting of toric and bitoric designs. A front toric lens has a spherical posterior surface and a cylindrical anterior surface. A back toric lens has a cylindrical posterior surface and a spherical anterior surface. A bitoric lens is cylindrical on both the posterior and anterior surfaces.

If the over-refraction is sphero-cylindrical and the K reading over the lens is spherical, then a front toric lens will be required. The amount of refractive cylinder is simply added to the lens Rx. For example:

Trial lens Rx: −3.00

Over-refraction: −1.00 −0.75 × 180

Rx to be ordered: −4.00 −0.75 x 180

The lab will manufacture the cylindrical correction on the anterior surface of the lens and incorporate a prism ballast of 1 to 1.5 D base down to enable stabilization of axis orientation.

In cases of corneal and refractive cylinder of 3.00 diopters or more it may be necessary to use a back toric design for the best possible vision, comfort, and stability of fit. The use of a back toric design will eliminate the flexure problem; however, some residual cylinder may be created.

When it is determined that a back toric is required, the initial lens may be determined through the use of the ¼ principle or rule. This simply suggests that the base curve of a back toric lens should be ¼ of the K reading difference steeper than the flattest K, and that the second posterior or toric curve should be ¼ of the difference flatter than the steepest K. For example:

> K: 42.00/46.00
>
> Total cyl: 4.00 D
>
> ¼ total cyl: 1.00 D
>
> Base curve: 42.00 D + 1.00 D = 43.00 D or 7.85 mm
>
> Second posterior curve: 46.00 D − 1.00 D = 45.00 D or 7.5 mm

The power of the lens will be calculated from the spherical correction of the spectacles, compensated for vertex distance if necessary. This power will then be adjusted so as to conform with the steeper-than-K relationship of the base curve to the flattest K. For example, if the Rx is −4.00 −4.00 × 180, and the spherical Rx is −4.00, add −1.00 for tear lens created by base curve 1.00 D steeper than K. Therefore, the Rx to be ordered is −5.00.

Using the principle of base curve radius equaling optic zone radius, the required optic will be 7.9 mm (BC = 7.85 mm). The peripheral curve width should allow for a well-blended tri-curve or toric PC as required. This will demand a total PC width of about 0.9 mm, which will add 1.8 mm to the lens diameter when added to the optic zone. The overall lens diameter would be 7.9 mm + 1.8 mm which equals 9.7 mm. The initial toric lens ordered for the example would be:

> Base curve: 7.85/7.5
> Diameter: 9.7 Rx: −5.00
> PC: .3/8.9 mm 3/10.00 mm .3/11.5 mm
>   will be blended

The toric posterior surface of the lens orientates on the toric cornea. Centration is improved and movement is reduced, thus improving the visual result to optimum levels. If there is residual astigmatism subsequent to the fitting of the back toric lens, then a bitoric design will be required. Over-refraction and K readings over the lens will once again determine any presence of flexure or residual cylinder. The presence of flexure would necessitate the fabrication of a new back toric lens with a flatter base curve just as in spherical-lens situations. The degree of residual cyl as expressed in the over-refraction can be incorporated directly onto the front surface of a new lens, which will, of course, be bitoric.

> Back toric lens base curve: 7.85/7.5
> Diameter: 9.7
> Rx: −5.00 VA20/30
>
> Over-refraction Plano −0.75 × 18
>
> Bitoric lens order base curve: 7.85/7.5
> Diameter: 9.7
> Rx: −5.00 −0.75 × 180

It should be noted that the axis of the cylinder will coincide with that of the base curve (flatter posterior curve) thus the posterior toricity will align it properly, negating the need for a prism ballast.

Some may argue that all back toric lenses induce about 30% residual cyl and therefore bitorics should be used as a first choice for any substantial amount of corneal cyl. In view of the fact that the most accurate assessment of a lens fit is through the trial use of lenses on the eyes to be fitted, we prefer using a simple step-by-step approach, which prevents overfitting.

AVAILABLE LENSES
Pure fluoropolymer lenses

Space does not permit discussing all the lenses identified in Table 26-1. The Advent™ lens developed by 3M and marketed through Allergan is unique in that it is a high-fluorine fluoropolymer contact lens with no silicone in the lens (Table 26-6). Its fluorine component is approximately 40% to 50% and is about 3 to 10 times higher than that of any other contact lens material. The physical properties and lens parameters are outlined below (Table 26-7). The lens is fitted either on K or 0.5 diopters flatter than K. The base curve selected should be approximately the flatter meridian or 0.10 mm flatter than K. Diagnostic lenses should be used. We generally start the patient on a four-hour initial wearing time and increase by one to four hours per day.

Table 26-6 ■ Interpretation of diagnostic lens fluorescein pattern is critical in achieving optimum fit

Descriptive	Analysis	Results
Too flat	Not desirable	Note central touch with too wide and excessive edge lift.
Flat	Acceptable option	Mild apical touch as alternate choice.
Uniform alignment	Optimal fit	Note even distribution of tear layer with moderate edge lift. Optimum lens movement, particularly for extended wear. Absence of mid-peripheral bearing.
Steep	Acceptable option	Slight apical clearance as alternate choice.
Too steep	Not desirable	Note excessive mid-peripheral touch. Additionally, you may see narrow, insufficient edge lift. May cause variable vision. May increase potential for binding. May limit tear pump action and trap debris and air bubbles.

Table 26-7 ■ Advent lens

Physical properties

Oxygen permeability .... 100×10^{-11} (35° C)
Refractive Index 1.39
Light Transmission .... 94% (370-740 nm)
Wetting Angle .... 43 degrees (receding)
Water Content .... <2% by weight
Oxygen-Permeability
*DK = 106×10^{-11} (cm²/sec) (mL O₂/mL × mm Hg); Brennan, Efron, Holden
DK = 170×10^{-11} (cm²/sec) (mL O₂/mL × mm Hg); Irving Fatt, Ph.D.
DK = 95×10^{-11} (cm²/sec) (mL O₂/mL × mm Hg); 1987 Revised Fatt.

Lens parameters

Diameter .... 10.1 mm
Center Thickness .... 0.18 mm
Base Curves .... 7.2 mm to 8.4 mm
Powers .... −0.25 to −7.00 diopters

Boston Equalens and Equacurve

These lenses have a UV blocker incorporated into the lens material. The UV blocker minimizes the amount of ultraviolet light entering the cornea, which provides some comfort factor from induced keratitis that results from movement of the contact lens on the cornea.

Newer designs such as Equacurve, a biaspheric that handles corneal toricity better, are being developed. Specialty solutions are recommended for the Boston Equalens (Table 26-8). Wearing comfort has been improved with these lenses because of their ability to reduce mucoprotein adhesion while attracting tear film mucin. A potential polymer-stiffening backbone itaconate™ is present in all Boston lenses and may reduce the degree of flexure in this material.

Table 26-8 ■ Recommended solutions for Boston Equalens and Boston Equalens RXD

Daily Cleaner	1. Boston Daily Cleaner
	2. Bausch & Lomb Concentrated Cleaner
	3. CooperVision HGP Cleaner
Soaking/Conditioning Solution	1. Boston Advance Conditioning Solution
	2. Boston Conditioning Solution
	3. Bausch & Lomb Wetting & Soaking Solution
	4. CooperVision HGP Conditioner
	5. Soaciens
	6. Boston Advance Reconditioning Drops
Reconditioning	Boston Reconditioning Drops
Other Solvents	Absolutely contraindicated

Boston Equalens R × D

This material was developed by Polymer Technology to give reduced silicone content to increase wettability and deposit-resistance while providing a higher DK than daily-wear silicone-acrylate materials. Its flexure-resistance makes it possible to design lenses that are 10% to 20% thinner to decrease DK/L or at standard thicknesses to mask a greater degree of corneal astigmatism. It also machines well in toric designs when required. The Rockwell Hardness of Boston Equalens R × D is 122 (as compared to PMMA 124). Reducing the silicone content and increasing the fluorine monomer by 50% over Boston Equalens has created a new daily-wear RGP lens with flex-wear potential in thin (<10CT) designs (Table 26-9).

Fluoroperm

As indicated by their suffix, the Fluoroperm line of materials is available in DKs of 30, 60, and 92 respectively. The Fluoroperm 30 is recommended for stability and wetting and is the most flexure-resistant lens of the group. The Fluoroperm 60 provides a higher oxygen-permeability for flexible wear while maintaining a good level of stability and wettability. The Fluoroperm 92 is recommended primarily for extended wear, and for high-oxygen demand corneas. The 92 material is the least flexure-resistant and will therefore require a thicker design when the corneal cylinder is moderate to high.

Quantum lens

This material developed by Bausch & Lomb is an aspheric design lens with a central 5 mm spheric design and an aspheric peripheral zone. The edge design is gently tapered posteriorly and gives greater comfort with reduced lens awareness. These lenses are available in a variety of stock powers, base curves, and diameters, with custom orders also possible.

Table 26-9 ■ Boston Equalens R X D material properties

DK	45×10^{-11} 35°C
Rockwell R hardness	122
Wetting angle	39°
Index of refraction	1.435
Specific gravity	1.27
UV absorber	Yes

Fluorex 700

This material manufactured by GT Laboratories has a high DK (70) and has proved to be quite stable. Of current interest is the T agent™ screen bifocal and trifocal, which has performed well in our hands. It has a low wetting angle (15°) and is very comfortable, with good oxygen performance and minimal flexure (Table 26-10).

3 AND 9 O'CLOCK STAINING

The presence of 3 and 9 o'clock staining has long been a problem in fitting rigid lenses. This area of the cornea tends to be the first to dry as a result of a rigid lens preventing the eyelid from sweeping over the 3 o'clock and 9 o'clock areas of the cornea by holding the eyelid out from the cornea. This is accentuated by the fact that the entire horizontal meridian of the cornea is exposed to the atmosphere the longest between blinks and is the driest portion of most eyes even in the absence of a contact lens.

The fluorocarbon and fluorinated monomer-containing lenses are somewhat helpful in this area in that the tear break-up action moves from the center to the edge of the lens, thus holding a tear meniscus at its periphery longer than a silicone acrylate lens. More important than this, however, is the actual fit and finish of the lens. Edges should be well tapered, rounded and polished. Thick blunt edges will cause discomfort and vault the eyelid too far from the cornea,

Table 26-10 ■ Property of Fluorex 700

Typical property	Test value
1. Hardness	85.8 ± 0.5 (Shore hardness units)
2. Water content	1%
3. Wetting angle	15.3%
4. Oxygen-permeability at 35°*	70.0×10^{-11} (cm$_2$/sec) (ml O$_2$/ml × mm Hg)
5. Dimensional stability	Stable
6. Refractive index	1.46
7. Light transmission (blue-tinted lens)	95%

*Oxygen permeability was measured by the polarographic method of Irving Fatt at 35° C.

causing poor blink action and subsequent drying, especially in the 3 and 9 o'clock areas. Sharp edges that are too posterior will become irritated and even abraded in the 3 o'clock and 9 o'clock areas. The ideal edge will have slight lift from the posterior peripheral curve to the apex of the edge. This will enhance the tear meniscus at the lens edge in such a way that 3 o'clock and 9 o'clock staining can be markedly reduced.

Flexure

As the generations of RGP materials evolved it became apparent that there were to be no gains without concessions. In general, the resistance to flexure decreased as the siloxyl content of the rigid gas-permeable lenses increased. This created the need for a new approach to fitting rigid gas-permeable lenses containing fluorocarbon silicone acrylate. Working retrospectively, we developed a step-by-step nomogram approach to achieving a high rate of first-fit success in fitting fluorocarbon silicone acrylate lenses.

At present our system to minimize flexure on corneas with cylinder is to fit as flat as possible and when necessary to increase the thickness of the lens. Generally, an increase of 0.02 for every diopter of cylinder is sufficient. Some fitters will flatten the base curve of the lens before increasing the thickness.

Factors affecting flexure are:
1. Base curve. The flatter the lens, the less the flexure.
2. Central position increases flexure.
3. Force exerted by the upper lid. If the lens is positioned under the eyelid, it eliminates with-the-rule flexure. The more the lens is under the eyelid, the less the flexure on with-the-rule astigmatism. Materials such as Boston Equalens R X D are more flexure-resistant and hold promise of becoming the lens of choice for solving flexure problems.

The lens should be positioned under the superior lid to minimize lens flexure and residual astigmatism, particularly in patients with astigmatism.

Decentration

If a lens is decentered downward, one might consider reducing its center thickness or the myo-edge to give lift.

In spite of all one's best efforts, problems can and will arise. Most are easily solved by making slight adjustments. Table 26-11 presents an oversimplified problem-solving formula.

Table 26-11 ■ Problem-solving steps

	Lens size, mm		
Problem	*≤8.8*	*9.0-9.5*	*≥9.6*
Tight lens	Flatten B.C.	Flatten B.C. and/or reduce size and O.Z.	Flatten B.C. and/or reduce size and O.Z.
No movement	Flatten B.C.	Flatten B.C. and/or reduce size and O.Z.	Flatten B.C. and/or size and O.Z.
Loose lens	Steepen B.C.	Steepen B.C. and/or reduce size and O.Z.	Steepen B.C. and/or size and O.Z.
Low-riding lens	Flatten B.C. and/or increase size	Flatten B.C. and/or increase size	Flatten B.C.
Low-riding lens	Use minus carrier lenticular	Use minus carrier lenticular	Use minus carrier lenticular
High-riding lens	Steepen B.C.	Steepen B.C.	Steepen B.C.
High-riding lens	Increase C.T. .10mm and use plus lenticular	Increase C.T. .10mm and use plus lenticular	Increase C.T. .10mm and use plus lenticular
3 o'clock and 9 o'clock staining	Increase lens size	Increase lens size, flatten B.C.	Flatten B.C. Steepen B.C.
Flare	Increase size and O.Z.	Increase size and O.Z.	Increase size and O.Z.
Poor VA (flexure)	Flatten B.C. and increase size	Flatten B.C. and increase size	Flatten B.C.

Key: B.C.-Base Curve   O.Z.-Optic Zone
      C.T.-Center Thickness   P.C.-Peripheral Curve
Courtesy of Paragon Optical, Mesa, Arizona

LENS MODIFICATION

Having a modification unit on the premises is most worthwhile for the average fitter. However, the high-DK materials handle differently. Our experience leads us to make the following suggestions:

1. Use established polishes that are recommended by the manufacturer for the specific material in question
2. Use slow spindle speeds
3. Use fresh velvatine tools
4. Avoid major modification of the lenses
5. Polish by hand whenever possible
6. Use generous amounts of polishing solution and keep the tool constantly moist
7. Avoid over-polishing—it may hinder wetting and can cause burns on the surface of the lens
8. Changing power diameter is probably best done by an authorized laboratory
9. Compared to silicone acrylates, more gentle pressure is required.

The surfaces of the high-DK materials are easily distorted and damaged through poor modification techniques. Many changes will require the manufacture of a new lens. Extreme care is important.

FLUOROCARBON LENSES AND CARE SYSTEMS

It is best for rigid gas-permeable lenses to be stored in a conditioning solution specifically formulated for that purpose. Conditioning solution not only acts as an antibacterial agent but enhances the "on-the-eye" performance of a lens by giving the surface of the lens a more hydrophilic character. This in turn increases the comfort and wearability of the lenses. We recommend lenses be stored wet prior to dispensing to help achieve a better initial reaction from the patient. This subject is covered more fully in the chapter that pertains to solutions and lens care.

It is important that patients be educated properly in the care of their rigid gas-permeable lenses. Incorrect or non-approved solutions may compromise the peformance of the lenses and subsequently result in complications, lens damage, or discontinuance of wear.

Enzyme treatment is less necessary with the FSA lenses; however, with heavy deposit formers, a Q-tip soaked in the surfactant may be necessary to clean the periphery of the lens.

There are a number of solvents that should not be used undiluted on FSA lenses. These are naptha, lighter fluid, ketones, ammonia, alcohol, and esters.

Success in fitting rigid gas-permeable lenses is dependent on proper fitting techniques, patient education, and follow-up. This chapter, which sets out some steps for lens selection and initial fitting considerations must be taken as a starting point. Fit evaluation and modification must never be forgotten because they are part of the formula for a successful contact lens practice.

SUMMARY

The impact and development of rigid gas-permeable contact lens materials has created the need for a better understanding of rigid lens-fitting. There is an entire generation of contact lens fitters who have received very little education on rigid lenses. The shortcomings of hydrogel materials combined with the vast improvements of the rigid lenses have caused many practitioners to re-think their approach to fitting. The "rounding out" of a contact lens practice through the use of state-of-the-art materials, designs, and fitting techniques makes lens fitting more pleasurable, proficient, and profitable. Since there are large numbers of rigid gas-permeable materials, it is impossible to detail a fitting system for each and every one.

Each material varies somewhat in terms of flexural resistance, oxygen permeability, specific gravity, and on-the-eye wetting performance. These factors will influence the way in which a lens fits on an eye. However, some basic considerations must be made for their successful use.

Fitting philosophies

The PMMA lens was an excellent optical medium with which to manufacture contact lenses that provided crisp clear optics. Its relative ease of machinability, stability, and resistance to flexure even with relatively thin lenses (0.10 center thickness) made it the material best suited to treat corneal astigmatism. Many fitters developed their own approach to fitting PMMA lenses. Large flat lenses, on K, steeper than K, and small steep designs using tricurves all were found to have their relative merits. The major problem with PMMA, however, was its lack of oxygen permeability, which soon became apparent, and the race was on as to which manufacturer would develop the most oxygen-permeable rigid gas-permeable material.

The human cornea has a life expectancy of some 200 years under normal conditions. A contact lens that inhibits the atmospheric oxygen that is available to the corneal, i.e., a PMMA lens, will alter the metabolic balance so as to effectively age the cornea. With the specular microscope, endothelial cell changes in the form of polymegathism (cell size change) and pleomorphism (cell shape change) are well documented in the literature. Even lenses made of low oxygen-transmissible materials have been shown to have this effect on the cornea when worn for long periods. Most clinicians agree that for lens wear on either a daily or prolonged basis, the lens with the highest possible oxygen availability is required for healthy corneal physiology.

Another factor that enhances the physiological response, especially in prolonged wear (extended-wear) or "over-wear" situations is the manner in which a rigid gas-permeable lens covers the cornea. In fact, it does not entirely cover the cornea. Since most corneas have an overall diameter of 11.0 to 12.5 mm and most rigid gas-permeable lenses have an overall diameter of 8.5 to 9.8 mm, the lens only covers about 65% to 75% of the cornea. Therefore, most rigid gas-permeable fittings will allow 25% to 35% of the cornea access to 100% of the total atmospheric oxygen that is available to that cornea at any given time. The result of this lens diameter/corneal diameter relationship is that the effective DK/L of a rigid gas-permeable lens is approximately tripled as compared to a hydrogel lens of equal transmissibility.

In addition, as compared to soft lenses, rigid lenses result in an exchange of 10% to 14% of the tears with each blink. This brings in more oxygen and removes debris.

27 ▪ RIGID ASPHERIC GAS-PERMEABLE CONTACT LENSES

Keith Harrison

- *Design compatibility*
- *Fitting characteristics*
- *Inferior orientation of aspheric lenses*
- *Lateral orientation of aspheric lenses*
- *Superior orientation of aspheric lenses*
- *High corneal cylinder*
- *Present developments*

Aspheric designs are not new to the North American marketplace, although they have never gained the widespread acceptance they enjoy in Europe. That may in part be due to the general lack of rigid-lens fitting on the part of the North American practitioners as compared to their European counterparts. North American practitioners who do fit a significant number of rigid lenses tend to use aspheric lenses of the multifocal variety (i.e., VFL II and APA II). The development of the new "superperm" rigid materials for daily and extended wear that lend themselves well to aspheric designs and fitting philosophies has caused a recent revival of interest in aspheric lenses. This interest is also the result of a desire to develop a rigid lens that will challenge a hydrogel lens in the one area in which it is superior to a RGP lens, namely initial comfort. Aspheric lenses can potentially meet this challenge through better approximation of the eccentricity of a cornea, thus improving fit alignment and increasing astigmatic correction.

DESIGN COMPATIBILITY

The new generation of fluorinated materials has achieved a measure of physiologic undetectability to the cornea while at the same time maintaining a highly biocompatible surface. The overriding key to success, however, is ensuring that the lens fits well. Design compatibility can only be achieved through refined lens geometry, which takes into account the fitting characteristics of the state-of-the-art materials.

Historically, aspheric lenses have had a poor reputation because of problems in manufacturing. Reproduction was poor and the polishing of the aspheric curves caused fitting and optical inadequacies. Vision was all too often compromised by relatively small (3 mm or less) optical zones. Recent developments in aspheric lens technology and lens-finishing through the use of computer-controlled lathes that are able to move in three axes have overcome these manufacturing problems. Aspheric molding techniques are also being refined to such an extent that they can be used in the near future.

FITTING CHARACTERISTICS

It should be understood that the same principles that apply to spherical lens designs are used also in the fitting of aspheric lenses. Therefore it is not difficult to relate the changes in base curve (radius) and sagittal depth to the basics of fitting regarding lens positioning and movement. However, each aspheric design will vary somewhat in actual practice from one design to another because of changing eccentricities and other factors.

It must be remembered that the asphericity of spherical lenses reduces their sagittal depth (except when negative E values may be used, as in post-RK fitting). Therefore, comparable aspheric contact lenses fit "flatter" than a sphere of the same "base curve" (Fig. 27-1).

The aspheric design is used to create a more evenly distributed tear interface and area of bearing thus increasing comfort through alignment. This holds true regardless of the corneal topography. The potential for success in fitting an aspheric lens is directly related to the degree of flattening (eccentricity) that the paracentral

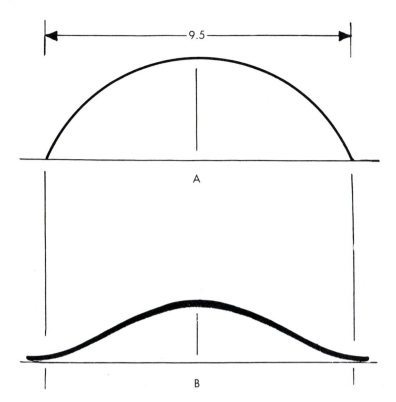

Fig 27-1 ■ Comparison of sagittal depth of spheric lens A to aspheric lens B of the same 8.0 base curve to 9.5 diameter. The aspheric lens has a reduced sagittal depth and therefore fits flatter than a spherical lens.

area of a cornea exhibits. In short, the more the eccentricity of a cornea increases, the more difficult it becomes to attain alignment of fit. Therefore, the peripheral curvature of a lens is probably even more important than its central curvature. This is illustrated by the high level of success claimed by aspheric lenses in fitting post-radial keratotomy, penetrating keratoplasty, and keratoconus patients. In all instances we consider the alignment of the lens in the periphery even more than we do its relationship with the central corneal topography.

The eccentricity of an aspheric lens mimics the peripheral flattening of a cornea, thus displacing the mass of the lens over a greater area (Table 27-1).

In simple terms, the eccentricity value is the degree of flattening or departure from a circle (Figure 27-2). Eccentricity is the degree of departure from a circle. The circle and the two elliptical curves all have a magnitude (radius) of 7.67 mm. The "base curve" is the same; how-

ever, the eccentricity of progressive flattening increases as the eccentricity increases.

Most aspheric single-vision lenses with a single E value have an eccentricity of 0.6 to 0.8. Biaspheric lenses have two different E values for the optical zone and the periphery. Aspheric bifocal lenses usually have higher eccentricity, which incorporates parabolic and/or hyperbolic eccentricities. It is this eccentricity value that affects the edge lift of the lens. The edge lift is determined by the relationship of the base curve to the eccentricity to the lens diameter as shown in Table 27-2. Initial comfort may be signifi-

Table 27-1 ■

Eccentricity	Shape
0	Circle
.0-.9	Ellipse
1.0	Parabola
Greater than 1.0	Hyperbola

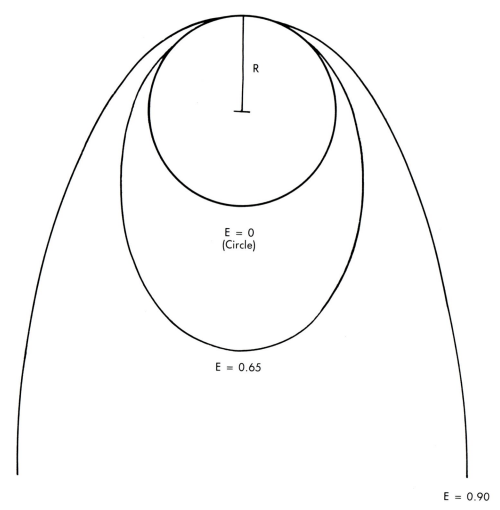

R

E = 0
(Circle)

E = 0.65

E = 0.90

Fig 27-2 ■ Eccentricity is the degree of departure from a circle. The circle and the two elliptical curves all have a magnitude (radius) of 7.67 mm. The "base curve" is the same; however, the eccentricity or progressive flattening increases (not to scale).

cantly better with an aspheric lens than with a spherical lens and long-term complications may well be significantly reduced.

We are now seeing the re-emergence of aspheric lenses in the new rigid gas-permeable materials as aspheric, biaspheric, and spherical-aspheric hybrid designs (Fig. 27-3). The high-flux materials lend themselves well to the larger (9.5 mm to 10.5 mm) diameters of the asphercs and, contrary to popular belief, they are relatively simple to fit. Using diagnostic lenses is most helpful and will enable both the fitter and the patient to develop a better "feel" for asphercs. As stated earlier, each aspheric, biaspheric, or hybrid design will exhibit slightly different fitting characteristics. It is therefore nec-

essary to follow the recommended diagnostic fitting procedure as outlined by the manufacturer.

The following is intended to be a basic guideline for proceeding through a diagnostic fitting when the manufacturer suggests starting with a mean K for base curve selection with a 9.5 diameter lens.

Step-by-step approach to fitting aspheric rigid gas-permeable lenses

1. For your trial fitting, use lenses of the same material and design as those that will be ordered, i.e., if an aspheric Boston Equalens is to be used, the trial lenses should also be an aspheric Boston Equalens.

Previous aspheric designs:

Aspheric optic and peripheral curve with constant rate of flattening (e value) from the center outwards

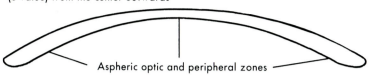

Aspheric optic and peripheral zones

Quantum design:

Spheric optic zone, aspheric peripheral zone with variable rate of flattening

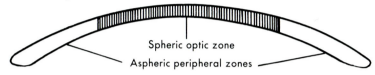

Spheric optic zone
Aspheric peripheral zones

Boston equacurve design:

Bi-aspheric and low eccentricity optical zone, higher eccentricity peripheral zone

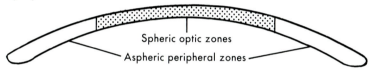

Spheric optic zones
Aspheric peripheral zones

Fig 27-3 ■ Quantum design: spheric optic zone, aspheric peripheral zone with variable rate of flattening.

2. The first lens used should be approximately the mean of the K's, i.e., 42.00/44.00 mean = 43.00 (7.85 mm) and a diameter of 9.5 mm.
3. Allow 5 minutes to settle.
4. Lenses should lag approximately 1 mm with each blink.
5. Lateral excursion with eye movement should be limbus to limbus.
6. Visual acuity with spherical over-refraction should be equal to or better than VA with spectacles.
7. Fluorescein pattern should appear as an even film under the lens with slight allowance for some pooling with the astigmatism and at the periphery of the lens.
8. If the comfort is poor or there is excessive edge pooling or movement, the next base curve (0.05 to 0.10 steeper) should be evaluated.

9. If little or no movement with the blink is observed or if there is no fluorescein at the periphery, the next base curve (0.05 to 0.10 flatter) should be evaluated.

Because of variations in design, it is impossible to regard this procedure as applicable to all aspheric lens-fitting. However, as a comparison, the following is an example of the same fitting using a Boston Equacurve (biaspheric) design, which recommends a "flatter" fitting philosophy.

1. If a Boston Equacurve aspheric lens is to be fitted, the trial set should be a Boston Equacurve.
2. The first trial lens should be at or flatter than the flattest K: K 42.00/44.00 flat K 42.00 D = 8.04 mm; the first trial lens would be 8.1 mm with a diameter of 9.5 mm.

Table 27-2 ■ Relationship of edge lift to base curve and diameter

Posterior apical radius (base curve)	Lens diameter	Edge lift
Constant	Larger	Increased
Constant	Smaller	Decreased
Flatter	Constant	Increased
Flatter	Larger	Increased
Steeper	Constant	Decreased
Steeper	Smaller	Decreased

3. Allow 5 minutes to settle.
4. The lens should lag approximately 1 mm with each blink.
5. Lateral excursion with eye movement should be limbus to limbus.
6. Visual acuity with spherical over-refraction should be equal to or better than VA with spectacles.
7. Fluorescein pattern should be even with allowance for slightly increased pooling with the corneal astigmatism and slight peripheral edge lift.
8. If the comfort is poor the next base curve 0.10 mm flatter or steeper should be evaluated (always try flatter first). Follow steps 3 to 7.
9. Slight upper-lid attachment without superior positioning is preferred; therefore, a diameter larger than 9.5 mm may be required to achieve this result.
10. If no movement is observed, select a base curve 0.20 flatter and follow steps 3 to 7.

Table 27-2 outlines the changes in lens-edge lift that result in altering the base curve and lens diameter. Aspheric basics such as this must be implemented in order to accurately evaluate what modifications need to be made to a lens fit.

The elliptic back surface of the lens eliminates the need for an exact mathematical relationship between the base curve and the diameter of the lens. The cornea has an eccentricity of 0.5 to 0.7 so that a posterior aspheric lens would match the cornea well and be parallel.

If the lenses do not center and move properly, visual acuity will be compromised. Whenever changes are made to the lens-fitting variables, i.e., the posterior apical radius, eccentricity, and diameter, the resultant sagittal depth of the lens is directly affected. Table 27-3 outlines the variables and their resultant effects on the sag of a lens.

All of the possible combinations and their results must be considered, otherwise changes can be made without there being any change in the sagittal depth. For example, if both the posterior apical radius and the eccentricity were steepened it would follow that the sag would be increased. However, if the two changes were made and the diameter were reduced, the resultant sagittal depth may remain unchanged from the original fitting.

INFERIOR ORIENTATION OF ASPHERIC LENSES

A lens may center well over the corneal apex; however, if that apex is centered at or below the inferior edge of the pupil, some of the optical quality of the lens will be lost. The apex of the lens can be changed by reducing its overall diameter by 0.2 mm to 0.4 mm. A lens with an overall diameter of 9.6 mm may be reduced to 9.2 mm, thus reducing its sagittal depth and enabling it to center better over the pupil. Another method to improve centering in this case would be to remake the lens to the same specifications with a minus carrier lenticulation. The upper lid will grasp the lens edge better and in

Table 27-3 ■ Variables and sagittal depth

Posterior apical radius (base curve)	Eccentricity	Diameter	Sagittal depth
Flatter	Constant	Constant	Reduced
Steeper	Constant	Constant	Increased
Constant	Constant	Smaller	Reduced
Constant	Constant	Larger	Increased
Constant	Steeper	Constant	Increased
Constant	Flatter	Constant	Decreased
Flatter	Flatter	Constant	Decreased
Steeper	Steeper	Constant	Increased

turn will position the lens more superiorly. This is especially helpful in hyperopic corrections.

If the inferior positioning is caused by a lens that obviously is too small, a larger lens should be made with a minus carrier lenticulation. The diameter increase should be 0.3 mm to 0.6 mm. The changes in the fit via sagittal depth will usually require a prescription modification also.

LATERAL ORIENTATION OF ASPHERIC LENSES

Most cases of lateral displacement will exhibit edge lift. Cases of against-the-rule astigmatism tend to have a higher incidence of lateral orientation. The lens diameter may be reduced by 0.2 mm at a time until the edge lift and displacement are eliminated. If this is not effective, a lens of 0.1 mm to 0.2 mm steeper base curve should be tried. If these steps fail to provide satisfactory positioning and alignment, a back or bitoric lens should be considered.

SUPERIOR ORIENTATION OF ASPHERIC LENSES

If the lens is positioned excessively high its diameter can be reduced in 0.2 mm increments and/or its edge can be thinned via a plus design lenticulation. Another treatment for this problem is to steepen the base curve by 0.1 mm and reduce the overall diameter by 0.2 mm. In nonresponsive cases, it may even be necessary to put a prism ballast on the lens.

HIGH CORNEAL CYLINDER

As previously discussed, large degrees of corneal astigmatism present problems of fit stability and lens flexure. This is no different for aspheric designs. In instances where there is a moderate-to-high cylinder or a keratoconus type of fitting, each eye must be assessed on an individual basis by the use of diagnostic lenses.

Nipple-type keratoconus cones are usually best fitted with steep designs of relatively small diameter. The oval and globus cones may be better fitted with a lens geometry more closely matching the flatter superior area of the cornea. This may cause the lens to exhibit what would normally be regarded as excessive inferior edge lift. It has been our experience that this attention

to the flatter superior corneal topography gives more satisfying results in terms of physical comfort and visual acuity.

The simplicity of fitting aspheric lenses includes some of our soft lens fitting systems, such as one or two diameters with varying base curve selection. This combined with the good performance of the high-permeability rigid gas-permeable materials may help in the re-emergence of aspheric lenses as a common rigid lens modality.

PRESENT DEVELOPMENTS

As stated earlier, rigid gas-permeable lens materials are beginning to reach the point of being physiologically undetectable and totally surface-biocompatible. In spite of all the forgiveness aspects of the materials, the lenses must be fitted well in order to be successful. Lens geometrics must combine with the state-of-the-art materials in order to attain maximum design compatibility. Edge profiles must be optimal to ensure a positive response both initially and in the long term.

In comparison to hydrogel lenses, rigid gas-permeable lenses must be improved so as to provide maximum comfort upon insertion and during adaptation, thus rendering the physical comfort factor a non-issue. At the same time, a scientific system of producing, reproducing, and fitting must be developed. This will probably incorporate posterior lens geometrics of more than one eccentricity produced by an axis-driven computer-controlled lathe or a molding process. This could create a bi- or multi-aspheric design, which while being highly reproducible, would reduce edge-lift requirements. The by-product of this would be greater correction potential of corneal astigmatism as compared to spheric multicurve designs.

Faster and more accurate systems of evaluating corneal topography will better enable us to project the best lens design for a given cornea. Improvements in photokeratoscopic and corneal mapping systems will probably render obsolete the keratometer as we know it. All these issues are presently being addressed in the research being done by lens manufacturers. The forthcoming developments from industry should render contact-lens fitting more of a science and less of an art.

28 ▪ KERATOCONUS

- Early detection of keratoconus
- Etiology
- Treatment with contact lenses
- Single-cut rigid lenses
- Soper keratoconus diagnostic fitting set
- Dura-T lenses
- Hydrophilic lenses
- Piggyback lenses
- Contact lens warping and keratoconus
- Gas-permeable lenses: types and application
- Summary

Keratoconus is a bilateral, progressive, conic deformity of the central or, more commonly, the paracentral cornea. It is a rare condition that affects an estimated 40,000 cases in the United States (0.015% of the population).

Three conditions have a relationship with keratoconus: (1) retinitis pigmentosa, (2) Down's syndrome, (3) atopic dermatitis.

In keratoconus, the apex of the cone is invariably located downward and nasally from the visual axis and may protrude 10 to 15 D or an additional 2 mm in relation to the normal height of the cornea, which is 2.5 mm (Figs. 28-1 and 28-2). The area of ectasia is generally limited to 3 to 6 mm in diameter; this characteristically is the zone of greatest thinning of the cornea. The condition is a non-inflammatory degenerative episode, but its etiology is not clear. It appears to occur in about 0.015% of the population.

The condition begins in adolescence, frequently in one eye, and then undergoes remissions and relapses until the age of 40 to 45 years, when it seems to stop. With repeated corneal breakdown the apex of the cornea becomes thin and scarred and loses the regularity of its front-surface optic properties.

The area of corneal protrusion is often surrounded by a superficial iron ring and may have tears and posterior folds, which result in high astigmatism.

Keratoconus generally affects both eyes but begins first in one eye and then several years later may be seen in the follow-up.

EARLY DETECTION OF KERATOCONUS

Early clues to keratoconus include (1) unusual scissor movement on retinoscopy, (2) increasing astigmatism on refraction, (3) irregular keratometry mires, (4) increasing myopic findings, (5) inability to improve vision on refraction to normal, (6) slitlamp findings including thinning of the cornea, (7) a partial thinning, (8) full Fleischer ring that encircles the cone at the lense of Bowman's membrane, (9) pachometry that measures evidence of corneal thinning. The diagnosis may be made with a Placido disc, which is a flat disc painted with alternating black and white rings that encircle a small, central, round aperture. The cornea is used as a front-surface convex mirror that reflects from the normal cornea a series of perfectly uniform, concentric circles. In a cone-shaped cornea the reflected target is distorted and the concentric circles are uneven, frequently broken and without symmetry (Fig. 28-3). The condition is often inferonasal or temporal but rarely in the center.

The limitations of the Placido disc in the diagnosis of early keratoconus should be appreciated. If the Placido disc on the keratoscope (an electric Placido disc) is tilted, the reflected circles may also be ellipsoid in a normal cornea, simulating early keratoconus. A slit-lamp diagnosis is difficult to make in the early phase, whereas in the late stages the diagnosis becomes obvious with apical thinning, Fleischer keratoconus ring, increased endothelial reflex, increased visibility of the nerve fibers, scarring of Bowman's membrane, and so on.

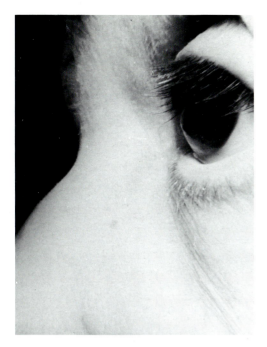

Fig 28-1 ■ Keratoconus. (From Hartstein J: Questions and answers on contact lens practice, ed 2, St Louis, 1973, The CV Mosby Co.)

Fig 28-2 ■ The apex of the cone and the visual axis are not in alignment. The cone is usually displaced downward and nasally.

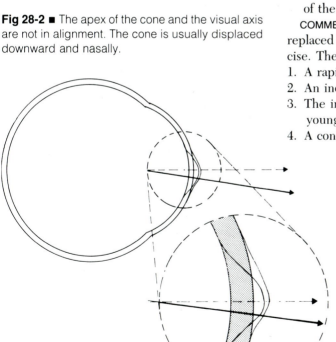

Keratometry is very helpful in the early phase of this disease since the mire images appear distorted and irregular. The two principal meridians are not at right angles to each other, and the dioptric value of the readings is quite high—48 D or higher.

Another instrument for diagnosis of keratoconus in the early stages is the retinoscope, which reflects irregular light reflexes from the surface of the cornea.

The diagnosis of keratoconus in the early stages is often elusive. It depends on the following:

1. The keratometry reading indicating high cylinder axes or irregular mires. Irregular astigmatism is one of the earliest signs of keratoconus. Characteristically, the major and minor axes are not at right angles to each other so the mires are inclined to each other.
2. Changing astigmatic refractive errors
3. Vision that is not correctable to 20/20 by spectacles
4. Scissor movement on retinoscopy
5. Placido-disc reflection
6. Slit-lamp findings including Fleischer's ring and evidence of corneal ruptures with scarring
7. Pachometric findings to indicate a thinning of the cornea

COMMENT. The Placido disc has largely been replaced by the keratometer, which is more precise. The earliest clues to the diagnosis are:

1. A rapid increase in myopia
2. An increase in astigmatism
3. The inability to correct vision to 20/20 in a young person
4. A confusing retinoscopy pattern.

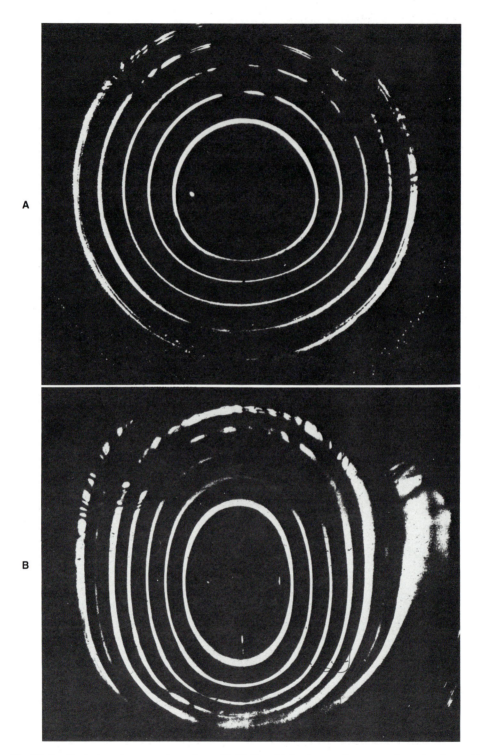

Fig 28-3 ■ Early keratoconus, less than 48.00 D, which shows, **A,** some distortion but within the variation of an astigmatic cornea. **B,** Moderate keratoconus, 52.00 D, which shows considerable distortion.

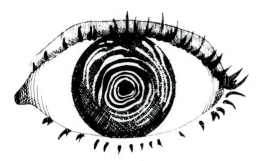

Fig. 28-3, cont'd. ■ **C,** Severe keratoconus with many distortions and breaks in the concentric circles.

Keratoconus may be classified by the stages of its advancement:

Stage 1: Oblique astigmatism with irregular keratometer mires. The Placido disc shows irregularities (Fig. 23-3).

Stage 2: Intensification of the above signs and vision not refractable to normal.

Stage 3: Pronounced conical shape with cor-

neal thinning can be identified on slit-lamp examination and pachymetry

Stage 4: Opacities at the apex.

More advanced stages include considerable scarring and hydrops of the cornea.

The area of conical protrusion is often surrounded by a superficial iron ring and even fine posterior folds. High irregular astigmatism often develops.

Keratoconus may be classified according to the degree of conicity of the apex of the cone. Classification is noted in Table 28-1. An example of an advanced keratoconus is indicated in Fig. 28-4.

Distinction should be made between three clinical types of advanced keratoconus. There is the round or nipple-shaped cone that lies most commonly in the lower nasal quadrant (Fig. 28-5 A and C). It is the most common type and is limited in diameter.

The third type is oval or sagging, is longer, and sags in the inferotemporal quadrant (Figs. 28-5 B and D). It is most prone to corneal hydrops. It is steeper than the round cone, having

Table 28-1 ■ Classification of keratoconus

	Mild	Moderate	Advanced	Severe
K reading	<45.00 D	>45.00 D	>52.00 D	>60.00 D

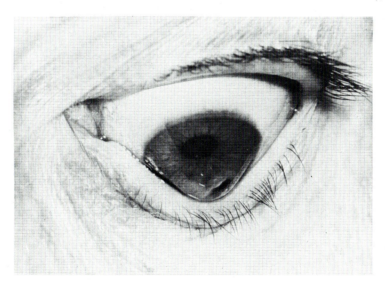

Fig 28-4 ■ Advanced case of keratoconus. (Courtesy Dr. Dean Butcher, Australia; in Stein HA and Slatt BJ: The ophthalmic assistant, ed 4, St Louis, 1983, The CV Mosby Co.)

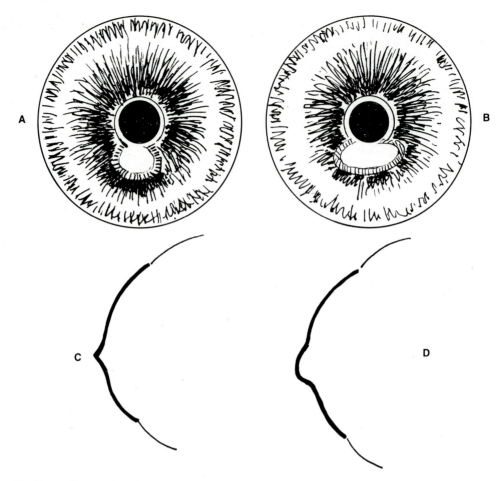

Fig 28-5 ■ Types of cones in keratoconus. **A** and **C** are illustrative of a nipple cone. **B** and **D** are illustrative of an oval or sagging cone. (Modified after Dominic Siviglia.)

an average keratometric reading of 68 D. The round cone is rarely greater than 65 D. There is also an ill-defined irregular cone inferiorly.

The round or nipple cone has the best prognosis in terms of contact lens fitting. Fortunately, it is the most common type. In another case, the globus cone is much larger and can involve three-fourths of the cornea. Fortunately, it is rarely seen.

ETIOLOGY

Many theories have been postulated on the etiology of keratoconus. Many clinical reports have linked it to various systemic disorders. Some have felt that the condition is inherited, others that eye-rubbing is a major cause because 66% to 73% of keratoconus patients reveal eye-rubbing in their history. Hormonal influences

have been implicated because the condition often starts at puberty. More females than males are affected and the condition worsens in pregnancy.

We personally feel the data on the above causes to date for the etiology of keratoconus is inconclusive.

COMMENT. There is some controversy whether rigid contact lenses cause keratoconus. Most authorities do not support this hypothesis because if it is true, the incidence of keratoconus should be much higher than it is in the general population. The starting age of a contact lens patient and the age of a keratoconus patient are similar. Also, in the early phases of keratoconus the person may be merely myopic, and so it is quite natural to assume that one causes the other. There are, however, some who believe that a rigid lens may accelerate the development of early forms of keratoconus.

There appear to be several episodes in a patient's lifetime when the disease arrests itself or becomes stable. This may last months or years. There is also no significant sex prediction but in our own practice it appears to predominate in females.

TREATMENT WITH CONTACT LENSES

The purpose of a lens is to cover the irregular astigmatism and the disordered anterior surface optic properties of an ectatic cornea by providing a regular, spherical optic surface before the eye. The lens does not retard the progression of the disease, which by itself may have long periods of natural remission. Spectacles are satisfactory only in early mild cases.

Several approaches using contact lenses may be used:
1. Single-cut small, gas-permeable lenses
2. Soper two-curved method of vaulting
3. Thin lenses
4. Scleral lenses (these are virtually obsolete now)
5. Soft lenses
6. Piggyback soft and rigid lenses

The first three approaches can be used with gas-permeable lenses.

SINGLE-CUT RIGID LENSES

Ideally, corrective rigid lenses should touch the apical cone lightly and rest on the peripheral cornea where there is little or no thinning (Fig. 28-6, A). Lenses fitted excessively flat eventually cause corneal abrasions (Fig. 28-6, B). Minimal

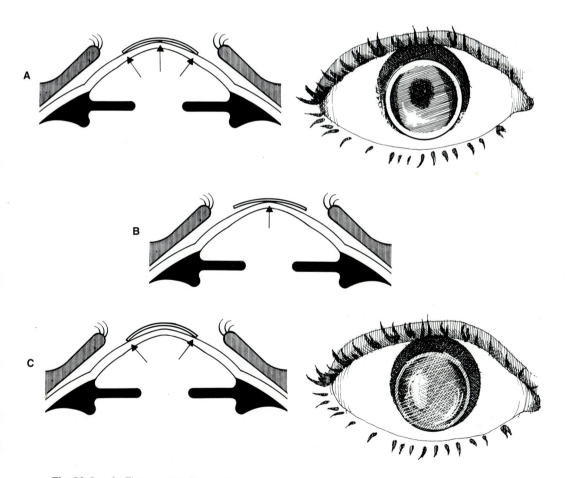

Fig 28-6 ■ A, Three-point fit—apical touch to the cone plus peripheral touch. Ideal for keratoconus because of the distribution of weight of the lens. **B,** Flat fit—apical touch but poor centration because of rocking on the corneal cap and edge stand-off. **C,** Steep fit—two-point touch with an air bubble between the lens and the cone. The apical cone is cleared.

Table 28-2 ■ Specifications of 10-lens keratoconus trial set

Scribed lens (D)	Radius (mm)	Diameter (mm)	Second curve (mm)	Power (D)
42.25	8.0	9.2	0.3 (12.25)	+1.25
43.50	7.75	9.2	0.3 (12.25)	+0.25
45.00	7.5	9.2	0.3 (12.25)	−2.00
46.50	7.25	9.2	0.3 (12.25)	−3.50
48.25	7.0	9.4	0.4 (12.25)	−5.25
50.00	6.75	9.4	0.4 (12.25)	−7.25
51.87	6.5	9.4	0.4 (12.25)	−9.25
54.00	6.25	9.6	0.2 (9.50), 0.3 (12.25)	−11.25
56.25	6.0	9.6	0.2 (9.50), 0.3 (12.25)	−13.50
58.75	5.75	9.6	0.2 (9.50), 0.3 (12.25)	−17.00

Courtesy Plastic Contact Lens Company, Toronto, Canada.

Table 28-3 ■ Dioptric curves for extended range of keratometer

High power (with +1.25 D lens over aperture)		Low power (with −1.00 D lens over aperture)		High power (with +1.25 D lens over aperture)		Low power (with −1.00 D lens over aperture)	
Drum reading (D)	True dioptric curvature (D)	Drum reading (D)	True dioptric curvature (D)	Drum reading (D)	True dioptric curvature (D)	Drum reading (D)	True dioptric curvature (D)
52.00	61.00	42.00	36.00	47.37	56.37	37.50	31.50
51.87	60.87	41.87	35.87	47.25	56.25	37.37	31.37
51.75	60.75	41.75	35.75	47.12	56.12	37.25	31.25
51.62	60.62	41.62	35.62	47.00	56.00	37.12	31.12
51.50	60.50	41.50	35.50	46.87	55.87	37.00	31.00
51.37	60.37	41.37	35.37	46.75	55.75	36.87	30.87
51.25	60.25	41.25	35.25	46.62	55.62	36.75	30.75
51.12	60.12	41.12	35.12	46.50	55.50	36.62	30.62
51.00	60.00	41.00	35.00	46.37	55.37	36.50	30.50
50.87	59.87	40.87	34.87	46.25	55.25	36.37	30.37
50.75	59.75	40.75	34.75	46.12	55.12	36.25	30.25
50.62	59.62	40.62	34.62	46.00	55.00	36.12	30.12
50.50	59.50	40.50	34.50	45.87	54.87	36.00	30.00
50.37	59.37	40.37	34.37	45.75	54.75		
50.25	59.25	40.25	34.25	45.62	54.62		
50.12	59.12	40.12	34.12	45.50	54.50		
50.00	59.00	40.00	34.00	45.37	54.37		
49.87	58.87	39.87	33.87	45.25	54.25		
49.75	58.75	39.75	33.75	45.12	54.12		
49.62	58.62	39.62	33.62	45.00	54.00		
49.50	58.50	39.50	33.50	44.87	53.87		
49.37	58.37	39.37	33.37	44.75	53.75		
40.25	58.25	39.25	33.25	44.62	53.62		
49.12	58.12	39.12	33.12	44.50	53.50		
49.00	58.00	39.00	33.00	44.37	53.37		
48.75	57.75	38.87	32.87	44.25	53.25		
48.62	57.62	38.75	32.75	44.12	53.12		
48.50	57.50	38.62	32.62	44.00	53.00		
48.37	57.37	38.50	32.50	43.87	52.87		
48.25	57.25	38.37	32.37	43.75	52.75		
48.12	57.12	38.25	32.25	43.62	52.62		
48.00	57.00	38.12	32.12	43.50	52.50		
47.87	56.87	38.00	32.00	43.37	52.37		
47.75	56.75	37.87	31.87	43.25	52.25		
47.62	56.62	37.75	31.75	43.12	52.12		
47.50	56.50	37.62	31.62	43.00	52.00		

Courtesy Bausch & Lomb, Inc.

apical clearance of the cone has been advocated, but this point of view represents a minority opinion. Attempting to obtain central clearance in even moderate cone cases will necessarily result in considerable pooling of tears around the periphery of the cone because of increased elevation of the conical area (Fig. 28-6, *C*). This pooling frequently leads to hazing, bubble formation in the vaulted area, and discomfort.

Trial lens-fitting (Table 28-2)

In the early phases of keratoconus, K readings are a guide to selecting a lens. As the condition develops, the mire image becomes irregular and the cone becomes steeper than 50.00 D so that the radius of curvature cannot be determined by ordinary keratometry. The only alternative is to fit the patient by trial and error.

The range of the keratometer can be extended to 61.00 D with an auxiliary +1.25 D lens (Table 28-3 and Fig. 28-7). However, because of the disordered mires, problems in fixation, and optic defects in the system, the results merely serve as a guide to trial lens selection. Fixation can be improved when one employs the viewing light of the topogometer.

A good fit should have a central touch of 2 to 3 mm centrally with a thin band of touch at the lens periphery, as determined by the fluorescein test. The three-point touch adds to the stability of the lens on the cornea and distributes the weight of the lens not only over the apex but over other bearing areas as well. The peripheral touch area corresponds to the zone of the intermediate curve. The initial lens selected, with the K readings serving as a guide, should have a base curve flatter than K. Then, with use of the fluorescein test, the lens is exchanged until one is found that results in slight apical touch of 2 to 3 mm or from 1 to 4 mm flatter than K. A light apical touch is desirable so that the lens can function as a pressure bandage on the thin, central corneal apex.

It is important to follow the keratoconus patient closely on a weekly basis because of progressive flattening of the cone by the initial lens. As the area of touch increases and the cone flattens, a new lens with a flatter base curve can be tried. Lens changes should be made until changes in the shape of the cornea are stabilized. With flattening of the cone it is not unusual to find that over a period of time as much as 4.00

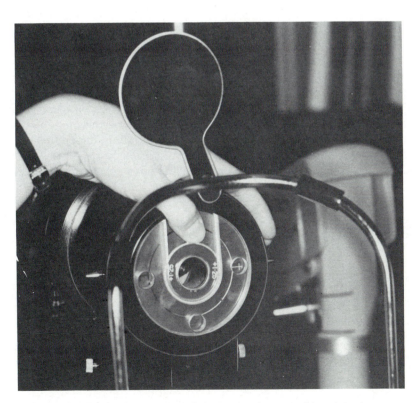

Fig 28-7 ■ INNS extension disc to extend range of keratometer.

to 6.00 D of plus power over the original lenses will be needed. Flattening may occur without a change in power if there has been a compensatory change in the lacrimal lens.

A guide to lens selection

Diameter. Large lenses with a diameter of 9 to 10 mm are generally used to provide stability and support whereas small lenses with diameters of 8 to 8.5 mm have been employed successfully for milder forms of keratoconus, that is, less than 52.00 D. A smaller lens may be used if it does not show excessive movement (Fig. 28-8). Basically small lenses are made quite steep and are employed when the cone is truly central. Small-sized lenses are lighter, so they can be fitted flatter. On the other hand this same merit can lead to loss of stability. Small lenses for keratoconus are usually bicurve with a narrow peripheral curve that rests on the apex of the cone end near its limiting border.

COMMENT. Small lenses were used only in cases of early keratoconus when PMMA was the only material available. With gas-permeable lenses, it is preferable to use larger lens for centration, comfort, and stability with blinking. Also a large-diameter lens invariably has a large optic zone.

Optic zone. The size is usually determined by trial and error with fluorescein. The size will depend on the site, protrusion of the conic deformity, and the amount of corneal touch. The optic zone should be larger than the pupil size in average illumination and should allow for the amount of decentration of the apex of the cone, which frequently is 1 mm nasally and 1 mm inferiorly. With a 5 mm pupil the average optic zone is approximately 7 mm.

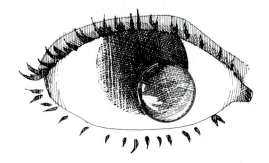

Fig 28-8 ■ Smaller lenses are used only for central cones, which are rare. If smaller lenses are fitted on an eccentric cone, they frequently slide off the cornea.

Peripheral curves. Peripheral curves can be tricurve or even pentacurve in advanced cases. The intermediate curve should be 1 or 2 mm flatter than the base curve. The peripheral curve is approximately 4 mm flatter than the intermediate curve.

In advanced cases additional peripheral curves are needed to avoid sharp blends. The difference in radius of curvature between the primary base curve and the peripheral curve is frequently considerable, as from 45.00 to 60.00 D to 35.00 to 40.00 D. These additional curves prevent abrupt changes in the radius of curvature as the lens undergoes radical flattening from the apex to its periphery.

Power. One can best determine the power by refracting the patient wearing trial lenses. A contact lens provides the cornea with a smooth and regular anterior surface so that light is evenly refracted. With spectacles, compensation cannot be made for the irregular astigmatism and distortion that accompanies keratoconus. The refraction through a contact lens can yield remarkable results with acuity improving from 20/200 to 20/30 or 20/25. The lens power usually has a range between −5.00 and −15.00 D. Sometimes a local anesthetic must be used for a trial-set refraction to reduce irritation and tearing during the examination.

Evaluating lens fit

1. A large bubble indicates the lens is too steep. Also vision is poor.
   TREATMENT. Try on a flatter lens. Gas-permeable acrylate lenses permit a flatter fit without compromising the epithelium.
2. Apical touch is indicated by the absence of fluorescein-stained tears at the apex of the cornea and indicates that the lens is touching the cornea at that area.
   TREATMENT. Try a steeper lens.
   COMMENT. Slight apical touch is acceptable.
3. The presence of fluorescein-stained tears under the central area but not under the peripheral curves near the edge of the lens indicates that the lens may be close to the desired central posterior curve, but too steep in the periphery.
   TREATMENT. The same-diameter lens could be ordered and wider, flatter posterior peripheral curves used. Over-refraction will reveal the lens power needed.
4. Refraction over the trial lens may provide

only poor vision. A small pupil test (accomplished by flashing a light in the opposite eye to create a small pupil by the consensual reflex) may improve vision. If so, the optic zone is too small.

TREATMENT. Try to order a larger-diameter lens. A larger lens is invariably tight, and so a flatter fit may be required.

5. A new lens may provide good vision and may have apical clearance, but may be too tight at the periphery as indicated by the absence of fluorescein-stained tears under the lens edge. A small bubble may be trapped under the lens.

TREATMENT. It is best to modify the lens. Use diamond radius tools (such as 11.50, 9, or 8 mm down to 1 mm flatter than the central posterior curve) to widen the posterior peripheral curves. Reapply to cornea and re-evaluate fluorescein patterns.

6. The lens may fit well, but vision may be improved with additional cylindric over-refraction.

TREATMENT. If the cylinder addition is large, incorporate the added cylinder in a spectacle.

Some people wear a soft lens and a rigid lens and spectacles but it is a little too much trouble for the average patient.

SOPER KERATOCONUS DIAGNOSTIC FITTING SET

The Soper lens (Fig. 23-9) is our fitting set of choice because we have had excellent results both in moderate and advanced cases of keratoconus. By concentrating on increasing or decreasing sagittal depth and by choosing an appropriate base curve or size one can fit most keratoconus patients with a minimal number of trial lenses (Table 28-4). Over-refraction is used to arrive at the best visual correction.

Progression of the cone can be detected by observation of an increase in apical staining and the presence of large abrasions. When this occurs, it indicates that the cone has moved forward, touching the lens. In such cases a new lens with greater apical vaulting must be ordered.

The Soper lens has been designed with a very steep, central posterior curve to accommodate the cone of the cornea and a much flatter flange

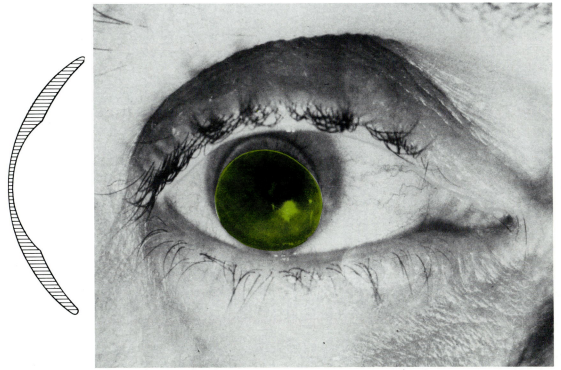

B

Fig 28-9 ■ **A,** Soper cone lens for keratoconus. There is a steep central posterior curve and a much flatter flange surrounding it. **B,** Soper cone lens over a moderate keratoconus deformity.

Table 28-4 ■ Soper keratoconus diagnostic fitting set

Cone	Try first	Sagittal depth (mm)	Central posterior curve (D)	Power (D)	Lens diameter (mm)	Thickness (mm)	Central posterior curve diameter (optic zone mm)
Moderate	A ·	0.68	48.00/43.00	−4.50	7.5	0.10	6.0
	B	0.73	52.00/45.00	−8.50	7.5	0.10	6.0
	C	0.80	56.00/45.00	−12.50	7.5	0.10	6.0
	D†	0.87	60.00/45.00	−16.50	7.5	0.10	6.0
Advanced	E	1.00	52.00/45.00	−8.50	8.5	0.10	7.0
	F	1.12	56.00/45.00	−12.50	8.5	0.10	7.0
	G	1.22	60.00/45.00	−16.50	8.5	0.10	7.0
Severe	H†	1.37	52.00/45.00	−8.50	9.5	0.10	8.0
	I	1.52	56.00/45.00	−12.50	9.5	0.10	8.0
	J	1.67	60.00/45.00	−16.50	9.5	0.10	8.0

*There must be at least a 5-diopter difference between the central posterior curve (CPC) and the flange curvature for the lens to be effective.

†The sagittal value (vaulting effect) of lens H (a 52.00 D lens) is *much* greater than lens D (a 60.00 D lens), which is attributable to the *much* larger diameter (9.5 mm) of the H lens.

surrounding it to rest on the more normal, surrounding cornea. The cornea is fitted from a trial set of lenses with base curves ranging from 48.00 to 60.00 D and lens diameters ranging from 7.5 to 9.5 mm. By varying the base curve and the size of the lens the axial depth can be increased or decreased. As the size of the lens is increased and the base curve held constant, the vaulting

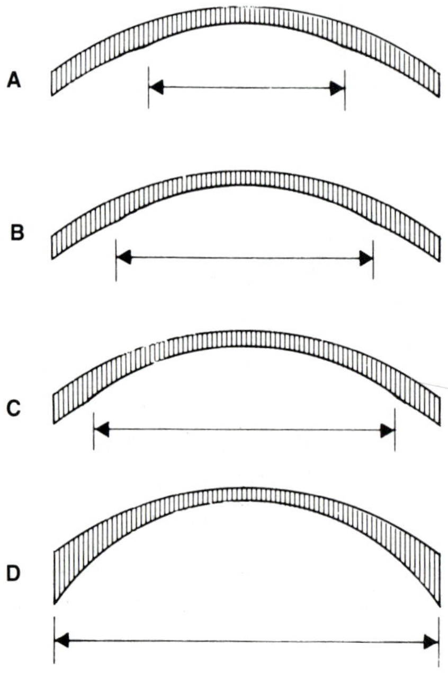

Fig 28-10 ■ The Soper lens. An increase in the sagittal depth can be made by an increase in the diameter of the lens. The base curves of **A** to **D** are the same.

effect is enhanced (Fig. 28-10). One of these two variables can be altered to obtain clearance. A good fit results when the lens has a slight touch or slight vaulting at the apex and a touch all around the periphery as detected by fluorescein. A central air bubble indicates that the lens is vaulting too much. A large central touch indicates that the lens is vaulting too little over the cone.

The Soper trial lens is best applied to the round (nipple) cone. The oval cone, which sags, is best approached with a large flat lens of standard design.

The course of keratoconus is changeable and unpredictable. As the cone progresses, a flat area of touch may occur and the cornea may develop abrasions and scarring. Patients then are seen every six months and modifications are made accordingly.

Sensitivity to light is often the first symptom of apical touch. Keratoconus patients should be informed of this fact and told to return when this symptom occurs suddenly.

Soper fitting procedure

If the patient to be fitted is wearing contact lenses, it is *absolutely imperative* that the lenses be discontinued at least 48 hours before refitting is started. Fitting these lenses takes only the time needed to try on several lenses and locate the lens that meets the criteria of a well-fitted lens. The first lens from the set tried is one that relates to the degree of conic progression. If the cone is moderate, lenses A to D are tried first;

if it is advanced, lenses E to G are tried; if severe, H to J are used first. If this lens has excessive apical vaulting, air will be trapped over the cone. In that case the lens with the next smaller sagittal values is tried, and if necessary, additional lenses are tried until the bubble is no longer observed. If, however, apical touch is observed, this indicates a need for a lens with a greater sagittal value and therefore the lens from the trial set with the next greater sagittal value is tried and the process is continued until the apical touch is alleviated.

The criteria for a well-fitted cone lens are as follows:

1. Apical clearance with circulation of tears between the lens and the apex of the cone and some lens movement. Apical touch should not exceed 1 mm.
2. Centration and no displacement.
3. Movement of the lens with blinking.

Interpolating the best fit

In some few cases the best fit may fall between two trial lenses; that is, the lens with the greater sagittal values demonstrates a small bubble whereas the lens with the lesser sagittal value shows a slight apical touch. In that instance the fitter must interpolate.

Example:
A 48/43 lens gives a slight touch.
B 52/45 lens produces a small bubble over the apex of the cone.
Interpolated lens to order: 50/45

COMMENT. Whenever it is possible, the lens central posterior curve (CPC) and the diameter ordered for the patient should be the same as the diagnostic lens. The lens made for the patient will fit exactly as the diagnostic lens. When interpolation between two lenses is done, some degree of guesswork is involved.

Calculation of patient lens power

One can determine lens power *only* by refracting over a trial lens. The lens used for this purpose should not have an air bubble over the visual axis.

Example:

Trial lens CPC	52/45	
Trial lens power		−4.50
Over-refraction		−2.00
		−6.50
Lens to order:	52/45	−6.50

If the central posterior curve to be fitted is 54:00 (by interpolation as previously discussed) and the trial lens and over-refraction are as above, the central posterior curve to be fitted will be 2.00 diopters steeper than the trial lens; therefore an additional −2.00 must be added to the power of the lens to be ordered. In this case the lens ordered would be 54/45 −8.50.

DURA-T LENSES

The use of Dura-T lenses has been advocated by Gasset. The major point in this technique is that the lenses are made thinner. The central thickness of these keratoconus lenses is only 0.08 mm.

The thinness of the lens reduces the weight of the lens by 30% approximately. The reduced mass assists patient tolerance and centration. It is especially useful with large inferiorly placed cones.

Fitting procedure

These lens are fitted from inventory. There are 30 lenses in a set, with a power range of −2.00 diopters in 0.5-diopter increments to −23.00 diopters and base curves from 47 to 60 diopters.

A −10.00-diopter soft lens is used as a base on the patient's eye. Select the proper K readings with this lens.

COMMENT. The soft lens is used to extend the readings of the keratometer. The power (−10.00 D) must be added to the final reading. Power is obtained by over-refraction.

This method is very simple. Only the base curve and power changes need to be considered. The other parameters, such as the size of the optic zone, peripheral curves, and blend, are all standardized.

The initial lens should have a base curve halfway between the flattest and steepest meridian; for example, if 52 and 58 are the K readings, select 55 as the initial base curve.

The fit should be assessed by fluorescein. A three-point touch is important—central and midperipheral touch with peripheral clearance. If the lens does not conform to this pattern, go flatter or steeper.

The refraction should be expressed in minus cylinders. Use the sphere and drop the cylinder. The over-refraction should then follow.

Example:
  $-12.00 +5.00 \times 90$
  Minus cylinder form, $-7.00 -5.00 \times 180$
  Power of the lens, -7.00 plus
  Over-refraction required, -4.00
  Total power, -11.00 D

The inventory method makes sense if a fitter has a large volume of patients with keratoconus. Besides being simple to calculate and evaluate, this method allows one to fit a large number of patients and to give them their lenses the same day.

A newer development is the Ni-Cone lens designed by Dominic Siviglia of Lancaster, Pennsylvania. This lens has 3 separate curves and is designed to fit all the areas of the cone at the same time. While the central posterior radius fits over the cone itself, the secondary vaulting system permits the lens to move freely. The third base curve is in the periphery and rests on normal cornea. The lens is lathe-cut and comes in four different gradations depending on the severity of the cone.

Aspheric design

Lens designs with asphericity ranging from 1.20 in the steeper base curves and 0.50 in the flatter base curves have been advocated by some fitters and the Formacon is an example of this lens for keratoconus.

HYDROPHILIC LENSES

Empirically it has been found that hydrophilic lenses are useful in the treatment of keratoconus. Although such a lens normally does not mask astigmatism, it has been shown to reduce by three to four times the amount of astigmatism present in keratoconus, making overcorrection with spectacles a simple task.

These lenses are comfortable and extremely useful for the patient who cannot tolerate a hard lens. Discomfort from hard keratoconus lenses is quite common; keratoconus patients rarely tolerate their lenses as well as person with myopia. The base-curve selection is usually flat, 8.1 to 8.4 mm, and the diameter is usually large, 13 to 14 mm, to provide lens stability.

A good fit is a lens that centers well with a minimum of movement. If the lens does not center, the diameter can be increased or the base curve made steepr. If there is an air bubble over the apical cone, a flatter lens must be used.

Fitting procedure

1. The diameter of the lens should be 2 mm larger than the corneal diameter.
2. Select a lens with a steep base curve as a starter lens. If it is too steep, an air bubble will be captured under the lens, there will be no movement, and the eye will be red because of compression and banking of the conjunctival blood vessels.
  Reduce the steepness of the lens until the fit is satisfactory.
3. Allow a few moments for the redness and tearing to subside. Wash the lens with non-preserved saline solution before insertion.
4. A properly fitted lens should have 1 mm of lens motion and no drag with lateral motion. The lens must be centered.

The reason why a soft lens works in keratoconus is poorly understood. However, it has been shown that a soft lens is able to reduce the amount of required cylinder by up to 5 diopters.

Another way to use a soft lens is to allow it to become the base for a rigid lens—piggyback style.

PIGGYBACK LENSES

To avoid the use of auxiliary spectacles, spheric, curved rigid lenses placed over the soft lens piggyback style work surprisingly well (Fig. 28-11; see also Fig. 28-1.)

This approach was introduced by Baldone. A soft lens forms the base lens and ensures patient comfort. A soft lens with an 8.4 mm base curve and 14 mm diameter will fit most corneas. The power range is between -5 and 15 diopters.

Over the soft lens a rigid lens may be either

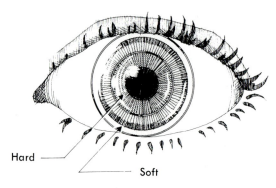

Fig 28-11 ■ A rigid lens riding piggyback over a soft lens.

placed to ride freely or placed into a depression to insert into the plastic that has been designed to hold a rigid lens. Usually, an 8.5 to 9.5 mm rigid lens is the best diameter to ensure centration and stability. Evaluation of the fit is standard.

Refraction over the trial rigid lens will give the power of the lens to be used.

If centration is a problem, an aphakic high-plus lenticular soft lens should be tried. The anterior lenticular bulge provides a convex surface, more appropriate to the fitting of a rigid lens.

COMMENT. This method should not be the first one tried. It requires double handling and double care systems—one for a rigid or gas-permeable lens and one for soft lenses.

An ultrathin permeable soft lens base with a gas-permeable rigid rider lens provides the best combination.

CONTACT LENS WARPING AND KERATOCONUS

It is important to distinguish corneal warping induced by contact lenses from true keratoconus. Corneal warping is a change in the contour of the cornea with resultant change in refraction. This may last days, weeks, or even permanently. Astigmatism does not persist once the lenses are discontinued. The condition is not as prevalent today with oxygen-permeable lenses as it was in the era of PMMA lenses.

Differentiation may be difficult. Keratoconus tends to progress and increasing myopia is common. Edema may be present with corneal warpage. Keratoconus induced by contact lenses is still controversial and has not been proved.

GAS-PERMEABLE LENSES: TYPES AND APPLICATION

These lenses, which include silicone and silicone resin lenses, CAB (cellulose acetate butyrate), the silicone-PMMA combinations (silicone-acrylates), styrene, fluorocarbon silicone acrylate, and pure fluorocarbon lenses, have been used with great success for fitting the patient with keratoconus. These lenses, which are fundamentally rigid, can be made 9.2 mm or greater and can still eliminate hypoxic changes because of their oxygen-permeability. Most patients with keratoconus have a corneal cylinder of 5.00 D or more. Most gas-permeable lenses can cover 5 D of astigmatism when spheric lenses are used. The large-diameter lens 9.2 mm or greater with an optic zone of 6.5 mm or greater permits this type of fitting without sacrificing centration and stability.

The fitting of such a lens requires a small fitting set with minimal selections available. Gas-permeable lenses can be fabricated to the Soper lens or any other lens chosen for keratoconus. The only problem with pure silicone is its brittle qualities and loss of dimensional stability. For best results, the composite lens with PMMA and silicone, the silicone-acrylate lenses, or the fluorocarbon silicone acrylate lenses are most appropriate.

We recently reviewed our management of patients with keratoconus who have contact lenses. We found that 55% of patients with keratoconus could be fitted with standard rigid gas-permeable lenses whereas 40% of the more advanced cases required a Soper-style gas-permeable lens and 5% required a piggyback lens.

Spectacles may work in mild cases of the *forme fruste* of keratoconus that does progress. Contact lenses may be the only treatment necessary for most patients with keratoconus, and they should be the first and preferred remedy. However despite the presence of contact lenses, many corneas continue to deteriorate. Keratoconus below 55.00 D generally lends itself to correction with lenses. Once the keratoconus exceeds 60.00 D, the use of lenses becomes difficult.

Keratoplasty should probably not be considered until there is pronounced corneal scarring reducing best corrected visual acuity in the better eye to 20/50 or less, acute corneal hydrops, conic thinning in the range of 0.3 mm where perforation is a distinct possibility, and a large eccentric cone greater than 5 mm in diameter. If a patient cannot tolerate a lens for at least 10 to 11 hours, keratoplasty may be the best alternative.

SUMMARY

Fortunately, keratoconus patients benefit significantly from contact lenses. Although fitting may be difficult and even frustrating at times, there is great satisfaction because most patients can maintain useful vision with contact lenses for most of their lives. Only a few require corneal transplants.

Although penetrating corneal transplants are the most popular method of keratoplasty, epikeratoplasty with an onlay graft is showing some promise. Epikeratoplasty does have one advantage: the fact that it may be reversible.

COMMENT. Fitting the patient who has keratoconus requires patience and expertise. Persons afflicted with this disease have fears about losing their sight every time they need a change or modification in their contact lenses. Success in fitting these persons requires the fitter to be optimistic, reassuring, and calm because the patient will be tense, agitated, and worried.

It is estimated that there are 40,000 keratoconus patients in the United States but only 500 become candidates for surgery. So only a few people out of a large keratoconus population cannot be treated by contact lenses alone. Fortunately, for those who come to surgery the results are excellent as over 90% will obtain a clear graft while 75% will have 20/30 vision or better.

29 ▪ *THE CORRECTION OF ASTIGMATISM WITH CONTACT LENSES*

Astigmatism occurs when the rays of light focus on two planes. It may be the result of a variation in the shape of the cornea, caused by a difference in the radius of curvature of the principal meridians of the cornea. It may also be the result of a different meridional refracting surface posterior to the front surface of the cornea. This form of astigmatism is called *residual astigmatism* because it persists despite the correct fitting of a lens to the cornea. It may be caused by a partially dislocated lens or a toric crystalline lens. It is important to distinguish between these two entities because the remedy for each is quite different (Fig. 29-1).

Residual astigmatism is that amount of astigmatism that remains after a lens has been fitted to the cornea. The most common source is lenticular astigmatism. In a previous lens wearer the appearance of a new astigmatic error invariable indicates warpage of the lens. A poorly fitted lens, especially one that is decentered, may also demonstrate residual astigmatism because of oblique incidence of light. At times a hard lens may mold the cornea, but such induced astigmatism is usually masked by the tear layer.

Most residual astigmatism is against the rule; that is, the meridian of greatest power lies nearest the horizontal meridian or the correcting plus cylinder is at 180 degrees. Actually it is

quite common—approximately 30% to 40% of patients will demonstrate some low order of an astigmatic defect of 0.50 D. However the vision of most of these patients is normal, perhaps not optimal, but does not require any special attention. It is only when the visual acuity declines to 20/30 or 20/40 with lenses or the patient suffers from visual distress that attention should be directed toward correcting the defect.

Over 25% of all patients interested in contact lenses demonstrated astigmatism over 1.25 diopters according to Holden (Table 29-1).

There are a number of options open to the fitter in correcting astigmatism; one may use a soft lens, either a spheric soft lens or a toric soft lens, or a rigid lens, either spheric or toric.

A gas-permeable lens, because it is larger than a PMMA lens, is more stable on a toric cornea and can mask up to 5 diopters of cylinder with a spheric lens design. The soft hydrogel toric lens can also correct a similar amount of astigmatism on those lenses in which the cylinder is ground on the anterior surface. Besides, the hydrogel lens, even in a toric configuration, has unsurpassed comfort. However, each system has

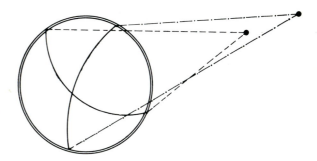

Fig 29-1 ▪ A toric cornea. The two curvatures have different focal points.

Table 29-1 ■ Distribution of astigmatism in prospective contact lens patients

0.25 D or more	0.50 D or more	0.75 D or more	1.00 D or more	1.25 D or more
76.5%	61.5%	45.4%	34.8%	24.8%
1.50 D or more	1.75 D or more	2.25 D or more	2.75 D or more	3.00 D or more
19.2%	15.8%	10.0%	6.0%	3.4%

From Holden, B: Aust J Optom 58:279-299, Aug 1975.

its flaws, and these, as well as the advantages, are reviewed.

TYPES OF CORNEAL ASTIGMATISM

With the rule: The cornea has a steep vertical meridian and a flat horizontal meridian. The contact lens rests on the flat meridian. If the lens is not fitted properly, it will tend to ride vertically up and down.

Against the rule: The cornea has a steep horizontal meridian and a flat vertical meridian. The contact lens rests on the flatter vertical meridian. If the lens is not fitted correctly, it will tend to ride horizontally from side to side.

Regular astigmatism: The two principal meridians are at right angles to each other.

Irregular astigmatism: The two principal meridians are not at right angles to each other; also, there is distortion of the keratometry mires when the corneal surface is irregular.

Residual astigmatism: This is the difference between corneal and total astigmatism. In contact lens fitting, it is the degree of astigmatism that remains after a hard contact lens has been placed on the cornea.

Soft lens correction

Spheric soft lenses. Spheric soft lenses can mask some degrees of corneal astigmatism. The astigmatism is not truly masked, but merely tolerated. The higher the spheric refractive error, the more this can be tolerated. If the total astigmatism is +1.25 D cylinder and the overall refraction is −6.00 D sphere, that degree of astigmatism may be tolerated. However, if the degree of spheric refraction is −2.50 D or less and the total amount of astigmatism is +1.25 D cylinder, in all likelihood that amount of astigmatism will not be tolerated. Thus the ability of the eye to tolerate the lack of any astigmatic correction depends primarily on its absolute value and secondarily on its relative value in relationship to the total refractive error. As a rule, if the astigmatism represents one third or greater of

the total refractive error, that degree of astigmatism needs to be corrected by means other than spheric soft lenses.

Frequently patients with 20/25 vision will complain bitterly of their vision with soft lenses. The addition of 0.75 D cylinder will improve their vision incredibly. In such patients, the addition of minimal toric corrections can be very helpful. The maximum tolerable astigmatic error, however, should be about 1.50 cylinder, regardless of the refractive error.

Standard-thickness lenses and not thin lenses should be used where possible for toric corneas. The use of ultrathin lenses will leave a considerable amount of cylinder uncorrected. If there is still defective vision because of uncorrected cylinder, one may wish to switch to a toric soft lens or a gas-permeable lens.

Toric soft lenses

The following are indications for astigmatism correction by toric soft lenses:
1. Corneal astigmatism.
2. Lenticular astigmatism.
3. Combinations of corneal and lenticular astigmatism.

The following are contraindications for fitting:
1. Irregular corneal astigmatism, as in a cornea scarred by previous herpes simplex infection.
2. Abnormal lid closure, as in partial Bell's palsy.
3. Any conditions that contraindicate the wearing of a contact lens in general.

Candidates for a soft toric lens include the following:
1. Rigid lens dropouts for any reason, such as induced toricity, discomfort, and corneal edema.
2. Soft lens dropouts, who were fitted with spheric lenses with poor visual results because the astigmatism component was not dealt with.
3. Patients with residual astigmatism. The front surface soft lens toric is ideal for the candidate

whose astigmatism is largely lens-induced.

4. Patients with large degrees of astigmatism, between 3 and 5 diopters.

The problems of fitting toric soft lenses are similar to those of fitting any soft lens, with the added difficulty of sustaining lens stability. It is this balance between a proper fit and alignment of lens axis to corneal toricity or to the zone of residual astigmatism that provides the challenge.

The major mechanisms for stabilizing the soft toric lens in either lenticular or corneal astigmatism and incorporating a toric surface include the following:

1. Prism ballast, 1 D or 1.5 D.
2. Truncation, either single or double.
3. Dynamic stabilization: the use of inferior and superior thin zones on the lens.
4. Aspheric back surfaces. This design sets up a drag phenomenon through a surface-tension zone between the lens periphery and the corneal periphery.
5. Posterior toric lenses.
6. An eccentrically placed lens that is weighted inferiorly, not being a prism but having a thicker inferior edge called a *bioflange*.
7. Combination of the preceding, that is, the Hydron lens uses an aspheric back surface with a central base curve with an eccentricity of 0.7 D, a prism ballast, and truncation.

Stabilization techniques

PRISM BALLAST. The amount of prism ballast varies between 1 and 1.50 diopters. The heavier prism ballast is required for eyes with tight lids, flat corneas, and an oblique axis of astigmatism. The prism factor adds weight to the lower portion of the lens, and its thickness precludes any significant oxygen-permeability in the inferior zone of the cornea. Hypoxic disturbances and arcuate staining of the cornea are occasionally encountered in the region of the prism. Manufacturers such as Bausch and Lomb and Hydrocurve presently provide lenses with pure prism.

TRUNCATION (Fig. 29-2). The contact lens is sectioned off 0.50 to 1.5 mm on the lower edge and occasionally on the upper edge as well. Smaller-diameter lenses of 13.5 mm use 1 mm of truncation, whereas the large diameters of 14.0 or 14.5 mm use 1.5 mm of truncation. A good truncated lens will be beveled so that edge compression of the cornea will not occur. Truncation tends to loosen a toric lens, which some manufacturers fix by making these lenses slightly steeper.

Truncation on the inferior edge permits the lens to rotate so that the lower flat edge comes to lie adjacent to the lower eyelid margin and thus stabilizes it. The lid configuration, which frequently varies from person to person, will affect the rotation of the truncated lens. A truncated lens may also be rotated if one edge, especially the lateral one, hits the lower lid before the other. A sloping lid that is higher laterally usually causes this to happen.

Truncation provides stability but is not a guide to the axis of the correcting cylinder. The 0- to 180-degree axis must be made with the slitlamp. The bottom of the truncated lens may not be parallel with the orientation of the lower lid, which frequently is sloping.

Often truncation is combined with prism ballast, so that the heavier dependent and thicker part is cut off. This also aids in reducing the overall lens weight of the contact lens. In addition, palpebral fissures that have sclera exposed inferiorly may require larger soft toric truncated lenses to permit the lower truncated edge to be in juxtaposition to the lower eyelid. Examples of these types of lenses are typified by the toric lens made by Hydron (Woodbury, NY) called the *Hydron T* and by Wesley-Jessen (Chicago) called *Durasoft TT*.

Truncation adds discomfort to the toric system. If the lower lid is in proximity to the truncated edge, lid impact occurs. Also there is displacement of the lens upward as the eyes are lowered to the reading position. Variable vision with reading results when upward decentration of the lens occurs.

THICK-THIN ZONES (DOUBLE SLAB-OFF LENS, DYNAMIC STABILIZATION). This lens system, patented by Fante in 1972, is perhaps the best for comfort because there is no lid impact on the inferior surface, but it does not offer as much lens stability as the truncated or posterior toric devices. The central body of the lens that lies in the palpebral fissure is thick, but the superior and inferior edges of the lens are thin (Fig. 29-3). When this lens is placed on the eye, the thinner zones align to come to lie under the upper and lower eyelids.

Many lenses, rigid and soft, rotate with blinking. However, such rotation is unacceptable with a toric lens system. Thus corrective cylinders are usually ground into this lens on the front

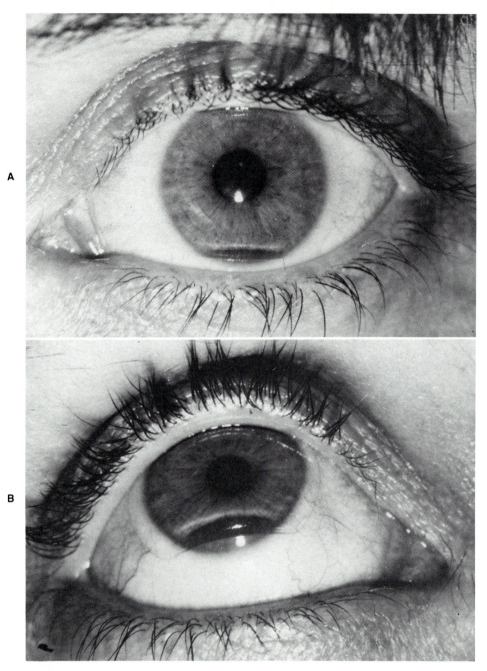

Fig 29-2 ■ A, Soft toric contact lens: a truncated-prism ballast lens in normal position. **B,** Looking up. The lens should stay in place with eye movement and yet be loose enough to move with a blink.

surface, so that the lens will stop rotating on the eye. Weicon (West Germany), CIBA-Geigy (Summit, NJ), and Dominion Contact Lens Company (Toronto) produce this type of thick-thin lens. These double slab-off lenses may also be combined with prism ballast to prevent dis-placement of the axis and rotation with blinking.

The thin-zone lens is best when the axis of astigmatism is in the major lines of power, that is, 180 or 90 degrees. Also it functions best when the drag between lids and lens is not excessive. The thin-zone lens is usually marked with etch-

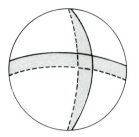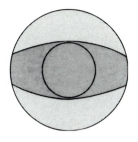

Fig 29-3 ■ Double slab-off soft lens used to correct astigmatism. The lens is made thinner superiorly and inferiorly so that the thinner portions tend to rotate and come to rest under the upper and lower eyelids.

ings on the 0- to 180-degree axis, which provide easy orientation to the axis of the cylinder.

POSTERIOR TORIC LENSES. Posterior toric lenses are perfect for patients with an imperfect corneal toricity because the axis of the lens can be aligned with the axis of the cornea that requires correction. This type of lens is stabilized by the toric correction being placed on the posterior side of the lens, which significantly reduces rotation and stabilizes the fit. It is valid for astigmatism that is largely generated by a toric corneal surface.

A number of manufacturers use this principle in the fabrication of their lenses.

The limitation of the system is that these posterior R toric lenses are available in only two power choices and work best with major meridional astigmatism. Also this system is not ideal for residual astigmatism, which does better with a spheric or aspheric lens and an anterior toric surface. Maltzman has pointed out that back surface toric lenses are the preferred soft lens when the cylindrical component of the refractive error is greater than the spherical component.

ASPHERIC LENS SURFACE. As aspheric lens surface aids in lens-axis stabilization by adding drag to the motion of the lens. It is not used as the primary force in lens stability but rather as an adjunct. Usually prisms or truncations are added to the system. Unfortunately such a lens becomes very tight with time, and so it is made flatter in the fitting, which reduces lens stability.

COMMENT. There is no best toric lens design. The lens must be chosen to suit the patient's needs. If comfort is paramount, choose a double slab-off toric lens. If stability is the foremost consideration, select a prism-truncated lens. There is no universal toric lens.

■
POSTERIOR SURFACE TORICS

Accugel
Hydrosoft
Kontur
Hydrocurve II Toric
Spectrum (CIBA)
Optifit (Wesley-Jessen)
Sunsoft

IDENTIFYING MARKS. Soft toric lenses may be identified by either etch marks or laser marks on the 3 and 9 o'clock areas of the lens, or at the 6 o'clock area. This will vary with the manufacturer.

QUALITY CONTROL. A toric soft lens design is an efficient correcting modality for astigmatism greater than 1.50 D. It is essential that the truncation is properly aligned with respect to the base of the prism.

To do this control, one uses a projection vertometer. The lens is mounted so that the truncation is positioned parallel to and adjacent to the observer doing the inspection. When observing the screen, the optic center of the mires should be in line with the central vertical line inscribed on the projection screen (90-degree axis); that is, the truncation is perpendicular to the axis of the prism. If the center of the mires is not in line with the central vertical line of the projection screen (assuming the lens has been centered) the cylinder axis will be off.

If this axis is not aligned correctly at this position of the lens, the lens should be rejected and remade. *Lens verification is critical for success when one fits the astigmatic patient with toric hydrogel lenses.*

One can check the power of the lens with a lensometer by blotting the lens dry with a piece of lint-free tissue paper and aligning the lens of 0- to 180-degree markings horizontally with the lens properly centered. The power can be read as one would for a spherocylinder spectacle prescription.

LENS FITTING. The toric lens has so many variables that trial-set fitting is used for best results. Only 60% of first fits can be achieved with a trial set of spheric lenses. With toric trial lenses results are better by 10%.

The fitting varies with the manufacturer and is dependent on the device employed for lens stability. For lenses stabilized by prism and truncation, the following method may be employed:

1. *Lens diameter selection*. Add 2 to 2.5 mm to the visible iris diameter.
2. *Selection of base curve*. The arithmetic mean of the K readings is taken and converted to millimeters of radius. For example, if the K readings are 40.25 × 180° and 42.50 × 90°, the mean radius would be 41.38 D. When this is converted to millimeters, the selected lens is 8.15 mm.

   A flatter base curve is selected and this is achieved when one adds 0.7 mm to the mean radius, which in this case would make the initial lens 8.75 mm.
3. *Over-refract in minus cylinders*.
4. *Record the vision of the back vertex distance*. One arrives at the cylindric component by doing a conventional over-refraction. The base curve of the final truncated prism-ballasted lens is compensated by the laboratory for the reduced vertical diameter that results from truncation.
5. The movement of the lens should be 1 to 2 mm with each blink. Check on the fit. The mires should be sharp and the retinoscopy reflex crisp.

To fit a double slab-off lens, we used as an example of this technique the Dominion Contact Lens, a Canadian lens. This is a lathe-cut double-slab-off lens made from the Toyo material. The lens has a front-surface toric design; the back surface is spheric and consists of two curves, a base curve and a peripheral curve, which varies with the base-curve radius. The meridional orientation of the lens is stabilized by a superior and inferior slab-off off the front surface and has 1.25 to 1.50 D prism ballast within the optic zone. The spheric power selection is unlimited up to −2.00 to +20.00 D, whereas the cylinder correction is limited to 0.50 to 3.50 D.

The recommended fitting set has 10 lenses that vary from 30.00 to 42.50 D in 0.50 D steps. The diameter is 14.5 mm for lenses 40.50 D and flatter and 14 mm for lenses 41.00 D or steeper.

The following method is used for double slab-off lenses:

1. The base curve is selected on the basis of a lens 4.00 D flatter than the flattest K.
2. Evaluate the lens-cornea relationship to position, movement, and quality of the K.
3. Over-refract and include the minus cylinders and the vertex distance.

The best candidates for selection are those with cylinders ranging from 1.00 to 2.00 D and those with regular astigmatism. Oblique cylinders between 30 and 60 degrees are difficult to orientate. Patients with tight lids and small palpebral fissures are screened out because of previous poor results with such patients.

Note that this particular lens, as opposed to others that use the same type of slab-off inferiorly and superiorly, has a toric zone only in the optic area of the lens. The lens has engraving at the 9 and 3 o'clock positions, and it is stabilized below as indicated by the presence of a blue dot.

COMMENT. Thick-thin-zone lenses are the least stable but most comfortable.

ASSESSING THE FIT. Once the lens has "settled" on the eye, always note the final lens orientation relative to the true 180-degree axis. At least 15 minutes is required for lens settling. If the lens orientation and stabilization is not achieved, a different stabilizing technique should be used.

CORRECTING THE AXIS. Axis corrections can be defined with etch marks, or laser beams, on all lenses at 0 to 180 degrees, a blue dot at the 6 o'clock position, or a vertical line. These marks are reference points to the orientation of the toric axis. A spectacle trial frame with axis lines is used. The lens is then rotated until the axis lines are in alignment with the prism base marked on the contact lens. The amount of rotation is directly read from the scale. The marks are usually in 5-degree intervals. For example, a lens at 5 o'clock will be rotated 15 degrees.

The 0- to 90-degree zone of the lens is regarded as the *subtractive inclination*. If the axis of the correcting cylinder toric lens is wrong, subtract the inclination in that zone. For example, if the minus cylinder axis is 20 degrees (which is in the 0- to 90-degree quadrant) and the over-refraction yields 15 degrees of axis correction, the final cylinder axis would be 5 degrees, that is, 20 degrees − 15 degrees.

The *additive quadrant* is between 90 and 180 degrees. So, if the axis is 140 degrees and the correct axis is 10 degrees, the final axis is 140 degrees + 10 degrees = 150 degrees.

COMMENT. We have adopted a mnemonic device, LARS, to help in axis correction. If the 6 o'clock position is used as the reference point, if the axis of contact swings to the left (when facing the patient) then "add" (LA = left add); if the axis swings to the right, then "subtract" (RS = right subtract).

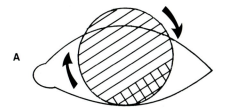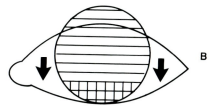

Fig 29-4 ■ **A,** Lens on immediate insertion. **B,** The heavy weighted lens combined with the torsional effect of the eyelid muscles, rotates the lens to a stable position.

VISUAL RESULTS. Visual acuity is not an absolute. Some patients with high degrees of astigmatism are content to have 20/25 vision, whereas others with low degrees of astigmatism are not content with this level of performance. However, as with all soft lenses, there are people with 20/20 vision who still complain of poor vision. Technically they are not rejects. In absolute terms 70% of our patients recieved 20/20 visual acuity with toric corrections, 80% of patients get visual acuity equal to or greater than the spectacle visual acuity, and 20% of cases required a second fitting to yield good visual results.

The results of soft toric lens fitting are directly proportional to the enthusiasm of the fitter. At best, 70% of patients are easy and require only one fitting. After a year an additional 20% may require refitting.

Protein on the lens can change the comfort of the lens, alter the lens contour, and interfere with visibility through the lens.

COMMENT. Oblique astigmatism is difficult to treat with soft toric lenses. These lenses are more difficult to manufacture and pose problems in lens stability. Blinking on an obliquely oriented toric lens causes lift and rotation of the lens.

FORCES ACTING ON A LENS. There are a number of forces that act on any given lens to provide stability. These forces are:
1. **Gravitational force:** Heavier lenses decenter inferiorly. In addition, if a prism is placed on one edge of a lens, the heavier thicker prism base of the lens rotates to the inferior portion on the lens.
2. **Hydrostatic force:** The hydrostatic force of the cornea draws the lens to the center so it rotates about the central axis of the cornea. If the lens moves off-center, a build-up of a suction force returns the lens to the center of the cornea.
3. **Lid action:** The eyelid muscle, the orbicularis oculi, has a significant effect on rotating the contact lens. If the lens edges are thick and thin, or prism-ballasted (wedge-shaped) then the rotational effect of blinking the lids is to rotate the lens so that the thin or thicker portion lies under the eyelids (Fig. 29-4). With truncated contact lenses, this effect is more marked.

PROBLEMS OF SOFT TORIC LENS FITTING

The causes of rejection of the toric lens are (1) discomfort, which can be created by foreign-body sensation of the lens, excessive movement of the lens, and awareness of the lens because of the abutment of the lens against the lower lid; and (2) poor vision, which can be attributable largely to rotation of the axis of the lens, which cannot be stabilized. This is particularly true with astigmatism of oblique axis 20 to 80 degrees and 110 to 160 degrees. Axis mislocation is a significant problem that was substantially reduced by the use of a truncated prism-ballast trial set. In some cases, the poor vision is related to variable vision symptoms of a tight or a flat fit and other visual defects that can confront any hydrogel lens wearer. There are cases in which poor vision is directly attributable to some diffuse corneal edema and the incorporation of fine subepithelial precipitates.

The signs of inadequate fit are:
1. Corneal edema or diffuse corneal stippling, especially under the thicker prismatic portion of the lens.
2. Inability to stabilize the lens axis.
3. Too much edge lift causing the lens to slip out of position.

4. Decentered lens or an inability to make the lens system flat enough to ensure adequate movement.
5. Discontinued lens wear because of limbal compression with engorgement of the limbal capillaries, which could eventually lead to corneal vascularization.

The factors that favor a good fit are:

1. Corneal astigmatism at the 90- and 180-degree meridians. If the astigmatism is oblique, say, at 60 degrees, the lids will create a rotational force on the lens with each blink. This movement is largely caused by the lens thickness not being the same on each side of the lens. As the lid moves down, it creates a greater drag or rotational force on the thicker side than on the thinner side.
2. Normal lid motion with small and tight palpebral fissures. Narrow palpebral tissues and tight lids create excessive movement of the lens and upset the toric alignment.
3. A lower lid that does not abut the truncated edge of a toric lens.
4. Use toric lenses for astigmatism greater than 0.75 diopters. Small amounts of astigmatism should be ignored.
5. Use of a toric-lens trial set to evaluate correction and rotational characteristics of the lens on the eye. The trial lenses have prism ballast, truncation, and toric surfaces.
6. Cylinders of about 2 diopters are ideal. The more the cylinder found in the treatment, the greater the difficulty in centration and the heavier the lens.
7. A minimally flat fit. If too loose, a lens will cause variable vision. A tight lens adds to stability but causes other undesirable signs and symptoms.
8. Lid configuration and lid tesnions are important considerations. The closure of the eyes on blinking, particularly if there is increased tension, or downward or upward sloping lateral canthi, will effect the performance and stabilization of toric lenses.
9. The double slab-off design is best for comfort.
10. Prism ballast plus beveled truncation is best for lens stability and precise axis correction.
11. Posterior toric lenses are best for a correction of moderate-to-high corneal toricity and particularly if the sphere component is small.

12. Aspheric lens design is a helpful adjunct to any lens system.
13. Large diameters, such as 14.5 mm, assist in centering the lens. One must compensate for the added tightness that a large-diameter lens confers by fitting the lens flatter.
14. Higher water content and thinner lenses aid comfort and oxygen permeability. Because lens thickness is usually measured at the optical center of a lens, the extra dimension of the prism in these lenses may not be included.

COMMENT. The fitting of a soft toric lens is not easy. One has to stay within the small zone of fitting too tight or too loose to ensure lens stability without adding complications. With the various lens modalities available today, a success rate of 90% can be achieved in the fitting of a toric lens.

Also, the frequency of lens replacements is higher than that of a spheric lens. With time, axis mislocation may occur because of protein debris in the lens, which can alter the fitting characteristics of the lens.

Unless the fitting criteria are present for a favorable hydrogel toric lens fit, a gas-permeable lens may be a better choice.

If residual astigmatism is present, we have found soft toric lenses better than rigid lenses because the large diameter permitted with soft lenses results in better stabilization. Also the extra power required can easily be ground on the front surface of the lens.

Some companies now manufacture toric lenses in extended-wear material. These lenses should be removed at least once a week and put through a care regimen.

It should be noted that the thicker edge of the prism ballast lenses does impair some of the oxygen transmission to the lower part of the cornea and may cause punctate staining.

RIGID CONTACT LENSES FOR ASTIGMATISM

Today, RGP material is the material of choice. PMMA has almost become obsolete in modern contact lens practice. Using the proper combination of RGP material and design, we have found almost 100% of patients with astigmatism can be effectively fitted and one need not resort to PMMA material. The gas-permeable rigid lens is preferred over PMMA because it is larger and therefore more stable. It also prevents hypoxic complications to the cornea.

Spheric rigid lenses

A spheric rigid lens should first be tried with any cornea of 3.00 D or less of corneal astigmatism. It is the lens of choice for toric corneas of small magnitude simply because a spheric lens is the easiest to fit, modify, and duplicate. A spheric lens is our choice of diagnostic lens to be used first, regardless of the degree of astigmatism.

It may be used in the following manner:

1. An ultrathin rigid lens may be used to correct low levels of residual astigmatism of 1.00 D or less. Such a lens will normally flex with blinking and will tend to nullify residual astigmatism against the rule. It is a good lens for residual astigmatism.
2. A conventional spheric lens may be used. One method is simply to "split K" so that the radius of curvature of the lens is *half-way* between that of the steeper and flatter meridians. Another approach is simply to ignore any astigmatism of 2.00 D or less. For each 0.50 D over 2.00 D of corneal astigmatism, fit 0.25 D steeper than K.
3. A large diameter lens of 9.5 to 10.5 mm fitted on K may be used. A large spheric lens provides stability on a toric cornea and is the lens of choice when a regular-sized lens fails to achieve adequate centration. Large lenses have also been used with success in some cases with astigmatism of 3.00 to 5.00 D. Only gas-permeable lenses should be used with large degrees of astigmatism where large diameters are required to ensure centration

and stability. In this case, PMMA lenses are a hazard.

4. Fitting characteristics should be monitored by fluorescein instillation, which can determine if the cornea-lines relationship is adequate (Fig. 29-5).

COMMENT. We have found that spheric rigid lenses account for over 90% of our rigid lenses used for correcting astigmatism whereas only 4% required a custom-ordered toric rigid lens. Some of the new aspheric and biaspheric designs have been extremely successful in fitting cases of low to moderate astigmatism (especially those who have with-the-rule cylinder). Such patients are extremely comfortable and exhibit excellent displacement of the lens mass in the areas of bearing.

THIN SPHERIC LENS. A microthin lens with 0.12 mm or less central thickness will flex on a toric cornea with astigmatism with the rule and will reduce an astigmatism against the rule. However, if the residual astigmatism is against the rule and the corneal surface has astigmatism against the rule, a thin lens will only augment the residual astigmatism.

SPHERIC EQUIVALENT. In patients with residual astigmatism of 1.00 D or less, the simple device of increasing the power of the spheric lens by an amount equal to the spheric equivalent of the remaining refractive error can be employed very effectively. For example, if the residual refractive error is −1.00 D cylinder axis 180 degrees, the spheric equivalent to be added to the spheric correction would be 0.50 D.

TORIC RIGID LENSES. The same basic principles of toric design PMMA lenses apply to the fitting of RGP torics. As always, on-the-eye perfor-

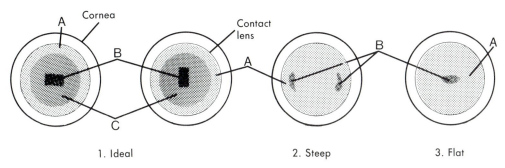

1. Ideal   2. Steep   3. Flat

Fig 29-5 ■ Fluorescein patterns on a toric cornea when fitted with a spherical rigid lens.

mance and material characteristics will vary from one fitting to another.

PRISM-BALLAST LENS. This lens has a spheric back surface, a prism base down of 1.5 prism D, and a toric front surface that provides the necessary correcting cylinder. Prisms greater than 2.00 D have such a heavy edge that they are seldom tolerated. For weaker power, -5.00 D or less, 0.75 prism D is frequently satisfactory. The bottom of the lens may be truncated to add stability and proper orientation. Truncation may produce problems however. It can weigh down the lens so that it overrides the lower limbus and can also irritate the lower lid by bumping it. Moreover, a truncated lens is difficult to fit for residual astigmatism against the rule because there is conflict between the gravitational movement of the lens downward and the need to contour the lens against a steep, horizontal meridian. Many fitters prefer a circular prism-ballast lens since it is easier to center and manufacture. One should use a trial lens for the refraction and determine the lens orientation by marking it with a grease pencil. This indicates the axis of the front-surface cylinder.

If one eye is fitted with a prism-ballast lens it is frequently necessary to fit the other eye in a similar fashion to avoid creating an intolerable vertical phoria. A prism-ballast lens should not be ordered unless absolutely necessary. What is gained by correcting residual astigmatism may be lost by the reduced optic quality of the lens imposed by the prism.

CORRECTING ASTIGMATISM WITH POSTERIOR TORIC RIGID LENSES

Sampson and Feldman have popularized the use of posterior toric lenses as a better alternative to bitoric lenses. These lenses are easily fabricated, have a spheric front surface that can be polished, rarely require any truncation or prism ballast for proper meridional orientation on the cornea, and will handle over 90% of all cases requiring toric lens design, residual astigmatism, or both.

In terms of corneal dioptric toricity, the total amount that may be generated on the posterior surface of a lens is about two thirds of the corneal toricity, which is given more accurately in Table 29-2.

To calculate such a lens consider the following example:

K = 42.00 D × 46.00 D × 90
Refraction -1.00 D with -2.50 D × 180
From Table 24-3, 1.75 D of corneal toricity is equal to 2.50 D of plastic toricity.
CPC = 42.00 D × 43.75 D
Lens = -1.00 D with -2.50 D × 180

Table 29-2 ■ Use of back toric contact lenses for high corneal toricity and residual astigmatism*

Cornea Cylinder of inside lens surface (D)	Lens Refractive cylinder values in air (D)	Cornea Cylinder of inside lens surface (D)	Lens Refractive cylinder values in air (D)
−0.25	−0.36	−4.25	−6.17
−0.50	−0.73	−4.50	−6.53
−0.75	−1.09	−4.75	−6.90
−1.00	−1.45	−5.00	−7.26
−1.25	−1.82	−5.25	−7.62
−1.50	−2.18	−5.50	−7.99
−1.75	−2.54	−5.75	−8.35
−2.00	−2.90	−6.00	−8.71
−2.25	−3.27	−6.25	−9.08
−2.50	−3.63	−6.50	−9.44
−2.75	−3.99	−6.75	−9.80
−3.00	−4.36	−7.00	−10.16
−3.25	−4.72	−7.25	−10.53
−3.50	−5.08	−7.50	−10.89
−3.75	−5.45	−7.75	−11.25
−4.00	−5.81	−8.00	−11.62

Courtesy Dr. Stanley Gordon, Rochester, NY.
*Corneal values based on refractive index = 1.3375; lens values based on refractive index = 1.490.

or
CPC = 43.00 D × 44.75 D
Lens = −2.00 D with −2.50 D × 180

Rule of quarters

One system of fitting the base curve for a posterior toric lens is to make one contact lens base curve one-fourth of the total astigmatism flatter than the steepest curve and one-fourth of the total astigmatism steeper than the flattest curve. Thus if the Ks were 42 × 46 × 90 and the total astigmatism was 4.00 D, then one-fourth is 1.00 diopter so the base curve of the bitoric rigid lens would be 43 × 45 or its equivalent in millimeters.

COMMENT. Gas-permeable rigid lenses are today's best method to correct high astigmatism. The family of gas-permeable lenses offers the benefits of an oxygen-permeable system and a large-diameter lens between 9 and 10 mm, which ensures axis stability. Also, these lenses can be fitted with a spheric lens of up to 5 diopters of cylinder, which adds to the ease of fitting.

The soft lens, however, is still the most comfortable lens, being flaccid, thin, and hydrated. It is more complicated than a gas-permeable spheric lens in that the fitter must contend with a system that requires a toric lens. The rigid gas-permeable lens offers better crispness of vision if the toricity is great or is found in an oblique axis. The best part of it is that a spheric lens can be used to handle most astigmatic corrections. When dealing with astigmatism that has to be corrected with a contact lens, the fitter should think first of a good gas-permeable lens and then of a soft toric lens.

CORRECTING ASTIGMATISM WITH BITORIC LENSES

A bitoric lens is used to fit a toric cornea when a spheric lens or a back-surface toric lens has been tried and found to be inadequate. It is usually required in any cornea if the toricity exceeds 4.00 D of astigmatism with the rule or 2.00 D of astigmatism against the rule. The spheric lens may center poorly and rock or cause poor acuity. For example, if the astigmatism is against the rule, the lens will rotate along the vertical meridian and slide either temporally or nasally. Such a lens will irritate the eye and will not be tolerated for full-time wear. A toric arc of touch is characteristic of the fluorescein pattern. Its prime purpose is to correct a physical disturbance in the cornea and not to remedy a refractive error.

A bitoric lens has cylinder correction on both the front and back surface. The back-surface cylinder is in relation to the toric shape of the cornea. The front-surface cylinder is used to correct the residual refractive error or the added astigmatism induced by the posterior cylindric correction. A toric, peripheral curve lens may provide the stability and centration for a spheric lens and should be considered before one uses back-surface toric lenses.

Occasionally a bitoric lens is needed when a prism-ballast, front-surface, cylindric lens is tried to correct residual astigmastism and the lens fails to center.

Fitting a bitoric lens (one-fourth practice)

Base curve. The lens is usually fitted as a back toric in the principle meridians. The flattest meridian is made steeper by one-fourth of the cylinder and the steeper one is made flatter by one-fourth of the cylinder. This is the rule of one-fourths.

Diameter. These lenses are generally made larger than 8.5 mm to avoid flare. The optic zone is generally 1 mm less in dimension. Some leeway in diameter size can be considered on the basis of normal factors such as corneal diameter, palpebral fissure size, and K readings.

Power. The power of a toric surface in plastic is considerably higher than an identical amount of toricity of the cornea because of the higher index of refraction of plastic. The power, measured in air, of a lens cylinder is approximately 1.45 times the cylindric power of a cornea of the same toricity. For example:

℞ −2.00 D −4.00 D × 180 = 41.00 D × 180/45.00 D × 90. If the full 4.00 D of cylinder were generated in a back toric lens, its power would be −5.81 in air at 180 degrees, which is −1.810 D of excessive cylinder. This requires a correction with a +1.81 D outside cylinder × 180.

The induced cylinder is independent of the corneal cylinder and is related to the outside toricity of the lens only.

$$n' - n: \frac{\text{Plastic} - \text{Air}}{\text{Tears} - \text{Air}} = \frac{1.49 - 1.00}{1.3375 - 1.00}$$
$$= \frac{0.49}{0.3375} = 1.4519$$

The induced cylinder is therefore 45% of the inside cylinder, when the inside cylinder is expressed in K diopters as usual (if the inside cylinder is expressed in millimeters the induced cylinder is 31%).

A simple method to arrive at the correct power is to trial-fit the patient with toric base curve, spheric, front-surface lenses. An over-refraction is done, and the added cylinder is simply put on the front surface of the lens.

The determination of the outside cylinder required (or, for that matter, whether an inside toric or bitoric is required) should be calculated by a competent laboratory because most practitioners do not have an understanding of the optics involved. The way it may be done is as follows:

Determine the predicted residual astigmatism or, for even greater accuracy, have the practitioner refract over a *rigid*, well-centered, spheric lens.

It should be evident that for the special case where the outside cylinder used is equal to and corrects all of the induced cylinder the power of the cylinder in air of this lens is equal to the K dioptric power of the inside cylinder. To illustrate, take the 4.00 D inside toric lens, which has a cylinder power in air of -5.81 D $\times$ 180. By placement of a $+1.81$ D front-surface cylinder on this lens D, the power in air now becomes -4.00 D cylinder $\times$ 180, and all of the induced cylinder is corrected.

A bitoric lens is difficult to manufacture accurately. Office modifications require great skill to avoid removing the peripheral toricity. The cost of these lenses is high, and they are difficult to reproduce for replacement. Frequently there is a power difference between the two toric surfaces, causing residual astigmatism. Move with caution and be sure that both you and the laboratory are capable of handling a bitoric lens before recommending one to a patient.

USE OF GAS-PERMEABLE RIGID LENSES

Gas-permeable rigid lenses include cellulose acetate butryate, silicone-acrylate, silicone resins, styrene, and fluorosilicone acrylate. There has been a dramatic increase in the use of gas-permeable lenses. With their use has come increased safety for the cornea, increased comfort, and better visual performance for the wearer. This has been discussed previously. Newer types of polymers with higher gas-permeability than before have entered the field. This change has

resulted in a dramatically wider use of the gas-permeable rigid lenses for correcting astigmatism.

Of more importance has been the increased size, which can be tolerated. This has enabled the fitter to use these lenses for the correction of astigmatism. The average diameter for non-toric spheric lenses should be 9.2 mm $\pm$ 0.2 mm. These lenses can be used in much greater diameter for larger corneal toricity. Even a 10, 11, or 12 mm gas-permeable lens may be required for corneal toricity greater than 5 diopters. These lenses are particularly useful for aphakic corneas and for distorted corneas with irregular astigmatism. The larger lenses permit better centration and vaulting over the corneal toricity. In addition to an increase in size, the gas-permeable lenses can be fitted flatter than PMMA lenses without induction of corneal hypoxia.

Tips for fitting gas-permeable lenses for astigmatism

1. A spheric trial set is needed for assessment of the fitting characteristics of the lens. Some fitters make up the trial sets in PMMA material because not only are they more durable but they also do not require any conditioning effect by solutions like some gas-permeable materials do. However, the most accurate trial set is one that is made of the same material as the lens that is to be ordered.

2. Because these gas-permeable lenses have a large diameter and their refractive power or cylinder correction may be large, attention must be given to the edges of the lens to ensure comfort. A high-minus lens should have a plus profile and a high-plus lens a myopic profile.

3. Fit first with spheric gas-permeable lenses. Our studies indicated that over 90% of cylinder may be corrected with a spheric ridge lens, which is the simplest type of lens to fit.

4. With high cylinders, one should have some thickness increase to the lens to prevent flexure of the steepest corneal meridian. Our rule of thumb is to add 0.01 mm extra thickness for every 1 to 2 diopters of cylinder to be corrected.

When the corneal toricity is 3 D or greater, a toric surface is ground on the back

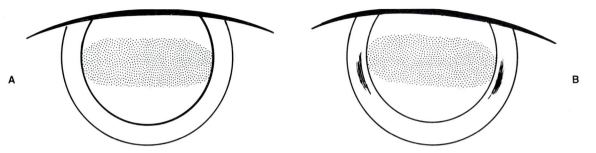

Fig 29-6 ■ **A,** With-the-rule astigmatism, which creates a flatter horizontal meridian in which the lens may decenter vertically. **B,** During blinking the lens may cause compression on the flatter horizontal meridian and may result in epithelial erosion (arcuate) at the 3 and 9 o'clock position.

surface of the contact lens so that the best surface of the lens is in alignment with the toric surface of the cornea.

Bitoric lenses are used for large amounts of corneal and residual astigmatism or if the back toric lens causes induced astigmatism. When cylinder is added to correct corneal toricity, it causes an excessive cylinder power effect because the index of refraction of plastic is greater than that of tears, which results in induced astigmatism.

Front toric lenses should be chosen when there is no corneal astigmatism but significant lenticular astigmatism. Stability is usually maintained by truncation and prism ballast.

5. If centering is a problem with the trial lens, one should go to a larger-diameter lens as first choice.

6. In with-the-rule astigmatism, one may develop vertical decentration because the lens rocks on the flatter meridian (Fig. 29-6, A). The rocking may cause corneal epithelial erosion at the 3 and 9 o'clock positions (Fig. 29-6, B). This problem may require a larger lens, and the lens must have perfect blend and thin edges.

7. Against-the-rule astigmatism may cause side-to-side decentration because of rocking on the vertical flatter meridian (Fig. 29-7). Also, with each blink corneal erosions may develop at the 6 o'clock position because the edge of the lens indents on the flatter part of the cornea inferiorly. This problem may require a larger lens or a steeper lens.

8. One should use a toric trial set if standard spheric lenses cannot be fitted. One is often surprised that a lesser degree of toricity is required than would be expected. One may have 5 diopters of corneal astigmatism as

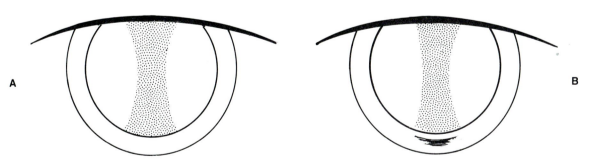

Fig 29-7 ■ **A,** Against-the-rule astigmatism, which creates a flatter vertical meridian in which the contact lens may decenter side to side. **B,** During blinking the lens may cause compression on the flatter vertical meridian and may result in epithelial erosion (arcuate) at the 6 o'clock position.

determined by K readings but only require a 3-diopter toric lens.

9. A gas-permeable lens does not function optimally unless it rides high. Low-lying lenses create discomfort because of lid impact, cause 3 to 9 o'clock staining with marginal episcleritis, and create variable vision. Because the diameters of these lenses must be large, the high-rising interblink position can only be achieved when one fits these lenses somewhat flatter and pays special attention to the edges of the lens and to the thickness so that the lids will lift the lens instead of pushing it down.

10. The gas-permeable lenses of larger refractive power and large diameter may ride low because the lenses are likely to be heavy. This means that the lenses may not function optimally, as in (9).

COMMENTS. In a retrospective analysis of correcting astigmatic errors over 1.25 D, we used the percentage of lenses as shown in the following:

Retrospective fitting analysis of cylinder > 1.25 D (869 eyes)

Soft lenses	
Spheric	30%
Toric	19%
Rigid lenses	
Spheric	48%
Toric	3%

In most cases a spheric or aspheric gas-permeable rigid lens will work to correct astigmatism and only rarely do we have to use a front, back surface toric lens or a bitoric lens.

Gas-permeable rigid lenses are preferred for clarity of vision and ease of fitting for toric corneas. They are preferred for large errors of cylinder over 4 diopters. Soft toric lenses, on the other hand, may be used for comfort and for residual astigmatism.

The lastest aspheric designs (spherical optic/aspheric periphery and bi-aspherics) may increase the use of RGP as a first-choice modality over soft torics because of their high comfort level and functional performance superiority.

30 ▪ *FITTING THE PRESBYOPE BIFOCAL CONTACT LENSES: RIGID AND SOFT*

Today, many contact lens wearers are reaching the age at which their eyes begin to lose the powers of accommodation. Those who are myopic and wear contact lenses begin to lose this ability at a younger age than the average hyperope. Added to this large group of potential presbyopes are the more than 70 million presbyopes who are over the age of 40. Each year, three to four million people become candidates for presbyopic correction, and more than half of the vision care population is presbyopic. Only about 2% of presbyopes wear contact lenses, although as more contact lens wearers become presbyopic this number will increase. The most important requirement for the successful correction of presbyopia with contact lenses is patient motivation. The success rate among motivated patients is well above 50% and, in the proper circumstances, may be as high as 70%.

SCREENING PATIENTS FOR PRESBYOPIC CORRECTION

The screening of patients who are suitable for presbyopic correction is the key to success. Those who are most likely to respond to presbyopic correction are those

1. who are highly motivated

2. who have an adequate tear film
3. whose jobs are not highly visual
4. who have no lid disease or abnormality
5. who have low hyperopia, and
6. affluent individuals who can afford the high costs involved.

Those who may not be successful are those with

1. any external ocular disease or abnormality
2. patients whose schedules are so busy that they cannot return for necessary check-ups and the small refinements that are required after the initial fitting
3. the high myope
4. dry-eye patients
5. those who have been fitted unsuccessfully once or twice before
6. patients with high astigmatism
7. ametropes whose vision at distance is somewhat compromised by contact lenses

There are a number of ways to fit the presbyope with contact lenses (see box). Fitting single-vision distance contact lenses and prescribing reading glasses, either full- or half-frames to

---

■

METHODS OF FITTING A PRESBYOPIC PATIENT

1. Reading glasses over contact lenses
2. Monovision
3. Bifocal contact lenses
   a) segmental bifocals
   b) annular bifocals
   c) aspheric bifocals
   d) central add bifocals
   e) diffraction bifocals
4. Modified monovision

be worn over the contact lenses is probably the method most commonly used today and it satisfies the needs of most presbyopes. This method, however, does not satisfy individuals who want to stop wearing spectacles altogether.

MONOVISION FITTING OF CONTACT LENSES

When monovision contact lenses are prescribed, one eye is predominantly fitted for distance vision while the other eye is predominantly fitted for reading. Monovision contact lenses offer numerous advantages: they provide a wider peripheral field of vision than do bifocal lenses; they provide acceptable distance and near vision; they provide comfortable vision; they offer extended-wear capabilities; and they are more convenient, simple to fit, and less expensive than bifocal contact lenses. The disadvantages of monovision contact lenses are that an adaptation period is required and headaches are common. Also, since night driving is difficult, patients may require driving glasses which frequently cause eye fatigue. Stereopsis studies on monovision patients and those who have the loss of depth perception have not yielded conclusive results. Some authors deny any fusion, while others say there is a reasonable degree of fusion. There is a strong individual patient variation but clinically patients do not appear to lose depth perception. However, one must take into account the patient's occupational requirement for stereopsis or the need for exacting near vision. Monovision lenses are our preference for correcting presbyopia when the patient's prescription is low or when the patient has some astigmatism.

Based on our experiences in fitting monovision lenses, we feel that the nondominant eye is not necessarily the one that should be fitted for near vision. We use the swinging plus test, in which a +1.5 D lens is held over one eye and then over the other. The eye that is the most comfortable with the +1.5 D sphere is fitted for near vision.

For hyperopia, while placing the add lens in one eye, we overplus the distance vision eye by a small amount to try to balance both eyes more effectively for near vision. This lessens the refractive disparity between the two eyes. Similarly, for myopia we undercorrect both eyes while placing the addition in one eye.

A consistent, reliable, effective rigid bifocal contact lens has not yet become a reality. The newer gas-permeable lenses, however, are of help in fabricating an adequate bifocal rigid lens. Higher-DK lenses will have a larger optic zone for distance and near vision, so that the shift in vision will be more readily accomplished. Also the permeability features may allow stabilizing devices such as prisms to be more readily tolerated. A strong desire to wear contact lenses is especially important for the patient who is a first-time lens wearer.

The soft bifocal lens has also made its way on the scene. Although not perfect, it eliminates the problem of discomfort for the middle-aged novice presbyopic patient. It is important to appreciate that, from a clinical point of view, the fitting of a bifocal lens may be an exercise in futility. Some fitters do better than others with bifocal lenses largely because of their expertise, enthusiasm, and motivation.

Every fitter has been confronted with patients who have worn rigid contact lenses for 20 years or more and who have become presbyopic. These people need contact lenses for general vision and are not happy using reading glasses. So despite the imperfections in the systems available for total contact lens application for distance and near vision, it is necessary to deal with the subject, like it or not. So it is important that the fitter learn bifocal fitting techniques.

Monocular over-correction with plus power

Over-correction is often a successful technique, especially in previous rigid-lens wearers who have become presbyopic. Despite a difference of 1.50 to 2.00 D between the lenses, there is sufficient vision in both areas to maintain binocularity. One eye sees well in the distance, whereas the other functions primarily in the near range. Over-correction is simple to implement, but about 20% of patients complain of headaches, disorientation, and lack of visual clarity.

Because of the great simplicity of fitting, this lens is what we first use for fitting persons with presbyopia. One can use trial lenses, which are not really practical for bifocal lens wearers. It is wise to choose the least myopic or the more hyperopic eye for the near correction. If the refraction is the same in both eyes, overplussing should be done on the non-dominant eye.

COMMENT. Baldone refers to this type of vision

as "Omni Vision". For the target shooter or Olympic shooter who has become presbyopic it is important that the dominant eye be over-plussed so that the front of the rifle, the sighting portion, is in sharp focus while the target may be slightly blurred.

BIFOCAL CONTACT LENSES

Although bifocal contact lenses have been available for the past 35 years, many fitters have shied away from advocating them because of the chair time that may be required and the number of disappointed patients.

However, today several newer types of rigid and soft bifocal lenses are available. There are two basic designs: one that permits *alternating vision* and one that permits *simultaneous vision*. The design of alternating vision contact lenses is similar to that of bifocal spectacles. With these lenses, the wearer uses one portion of the lens for distance vision and another portion for near vision, making it essential that the lens move well on the eye. As the eye moves down to read, the lower eyelid moves the contact lens up, so that the reading segment lies in the pupillary area (Fig. 30-1). We instruct patients to blink on downward gaze just before reading. This dislodges the lens and moves it to a position suitable for reading. Truncation, prism ballast, or a combination of these two methods stabilize the lens against rotation (Fig. 30-2). We have found that the truncated portion is uncomfortable in rigid lenses.

Simultaneous vision occurs when both fields of vision, distant and near, are focused on the retina but the individual learns to ignore one field and concentrate on the other.

The same variation in designs is available in soft lenses. In this situation these are all built into the finished product and there is no opportunity for the fitter to make any modifications. Lenses like the Bausch & Lomb PAI (seg-

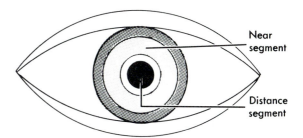

Fig 30-1 ■ Annular bifocal lens. The near segment is pushed up by the lower lid.

mental type), the Ciba Bisoft (annular type), the Hydrocurve aspheric lens and the Alges central addition bifocal are representative of their type.

Patient selection for bifocal lenses

1. Patients who are difficult to fit should be avoided if possible. This includes people with lax or low lids because of the lack of support of the heavier bifocal segment, those who are poorly motivated, and those with severe or residual astigmatism.
2. Persons with hyperopia do better than those with myopia. Hyperopic patients need less bifocal addition than persons with myopia of equal power. A minus lens requires more prism ballast than a plus lens does.
3. Patients who require bifocals for both distance and near range are preferred over patients who primarily need reading glasses. A previous single-vision lens wearer is also a good candidate.

Of prime consideration are the present refraction and the type of work required to be done by the patient. *Ideally:*

1. The addition required should be between +1.00 and +1.75 D.
2. The spheric-equivalent addition should be between −4.00 and +2.00 D with the minus

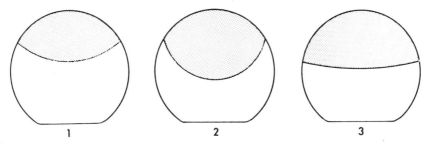

Fig 30-2 ■ Segmented bifocal contact lens with rotation prevented by truncation.

cylinder deleted, not being greater than 1 D.
3. The patient should understand the limitations of the bifocal system and still be motivated to want bifocal lenses, because for very small print and reading in poor lighting a reading glass may still be required. To eliminate "readers" entirely, overplus one eye, perhaps up to +0.75 D.

Fitting procedure

One obtains the distance correction by using the spheric equivalent and adding −0.50 D to this power; for example, a −3.00 D lens would require a −3.50 D lens as the initial selection of power. An over-refraction is done to achieve the best vision.

Near vision is estimated with the appropriate lens, that is, −2.50 D. In other words, using the above example, choose the addition that requires the smallest prescription commensurate with normal reading requirements. If this lens does not satisfy the near visual needs of the patient, additional plus power is added. The maximum amount of plus power to be added is the power that does not affect the distance vision. If vision is barely adequate, +0.75 D can be added to the nondominant eye. This technique borrows from the monovision device to achieve satisfactory vision.

Problems in fitting

The problems that can occur with bifocal lenses are ghosting, doubling, haloes, poor visual acuity, some distortion on gaze to the right or left, and troubles caused by the effects of changes in ambient light. Some of the causes of poor near vision and ghosting are outlined in the boxes on this page.

Decentration of the central zone will usually cause fluctuating vision or ghosting. The lenses can be made larger or tighter if this occurs. One can stabilize lathe-cut lenses by adding truncation and prism. Spin-cast lenses are stabilized with an aspheric posterior surface.

Fluctuating vision can be attributable to excess lens movements. These lenses should not move more than 0.5 to 1.5 mm.

Hyperopes require less power addition than myopes to achieve the same results. Also patients will not tolerate more than 0.50 D of uncorrected cylinder at near range. These restraints of optic correction should be appreciated before one fits such a lens.

CAUSES OF POOR NEAR VISION

Excessive lens movement
Incorrect segment height
Improper blinking
Lens too flat or steep
Residual cylinder
Lack of pupil constriction at near
Reduced illumination

CAUSES OF GHOSTING OR DOUBLING

Excessive lens movement
Superior riding lens
Improper central optical zone for pupil size
Too much rotation of segment
Too flat or steep
Poor segment blending
Residual cylinder

CAUSES OF POOR DISTANT VISION WITH BIFOCAL

Wrong power
Incorrect segment height
Large pupil with small optical zone
Small pupil with central add

Patients with low lower lids do poorly on those lenses with truncation and require the lower lids to push up the lenses with reading.

The spin-cast bifocal lens is designed so that there is a gradual increase in power of the lens. But both the distance and reading portions lie within the pupillary diameter permanently. This position produces two images all the time, one from each part of the lens. The patient soon learns to disregard the more out-of-focus lens. This lens requires minimal movement and so has to fit relatively tightly. The simultaneous-vision lens requires maximum correction to achieve adequate power. Simultaneous-vision lenses function best on patients with large pupils. Elderly patients and glaucomatous patients on miotic drugs do poorly.

COMMENT. The best candidates for these lenses are people who have worn soft lenses for distance in the past. Persons, such as architects, with occupations that require sharp acuity may not have sufficient clarity through soft bifocal lenses.

Our best success is using the soft bifocal lens and overplussing the more hyperopic eye, or the nondominant eye. With good patient selection, successful results were obtained in approximately 65% of cases. By success, we mean that the patients were satisfied with their vision through these lenses. It does not imply 20/20 vision in each eye for both distance and near range. Also we took our sample 1 year after the bifocal lens was worn.

In our review of 100 cases, only previous lens-wearers were selected, with 100 patients having soft lenses, and 100 patients having rigid lenses. The results were about the same.

The use of the lathe-cut bifocal lens is hampered by the prism, which can cause the lens to be quite thick at the base. This design can create discomfort. Also, if the line of truncation is not contoured to the lower lid, rotation of the lens will occur when the eyes look down.

So far, our best results have been with two lens types (a) the aspheric variable-focus design in which there is a power change from the lens center to the lens periphery and (b) the Alges central add bifocal. The optic principle is that the pupil changes its position relative to the lens center on down gaze into a greater plus zone.

Finally, required additions of +2.00 D or greater in myopic patients do not have a good success-performance ratio. It is better to exclude these people from consideration.

COMMENT. Better results are obtained with the newer rigid gas-permeable lenses than with PMMA. The size of the optic zone for distance and near range can be made larger. With soft lenses, durability is often a problem because these lenses become more quickly coated in an older person than a lens on an eye that is 20 years younger. In all probability the increased incidence of deposit formation in the middle-aged person is related to increased vicosity of and changes in the tear film. Perhaps increased lipids in the blood stream, dryness of the eye, and diet play a role.

TYPES OF BIFOCAL CONTACT LENSES
Annular bifocal lens

This lens is designed with the distance power ground into the center portion and the near power ground into the periphery of the lens. The power of the lens may be incorporated into the front or back surface. Vision may be simultaneous with the eye seeing clearly at distance and out of focus at near range or alternating with the lens designed to shift its position if sight is directed from distance to near range (see Fig. 30-1).

This lens is not popular in rigid form. Using the principle alternative vision, the patient always experiences one out-of-focus image. With this method of using the bifocal lens there is difficulty in producing a lens that moves up adequately for clear near viewing. This lens is pupillary-dependent and dependent on lighting conditions.

COMMENT. When annular bifocals are worn, ghosting and blurring for distance is not uncommon. These lenses, however, are easier to fit and very comfortable when made of the soft-lens material. They provide good near vision.

Segmental bifocals

Prism-ballast bifocal lens. This bifocal lens is stabilized in one of two ways: (1) it is made so that the lower portion is heavier and wider than the upper, or (2) the bifocal segment is made in the form of a prism by fusion of an insert on the distance lens or by grinding of the segment on the front surface of the lens.

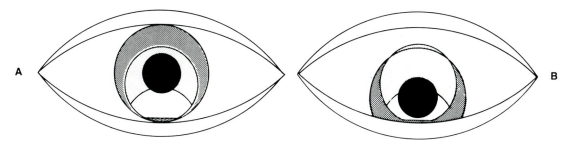

Fig 30-3 ■ **A,** Camp bifocal lens. The bifocal segment is pushed up, **B,** for reading.

Specifications for annular bifocal lens	Specifications for fused bifocal lens

Front surface
    Diameter: 9mm
Bifocal addition
    Base curve: fit on K to allow movement
    Optic zone: 3.5 mm—relative to pupillary size for distance power only
Back surface
    Diameter: 8.5 to 10.5 mm
Bifocal addition (de Carle)
    Base curve: tight fit—0.50 D steeper than K
    Optic zone: smaller than pupillary zone; approximately 3 mm size
	Bifocal segment: 6.5 mm
	Diameter: 8.5 to 9.5 mm
	Prism ballast: 1.5Δ
	Segment height: fitted 1 mm higher than the pupillary margin for plus lenses and 1 mm lower for minus lenses
	Truncation: 0.4 to 0.5 mm

The segment may be fused into an insert on the distance lens. The added power is derived from the fused segment having a higher index of refraction than the upper portion of the lens.

Fused segment bifocal lens. The fused bifocal lens (Fig. 30-3) is thinner, with a sharp division between distance and near vision and with a front surface free for a cylinder correction. The functional area of the fused segment is frequently of poor quality and becomes an area of optic distortion (Fig. 30-4).

The one-piece monocentric bifocal lens in which the segment has been ground on the front surface of the lens has the advantage of a segment selection and no image jump (Fig 30-5). The bifocal addition can be shaped to suit any purpose.

Generally, if someone has been wearing distance correction, we order a lens 0.2 mm larger in diameter and specify that the segment be 4.0 mm in height. It is, however, better to have a fitting set to verify.

The *Tangent Streak*™ bifocal is a fused bifocal with a very large reading segment. The lens is prism ballasted. It is custom made and available with variable segment heights and a variable optic zone. It is manufactured in high-DK rigid gas-permeable material with a DK of 70. This lens is a "no-jump" bifocal with a smooth junctional zone and a large distance and reading area. The lens is designed so the reading addition is 1.3 mm below the visual axis and it requires slightly more prism ballast in the RGP material than PMMA lenses. Table 30-1 presents some of the parameters currently available. Fitting is performed with a base curve that is usually 0.50 to 0.75 flatter than K to permit good movement. One should measure the corneal diameter, which should range from 10.5 mm to 12.5 mm and make the lens about 2 mm less than this. The lens should lie about 1.3 mm below the visual axis. These lenses are currently available

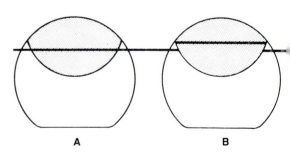

A   **B**

Fig 30-5 ■ Monocentric bifocal lens. Each lens is calculated so that no image jump occurs along the segment line. It is a one-piece lens, truncated at the bottom. If a bifocal lens is not monocentric, a line seen through the lens will be displaced as in **B**.

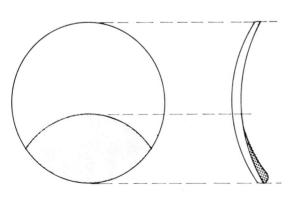

Fig 30-4 ■ Camp fused bifocal lens.

Table 30-1 ■ Tangent Streak℠
parameter ranges*

Distance power	+12.00 to −20.00 diopters
Base curve	6.50 mm. to 8.50 mm.
Horizontal lens size	8.0 mm. to 10.50 mm.
Add power	+0.75 to +3.50 diopters
Prism	1.75 to 4.00 prism diopters
Centers thickness	

*Courtesy Fused Contact Lens Corp, Chicago, Ill.

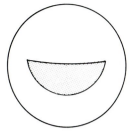

Fig 30-6 ■ Crescent (Black) bifocal lens.

in Fluorex-700 DK material, which wets well and is stable.

One-piece bifocal lenses

CRESCENT BIFOCAL (BLACK) LENS (Fig. 30-6). The crescent bifocal (Black) lens is a crescent-shaped bifocal lens with the flat surface on the top. This lens offers minimal image jump as compared to the round-top bifocal lens. It is necessary to fit the segment so that it is in the lower pupillary border, since it induces diplopia if it is above or below it.

MONOCENTRIC BIFOCAL (MANDELL) LENS (Fig. 30-7). The monocentric design of this lens eliminates image jump because the distance and near vision sections lie in the same focal plane. The top of the bifocal segment should be slightly higher than the lower margin of the pupil.

COMMENT. The monocentric bifocal lens does not have a prism on the lens blank. It is ground on the front surface. The absence of a prism in the basic segment eliminates such visual problems as monocular diplopia and ghost images. Its concave shape affords a wider range for near viewing (see Fig. 30-2). It is superior to the fused bifocal lens because of its better optic properties and wider field of near vision.

TRUNCATION. Truncation serves to provide a flat edge for better contact with the lid and reduces overall lens weight (Fig. 30-8).

The truncation should be flat with rounded corners and tapered evenly on both surfaces. The bevel is usually 0.4 to 0.5 mm in diameter. The truncated edge should remain on the lower lid as the eyes shift down. With the lenses on the lower lid the upper pole of the lens should not override the upper limbus. Adding truncation has the same effect as adding more prism ballast: it adds stability to the lens and stops rotation.

Difficulties with near vision with segmented bifocal lenses. The principle of the segmented bifocal is that the reading segment moves up when the patient looks down to read. (Fig. 30-9). If the lens is too tight, it may not shift upward in the reading position. With the patient looking straight ahead, the lens should be lifted up 1 to 2 mm in the blink and then dropped back to a lower position. A lens that fits too tightly may be improved if one flattens the peripheral curve, reduces the diameter, or flattens the base curve.

If the lens drops too low (Fig. 30-10), one may solve this problem by broadening the truncation area, increasing the base curve of the lens, or decreasing the prism by 0.50 D.

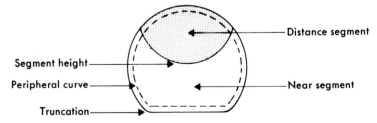

Fig 30-7 ■ Monocentric (Mandell) bifocal lens. The advantage of this lens design is that the entire pupil is covered by the bifocal segment as the lower lid pushes the lens upward during the act of reading.

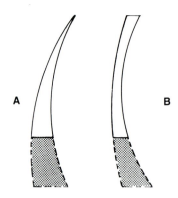

Fig 30-8 ■ Truncation provides lens support, reduction in lens weight, and a wide edge of contact to engage the lid. The effect of truncation depends on the refractive error. It adds ballast on a plus lens, **A,** and reduces ballast on a minus lens, **B.**

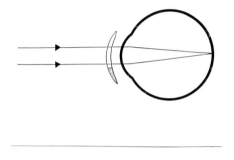

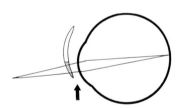

Fig 30-9 ■ Translation of a segmented bifocal contact lens. (From Stein HA, Slatt BJ, and Stein RM: Ophthalmic assistant, ed 5, St Louis, 1988, The CV Mosby Co.)

If the vertical diameter is too great, the lens will not be able to move up with reading (Fig. 30-11). The solution for this problem is to reduce the lens diameter.

Specifications for monocentric bifocal (Mandell) lens

Monocentric diameter: 9 to 10.5 mm
Optic zone: 1.2 mm less than diameter
Prism ballast: 1.5Δ
Truncation: 0.4 to 0.5 mm

Insufficient height of the reading segment to cover the pupil for all positions of gaze inferiorly can be solved when the height of the segment is increased. Irvin Borish describes a method of coloring the bottom portion of a trial lens to determine the effect of segment height on a person's activity or vocation.

If the distance vision is impaired, this problem may indicate that the bifocal segment height is too high (Figs. 30-12 and 30-13). It can be solved in two ways: one can prescribe a new lens with a lower segment height or reduce the diameter of the lens, especially at the truncated edge. It may also indicate that the lens is too tight and is not positioning low enough. Reducing the diameter of the lens, flattening the peripheral curve, or adding 0.50 D more prism will solve this problem. Achieving suitable power requires over-refraction for distance.

ASPHERIC LENSES

A third type of bifocal contact lens is the aspheric design, which provides simultaneous vision by allowing the lens wearer to select preferential rays from either distant objects or near. This is a progressive—addition type of lens, formed with alterations in the anterior and posterior curvature of the lens. Aspheric lenses create retinal images from different points on the

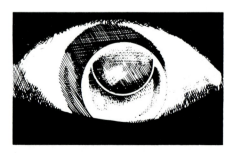

Fig 30-10 ■ Bifocal lens is decentered. The lens is too small.

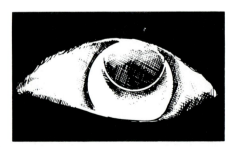

Fig 30-11 ■ Bifocal lens. The diameter of this lens is too large—the lens touches the upper lid.

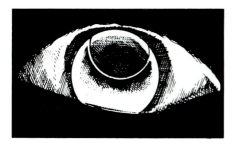

Fig 30-12 ■ Bifocal segment too high.

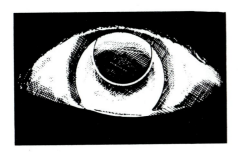

Fig 30-13 ■ Bifocal segment correct height.

lens. Because of this, the power can be uniformly increased in the periphery by the degree of asphericity. Modern technology with automated lathes has permitted great refinement of this lens type during the past few years.

The multifocal rigid lens is an aspheric, variable-focus, corneal lens that provides clear distance and near vision. It has no segments or prisms. The power of the lens increases from the central area of the lens to the periphery. This produces an increase in plus power toward the edge of the lens. The central rays from a distant object are focused on the retina, whereas the paraxial rays are focused in front of the retina. To achieve a +2.00 D effect for reading, the posterior aspheric base must flatten approximately 6.00 D within the pupillary area.

Spheric aberration is greatly increased by the shorter focal length toward the periphery provided by an aspherically based multifocal lens. This increase in spheric aberration reduces the effective aperture and increases the depth of focus of the lens. The base curve is aspheric but should be fitted steeper than the flattest corneal curvature by 0.35 mm. The front surface is spheric.

This lens can be fitted using diagnostic lenses. The advantage of aspheric lenses is their thinness and the fact that they do not require any specific orientation. However, these lenses must be precisely centered, which often means a tight fit and possible physiologic compromise of the cornea.

How to fit

1. Select a diagnostic lens 0.30 mm steeper than the flattest radius of corneal curvature. For example:

   42.75 D Flatter corneal curvature
   7.89 mm Diameter value
   −0.30 D Subtracted variable
   7.59 mm Adjusted value
   7.6 mm Diagnostic lens selected

2. Make sure that the lens centers well with a minimum of movement—1 to 2 mm.
3. Over-refract through the trial lens to obtain the best distance correction. Initially the patient may report that the vision is blurry and that a short rest period is frequently needed to adapt to the lenses.
4. Instruct the patient to look at a near-vision card. Add 0.25 D at a time until the print J_2 can be read. Do not overplus the patient; doing so can be quite easy. The best guard against this problem is to have the patient look alternately at the distance chart to ensure that vision at 20 feet still remains clear.

   The final power should be
   −4.50 D—distance refraction
   +0.75 D—near over-refraction
   −3.75D—for total lens

5. If vision is blurred at near range, check the centration in the reading position. If the lens is displaced by the lid so that the patient is looking through the peripheral portions of the lens while reading, the acuity will be poor and variable. One can verify this displacement by determining whether the vision clears when the reading card is held at eye level. In such a case a steeper or larger lens might be used.

   Base curve. Because 55% of the lens rests on a paracentral position of the cornea, the degree of flattening of the cornea should be known. Because each cornea has a different topography and is even different from temporal to nasal sides, only an approximation value can be assigned to the peripheral contours of the cornea.

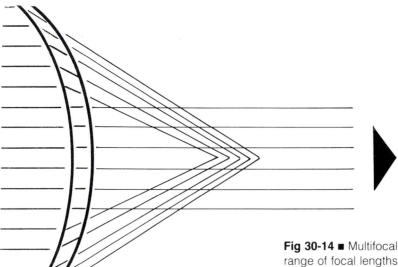

Fig 30-14 ■ Multifocal spectacle lens with a broad range of focal lengths.

K reading	Curve values of paracentral cornea (diopter flatter than K)
7.20 to 7.50	5.00 to 8.00 D
7.60 to 7.90	4.00 to 7.00 D
8.00 to 8.40	3.00 to 6.00 D

The optic section is generally 3 to 4 D steeper than K. To give an adequate range of reading, add 2.50 D or more. With an aspheric lens, the rest of the lens is in alignment with the paracentral cornea even though the optic zone is 4.00 D steeper.

Diameter. Most lenses are fitted with a diameter that averages 8.8 mm.

Power. The spheric power of the refraction is the base power. But an equal amount of minus must be added to the base reading to neutralize the amount of steepness over the flattest K.

Example. The base curve is −4.00 D steeper than K; add −4.00 D to the spheric power. If corneal astigmatism is present, one half of the corneal cylinder over 1.00 D should be added to K for better alignment.

Optic zone. There is a Catch-22 situation with the optic zone. If the optic zone is too small to engulf the pupil in dim illumination, the patient will suffer from flare and glare, that is, ghost images, stars around lights, and so on. However, if the optic zone is made too large, it rests on the flatter paracentral cornea and tight symptoms are produced, since this problem causes corneal edema. With an aspheric lens, there is no junction between the optic zone and the peripheral segment of the lens. Flare is not a problem, and so an 8.8 mm lens is sufficient to cover a 6 mm pupil, which is considered large.

The lens. The anterior surface is spheric. The posterior surface is both spheric in the range of the corneal cap and aspheric in the periphery. The geometric center of the lens houses the distance correction. As the lens begins to flatten

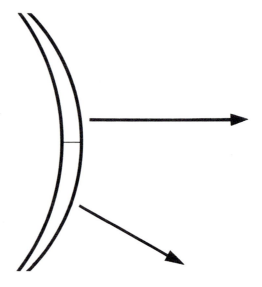

Fig 30-15 ■ Traditional bifocal lens with distance and near focal lengths.

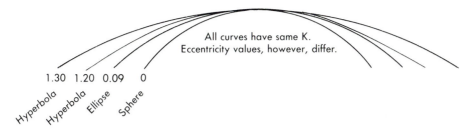

All curves have same K.
Eccentricity values, however, differ.

1.30   1.20   0.09   0
Hyperbola Hyperbola Ellipse Sphere

Fig 30-16 ■ Each curve has the same base curve. They differ only in the rate of flattening. An aspheric curve is determined by its central curvature and its **E** value, that is, peripheral curvature. Represented are a sphere, ellipse, and hyperbola.

(Figs. 30-14 and 30-15), 0.10 D extra power is added in a gradual fashion in 0.10 D gradients. The aspheric optic section has an individual focal zone. The gradual increase in power toward the periphery creates a smooth transition of power without image jumps. This effect can be measured in terms of eccentricity values.

Eccentricity values. This value of eccentricity is determined by the measurement of the rate of flattening of the curve in the distance. The value is measured with an optic spherometer (Radiuscope; Fig. 30-16). The following formula is applied:

$$\text{Eccentricity} = \frac{1 - \dfrac{TR}{MR}}{\sin \theta}$$

TR is the transmeridian radius.
MR is the meridian radius.
The angle theta (θ) is the tilt of the lens on the off-center reading.
This is measured on the Radiuscope-eccentroscope.

Measurements required for ordering a lens include K reading including the axis, spectacle prescription, spectacle addition, diameter of cornea, diameter of the pupil in dim illumination, and palpebral fissure.

Patient selection: Who to fit. Those patients least likely to succeed with bifocal contact lenses are:
1. Patients with flat spheric corneas
2. Patients with astigmatism greater than 2.00 D
3. New lens patients and previous contact lens failures
4. Patients with low distance refractive errors ±1.00 D
5. Patient with dry eyes
6. Patients with narrow palpebral fissures.

The best candidates for bifocal contact lenses are:
1. Those who were successful single-vision lens wearers
2. Those who are highly motivated and have a highly motivated fitter
3. Those who have an occupational need for bifocal contact lenses, such as waiters and people in the media (including films)
4. Those whose occupations have low visual demands
5. Those with pupils that do not demonstrate large variations in size with ambient light
6. Those whose lower eyelids are in the normal position.

COMMENT. The results of this lens system is not apparent at the first fitting. A vision of 20/30 to 20/40 may improve to 20/20 in 4 to 5 days. Changes in refraction and lens changes should not be made until refraction is stable over two visits. Patience is essential. Our studies indicate a success rate of over 64% (Table 30-2).

We recently collaborated with Dr. J. Josephson in a study using the Barnes-Hind Hydrocurve bifocal contact lens. This aspheric bifocal lens, which is designed with a center eccentricity (E) value of 1.3 (hyperbolic curve), reduces gradually from a parabola to an ellipse, and finally to an E value of 0 (spherical) in the periphery (see Fig. 30-16). Of the 34 presbyopic

Table 30-2 ■ Successful with aspheric bifocals

Aspheric bifocal	Total fits	Successful fits (>6 months)
B & L—PAI	75	55 (73%)
Hydrocurve	70	45 (64%)
VFL design RGP	35	26 (74%)

patients fitted with these lenses, 60% achieved success in wearing them.

Josephson et al also performed a study in which 10 presbyopic patients were fitted with monovision lenses and another 10 with aspheric bifocal lenses. At the end of a month, these two groups were reversed; that is, the subjects in each group were tried on the opposite lens system. These were highly motivated patients. What was surprising was that more than 80% preferred aspheric bifocal lenses, whereas only 20% were happier with monovision lenses.

The aspheric lens works, but only with lower adds; higher adds produce some distortion.

Special problems in fitting relevant to the aspheric bifocal lens. *Decentration of the lens* will cause blurred vision. This error can be fixed in routine ways. The lens base curve must tighten as the diameter of the lens is increased.

Poor vision at near range is usually caused by a lack of tear pooling. The central vault must be 3 to 4 D steeper than K. Optimum results are obtained in a lens with 2 to 4 mm of central pooling and a thin tear-bearing area peripherally. The tear film is best appreciated through a fluorescein test. A narrow bright-green pool at the very edge should be present to reveal a meniscus tear accumulation at the bevel.

With *variable vision*, the movement of the lens should be fast, not slow. A distance of 0.5 to 1.5 mm is ideal. With the soft lens only 1 mm of lens motion should be tolerated. Excessive movement is often caused by tear pooling. This is most evident on insertion of the lens. The lens must settle before it is assessed.

COMMENT. The VF-II Silicon lens has proved to be a reasonably good presbyopic lens for most of our patients. (VF means *variable focus*)

Central addition bifocal. A fourth type of bifocal lens, one with a central add, has been very popular in our experience. Currently, the Alges® bifocal contact lens is the leading name in this type of lens. Lenses with small central adds in diameters of 2.12 mm, 2.35 mm, and 2.55 mm are available. For the wearer, the effect of this type of lens is similar to seeing around a small posterior subcapsular cataract. The patient simultaneously uses the outer portion of the lens around the central add for distance vision and uses the central addition portion to focus for near vision. The induced miosis that occurs physiologically during reading and close work is an additional help in these activities. Changes in pupil size as a result of changes in ambient lighting can have a major effect on this type of lens (Fig. 30-17). If the pupil is normal, then the 2.35 mm optical zone is generally adequate, allowing the individual to see around the central addition portion of the lens. However, when the pupils are dilated or constricted in response to ambient lighting conditions, abnormal ghosting and blurring can occur. We are currently investigating use of the 2.55 mm optical zone central add, which appears to give excellent results. The Alges bifocal contact lens is made by a computer-driven lathe guided by a laser interferometer, a process that yields exquisitely reproducible lenses.

DIFFRACTION BIFOCAL CONTACT LENSES

The diffraction bifocal, first introduced by Pilkington Glass and called the Diffrax™ bifocal and later, Allergan, is made up of concentric rings with small facets, something like a prism that diffracts 50% of the light rays into a separate

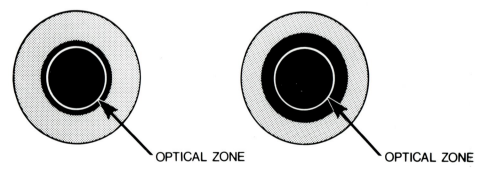

Fig 30-17 ■ Effects of ambient light by which the pupil becomes larger than the optical zone of the contact lens producing ghosting. (From Stein HA: Specialty contact lenses, CLAO J 13:5, September 1987.)

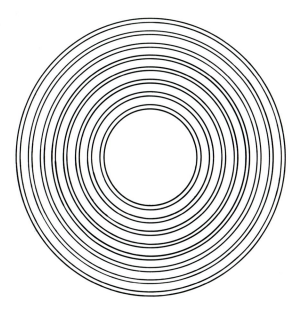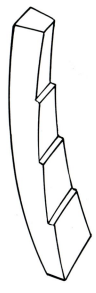

Fig 30-18 ■ The diffraction type of bifocal lenses provides simultaneous vision. The facet on the back surface diffracts some of the rays of light to a second focal point.

point (Fig. 30-18). The higher the addition required, the more the number of rings required.

The many prism-like facets are on the corneal side. They are smaller and finer than normal lathe marks and although they lie on the corneal side of the lens, they do not irritate or cause abrasions of the cornea.

Currently these lenses have been investigted by us from two sources:

1. Pilkington/Hydrocurve manufacture their Diffrax bifocal in a gas-permeable rigid material with diameters of 9.0 and 9.5 and a base curve of 7.2 to 8.4. Powers range from +5.00 D to −7.00 D. At present they are made in the Polycon II material with 0.07 thickness, with adds from +1.00 to +3.00 in steps of 0.5.
2. Allergan diffractive lens powers range from +4.00 to 6.00 D and a diameter of 13.8, with adds of +1.50 and +2.00. This is a soft HEMA material.

Both these lenses have had excellent results in our hands. The soft lens is more appealing with those who desire comfort. The rigid lens is more appealing for those who desire sharper vision. The lenses represent simultaneous vision in that the individual selects the area of regard that he prefers.

COMMENT. At the time of this writing, the diffraction principle seems to be a real improvement in bifocal design with ready patient acceptance. There is some ghosting with some patients and some debris accumulation in the little facets on the back surface; however, this does not appear to be a significant problem. On the introduction of this lens there was some concern that the facets on the back surface would irritate the cornea. This has not occurred in our experience. This lens is not pupil-size dependent. Because of this, perfect centration is not essential and greater lens movement and tear exchange is possible.

MODIFIED MONOVISION

We also use another system that we call *modified monovision* for patients who have tried bifocal contact lenses but who, for one reason or another, have had difficulty obtaining good distance or near acuity. In this system, one of the patient's bifocal lenses is replaced with a single-vision lens. Thus, one eye has a standard distance lens and the fellow eye has a bifocal lens.

SUMMARY

Bifocal success depends on
1. Screening carefully

2. Understanding the strengths of each lens system
3. Using these strengths to the best advantage
4. Good patient motivation and education

With this in mind, the motivation of the patient and the enthusiasm of the fitter is of utmost importance. The patient must return for visits to ensure optimal performance and the fitter must in turn be prepared to make changes in the lens to obtain maximum vision at both distance and near.

31 ▪ *SPECIAL USES FOR RIGID AND SOFT LENSES*

- X-CHROM lens
- Piggyback contact lens system
- Lenses for sports
- Nystagmus
- Contact lenses for children
- Orthokeratology
- Radial keratotomy

X-CHROM LENS

Persons with normal color vision can see all ranges in the spectrum of white light in wavelengths from 380 to 760 nm and can differentiate a wide range of hues of color ranging from red to blue. However, 8% to 10% of males and 0.5% of females have some impairment in color vision ranging from mild to almost complete impairment. This failure of differentiation is for the most part in the red-green area and to a much lesser extent in the blue-yellow area.

An X-CHROM corneal lens, which transmits light in the red zone from 590 to 700 nm, has recently been introduced. This lens can improve color discrimination for the individual who is partially blind in the red-green area. A red lens is fitted to the nondominant eye of a person with red-green partially defective vision. The other eye remains uncovered. The uncovered eye will perceive a red or green object as usual, but the eye with the red lens will perceive the red wavelengths of light and will absorb the green wavelengths. The brain now receives two different intensities; by a rapid self-learning process the patient can identify both colors properly.

The manufacturer claims that the person wearing a single X-CHROM lens can read the numbers in Ishihara's test and can identify traffic signals and color-coded wires and that the rapid self-learning process with the single red lens

permits the individual to perceive the world more vividly than ever before.

The American Committee on Optics and Visual Physiology has offered the following statement on the use of the X-CHROM lens:

A red tinted contact lens worn over one eye may help color defectives to discriminate colors by changing the relative intensities of red and green objects viewed through the filter. Examiners should measure color vision of each eye separately as well as together and compare the color test scores achieved with and without the use of the lens. In evaluating color vision qualifications, particular attention should be given to the ambient light levels under which the activity is carried out and the level of color recognition required by the task. Consideration must also be given to the detrimental effects of wearing such a lens on space localization of moving objects and other aspects of binocular vision. Persons operating moving vehicles wearing a tinted lens over one eye may experience hazardous distortions of the positions of perceived objects and may, therefore, be dangerous drivers in certain circumstances. Conservative judgments are justified until the extent of these hazards is better understood.

How to fit

The lens must be thin to permit adequate vision, must be large to avoid edge awareness (8.5 to 9.3 mm), and must center well. The lens should be fitted steeper than usual to achieve reduction in movement.

COMMENT. We have had some experience with this lens and it seems that the motivation to correct the color defect must be extremely high to overcome the cosmetic disadvantage of the person's appearance while a single red lens is worn. On the other hand, parents of children with color-defective vision should be made aware that congenitally inherited color defects of vision can be altered. If the child's vocational or avocational direction is toward a field requiring good color discrimination, such as marine navigation or aviation, this type of lens is available. We have fitted a few art-college students with this lens, which aids them with art work. Although it does not correct the color defect, it does permit them to make a discriminatory judgment of color. This lens also has value for electricians in detecting the color-coding of electrical wires.

PIGGYBACK CONTACT LENS SYSTEM

The piggyback lens is basically the wearing of a soft lens against the cornea to provide comfort and a rigid lens over the soft one to attain useful vision (Fig. 31-1). A standard soft lens is applied to make the new anterior surface of the lens-cornea combination have a smooth anterior spheric surface.

On the surface of the soft lens is placed a cone lens, which has a steep central posterior curvature surrounded by a much flatter peripheral zone. The steep zone is stabilized over the corneal cap and the flatter zone rests on the periphery of the lens.

In corneal grafts, the steep zone vaults over the astigmatic graft. A set of cone lenses is required to see which lens provides optimum clearance, centration, and movement. After the lens has been fitted, a manifest refraction is done over the selected diagnostic lens to determine the final power.

A lenticular soft lens with its high-plus power is used for the base lens whether the eye is aphakic or not. This provides compensation for the myopia induced by the steep-fitting cone lens and provides a better base for fitting.

In patient selection these lenses can be used for the following conditions:
1. Postoperative corneal keratoplasty
2. Aphakia
3. Keratoconus
4. Traumatic induced irregular astigmatism
   Problems with the system are as follows:
1. Inability to center the rigid lens
2. Inability to handle the combination of lenses
3. Confusion over rigid and soft cleaning and soaking solutions.

Two separate systems are required. The time and cost of two separate lenses may be a burden. Also the handling of two lens systems must be

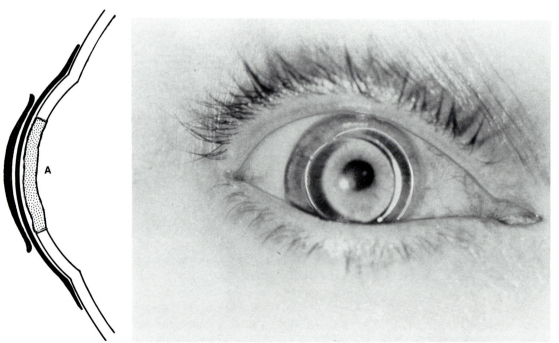

Fig 31-1 ■ **A,** Piggyback system of soft contact lens riding on a corneal transplant with a surface rigid lens to provide optical correction. **B,** Piggyback contact lens system with a gas-permeable lens resting on a larger soft lens.

taught, and so patient compliance must be exceptional.

Some laboratories will custom-create an anterior depression in the soft lens in order for the rigid lens to fit. This feature permits better centration because the rigid lens fits into the shallow depression of the soft lens.

COMMENT. This system, first introduced by Dr. Joe Baldone of New Orleans, should be used only as a last resort. It is applied to those patients who have been failures in wearing of rigid gas-permeable lenses and soft lenses.

Although the results are good in the majority of problem cases reported, the system is too cumbersome and expensive for routine use except in complicated cases. One really ends up with a mixture of soft and hard lens problems, plus the difficulty of having one lens ride over the other.

LENSES FOR SPORTS

Generally a soft lens is preferred for any contact athletics because of the danger of a lens being jolted out of the eye. So frequently has this happened that the National Basketball Association has passed a ruling that games cannot be stopped to look for a lens that accidentally pops out of a team member's eye.

Athletes, like everyone else, can have astigmatism and frequently need a rigid lens. A hockey player, such as a goalie, who is trying to follow a puck traveling 50 miles per hour needs the best vision attainable.

There are two ways to handle the problem. The rigid lens may be fitted steeper than K by 1.00 to 1.50 D so it fits tightly. This lens cannot be tolerated for full-time use because tight symptoms frequently develop after 4 or 5 hours of wear. Alternately the lens may be increased in diameter over its regular size by 2 mm. Additional peripheral curves must be added to reduce the apical vaulting produced by the larger-diameter size. An aspheric lens is a perfect choice for this situation. Its elliptic design ensures a good peripheral contour, and it comes in rather larger sizes—up to 10 mm.

COMMENT. If there is a high-degree of astigmatism, that is, 7 rather than 3 D, a gas-permeable lens of large diameter, 9.2 mm or more, is the lens of choice. A toric design may be required. Dynamic visual acuity, the ability to see clearly a moving target, is enhanced with rigid lenses in comparison to soft lenses.

Which lens to choose for sports

The rigid PMMA lens has been rendered virtually obsolete for sports by the gas-permeable lenses and the soft lenses. Gas-permeable lenses offer the following advantages:
1. They are larger than PMMA lens and so center better and are not easily displaced.
2. They are more comfortable.
3. They do not need to be specially designed for most sports.
4. They are less likely to cause photophobia because they move less and have a larger optic zone than PMMA lenses do.
5. They are better tolerated with fatigue.
6. They are more likely to be worn on a regular basis. If a contact lens is worn intermittently for sports, the player will always have to adjust to a size difference, which will affect his or her eye-hand coordination.
7. The optic characteristics of rigid gas-permeable lenses are excellent.

Soft lenses have other features:
1. They are best for body-contact sports because they move the least and are almost impossible to knock out.
2. They create the least photophobia.
3. They are the most comfortable lenses and can be worn full time.
4. They are always centered with eye movement. Their displacement is rarely more than 2 mm with a blink.
5. They are best in situations in which there is irritation to the eyes because of dust, wind, and sun because they cover the entire cornea and a few millimeters of the sclera. This feature makes them the lens of choice for soccer, football, tennis, rugby, cricket, lacrosse, and polo.

The major disadvantage of a soft lens is that the contrast sensitivity is not as good as that of PMMA or gas-permeable lenses.

Tennis

For tennis, a soft lens is preferred. In the service shot, the head and eyes go up to watch the ball. A soft lens has very little drag and drop. So centration and stability are maintained in the up position. With a rigid lens, the lens frequently drops as the eyes move up.

Also, a rigid lens is more likely to cause photophobia and glare. This problem is especially true on outdoor courts under a sunny sky. These effects can be ameliorated with sunglasses. However, tinted lenses reduce contrast, which in a moving game is essential. Dynamic visual acuity is largely predicated on contrast. Note that the professionals rarely use sunglasses during play even during day matches.

Squash and racquetball

It is important to remember that a contact lens does not provide any special safety over the naked eye. Eye protection is mandatory because the incidence of eye injuries is high, especially for the creation of a hyphema with severe damage. With the use of high-speed photography, ball speeds in racquetball have been reported at 78 mph for the novice and 127 mph for the A-level player. Professional squash and racquetball players move the racquet at speeds of 108 to 125 mph.

A lens 3 mm thick or a polycarbonate plano lens is best over the contact lens. Again a soft lens is preferred because of the dynamics of the serve and the high illumination from direct and reflected light (Fig. 31-2).

Skiing

Most skiers can tolerate any lens because the cold weather depresses the basal metabolic rate

of the corneal epithelium. Thus the oxygen demands are reduced. This advantage is partially reduced by the decrease in oxygen tension that prevails at high altitudes.

Tinted rigid lens do not offer protection against ultraviolet rays because the central surface of the cornea is not protected. Gas-permeable lenses are better than PMMA lenses and can now be tinted. Soft lenses are comfortable and can be tinted.

Actually, all these lenses are tolerated well. The soft lens is preferred because there is less photophobia, more protection against the wind, and good oxygen permeability if a thin lens is used. Goggles that are polarized and tinted are still recommended regardless of the lens type employed for better protection against direct and reflected ultraviolet rays.

The gas-permeable lens is an excellent alternative for those people with astigmatism. The lens is large and not likely to be displaced by tearing. Also its permeability features make the tolerance of this lens excellent. Its optic characteristics are better than those of a soft lens especially in the area of contrast sensitivity. When a large-sized lens is used, 9.2 mm or greater, the chances of it being lost in a fall are

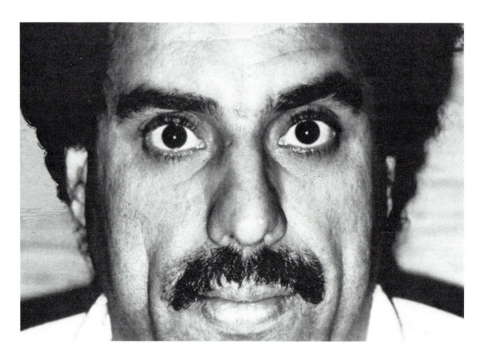

Fig 31-2 ■ Sharif Khan, world-famous squash player, who wears soft contact lenses that permit him to excel in squash because of minimal lens movement.

negligible. A properly fitted gas-permeable lens should fit under the upper lid margin. In a spill, the upper lid should retain the lens.

Football, hockey, and basketball

Obviously in these rough sports dislodgment by bodily contact is the major issue. The most desirable lens must be the soft lens; it will not pop out because of a hard body check into the boards or an aggressive tackle or a basketball giant pushing another player to the side. Besides, a soft lens can be worn intermittently because many professionals only wear lenses while playing.

We must emphasize once again that a contact lens of any type offers no protection from trauma to the eye. Children playing hockey or football *must* wear eye protection. On the other hand, the wearing of a contact lens does not add any special liability to the eye either.

Swimming and soft contact lens

Although we have reported on the literature on the use of contact lenses in swimming, the recent outbreaks of acanthoemeba corneal ulcers have made us come full circle and condemn the use of contact lenses for swimming. Despite the fact that contact lenses can be worn in fresh lake water and swimming pools without loss, the risk of contamination of these waters with bacteria and acanthoemeba is too great. If extended-wear lenses are used, protective water-tight swim goggles or face masks can be used. Ideally, the lenses should be removed before swimming and reinserted afterward.

COMMENT. Samples of water from lakes and swimming pools that we have tested personally by cultures were full of contamination. All contained microbial contamination; the more serious was *Pseudomonas aeruginosa*. Small punctate erosions that may be present in the swimmer's eyes could develop into a devastating infection. Water-tight goggles or masks worn with contact lenses may be used to relieve swimming blindness in those with high refractive errors.

Soft contact lenses for scuba divers

Over 2 million people in Canada and the United States are aficionados of scuba diving. The use of soft contact lenses has been tested and approved for scuba diving. They give good vision in divers and do not present any hazards.

There is only minimal lens loss, which seems to occur at shallow depths. At 30 feet, no lens loss is encountered. There is tolerance for these lenses despite the low water temperatures in which they are used. Bacterial contamination of these lenses has not been a problem because the diver's eyes are protected by the face mask worn during diving.

NYSTAGMUS

Persons with nystagmus, particularly of the congenital type, see very poorly with glasses. The oscillations of the eyes under the spectacles produce a constant parallax. With contact lenses, vision disturbance that was created by eyes constantly in motion against fixed spectacle lenses is vastly improved.

The visual gains are truly remarkable; frequently visual acuity can be improved from 20/200 to 20/50 or 20/30.

As fixation is improved by the corrective lens moving with the eye, the actual amplitude of oscillations is decreased. This is particularly noticeable under dim illumination. Also many people with nystagmus seem to have a large degree of astigmatism, which makes correction by anything but a rigid lens a futile endeavor.

The only precaution in the fitting of such lenses is to use larger-diameter lenses that are gas-permeable.

COMMENT. Improvement is most apparent in those persons who have pendular nystagmus without foveal aplasia. Those with albinism, aniridia, and achromatopsia do not make good visual gains with contact lenses.

CONTACT LENSES FOR CHILDREN

Contact lenses are being used to treat children under 1 year of age. These children are usually aphakic, and lenses are a must if their aphakia is monocular.

They have also been used as an occluder in which the lens is overplussed to create blurred vision in the fixing eye.

Other medical uses of contact lenses in children include the treatment of aniridia, albinism, and achromatopsia. These lenses usually have a deep peripheral tint outside the optic zone to partially offset the effects of photophobia and glare.

With aniridia there is no iris. With achromatopsia, there is an absence of a cone population, and so protection against excess light is mandatory. With albinism, the iris pigment is missing as shown with transillumination, and these children are virtually incapacitated by light. At times, a contact lens is worthwhile for the treatment of unilateral myopia with amblyopia.

If the child is aphakic, K readings can be performed in the operating room by using a Terry keratometer while the patient is under anesthesia. The K readings are helpful but not crucial, and one need not submit the child to a general anesthetic just to obtain a K reading.

These lenses should be fitted flat so that there is adequate movement. Small lenses must be custom ordered so that they may be inserted into the narrow palpebral tissues. The power of the lens is estimated by retinoscopy. If there is frequent lens loss in infants, the lenses ordered should be 15 to 16 mm in diameter.

Gas-permeable lenses and soft lenses are both advocated. The rigid lenses are more easily handled by parents, and one can use devices that aid in insertion and removal. Also, these lenses have superior optic properties and are more durable. They do not tear and spoil because of protein accumulation the way a soft lens can.

To go through this exercise, the parents must be highly motivated and intelligent. The failure rate under the best of conditions is high. Part of the reason is the very early date at which some children are fitted. For infants with congenital cataracts, surgery in some centers with the application of a contact lens is now being done on the first day of an infant's life. Special custom-ordered lenses of 25 diopters or more are often required for the infant.

There is great difficulty in fitting contact lenses for children. Despite gloomy reports of the past, better fitting techniques on very young children, even 1 month old, have yielded new triumphs with this disorder.

It is reasonable to ask, Why not use intraocular lenses on children? They would eliminate handling problems, the high cost of maintaining lenses through loss or breakage, infection, and the unending commitment of parents to an eye. Indeed, this method may be the best route to choose for long-term correction and comfort. However, there are no 40- or 50-year-old studies to use for guidance. Therefore there is some risk that these lenses used safely in adults for 20 to 25 years may not be adequate for children. Also a child's eye grows in size developmentally with the rest of the body.

Fitting

The fitting of any type of contact lens may be done on infants and small children in the operating room with the Terry keratometer while the child is under general anesthesia. In this manner, a lens fitted close to the topography of the cornea can be selected. Because these lenses are thicker and larger than regular lenses, the fitting should be flat so that the lens will move. An aphakic lens dropped by gravity and hanging low on the lower limbus and beyond is unacceptable. The lens should move freely so that molding of the cornea does not occur, and the lens should be properly centered so that the pupil is directly under the optic section of the lens.

COMMENT. In children under 18 months of age, a general anesthetic may not be needed. The child can be restrained for both the keratometer and the final over-refraction by retinoscopy.

With silicone lenses still available for pediatric use, a suction force is created by the flat-fitting lens and the cornea. To remove the lens, one must move it over to the limbus where the suction effect is released. The lens can then be removed with a suction cup. It is applied to the surface of the lens, which now can be safely removed from the eye.

Hydrophilic lenses have been used on children. They are flaccid so that the likelihood of abrading the cornea is minimal. Also their suppleness and hydration makes them very comfortable, and so tolerance is not an issue. The range in which a single lens can fit many eyes makes precise measurements of corneal topography unnecessary. The lens is fitted flat and if 1 to 2 mm of lens motion is found, no further fitting alterations need be done. The recent extended-wear hydrophilic lenses that are permeable to oxygen either by virtue of their thinness or higher water content, which is about 70%, relieve the burden of parents having to insert or remove these lens on a daily basis.

Yet, despite these advantages, there are complications even with extended-wear hydrophilic lenses. Spheric lenses do not correct astigmatism, which may require a spectacle overcorrection or an acceptance of smaller visual-acuity goals. Toric soft lenses are too complicated to regulate for an infant. The large size of these lens make them difficult to insert and remove in a child. Despite being intended for extended wear, these lenses must be removed and cleaned periodically. One hazard of wearing them is that corneal edema with vascularization can occur without any visible evidence of it happening. Periodic slit-lamp assessments are vital either directly or while the patient is anesthetized. Practical objections also include the high initial cost, a greater loss and breakage rate, and the need for frequent changes because the cornea changes its size in the first 4 years.

Hydrophilic-lens enthusiasts point out that the astigmatic portion of visual loss is minimal and it is not common under the best of circumstances to achieve 20/20 vision in a unilaterally aphakic child. Pediatric lenses are available and present in most power selections. The need to change the lenses in terms of fit and power would exist despite the type of lens and plastic used. Inflammation in soft lenses is usually related to soft-lens solutions, particularly contaminated distilled water, and nonpreserved saline solution that has not been changed daily. Dirty cases and screw-top vials are also a source of bacterial contamination. The likelihood of infection occurring in an adult-supervised soft lens is minimal because the care systems would be closely monitored.

COMMENT. If autoclaving of the lenses is done periodically, the infection rate is minimal. We have not had any infections, but we have only run a small number of cases with a pediatric hydrophilic lens.

The ease of fitting and the ability to use the hydrophilic lenses over an extended time makes this lens a top choice. The use of intra-ocular lenses in aphakic infants has been confined to a handful of investigators and their results have been equivocal. The development of epikera-tophakia for infants with monocular cataracts has demonstrated a higher success rate and, at the time of this writing, may be the route to go with infants.

Fitting without K readings

One can fit both soft and rigid lenses without K readings by noting the fluorescein patterns and lens movement using high-molecular weight fluorescein.

A trial lens of power $+10.00$ to $+11.00$ D is used. Fluorescein is placed in the lower cul-de-sac. Apical touch means the lens is too flat, and a bubble under the lens indicates that the lens is too steep. Err on the flatter side. The lens movement with the lens passively rotated by the patient's lids should be free and unencumbered.

Refraction should be done with the lens in place. This eliminates vertex calculations and takes into account the positive tear meniscus, which can result in 2.00 D of power or more. Our best results occur when the lens is freely movable. Some fitters fit steeply and so obtain a larger tear pool effect, giving extra plus power.

The final lens should be over-powered by 1.50 to 2.00 D to provide the child with best vision at the near range because this is the most useful distance.

Silicone lenses may be preferred because they provide better optic characteristics than soft lenses do and can be worn in an extended fashion because of high oxygen-permeability. With the newer RSP lenses it is important to use only those lenses with a high silicone content that are permeable to oxygen at the thickness required for an aphakic lens.

SILICONE LENSES FOR CHILDREN

Advantages
Best permeability and best thermal conductivity
Better acuity than with hydrogel lenses
Stable in power
Medications can be given with the lens in place
Minimal lens loss because of the tighter fitting characteristics
Minimal flexure
No interstices for bacterial growth in the lens itself

Disadvantages
Protein debris on the lens can be excessive
Loss of surface coating, which makes the lens hydrophobic
Corneal vascularization
Corneal infiltrates
Flat fit makes removal of lens hazardous if done the regular way

Which lens to choose

Obviously each lens system requires parental management. The rigid lens system is the most demanding because of daily routines. The parent must accept the long-term duty of caring for the lens until the child is able to do this job without assistance.

The intra-ocular lenses should solve most of the problems of any aphakic contact lens system. At this moment, no one is advocating this method for routine use until more data are accumulated. We are waiting for the development and results of epikeratophakia on infants because this approach seems most promising.

We like the pediatric hydrogel extended-wear lens. It relieves the family of the daily task of handling lenses. Its lack of durability is a problem because in many cases the lens may survive for only 6 months to 1 year. Cost is also a consideration. Yet, despite these imperfections, our best results come with the use of large hydrogel lenses. The lens should be large enough to avoid the customary night-time loss that may occur in infants who rub their eyes.

It is important to remember that despite poor acuity, such as 20/60, the overall visual gains make the enterprise still valid.

COMMENT. We have used the hydrogel lenses for extended wear and then switched to gas-permeable lenses when the child was old enough to handle a daily-wear lens without difficulty.

ORTHOKERATOLOGY

Orthokeratology has been advanced as a system for "sight without glasses." The premise behind the system is that progressive flattening of the cornea through the use of a series of flatter-fitting lenses will eliminate myopia. The assumption is made that the degree of flattening will be uniform in all meridians. Certainly this is not always the case because there are many instances of flat-fitting lenses worn over a long period of time resulting in a toric cornea.

The advocates of orthokeratology point to its usefulness in treating certain groups of people who require good vision but cannot wear contact lenses. This group includes pilots, airline stewardesses, fire fighters, athletes engaged in competitive sports, policemen, and people who do a great deal of swimming. This method of doing away with glasses is certainly not any bolder than thermokeratoplasty or Barraquer's surgical keratoplasty (keratomileusis) or serial radial cuts in the cornea (radial keratotomy).

Orthokeratology fitting sets are available. American Optical Corporation employs the May-Grant method, which uses a fitting set of 370 lenses with a base-curve range of 38.00 to 47.00 D and a power range of +0.50 to −4.00 D. Corneal curvature changes are effected when between 70% and 80% of the corneal surface is covered. Larger-diameter lenses are used with a range varing from 8.5 mm for the steepest curves to 10.2 mm for the flattest base curves. The thickness of the lens is within the ordinary range of rigid lenses, that is, about 0.15 mm, depending on the power of the lenses. At present, gas-permeable lenses are being used to relieve the effects of corneal hypoxia. These lenses have made the procedure safer and the wearing of these lenses more comfortable.

The lenses are reassessed approximately every 6 weeks with particular attention given to refraction through the lenses, new corneal readings, and slit-lamp evaluation of the cornea. When changes of corneal curvature occur, a new lens is given, predicated on the new, flattest corneal curvature. An appropriate power reduction should normally ensue. A patient may need five or six pairs of lenses the first year, three or four the second year, and two or three more the third year.

A proper fit is one in which the lens has a tangent touch to the flattest meridian of the cornea. As a general rule, five to seven pairs of lenses are required to achieve a flattening effect. Among persons with myopia who practice this technique it is estimated that 85% with 20/100 vision will develop 20/20 vision in 1 year, 70% with 20/200 vision will develop 20/20 vision in 2 years, and 55% with 20/300 vision will develop 20/20 vision in 3 years. The procedure is most applicable to myopic people and is only practical with those with moderate degrees of myopia, −3.00 D or less.

A retainer, plano lens has to be worn during the day with a minimum wearing schedule to keep the cornea flat. Some patients can eventually be weaned from the retainer, whereas most require it indefinitely once a week or once a day. A study of 150 Air Force cadets in Colorado Springs who had orthokeratology performed on them and were followed revealed that none of them showed significant permanent changes. It was not uncommon for the cadets to have their vision improved from 20/100 to 20/40. However, most of these changes were transient unless a retainer contact lens was employed. But induced cylinder and corneal abrasions were no more frequent than in the average contact lens wearer.

Most ophthalmologists have limited experience with orthokeratology. Such complications as overwear reactions, corneal abrasions, induced corneal astigmatism, and ocular discomfort from the wearing of such large, flat lenses are possible. In fact, in medical studies done, the rate of corneal complications was no greater than with ordinary rigid lenses. So the added risk, in terms of the health of the eye, may be exaggerated. More experience with this technique is needed. The main objections to the procedure are as follows:

1. The length of time required for results is high, and so the procedure is costly.
2. The effect is not predictable. There is no way to screen who will benefit and who will not.
3. A retainer contact lens is usually required to maintain the flattening effect. The treatment does not offer sight without glasses or contact lenses.
4. The scope of people who can be helped is limited to moderate myopes.
5. The improvement is not uniform. A patient frequently will obtain 20/20 vision in one eye and 20/40 vision in the other.

Medical evaluation of this technique has recently been done in which an ophthalmologist (P Binder) and two optometrists who practice orthokeratology (CH May and SC Grant) worked together on a series of cases.

Their conclusions were as follows:

1. The procedure is essentially safe. No adverse effect was found in the orthokeratology group.

   There was some mild distortion of the keratometric mires but nothing really serious. None developed corneal warpage, and there was no increased incidence of corneal abrasion, punctate staining, or other signs of corneal disease.

   There were some optic surprises. A third of the group studied required reading glasses. Also, the quality of unaided visual acuity was worse than that obtained through glasses or contact lenses.
2. Refractive errors beyond 4 D were not significantly aided by this technique. Also, it was difficult to predict which patient would do well once therapy was initiated.
3. Reduction in refractive errors of 1.5 D could be done with eyes with moderate myopia

(2.00 to 4.00 D) but not in eyes of minimal myopia (-1.25 D or less).

4. There was no correlation between the change in corneal curvature and the change in refraction. An analysis of peripheral corneal contours and refractive change yielded similar results.
5. The retainer lens stage was not reached by the majority of patients. Those who achieved this plateau did so after 24 months.
6. In three of the four patients who reached retainer levels, the corneas promptly resumed their prefitting shape once the retainers were discarded.
7. A high rate of failure was attributed to patients who failed to keep appointments.
8. Disturbing optic features include a high incidence of spectable blur, induced with-the-rule astigmatism, myopia, and a poor quality of unaided vision, often 20/40.
9. The results were unpredictable, with the maximum benefit taking place with 9 months. There were no stable parameters to predict which patients would benefit from this treatment.
10. Best results occurred with myopia of 2 D and worsened as the refractive error increased, especially beyond 4 D.

COMMENT. Despite the rather negative tones of this report, the subject requires some analysis. There are very few medical reports on the effectiveness of orthokeratology. We need more testing to evaluate this technique.

In terms of safety and expense, orthokeratology is cheaper and safer than surgical techniques, such as radial keratometry. As the demand for sight without a device exists, it behooves us to look at this procedure and try to improve it, rather than discard it. If it can be made to function so that the effect is permanent, it just might make surgical efforts obsolete.

There is very little orthokeratology practiced among ophthalmologists. It is limited even among optometrists because there is considerable chair time involved. The limitations of this procedure as it stands today do not make the enterprise clinically worthwhile.

RADIAL KERATOTOMY

The ultimate goal of radial keratotomy is to achieve emmetropia or at least a reduction in myopia that appears close to emmetropia so that spectacles are not required. However in at least 30% to 50% of cases this does not occur despite

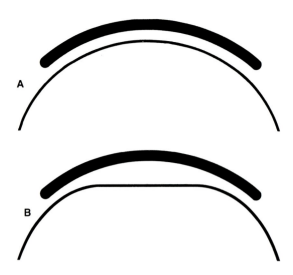

Fig 31-3 ■ A, Contact lens over a normal cornea. **B,** Contact lens over a postradial keratotomy cornea. The contact lens may irritate the knee of the cornea. In addition, a large plus tear layer is created.

a repeat procedure. Thus for those with residual myopia of 1 D or more, contact lenses may be necessary. The problem of fitting contact lenses in post-radial keratotomy can be challenging. The patient is often resistant to trying contact lenses or has been a chronic contact-lens failure in the past. In addition the patient's corneal topography may have changed. With the increased central flattening of the cornea (Figs. 31-3, *A* and *B*) there occurs a knee at the mid-periphery that creates a problem because this knee rubs against the contact lens. The central flattening, similar to a flattened corneal transplant, often leads to decentration of the lens. The contact lens tends to center on the highest point of the cornea, which in this case is the mid-peripheral zone, which is about 3 to 4 mm from the center.

In our experience it is best not to use the new central flat K readings but to return to the original presurgical Ks and design the lens accordingly. A large diameter lens is also advisable. High-DK lenses as large as 10 to 10.5 mm will provide better stability.

The power of the contact lens will not be the same as the refractive error. This is because there occurs a large plus lens tear film in the central flat area. Thus the new lens required will be much more myopic in power than would have been expected. An over-refraction over the contact lenses is most important in determining the final lens power.

Trial fitting becomes very important. A modification unit is most helpful in making a tight lens looser. The use of fluorescein is important in assessing the fit.

For those patients who find the contact lens irritating, a piggy-back system can be very helpful. Here a soft lens with a flat base curve is applied to the cornea before a suitable rigid lens is placed on top of the soft lens. The soft lens may be of the extended-wear type so the individual has to remove and care for the rigid lens on a daily basis and the extended-wear lens on a weekly basis.

Complications

1. Neovascularization. Because radial cuts at surgery have been made near the corneal limbus (perhaps some of the cuts have inadvertently crossed the limbus), neovascularization may occur. It should be carefully watched.

2. Bubbles and debris. Air bubbles and debris may occur in the central portion because of the greater separations of the cornea from the contact lens. The mid-peripheral knee prevents the venting of the debris and tear exchange from taking place. One may have to fenestrate the lens to eliminate debris and tear entrapment centrally.

3. Epithelial defects. The hypoxia induced with contact lenses and the accumulation of debris may be a sufficient insult to the corneal epithelium to create corneal erosion in an isolated spot of the linear surgical cuts.

COMMENT. In our experience at least 3 to 4 contact lenses and considerable chair time is required to achieve good results from post-radial keratotomy. Decentration, poor venting, and edema of the mid-peripheral knee are common problems that need to be solved.

32 ▪ APHAKIC AND PSEUDOPHAKIC RIGID AND SOFT LENSES

CONTACT LENSES VERSUS INTRA-OCULAR LENSES

Effective functional visual return and patient satisfaction are the first considerations for the cataract patient.

Cataract patients today demand better methods of visual rehabilitation than aphakic spectacles provide. Aphakic spectacles with all their inherent aberrations, distortions, and field limitation leave much to be desired (Fig. 32-1). The method of operating on some persons for cataracts and fitting them with spectacles afterwards immobilizes their daily activity to such an extent that it often ages them considerably and substitutes one disability for another. Fortunately this era is now over thanks to the early pioneers in contact lenses and later to surgeons like Harold Ridley, Edward Epstein, Peter Choyce, and others who began implantation with cataract surgery.

Today intra-ocular lens implantation is the procedure of choice for most new cataract patients. With the increased number of intra-ocular lenses available today, the ophthalmologist is able to provide a more natural type of vision for the cataract patient. At one time intra-ocular lenses were indicated only if the patient was very elderly or had macular degeneration. Such a patient was offered the procedure in one eye only.

The indications have broadened, to say the least, to include almost every cataract patient, with a few exceptions.

In conditions or situations in which an intra-ocular lens is contraindicated such as for those patients reluctant to have an implant or those with chronic uveitis, a contact lens may provide a safe effective alternative method for visual rehabilitation.

Despite the shrinking number of people using contact lenses for therapy of aphakia, a sizable percentage of existing patients will need aphakic contact lenses to give them the best vision. Today, however, secondary implantation has become quite popular. Patients discontented with their spectacles or contact lenses a few years after surgery are now seeking this implantation so as to be more like other people they know who have just had the operation performed.

In this chapter we basically cover the daily-wear aphakic lens and leave the detailed use of extended-wear lenses to a later chapter.

SELECTION OF LENSES

Every ophthalmic resident learns early the enormous visual advantages that contact lenses possess over a spectacle correction for the treatment of aphakia.

The rigid lens offers good optic performance and can mask astigmatism. Since the prime purpose of doing a surgical procedure on a cataractous lens is to improve visual acuity, the superior vision of a rigid lens makes it most desirable. Another advantage of a rigid lens is its small size, which makes it easier to insert into the small, recessed palpebral openings of the aphakic patient. A rigid lens can be felt, a feature of great importance to the bilateral aphakic patient, and can be removed with lid manipulations rather than by grasping the lens as in the case of a soft lens.

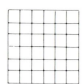 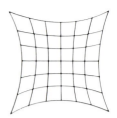

Fig 32-1 ■ Distortion by a strong convex aphakic lens that distorts a square to a pincushion shape. (From Stein HA, Slatt BJ, and Stein RM: The ophthalmic assistant, ed 5, St Louis, 1988, The CV Mosby Co.)

A soft lens is difficult to see swimming around in a solution, is likely to flip inside out when it is applied to the eye, and must be removed directly by pinching it off the cornea, a task that many elderly patients are frightened by. What makes the situation worse is that these lenses are not very tactile. In essence, what an ophthalmologist does when prescribing an aphakic soft lens for both eyes is to ask elderly persons to use their fingers for removal.

The major disadvantage of any lens, be it rigid or soft, is that it must be handled. For the elderly patient with arthritis, a tremor of the head or finger, Parkinson's rigidity, or poor central acuity resulting from macular degenerative changes, an intra-ocular lens is perhaps the only choice. For the elderly patient over 70 years of age an intra-ocular lens is a better alternative because it is well known that the number of lens dropouts increases dramatically with increasing age. Elderly patients cannot cope with lens insertions, running out to purchase solutions, or the fear, especially if they live alone, of one day being unable to remove their lenses. Also elderly people who have never worn contact lenses view such an enterprise with considerable apprehension and repugnance. Bilaterally aphakic patients, unless they use a special spectacle accessory device, cannot see well enough to look for their lenses.

COMMENT. Our preference for daily-wear contact lens when required is a gas-permeable rigid aphakic lens. The optic performance is better, the handling is easier, and the touch of the lens is more sure. The only thing the practitioner has to know is the oxygen permeability of the lens selected at aphakic levels of lens thickness.

DAILY-WEAR APHAKIC SOFT LENSES

The daily-wear soft lens is best used for the unilateral aphakic. If the aphakic person is soon to become bilaterally aphakic, extended-wear lenses or a lens implant should be considered.

Prefit evaluation

The time to fit a lens can vary because the cataract surgical procedures are no longer uniform. An eye with a small incision from phacoemulsification can be given a soft contact lens in the first week after surgery. An extracapsular cataract extraction done with a larger incision will have to wait until the inflammatory reaction and the corneal parameters have settled.

A good guide to the fitting time is to wait until there is no further corneal edema. Corneal edema may be assessed with the optical pachometer. The measurement consists of aligning the displaced image of the anterior corneal surface with the image of the posterior surface. The simpler electronic ultrasound pachometer reveals the corneal measurements directly; the readings are usually made in millimeters. The average central corneal thickness is 0.507 to 0.505 mm. A thickness of 0.6 mm should be considered as suspect and more than 0.7 mm as showing pronounced corneal edema.

A contact lens by itself can cause corneal edema. An aphakic lens placed on a normal non-operated cornea can cause a 4% to 8% increase in corneal thickness. One must keep in mind that an aphakic lens is the thickest contact lens used. While a − 10 D myope has the thin portion over the visual axis, a + 10 D hyperope or aphakic person has the thickest portion of the lens over the corneal cap and visual axis. So a soft lens used for aphakia causes an increase in corneal edema over the most critical part of that structure, that is, the central optical cap. Even if highly permeable lenses are used, the permeability at aphakic levels of lens thickness may not be great.

Because most private ophthalmic offices do not have a pachometer, there are other methods to consider. The corneal keratometer measurements should be clear, undistorted, and stable with two readings taken 1 week apart. The aphakic person often is unable to fixate well, and a small fixation light attached to the keratometer or the light attached to the keratometer or the light of the topogometer may be helpful to obtain central K readings. The retinoscopy reflex should be undistorted and the refraction stable over a 2-week span. Slit-lamp findings of vertical striae, dry spots on the cornea, and epithelial edema shown with sclerotic scatter or retro-illumination can also yield good data as to the state of corneal repair.

Another problem with the early fitting of an aphakic contact lens is loss of endothelial cells. It has been shown that an aphakic soft lens placed on an eye can cause a dropping or loss of endothelial cells after one day's wear. So, when one is fitting the lens, it is important to begin when corneal edema is virtually absent.

COMMENT. Persistent corneal edema should be detected and treated. It may be attributable to endothelial cell loss, vitreous touch, and so on. A contact lens placed over such an eye can only aggravate the condition and should not be used.

Fitting technique

The vertex distance of the refraction should be recorded, since a proper account of this must be taken into consideration in determination of the power required in the final lens. In general, because of the greater weight of the aphakic soft lens, the diameter of the soft lens must be made larger to stabilize the lens for proper centration. This fact is particularly true if there is significant astigmatism present.

As with most lenses, the prescription should be converted to minus cylinders. If the cylinder is less than 0.50 D, it can be disregarded. If the cylinder is greater than 0.50 D, take one half the cylinder and add it to the sphere (the spheric equivalent). If the cylinder is 1.50 D or greater, incorporate this additional cylinder into the bifocal spectacles. The vertex distance must be accounted for because it can change the final power by as much as 1.00 to 1.50 D. Convert the patient's K reading into millimeters. The initial K reading is only a guide to lens selection. The lens should be placed in the eye and allowed to settle for 20 to 30 minutes. At this point an over-refraction can be done to yield the final prescription.

If the lens does not move 1 to 2 mm with a blink, a flatter lens should be chosen. The regular soft aphakic lens does not have great permeability features, and so adequate tear exchange must be present. Also with time, deposits tend to tighten a lens by increasing its radius of curvature and making its contour steeper.

The base curves most commonly used for aphakic patients are 8.1 to 8.4 mm. The base curve should be flatter than the radius of curvature in the central region. The lens should rest on the apex of the cornea, vault the region of the limbus, and rest again on the peripheral portion of the sclera.

Myths about soft aphakic lenses

The soft aphakic lens is as durable as its rigid counterpart. The soft aphakic lens does well to last 1 year. The deposits are heavier and more varied and include mineral and lipids as well as protein. A rigid lens does not accumulate tenacious adherent deposits that are hard to remove with simple cleaners.

The incidence of infection is the same for an aphakic person wearing a soft lens as it is for a phakic person. The aphakic person has a higher incidence of bacterial conjunctivitis. The tear film is likely to be reduced and have an increased number of minerals due to concentration increase. There may be corneal erosion from xerosis. The concentration of the tear antibacterial enzyme, lysozyme, is also reduced. With increased protein precipitates and lower defense mechanisms, the setup is for a greater incidence of bacterial conjunctivitis.

Because the soft lens is so thick in the aphakic person, vision is good because the astigmatism is masked. If there is significant astigmatism, 2.00 D or greater, the aphakic person with a healthy retina will not have 20/20 vision. In fact, if there is no astigmatism, the aphakic person with a soft lens will not see as well as an aphakic person with a rigid lens. The contrast gradient with any soft lens is reduced when compared to vision yielded through a rigid lens.

Vision with a soft lens may be brought up to rigid-lens efficiency with the use of spectacles. Patients who switch from rigid lenses to soft lenses will invariably complain of hazy vision even if the recorded vision is 20/20 in each eye with both sets of lenses.

An aphakic soft lens may last 6 months to 1 year. Its life is shortened by the following:

1. Deposits, which interfere with clarity of vision.
2. Splitting by the fingernail or poor placement in the case.
3. Loss because this lens is impossible to see or feel, especially when stored in a liquid medium.
4. Displacement because this lens can be decentered without causing pain, and so this event may not be noted early.

The success rate for a soft aphakic lens is high. This is true in a 1-year projection, but it is dismal 5 years later. From an 80% rate of satisfaction in the honeymoon year, the rate of wear drops down to 30% in good hands. This occurs with bilaterally aphakic people.

Extended-wear soft lenses solve one of the problems of daily-wear lenses. They eliminate some handling, and that is their greatest advantage. Complications are abundant if the lenses are not removed and cleaned weekly and replaced regularly. Deposit formation may be so intense and rapid that a lens may have to be replaced every 3 months.

Neovascularization of the cornea is the same whichever lens is applied. The aphakic soft lens wearer is the most prone to neovascularization of the cornea. This is true whether a patient wears daily or extended-wear lenses. Corneal edema under a soft lens can be as much as 10%. With a rigid lens, corneal edema is apical in location and so limbal blood vessels cannot penetrate the compact peripheral stroma. With a soft lens, the entire cornea is edematous.

The success rate of hydrogel fitting is directly related to the motivation and patience of the fitter and his patient. Although this is true, motivation alone will not eliminate handling problems, mucous strands, xerosis, infection, vascularization of the cornea, cleaning problems, cost, and repetitive visits to the fitter.

DAILY-WEAR RIGID APHAKIC LENSES

An aphakic lens can be fitted when the K readings and refraction have stabilized. At least two similar K readings should be obtained before a lens is ordered. With the present refinements in surgery, measurements can frequently be made by the fourth week after surgery, with patients obtaining the lenses by the fifth or sixth week. It is well to remember that a round pupil extraction eliminates the flare often encountered after keyhole or full iridectomies. With phaco-

emulsification techniques a lens may be applied to the cornea within a week. In general the smaller the size of the surgical wound, the earlier the lens can be applied to the eye.

Motivation of the aged patient may be enhanced when patients are given their spectacle correction in a trial frame and are allowed to take a short stroll with assistance. The same procedure should be done with a trial contact lens. The results are most gratifying.

Fitting technique

Aphakic lenses are best ordered through a trial set. Some of the advantages are that patients can be introduced to a lens without having to make a firm commitment to order one. Since the initial discomfort of a rigid aphakic lens is ont so severe as a cosmetic lens fitted to a normal cornea, patients gain confidence as to their suitability for lens wear. The fitter gains a more dynamic overview of the lens-cornea relationship. Vertex-distance allowances do not have to be made because they are taken care of in the over-refraction. Also, the effects centration can all be assessed at a glance with trial lenses.

The guide for lens selection is keratometry. This is somewhat difficult in the aphakic patient because fixation is not accurate and because of the poor, uncorrected visual acuity. However, a lighted fixation target mounted on the keratometer overcomes this particular problem (Fig. 32-2). Before a lens is ordered, the mires should be clear and free of distortion and the K readings should be stabilized.

It is important that measurements of power of aphakic lenses be done in the same way in the office as in the laboratory. Front-vertex power is measured when the concave surface faces the examiner in the lensometer. The back-vertex power is assessed when the convex surface faces the examiner. With aphakic lenses over 10.00 D there may be up to 2.00 D of difference between the front-and back-vertex powers.

Many fitters advocate overplussing one eye by 0.50 D to give the patient good vision in the intermediate zone and adding excessive power in the other eye by +1.50 D to facilitate reading. This is an excellent idea for many elderly patients whose functional distance vision is no greater than the size of a room. Of course, if the patient drives a car, he or she should be given the best possible distance correction.

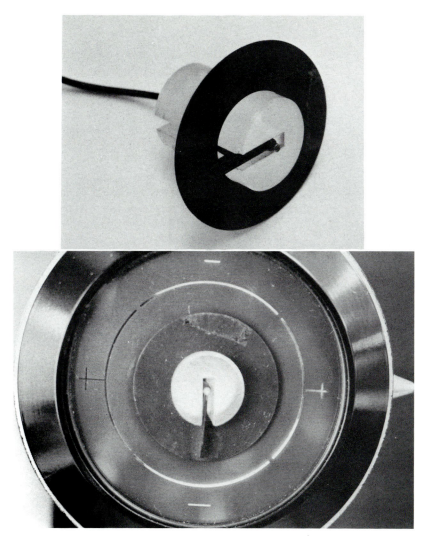

Fig 32-2 ■ A lighted fixation target mounted on the keratometer adds guidance for fixation for the bilateral aphakic patient.

If the astigmatism exceeds 1.50 D, the lens should be fitted about 0.1 mm steeper than the flattest K. If the astigmatism is 3.00 D or greater and centration is poor, a toric peripheral curve is best, since toric base-curve lenses are generally unsatisfactory.

The choice of final lens should be based on the centration, movement, and fluorescein pattern. The lens should center well, ride up slightly after the blink, and then gradually drop 1 to 3 mm.

Problems in fitting

The proper fitting of the person with aphakia is a highly complex matter because of

1. the tendency of high-plus lenses to ride down and be moved excessively by the lids because of their greater thickness and weight and their more forward center of gravity,
2. the often flaccid or lax lower lids of older patients, unable to support the weight of some low-riding lenses, that may allow the lenses to dig into and irritate the lower limbus,
3. pupillary irregularities such as keyhole or upward-displaced pupils, which are still quite common, and
4. high degrees of corneal cylinder astigmatism against the rule often found after cataract surgery.

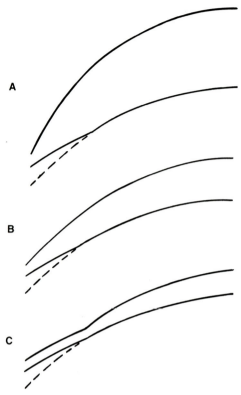

Fig 32-3 ■ **A,** Single-cut plus lens; **B,** regular lenticular construction for plus lenses; **C,** minus-carrier lenticular construction for plus lenses. **A** through **C** have the following common parameters: central posterior radius (base curve), 7.5 mm; posterior optic zone, 7.5 mm; posterior peripheral radius, 9.0 mm; lens diameter, 10.0 mm; central anterior radius, 6.0 mm; edge thickness, same for all. **B** and **C** have the following similarities and differences: (1) The anterior optic zone is 7.5 mm for both, and both are of a lenticular construction with the carrier radius (anterior peripheral radius) flatter than the anterior central radius. (2) The carrier radius of **B** is concentric to the posterior central radius (7.5 mm), whereas the carrier radius of **C** is concentric with the posterior peripheral radius (9.0 mm). The relationship of the carrier radius of 9.0 mm to the base curve radius of 7.5 mm is approximately −10.00. The major advantages of the minus-carrier lenticular construction over the regular lenticular lens construction are (1) minimum thickness, **A** through **C;** (2) more upper lid "hold" on the lens resulting from the flatter carrier; and (3) diameter reductions that can be made without affecting the edge thickness or the posterior curve. By consistently making the carrier radius concentric to the posterior peripheral curve(s) the only variables that affect the thickness are the power and the anterior optic zone.

To avoid visual disturbances such as flare, ghost images, or double vision, it is imperative to position the lens so that the optic zone covers the entire exposed pupil at all times.

Types of rigid aphakic lenses

There are basically two types of rigid aphakic lenses: the minus-carrier lenticular lens and the single-cut lens. The correct selection depends on the pupil and the lid characteristics of each individual case. For example, a keyhole pupil requires a lens, which usually rides somewhat above center, to completely cover the exposed pupil. If there is a mild postoperative ptosis so that the upper lid extends down far enough to cover virtually all the exposed superior pillars of the cut iris, this factor need not be considered.

Lenses with larger optic zone are necessary for large pupils and for conditions such as astigmatism against the rule or decentered corneal apical caps that tend to displace lenses laterally.

For flaccid lower lids, thick lens edge may be desirable to better support the weight of low-riding lenses or the lenses may be designed to ride up held there by the upper lids.

Minus-carrier lenticular lens (Fig. 32-3)

INDICATIONS. The following are indications for minus-carrier lenticular lenses to give lift to the lens.

1. Low-riding aphakic lens
2. Corneal curvature flatter than 45.00 D
3. Astigmatism against the rule greater than 1.50 D
4. Large palpebral apertures, especially accompanied by lax lower lids
5. Round pupil extractions

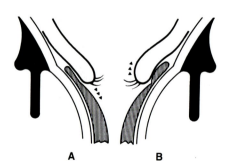

Fig 32-4 ■ **A,** A lenticular lens has a convex peripheral ridge, which the lid tends to push down. **B,** A minus lenticular lens. The lid tends to lift such a lens by its hold on the peripheral wedge.

Specifications for minus-carrier lenticular lens

Base curve: Trial set best; starting base curve should be 0.25 to 0.50 D steeper than K for initial lens; for each diopter greater than K 0.25 D should be added to base curve

Diameter: 9.0 to 9.5 mm; diameter should be increased for (1) flatter corneal curvature, (2) large corneas, and (3) lax and low lower lid margins

Edge thickness: 0.3 to 0.45 mm; varies largely with diameter and size of optic zone

Optic zone: 7.0 to 7.5 mm; smallest size consistent with good vision is best; optic zone should be 2 to 3 mm larger than pupil size and usually 1.5 to 2 mm smaller than diameter

Peripheral curve: 5.00 to 6.00 D flatter than the primary base curve

Power: Best determined by refraction over a trial lens

Radius of carrier: 1 to 3 mm flatter than base curve

These lenses have a flat carrier curve that increases the upward vector component of the upper lid pull on the lens. The flat carrier curve functions to reduce the weight of the lens, and as a result the tendency to sag is diminished (Fig. 32-4). This lessened tendency to sag is achieved when the lens is designed with a small, anterior optic zone, preferable 7.0 mm in diameter.

Such an expedient is helpful to compensate for the excessive center thickness of the lens, which, of course, is determined by its power. For example, a +2.00 D lens, 8.5 mm in diameter, would have a center thickness of 0.045 mm as compared to a +10.00 D lens, 8.5 mm in diameter, which would have a center thickness of 0.22 mm. An aphakic lens is frequently five times thicker than a corresponding low-powered plus lens.

The ordinary lenticular lens has been pushed into obscurity by the minus-carrier lenticular lens (Fig 32-5). The former lens was difficult to manufacture, and it frequently caused lid irritation as the upper lid passed from the relatively flat curve of the carrier portion to the steep curve of the option portion of the lens. Also the downward force exerted on the lens as the upper lid collided with the steep curve of the anterior optic zone tended to push the lens down.

The minus-carrier lenticular lens is well supported by the upper lid and can be held in position about 1 mm above the corneal center. Since this lens is much thinner than a conventional lenticular lens, there is less tendency for it to drop over the lower limbus (Fig. 32-6).

COMMENT. This relatively large lens is most suitable for large, flat eyes. One advantage of its size is that insertion and removal are easier for

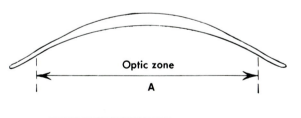

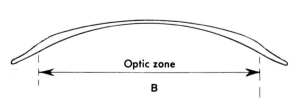

Fig 32-5 ■ Lenticular lenses. **A,** High-plus lenses tend to ride low because of their bulk and weight. **B,** The minus-carrier lenticular lens is thinner than a conventional lenticular lens and is well supported by the upper lid acting on the peripheral carrier.

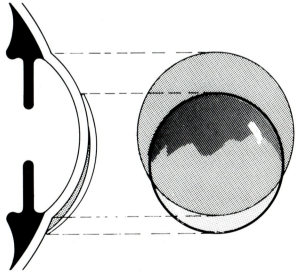

Fig 32-6 ■ A major disadvantage of any lenticular lens is that it tends to ride low. When the person reads, the depression of the lens over the limbus is accentuated.

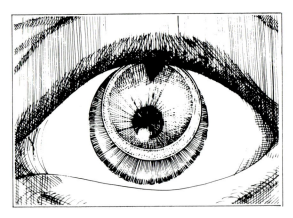

Fig 32-7 ■ The minus-carrier lenticular lens is best used for round pupil extractions. The peripheral portion of the lens creates flare in patients with sector iridectomies.

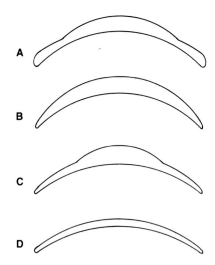

Fig 32-8 ■ Aphakic lens designs. **A,** Minus-carrier lens; **B,** single-cut lens; **C,** lenticular lens; **D,** microthin single-cut lens.

the aphakic patient. It centers well, an asset to the elderly patient with lax lower lids.

Tinted lenses are quite helpful for aphakic patients. Blue or gray tints are usually recommended. Aphakic patients frequently complain of halos around lights and reflections from artificial illumination. The annoying sensitivity to light may be caused by poor lens optic properties or internal lens reflections of the lens and the absence of the patient's own lens, which previously absorbed most of the visible wavelengths of incident light. The crystalline lens of the eye is a light filter; when it is removed the retina is struck by light never before experienced.

Single-cut lens. The single-cut lens should be used for patients with full or keyhole pupil in

order to diminish flare (Fig. 32-8). There is no carrier segment on the periphery of the lens that can create ghosting and flare with keyhole pupils (Fig. 32-9). The small dimensions of this lens also mean that the edge thickness can be made smaller than the edge of any lenticular lens. This is quite desirable since it makes the lens more comfortable. Though smaller in overall dimension, the optic zone of the lens is quite large and compares favorably to that of a lenticular lens. A key advantage of this lens is the absence of a sharp juncture between the central and carrier front-surface curves, which eliminates the annoying lid bump.

The following are indications for the single-cut lens:

1. Small palpebral apertures
2. Steep corneas—more than 45.00 D
3. Low-riding lenses

One difficulty with the single-cut lens is its convex edge, which is easily pushed down by the descending lid. This lens also tends to drop with astigmatism with the rule. The major disadvantage is lens removal; the elderly aphakic patient experiences great difficulty in removing this small, steep lens from the cornea.

Modification. A modification of the single-cut lens is the 7.5 mm diameter aphakic lens designed by Dr. Rober Welsh. This lens is particularly successful when the steepness of the cornea is 45.00 D or greater. This lens centers well,

---

■ ────────────────

Specifications for single-cut lens

Base curse: Fit steeper than K by 0.50 D; fit spheric lens for 1.00 D or less of astigmatism
Central thickness: 0.35 mm centrally
Diameter: 7.5 to 8.5 mm; the difference between a 7.5 and an 8.5 mm diameter lens can mean a difference in 40% of the weight of the lens
Edge thickness: 0.1 to 0.2 mm thick; the average is 0.125 mm
Optic zone: 7.0 mm; this varies with the pupillary size; with complete iridectomy an 8.0 mm size may be optimal
Peripheral curve: Usually only a single peripheral curve is needed that is 6.00 to 7.00 D flatter than the base curve
Power: Best determined by refraction over a trial lens

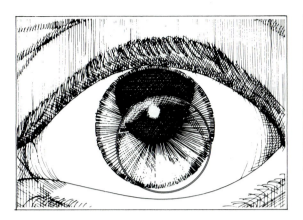

Fig 32-9 ■ Single-cut lenticular lens. This lens should be used in patients who have had a sector iridectomy.

is quite comfortable, and creates a minimum of spectable blur. This small, lightweight lens can be worn continuously by selected patients, who must be previously day adapted before full-time wear and seen on a daily basis initially to ensure that the cornea tolerates the lens. Some persons with aphakia learn to displace their lenses onto the sclera and wear their hard lenses continuously on this basis.

This lens is often fitted steep to make the fit tighter. If the total power is 10.00 D, by making the base curve steeper than K by +2.00 D, one can create +2.00 D of power in the lacrimal layer, and the final lens power need only be +8.00 D.

The small, thin lens frequently creates handling problems, particularly upon insertion and removal. The thin edge, which makes it more pleasant to wear, also makes it more difficult to remove. Frequently a second party is required to assist the aphakic patient in manipulating the lens. It is also more prone to warp. Despite these drawbacks, the single-cut lens is the lens of choice for a steep cornea, that is, any cornea greater than 44.00 D. This lens is comfortable, and because of its light weight is less likely to cause corneal edema or sag.

COMMENT. Single-cut lenses are thinnest at the edge and may tend to break or chip at this point. Handling problems in the aphakic patient increase the possibility of breakage. A common mishap is fracturing the lens at the edge when one is placing the cover on a decentered lens in the storage case.

■
Specifications for aphakic (Welsh) lens

Central thickness: 0.35 mm, approximately, depending on the power
Diameter: 7.5 mm
Edge thickness: 0.125 mm
Flat peripheral curve: 12 to 13 mm radius and 0.2 mm from the edge
Minimal blend: 0.1 mm to smooth the junction
Optic zone: 6.7 mm

INSERTION OF APHAKIC LENSES

As mentioned previously, aphakic lens candidates are more likely to be successful if they are less than 70 years of age because they are usually better able to handle a lens. After the age of 70 years the elderly patient is more likely to have osteoarthritis, a tremor of the hand, and some loss of proprioceptive facility, which make manipulation of a lens exceedingly difficult and frustrating.

The bilaterally aphakic patient has a real problem in finding the lens. Unless the person is guided by spectacles, the lens must be found by feel. This is really not much different from giving a blind person contact lenses.

For those patients who cannot manage a lens by conventional techniques, using reading aphakic spectacles with one frame blank or the aphakic lens attached on a flip hinge (Fig. 32-10, *A*) is helpful. The patient can insert the lens through the blank side of the frame while guided by the other eye, which has the advantage of a spectacle correction of +12.00 to +16.00 D.

Insertion aids, such as magnification mirrors, are helpful as plastic fingers are. The best technique is the blind one. The patient should be shown that the eye can be found with one's proprioceptive abilities and not with vision; that is, it is quite easy to touch the tip of one's nose with the eyes closed. At times the upper lid will have to be lifted to allow enough room for the bulky soft lens.

For the patient with a tremor the lens can be placed on the middle finger while the index finger below retracts the lower lid. The index finger then gives support to the lens-carrying finger.

REMOVAL OF APHAKIC LENSES

Removal of the lens is also a chore. The lids are lax and the lid margin of the upper lid may

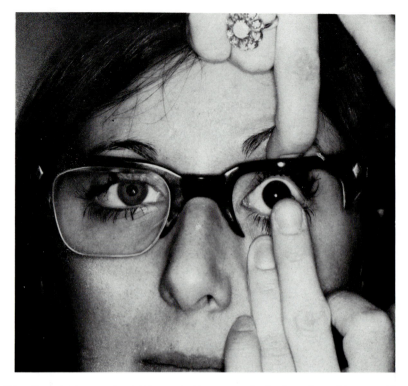

Fig 32-10 ■ Special frames to aid the aphakic person in the insertion of lenses. The glass is removed from one side and the plastic is bowed forward to permit the finger to grasp the upper eyelid.

buckle when the lid is laterally snapped to remove the lens. Also, since many elderly people frequently live alone, secondary aid is not always available. Ancillary services may be more of a hazard than a help. For example, a suction cup is a dangerous aid for elderly patients living alone because they may apply the cup directly to the cornea when without their knowledge the lens has become decentered. An eyecup with water inserted in the lower fornix can be the

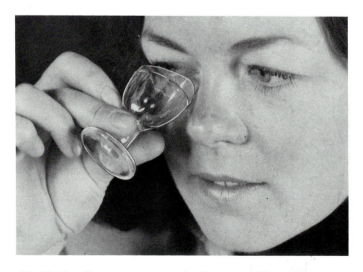

Fig 32-11 ■ Emergency removal with eyecup filled with water.

Table 27-1 ■ Aphakia trial set for the silicone-acrylate lens

Diameter (mm)	Central posterior curve (mm)	Power (D)	Intermediate optic zone (mm)	Design-carrier
8.7	7.20-8.20	+14.00	7.7	Single cut
9.2	7.20-8.20	+14.00	8.0	Single cut
9.8	7.30-8.50	+14.00	8.2	Lenticular EOZ* 8.0 mm—6.00 D
11.0	7.50-8.50	+14.00	9.0	Double lenticular EOZ 8.0 mm—3.00 D EOZ 9.5 mm—15.00 D

*EOZ, Exterior optic zone.

salvation of patients with lax lids trying to get lenses out of their eyes (Fig 32-11). The lens can also be washed out with saline irrigation or by dunking the head in the basin of water with the drain closed.

Make up office pamphlets with information on what to do if emergencies arise because an elderly patient may not retain the instructions he is given in the office. The pamphlet may help the patient cope with red eyes, abraded corneas, signs of infection, lost lenses, and so on.

COMMENT. There are two anachronisms in this section. The keyhole pupil, or full iridectomy, is virtually obsolete. Usually all cataract extractions have round pupils with intact sphincter. Also rigid PMMA lenses have given way to rigid gas-permeable lenses.

GAS-PERMEABLE LENSES FOR APHAKIA

Our favorite aphakic gas-permeable lens is made of the silicone-acrylate combination material, or the fluorocarbon silicone acrylate, which is described in detail in Chapters 21 and 22.

One of the major disadvantages of using a gas-permeable lens is that the lens may become tight and adhere to the cornea. A negative suction cup effect is introduced. A cycle of events is begun because the pressure on the tear film by the lid and lens only serves to squeeze out more tears. When the lid is in the up position, the lens shapes itself in the cornea and blocks the inflow of tears, producing a one-way valve effect.

Also some gas-permeable lenses do not permit sufficient oxygen-permeability at the thickness required for an extended-wear aphakic lens. For example, the CAB lens at 0.30 mm center thickness really cannot support the oxygen needs of the cornea under the closed lid. If these lenses

are to be used for extended wear, the lens should have adequate gas-permeability with respect to the thickness of the lens, the temperature zone in which it is going to be worn, and the adequacy of the tear film.

A problem with aphakic lenses of any material that is rigid is that these thicker lenses tend to ride low. If the upper edge of the lens is not covered by the upper lid, the major remedy for discomfort is lost.

Fitting the silicone-acrylate lens* (Table 32-1)

Although single-cut and lenticular designs may be equally effective in many patients, the elderly aphakic patient will find the larger lenticular contact lens easier to handle. Therefore, the initial trial lens should have a large-diameter, lenticular myoflange (minus carrier) design

*Modified from Rosenthal P: The Boston Lens: theory and practice, Wilmington, Mass, 1979, Polymer Technology Corp.

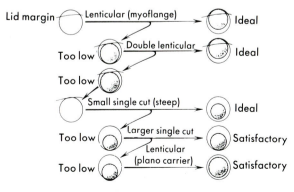

Fig 32-12 ■ Fitting the aphake. (Courtesy Polymer Technology Corp., Wilmington, Mass.)

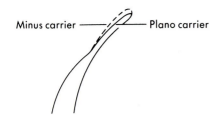

Fig 32-13 ■ Profile of lenticular-design aphakic or hyperopic contact lens. (Courtesy Polymer Technology Corp., Wilmington, Mass.)

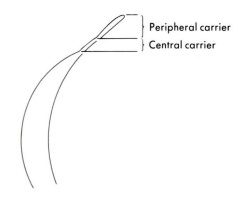

Fig 32-14 ■ Double lenticular design for aphakic contact lens. (Courtesy Polymer Technology Corp., Wilmington, Mass.)

(Fig. 32-13), and a base curve that provides the fluorescein pattern of minimal apical clearance.

1. If the initial trial lens position sufficiently high so that the upper lid covers the superior portion of the carrier throughout the blink cycle, it is the design of choice.
2. If the initial trial lens slips below the margin of the upper lid despite the fact that the upper lid covers the superior portion of the cornea, evaluate a larger double lenticular design (Fig. 32-14). If the superior portion of the carrier remains tucked under the upper lid, it is the design of choice.
3. If the lenticular and double lenticular designs position too low or if the upper lid does not cover a sufficient area of the cornea to hold a lenticular lens in a satisfactory position, evaluate the fit of steeper single-cut lenses.
4. If single-cut lenses, regardless of diameter, position too low for satisfactory vision or slide off the cornea as the patient blinks in upward gaze, a lenticular design having a tapered plano carried or tangential periphery may be the best lens for that patient.

Silicone lenses for aphakia

The silicone lens is potentially the best candidate for extended wear. For the past several years it was the lens of the future, but at this writing, the time has come for extended-wear lenses to be used in children.

This lens is ideal because it is at the top of everyone's oxygen-permeability charts. Even at 0.3 mm thickness, it provides almost 20% equivalent oxygen performance, which is way above the level required for maintaining the oxidative need of the cornea under a closed lid.

The good features are its optic performance and its ability to render the cornea free of any hypoxic changes. Today there is only a limited number of soft silicone lenses manufactured by Bausch & Lomb in powers of +12 D to +20 D for the elderly aphake and +23 D to +32 D for pediatric use. These lenses are used extensively in pediatrics where they are a welcome addition in the management of infants and young children. Bausch & Lomb is to be congratulated for maintaining the production of this lens.

PSEUDOPHAKIA AND CONTACT LENSES

Today intra-ocular lens implantation that results in pseudophakia or the implantation of an artificial lens as compared to aphakia (no lens) is the state of the art. Almost 1 million patients in North America undergo this procedure annually, in which a posterior chamber intra-ocular lens is inserted.

However, there is still a small number of unhappy patients who cannot regain binocular fusion and stereopsis with the naked eye or cannot be suitably fitted with spectacles.

The reasons for this lack of stereopsis in pseudophakia is:

1. Anisometropia—a marked difference in the refractive error of the newly operated eye over the fellow eye
2. High astigmatism in the newly operated eye
3. Aniseikonia because of a difference in the image size between eyes
4. Meridonial aniseikonia because of the difference of astigmatism in one axis between eyes

We have had a number of these unhappy patients referred to us by our colleagues. Our experience has been to fit them with rigid gas-permeable lenses of the highest DK on a daily- or extended-wear basis, depending on the manual dexterity of the patient.

Details of fitting these lenses will be found in Chapters 25 and 26. However, the same basics apply as outlined above. The heavier lenses may require a myoedge to lift the lens up under the upper eyelid. Lenses should also be made larger in diameter.

Our success in using contact lenses for pseudophakia has been most encouraging. This treatment approach is a necessary part of our armentarium for the patient who does not have binocular vision after cataract surgery.

SUMMARY

The era of contact lenses for the management of aphakia is rapidly coming to a close. There still remain a few million aphakes wearing spectacles. These are patients who were operated on either prior to the years of intra-ocular lenses or when the indications for lens implantation were more stringent. Only a few years ago many individuals were denied lens implantation because of their age or medical conditions such as diabetes, glaucoma, etc. Thanks to improved surgical techniques and improved intra-ocular lens implants, these individuals can now have implants inserted at the time of cataract surgery. In time, there will be very few indications for contact lenses for aphakia.

33 ▪ EXTENDED-WEAR LENSES

- Physiologic considerations
- Oxygen characteristics
- Aphakic versus myopic extended-wear lenses
- Patient selection
- Safety of extended-wear lenses
- Available lenses
- Fitting
- Managing an extended-wear practice
- Care
- Complications and problems with extended-wear lenses
- Further complications and why they occur
- The disposable system
- Conclusion

Today advanced lens technology is addressing itself to the problem of improving lenses that can be worn for extended periods of times without the need for daily handling. Advances in lens material and design combined with more sophisticated techniques in determining the response of the cornea to a lens worn on a 24-hour basis have made this possible. The news media have perhaps helped in increasing the demands of the public by making them aware that there are methods that will permit them to see without the trouble of insertion and removal of lenses and the accompanying care required. These methods are radial keratometry, surgical refractive keratoplasty and extended-wear contact lenses.

Extended-wear lenses have become a reality since 1984. Three factors have influenced this development. One is the manufacturing technologic advance in producing increasingly thinner soft lenses to provide a more comfortable lens with thinner edges that do not irritate the eyelid. This has resulted in the ability of the lenses to transmit oxygen. It has been clearly shown that if one halves the thickness of a soft lens, one will double its oxygen transmission. A second factor that has resulted in the availability

of extended-wear lenses has been the ability to polymerize soft lens materials and manufacture lenses that will absorb more water in their substance. For every 10% increase in water absorption of these materials there is a corresponding 50% increase in oxygen transmission; thus if water content increases 20%, the oxygen transmission doubles. A third factor has been the development of disposable contact lenses. The throw-away lens (weekly or biweekly) has become a succesful and practical reality.

Unfortunately the news media ignore the problems and attendant risks involved and appeal only to the imaginative, emotional response of the individual. This produces considerable pressure on the surgeon and contact-lens fitter.

The use of extended-wear lenses for the correction of the aphakic patient has become a historical curio. Intra-ocular lenses are used for the correction of aphakia whenever possible. This approach has become so satisfying for the patient that the debate of contact lenses versus intra-ocular lenses has long been won by intra-ocular lenses.

The overwhelming evidence is that intra-ocular lenses are much more gratifying, easier to use, and offer better visual results than soft extended-wear contact lens. The patient does not have to worry about the handling, management, or hygiene of the lens nor is the patient beset with the complications of extended-wear use. These complications are considerable. They include vascularization of the cornea, corneal ulcers, and multiple corneal infections. The intra-ocular lens-contact lens debate for all intents and purposes is over. Intra-ocular lenses are the method of choice for use after cataract surgery.

To some extent the growth and popularity of extended-wear lenses have been delayed by adverse publicity, by the practitioners' reluctance to handle the extra visits required, by the patients' reluctance to accept the higher fee necessary, by the fitters' reluctance to be faced with some medical problems that he or she may not be able to handle, and by the risk of the rare sight-threatening complications.

The safety of extended-wear lenses has been challenged. The major problems have been reports of infective keratitis, autoimmune responses, inflammatory reactions, neovascularization of the cornea, endothelial polymegathism, and epithelial problems.

The popularity of extended-wear lenses reached its zenith with lens manufacturers actually advertising on public television the wonders of the thirty-day lens. This lense could be worn for almost a month without fear or risk! Later this message proved to be embarrassingly inaccurate as reports came in regarding complications such as acanthamoebic keratitis, corneal ulcers, and severe vascularization of the cornea. Many experts and contact lens authorities said that these lenses were unsafe and should be banned. Opinions on extended-wear lenses shifted from one extreme to the other, from acceptance to overt hostility. Where was the truth? The evidence was not clear cut. Wearing these lenses obviously could cause havoc in the eyes. The severity of complications was directly related to the length of time that extended-wear lenses were worn. Two weeks of wear was better than four weeks of wear in terms of frequency of complications. One week was a still better time span for lowering complications, and not wearing the lenses on an extended basis was the safest. But is it possible for extended-wear lenses to be used in a limited form with minimal or acceptable risk? The body of opinion is still divided. The fundamentalists say that this is not possible while the more liberal authorities say that it is. Consent is given to those people who limit their wearing time to one week and agree to be followed every three months and are free of allergies, dry-eye syndrome, or blepharitis. Patients are also warned about symptoms that should alert them to possible danger; i.e., red eye, pain, blurred vision, etc. Thus, the use of extended-wear lenses has been restricted or curtailed. Despite this, the disposable or so-called "throw-away lens," initially introduced by Johnson & Johnson (Accuvue™) gives us reason for optimism and will be discussed later.

PHYSIOLOGIC CONSIDERATIONS

Significant advances have been made in corneal physiology with hydrogel lenses. Informa-

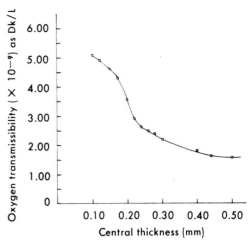

Fig 33-1 ■ Curve to illustrate the nonlinear relationship between the central thickness and the oxygen permeability of hydrophilic lenses at 20° C. The thinner the lens, the greater the oxygen transmission. (From Feldman G and associates: Contact Lens J 10(3):13-20, Dec 1976.)

tion on corneal physiology has shown that the oxygen requirement of the cornea during sleep is less than one half that required when the eyes are open. It has also been shown that a change of dimension lens thinness and water content results in better oxygen transmission of a lens (Fig. 33-1). Measurements show that the oxygen transmission of a lens measured at body temperature is 15% to 40% greater than that of a lens measured at room temperature (Table 33-1); consequently, laboratory methods of measuring gas transfer of a lens do not truly reflect its behavior on the eye.

Generally lenses that have power are constructed with either a thicker center or a thicker periphery depending on whether they are plus or minus lenses. Thus any given contact lens will have a variation of oxygen being transmitted across its surface. Because of this, the information that is truly significant is how much total oxygen reaches the corneal side of a contact lens. This is based on the average thickness of the lens. The factor of tear exchange and venting comes into play in which additional oxygen is provided from the tear film on flexure and movement of the lens.

The thickness of an aphakic lens often causes problems. In order to incorporate adequate power into a lens of +10.00 D the lens must be at least 0.4 mm thick in the center, whereas a

Table 33-1 ■ Comparison of expansion rate and oxygen permeability of four polymers of varying water content as hydrogel lenses at a standard thickness of 0.2 mm*

Polymer	Average water content (%)	Average expansion rate (%)	Oxygen permeability, DK ($\times 10^{-11}$)		
			21° C	27° C	35° C
A	43.8	18.6	2.50	3.33	4.30
B	53.1	25.8	6.81	8.23	10.21
C	63.2	36.4	9.71	11.82	14.24
D	71.3	46.7	14.28	15.33	17.77

From Feldman G and associates: Fitting characteristics and gas permeability of thin hydrogel lenses, Contact Lens J 10(3):13-20, Dec 1976.
*Note that the higher the water content the greater the oxygen permeability.

−4.00 D power can have a central thickness of only 0.03 mm. This also means that the aphakic lens is ten times heavier and must be made in a larger diameter for stabilization. Its thickness also makes it less permeable to oxygen (Fig. 33-2). Thus to create an ideal oxygen-permeable hydrogel lens, one cannot significantly reduce the thickness of an aphakic lens because of the power requirement, which makes it necessary for the lens to be thicker than a myopic lens.

Two types of hydrogel lenses have evolved: (1) those with water contents less than 50% that are designed for daily wear and (2) those with higher water contents that are designed for extended wear. The added water composition provides two elements that favor extended wear: (1) increased oxygen transmission so that there is adequate oxygen to a thermally elevated cornea lying under a closed eyelid, and (2) greater heat dissipation from the cornea.

Both the thinner, myopic, hydrogel lens and the thicker, hydrogel, aphakic lens can be safely worn on an extended-wear basis by certain persons, regardless of the water content of the lens. The problem is how to identify which persons are at risk. Even after daytime adaptation and continual monitoring, significant lens deposits and corneal changes will occur in a number of patients.

Although corneal changes are minimal with well-fitted lenses, coating of these lenses does become a significant problem in the elderly. With coating of lenses, there are some physiologic factors that decrease vision, impair corneal performance, and irritate the tarsal conjunctiva. Consequently, extended-wear lenses are not "fit-and-forget" lenses. The patient must be routinely monitored to avoid medico-legal implications if problems arise.

The cornea receives most of its oxygen from the atmosphere, which has 21% oxygen when the eye is open. When the eye is closed, this reduces to 8% as the oxygen is supplied by the perilimbal and tarsal vessels.

The desire to wear lenses for 24 hours of the day for several days must take into consideration that there is no longer adequate tear exchange through blinking. In this situation, with the closed eyelid, atmospheric oxygen is snuffed out and the cornea must obtain its oxygen supply directly from the overlying tarsal conjunctival

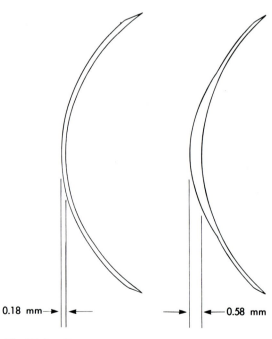

0.18 mm—►

◄—0.58 mm

Fig 33-2 ■ Comparison of a regular soft lens, *left,* with an aphakic lenticular lens, *right.* Note the considerably thicker central portion of the aphakic lens that contributes to corneal edema.

plexus of vessels and the limbal vessels. At least 5% of atmospheric oxygen equivalent is necessary for adequate oxygenation of the cornea in order to maintain corneal glucose reserves at an adequate level.

Some nocturnal changes that occur when the eye is closed are outlined below:

1. Richard Hill has pointed out that normally the oxygen supply is decreased by a third in the nighttime closed-eye environment compared to the oxygen supply in the daytime closed-eye environment. Furthermore, there is still further oxygen reduction to the cornea under a contact lens.

2. There is nocturnal swelling of the cornea as supported by pachometric evidence (Fig. 33-3). As the cornea thickens, the lens may no longer fit with a thicker cornea and may reveal tight signs.

3. Even during the waking day, with normal blinking there is only 1% to 5% tear exchage under a soft lens as compared to 20% tear exchange under a rigid lens. Thus one is most dependent on the oxygen transmission of the material of extended-wear lenses.

4. The temperature of the cornea increases by 3 to 4 degrees C with closed eyelids. The cornea in turn requires more oxygen with a higher temperature.

5. There is diminished tear production during sleep. As a result, the soft contact lens dries out, leading to edge lift-off and ejection of the lens by the lower eyelid. Consequently there is a higher loss rate in the elderly and in children who frequently rub their eyes.

6. The pH of the tears shifts to acid at night because of the buildup of lactic acid. The soft lens shortens it radius and tightens up when in an acid medium. This can be shown in tests in a beaker with changing pH. The significance of this is that a well-fitting lens may become too tight at night and when one rises in the morning. This may account for the tight lens syndrome described under the discussion on complications.

7. In dry environments, a lens can lose 20% of its water content. This is more significant in the low water and thin lenses. Not only may the lenses steepen, but also Hill has shown that there is a decrease in equivalent oxygen performance and a resulting corneal edema.

8. Korb and Holden have shown that the aphakic cornea requires only about 50% of the oxygen that a phakic cornea requires. Consequently, aphakes can get by for extended wear with the thicker lenses required for aphakic power considerations.

9. The tear pump action, even with extended-wear lenses, plays a role in corneal oxygenation. Although the eye does not blink at

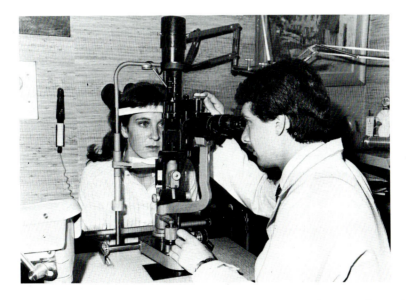

Fig 33-3 ■ The thickness of the cornea may be measured with a pachometer. Corneal swelling over 6% to 8% is usually pathologic. (From Stein HA, Slatt BJ and Stein RM: The ophthalmic assistant, ed 5, St Louis, 1988, The CV Mosby Co.)

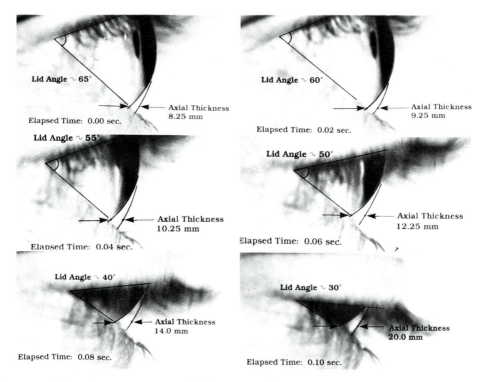

Fig 33-4 ■ Softcon lens photographed by high-speed film sequences (50 frames/sec), showing lens tear pumping action. (Courtesy Dr Lester E Janoff and American Optical Corp, Southbridge, Mass.)

night, there are still roving and rapid movements of the eye, at least during sleep, that will result in tear exchange and removal of debris. During the day, the beautiful high-speed photographs of the eye (Fig. 33-4) illustrate that during blinking the tear reservoir at the periphery of the lens and cornea is expelled, creating a partial vacuum in the area of the vault.

OXYGEN CHARACTERISTICS

The greater the oxygen transmissibility of a lens, the better the lens performance will be for achieving extended wear with minimal corneal interference. However, one must look at terminology carefully. The oxygen transmission of a lens represented by $\frac{DK}{L}$, where D is the diffusion coefficient of a material, K is the solubility constant, and L is the lens thickness. This is a laboratory measurement and is a satisfactory way to compare one material over another (Fig. 33-5). Of more importance clinically is the EOP, or *equivalent oxygen performance* (Fig. 33-6). This is a value relating the percentage of oxygen

reaching the cornea to atmospheric oxygen percentage. One can see from the illustration that in high-minus lenses, there is inadequate oxygen transmitted through the lens through the thicker periphery. Similarly with high-plus lenses, less oxygen passes through the lens centrally.

Another factor to consider is tear exchange—the extended-wear lenses, particularly the thinner lenses, may have to be fit just perfectly to prevent wrinkling and visual aberrations. If the permeability of the lens is adequate, this can be performed without difficulty or compromise to the cornea. Generally speaking, however, one always should be on guard for a situation of stasis of the lens because of tightening and dehydration.

With many of the soft hydrogel lenses there is a trade-off as to how thin they can be made with the high- or low-water-content variety without breakage and damage easily occurring to the lenses. However, the lenses are better polymerized today so that lens damage is not a major factor even with the very thin or high-water-content lenses.

Remember that for every halving of the thick-

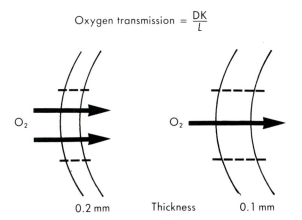

Oxygen transmission = $\dfrac{DK}{L}$

0.2 mm   Thickness   0.1 mm

Fig 33-5 ■ Oxygen transmission of any contact lens will vary with the thickness of the material. The thinner the lens, the more oxygen will be transmitted. This is directly proportional.

ness of a lens, the equivalent oxygen performance (EOP) is doubled. On the other hand, for every 10% increase in water content of a soft lens, the oxygen performance is increased by 50%. So a 60% water-content lens has 50% more oxygen performance than a 50% water-content lens, and a 70% water-content lens has double the oxygen performance that a 50% water-con-

tent lens has. This factor may be very significant in the thicker parts of a lens such as the center of a high-plus lens or the periphery of a high-minus lens.

COMMENT. Inadequate tears can really spoil extended-wear lenses. There is often a shift of residual tears to the lens based on osmotic flow. Lack of tears causes great protein deposition, which in turn may change the shape of the lens, make it tighter and more myopic than before, reduce the oxygen permeability of the lens, and reduce visual acuity.

APHAKIC VERSUS MYOPIC EXTENDED-WEAR LENSES

The therapeutic need for a contact lens for visual rehabilitation of an aphake is markedly diminished. Even with the explosive influence of the intra-ocular lens in today's management of aphakia, there still exists a real need for an extended-wear lens that can rival the intra-ocular lens for visual effectiveness and safety. Of the 1 million cataract operations performed annually in the United States, only about 40% to 50% had intra-ocular lens implants in 1981, with many of the remainder consisting of one-eyed patients, patients with corneal and anterior segment disorders, advanced diabetes or glaucoma,

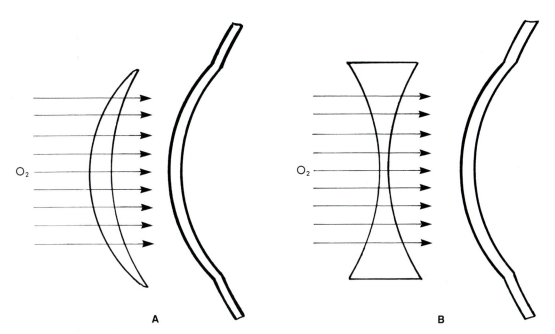

A   B

Fig 33-6 ■ Equivalent oxygen performance (EOP) represents the total amount of oxygen passing through the entire contact lens. **A,** EOP of a plus lens, which is thicker in the center. **B,** EOP of a minus lens, which is thicker in the periphery.

and a host of other absolute and relative contraindications. Today 95% of such cataract procedures will be given an intra-ocular lens. Yet there is still a group of patients in whom the extended-wear lens offers an alternative to the hazards of wearing aphakic glasses.

Considerations for the aphakic person are different from those for the myope. Usually the aphakic patient is much older, with poor tear function and inadequate tear constituents. In addition, slight tremors of the hands and poorer visual acuity may make insertion and removal more difficult for the elderly. The aphakic lens is usually three times thicker than the myope's lens, and it transmits less oxygen. Studies by Korb, however, have shown that the cornea of an aphakic requires only half as much oxygen as that of a phakic individual. Thus one may get by with a lens that is not so oxygen-permeable for aphakia.

Success for extended-wear lenses is enhanced in aphakia with careful selection of patients. The following persons are best suited to the lenses:

1. Poor sleepers who wake up several times during the night
2. Persons who are previously adapted
3. Persons with good tear production
4. Persons with low-power aphakic prescriptions so that the lens can be made thinner centrally.

COMMENT. Aphakic persons have a greater need for an extended-wear lens than a young myope does. Today their use is probably confined to pediatric ophthalmology.

In myopia, the problems are much simpler. The lens may be made extremely thin (0.035 mm). Generally, these persons are young, have healthy tear constitutients with adequate tear flow, do not have marginal corneal degenerative or dystrophic changes, and generally are alert and sensitive enough to recognize and report early signs of irritation. In addition, they tend to be more skillful in following the routines of care and being able to remove the lens in case of trouble. Wilson has outlined some of the reasons why myopic extended-wear lenses are much more successful than aphakic extended-wear ones.

Advantages of myopic cosmetic lenses over aphakic extended-wear lenses

1. Initial fit equals final fit
2. Easier to handle

3. Lens thinner and has better oxygen performance
4. Healthier cornea
5. Better tear constituents
6. Better tear flow
7. Less prone to infection
8. Fewer failures with selected patients

PATIENT SELECTION

For myopic extended-wear lenses our first choice for patients are those who have already been soft contact lens wearers. These patients are well motivated, know how to take care of soft lenses, and are most appreciative of the minimal care requirements for extended-wear lenses. They are also so indoctrinated with the care of contact lenses that they are not likely to forget the care routines once fitted. In the event of irritability from any source, such as fitting change, dust, or foreign body, they are usually sufficiently aware of how to remove the lenses.

Other persons suitable for myopic extended-wear lenses are those that have some hand abnormality or medical condition that makes putting on and taking off a pair of spectacles a real chore. We have seen patients with multiple sclerosis who have almost injured their eyes when putting on spectacles.

There are three types of patients who may develop problems with extended-wear lenses:

1. Dry-eyed patients
2. Patients with lid-margin disease
3. Patients with ocular infections

The eyes dry more frequently during sleep and may cause more of a problem with extended-wear lenses than with daily-wear lenses. If mild, this may be overcome by the use of artificial tears. If unmanageable, it indicates that extended-wear lenses should be discontinued.

Nocturnal lagophthalmos or lagophthalmos occurring after ptosis or blepharoplasty surgery may result in drying. Dry climates such as in Arizona may further produce a problem and compromise extended-wear fitting.

Blepharitis or meibomianitis may also compromise extended-wear lenses, since *Staphylococcus*, frequently a causative organism, may produce conjunctivitis, keratitis, and corneal ulceration. Extended wear can be undertaken only when the lid margins are clear.

COMMENT. Evaporation of water from a hydrogel lens is common in an arid environment. Places like Arizona, the interior of an automobile, some older office buildings and schools, and so on can cause the anterior surface of a lens to lose some of its hydration. Instead of having regular anterior surface optic characteristics, the surface becomes wavy and vision becomes variable. It is a common cause of 4 pm visual focusing problems.

SAFETY OF EXTENDED-WEAR LENSES

The safety of extended-wear lenses has been challenged. There have been many reports of infections that are so rampant that many practitioners have abandoned extended-wear lenses altogether. Some of this has been because of lens deposit formation that interferes with the oxygen performance of a given contact lens after a period of time. The most significant cause, which is corneal insult, has been small microcysts of the cornea that break down to form a punctate keratopathy. This produces a nidus for infection for any bacteria that may be lingering in the conjunctival sac or that may be adherent to the contact lens surface. In different centers corneal ulcers have been reported ranging from 30% to up to 70% of contact lens wearers. The most common ulcers have been caused by *pseudomonas*, *staphylococcus*, and *acanthaomoeba*. Even fungi have been implicated in disaster areas of scarring keratitis. In 1980 there was less than 3% of infections associated with extended-wear soft contact lenses. However, in recent years as many as 25% of contact-lens wearers have been associated with some degree of infection. This may be because there are many more soft-lens wearers today than there have been in the past. Policy statements have been made by many learned societies.

AVAILABLE LENSES

Up to now, there have been a number of lenses that appear to have a capability for extended wear, listed as follows:
1. Hydrogel lenses
   a. High-water-content lenses, <70%
   b. Ultrathin lenses, <0.05 mm
2. Silicone soft lenses
3. Gas-permeable rigid lenses
   a. Silicone-acrylate lenses
   b. Silicone resin lenses
   c. CAB (cellulose acetate butyrate) lenses
   d. Styrene lenses
   e. Fluorosilicone polymer lenses
   f. Fluorocarbon lenses

Any or all of the above lenses may be used effectively. One must learn to develop experience with one or more of the lenses, recognize the problems that arise, and learn how to correct them. The fitting and the selection of patients has to be ideal so that one can maximize the number of patients wearing extended-wear lenses and minimize the number of unscheduled return appointments.

Our preference for an extended-wear lens at present is for a high-water-content lens, such as

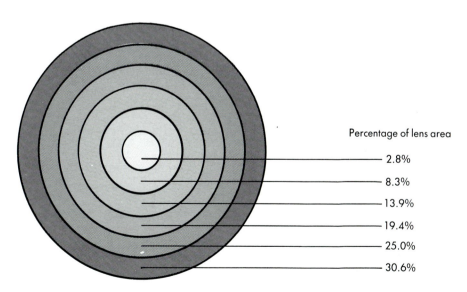

Percentage of lens area

- 2.8%
- 8.3%
- 13.9%
- 19.4%
- 25.0%
- 30.6%

Fig 33-7 ■ Relative percentage of the cornea covered by a soft contact lens. Note the high percent of the peripheral corneal cells, which may be embarrassed further if there is insufficient peripheral oxygen transmissibility. (Courtesy CooperVision Inc, Optics Division, Irvine, Calif.)

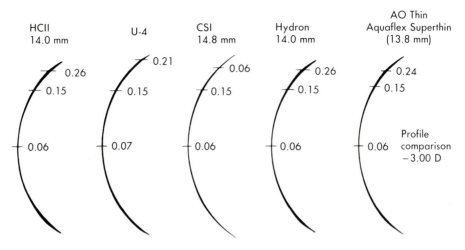

Fig 33-8 ■ Profile comparison of a −3 D lens. All lenses have the same center thickness, but the CSI lens has a thinner periphery.

Permalens, Sauflon, or Duragel, or the very thin lenses with 0.03 mm center thickness. Remember that one must be concerned with oxygen flow through the peripheral portion and not just the center of a contact lens. Fig. 33-7 illustrates the larger percentage of corneal cells in the periphery of a cornea. If the lens is myopic, in the higher powers there will be a thicker lens profile in the periphery. The CSI lens designed by Korb was essentially designed to provide a thinness to the periphery of the lens (Fig. 33-8). New molded high-water-content lenses appearing on the market today offer increased durability.

COMMENT. Although new systems of molded soft lenses may provide an increased durability to the lens and a reduction in cost, the ultimate achievement will occur when the material can be made resistant to anterior and posterior surface debris.

FITTING

Because lens designs, series, diameters, and base curves change so frequently, the practitioner is advised to consult the manufacturer of the lens of his choice for detailed parameter information.

Certain basic principles and guidelines to follow are:

1. Decide whether one is fitting high-water-content lenses, such as Permalens, Duragel, TC 75, and Scanlens 75, or low-water-content thin lenses, such as O_4, CSI, Cibasoft thin, Hydrocurve II, and Hydron, or whether one wishes to use the gas-permeable rigid lens.
2. Fit the flattest lens that will give good comfort and vision.
3. No matter how sloppy and loose the lens may appear, if the patient sees well and is comfortable it is safer to leave it. Ultimately there may be a tightening up of the lens.
4. Avoid fitting a lens too tight with little movement. Although with extended-wear lenses during daytime use one may safely get away with this, bear in mind that the buildup of lactic acid during sleep may tighten the lens and produce limbal compression.
5. In case of a red eye be sure to give adequate instruction in removal of the lens. Serious complications can be avoided by early lens removal.
6. Be sure the patient can handle the lens well and knows the care systems for looking after the lenses.
7. In aphakia, if poor vision is a problem, try to select a lens with a large optic zone. Frustration with one manufacturer's lens because of the optic zone or edge design does not mean another lens will not work.
8. In myopic extended wear, the initial fit is usually the final fit. In aphakia, there may be a tightening up of the lens within a week, and so the lens may have to be changed in fit.
9. The myopic lens, being thin, may drape over the periphery of the cornea and entrap

tears centrally. This may produce a plus tear film (Fig. 14-8) requiring more minus power for correction. If this occurs, a flatter lens rather than a change in power is required.

10. In power, the thicker hyperopic lens may stand away from the paracentral portion of the cornea, creating a minus tear film (see Fig. 14-8, *B*). This may result in 1 to 2 D more plus power required after the patient has been wearing the lens a week.

11. Lenses may give a pseudotight appearance on gross observation. One may apply, under slitlamp observations, light finger touch on the lower lid to displace the lens upward. The lens should move easily and drop quickly, an indication of a safe fit. The old rule of a 0.5 to 1 mm lag may not necessarily apply to the extended-wear lenses, which require only minimal tear exchange.

Characteristics of a flat fit

1. Excessive movement and frequent dislocation of the lens occur.
2. Through a dilated pupil, a retinoscopic reflex is crisp centrally and distorted peripherally.
3. There may be conjunctival injection.
4. There is awareness of the lens.
5. Visual acuity is variable.

Characteristics of a steep fit

1. There is no movement of the lens when blinking.
2. The lens does not move easily when one attempts to move off center.
3. The limbal vessels may be congested.
4. The cornea may show microcystic edema or even gross edema.
5. If the pupil is dilated, the retinoscopic reflex will be distorted on blinking.
6. There is lens awareness.
7. The vision acuity is variable and will change with blinking

MANAGING AN EXTENDED-WEAR PRACTICE

There are two basic systems in managing an extended-wear lens practice. Until recently, the majority of practitioners chose the method in which a single lens per eye is purchased, the patient either wears the lens for a definite period (such as 1 week) or wears the lens without changing it until the lens is sufficiently coated or problems arise so that a change of lens is required.

This is no longer an acceptable system in light of the number of serious complications that have occurred. An alternate method is to provide two lenses per eye initially and when the patient returns for monitoring, the unused one is inserted and the previous lens is kept to be professionally cleaned. This method may be suitable for the elderly.

The disposable lens, which is discussed later, is another system in which lenses are discarded every week or every two weeks and replaced with new lenses.

Once one has arrived at the initial lens selection either through an ordering system for diagnostic lenses or from an inventory system, one has to then decide on whether one will engage the patient in care systems for his or her, extended-wear lenses. We believe in removal and cleaning every week. Our studies on 386 lenses showed that lenses with no cleaning lasted on the average 5 months, lenses cleaned monthly or every 2 months lasted 9 months, and lenses cleaned weekly lasted 1 to 2 years. We believe a clean lens significantly improves comfort, clarify of vision, and prolong lens life.

Our routine for a new extended-wear lens patient, where possible, is to select the correct extended-wear lens from our inventory of lenses. The patient is then started on a daily wear handling routine for 7 days and then reports to the office on the morning of the eighth day, having slept with the lenses on the night before. By going on a daily-wear routine first, the patient, we believe, complains less because of corneal and lid adaptation and learns how to insert and remove the lenses while being still sufficiently motivated. Myopic lenses are generally stable in fit and power and require no change.

At the 24-hour overnight check, visual acuity should be noted. A slit-lamp examination will evaluate the fit, the movement of the lens, and the state of the cornea. Careful attention to corneal clarity is important. Epithelial edema with a drop in vision can best be visualized by retro-illumination with a slitlamp beam. Stromal edema can best be detected by wrinking of Descemet's membrane, particularly in the central part of the cornea. The limbal vasculature should be examined carefully.

Once the patient is examined on the eighth day after overnight wear, he is permitted to wear the lenses for 2 weeks and visits us at the end of this period provided that there is satisfactory ocular performance of the eye lids. Lenses are then examined along with the eyes, and the patient is permitted to continue wearing lenses as long as he continues with the recommended care systems. Patients return at 3- and 6-month intervals. All are informed that we are problem oriented, and so they are asked to return, particularly if vision has decreased, they develop a red eye, or if the lens becomes uncomfortable.

COMMENT. The merit of keeping the lenses in as long as possible is freedom from hand and chemical contamination. But why wait until the lens is cloudy and the eye red?

Fitting of the lens

The best device to fit a lens is to use a diagnostic lens. Since keratometers measure the anterior corneal curvature within a 3 mm chord diameter and extended-wear lenses are 13.5 mm or greater in diameter, the K readings should only be used as a guide in lens fit.

After a twenty- to thirty-minute settling period, the lens is evaluated according to sagittal depth. If the lens is too loose, it requires a larger or steeper lens (increased sagittal depth). If the lens does not move, a tight fit, then a smaller or flatter lens should be employed (decreased sagittal depth). The lens must center on the cornea and move 1.0 and 1.4 mm for blink.

Signs of a tight lens are absence of lens movement, trapping of mucous and cellular debris under the lens, compression of limbal vessels, corneal infiltrates, and mild corneal edema. Signs of a loose lens are excessive movement with blinking or eye movement, lag with eye movement, conjunctival hyperemia, and centration that is easily lost.

CARE

The extended-wear lens should have some form of cleaning. Adequate cleaning followed by distinfection increases the life of any lens and in particular extended-wear lenses.

The effects of coating of a lens are multiple:
1. Vision is decreased, often significantly, in the aging process of the lens and in the aged.
2. The increase in the mass of the lens alters the heaviness of the lens and so it rides low. This is more predominant with the high-plus lens.
3. The adhering deposit produces an antigen, which in turns gives rise to giant follicular conjunctivitis.

4. With deposits there may be a tightening of the lens and thus a change in parameter. Vaulting at the corneal apex occurs, and so the power of the lens is reduced. A hyperopic lens requires more plus whereas a myopic lens requires more minus.
5. There is a decrease in the oxygen transmission of a deposit-ridden contact lens according to some observers.

A number of systems for cleaning an extended-wear lens available:
1. Enzymatic cleaning may be used. With high-water-content lenses there may be residual enzymatic activity in the lenses that may be mildly toxic to the cornea. We recommend reducing the enzymatic contact time to perhaps only 1 hour, cleaning with surfactant, rinsing well, and storing in normal saline solution.
2. Hydrogen peroxide, 3%, is an effective oxidation method that disinfects and also helps in cleaning the lens. The hydrogen peroxide penetrates the lens matrix, causes lens expansion, and loosens particles within the lens and on the lens surface. There are varying neutralization times recommended by different manufacturers.
3. Ultrasound acts as a catalyst in speeding up any chemical used on a contact lens. It also generates heat, which also accelerates the cleaning process. Currently we recommend the ultrasound cleaner manufactured by BPI,* a biphasic unit that is gentle enough to clean a soft lens without damaging the plastic. This is an in-office unit to rejuvenate old lenses. Home units for prophylactic cleaning are available. Our system is to use any surfactant cleaner and place the lens in 3% hydrogen peroxide with ultrasound, followed by a further 10 minutes in a weekly cleaner or enzymatic tablet for 10 minutes, followed by 10 minutes in normal saline solution (Fig. 33-9). Ultrasound cleans the surface of the lens unevenly. Usually deposits return after three months. Generally, we now favor replacing the lenses as opposed to ultrasonic cleaning.
4. A variety of surfactants for soft lenses is available. These agents solubilize the residue accumulated and mobilize the surface deposits that have accumulated. We have been especially pleased with some of the more recent

---

*Brain Power Inc., Miami, Fla.

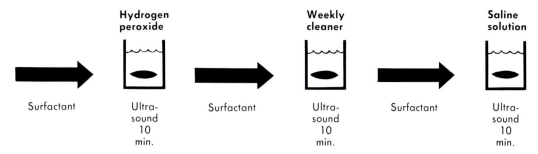

Fig 33-9 ■ Ultrasound method of cleaning a heavily coated lens through a system using hydrogen peroxide followed by cleaning in a weekly cleaner or enzymatic cleaner followed by purging with ultrasound in a saline bath.

all-purpose surfactants, which appear to give superior cleaning results for all lenses and reduce the need for the enzyme tablet.

Although the cleaning system is only minimal for extended-wear as compared to daily-wear lenses, there has been a considerable decrease in the adverse response, toxic and allergic, that so frequently arises from daily use of thimerosal- and chlorhexidine-based products. It is most uncommon to see this phenomenon with extended-wear lenses.

COMPLICATIONS AND PROBLEMS WITH EXTENDED-WEAR LENSES

The majority of problems that were initially seen in the early days of extended wear have, in fact, faded with improvements in lens plastic, lens designs, and better care systems for extended-wear lenses. With the development of high-water-content lenses, very thin lenses, silicone lenses, silicone-acrylate lenses, and the fluorocarbon silicone acrylates, all possessing reasonable permeability (DK) values and adequate oxygen performance, we have today reasonably successful lenses for extended wear. We also have a better understanding of who should and who should not use extended-wear contact lenses.

In fitting extended-wear lenses one should be alerted to the following possible complications. Some possible early complications are:
1. Blurring vision
2. Acute keratopathy
3. Diffuse corneal edema
4. Tightening of lens, and
5. Lost lenses.

Some possible late complications are:
1. Lens problems

   a. Protein, lipid, or mineral buildup (hazy vision, corneal edema)
   b. Lens displacement
   c. Fungus invasion
   d. Glued-on lens syndrome
2. Patient problems
   a. Corneal vascularization
   b. Keratoconjunctivitis
   c. Corneal edema
   d. Corneal steepening
   e. Patient dropouts

Early complications

The following problems are sometimes seen with extended aphakic hydrophilic lens wear:

Blurring vision. A decrease in vision and morning blur may initially be adaptive symptoms caused by corneal hydration in the early days. This can be tolerated for 1 to 2 weeks because it is often a normal adaptive system, but, if it persists, a lens change in either a flatter fit or a new material is required. This early blurring of vision may also be caused by relative dehydration of high-water-content lenses during the usual dry state when the patient is sleeping and may be helped by a nighttime and morning lubricating drop. The early manifestation of blurring may be fine vertical striae in Descemet's membrane (Fig. 33-10).

The most common cause of blurred early morning vision is the accumulation of debris and protein deposits in a mucoid strand that covers the lens. The mucoid accumulation rapidly disappears with blinking and is not a serious problem. It occurs more often in the contact-lens wearer who is over the age of 35.

Acute keratopathy. Acute keratopathy is a serious complication that can occur at any time

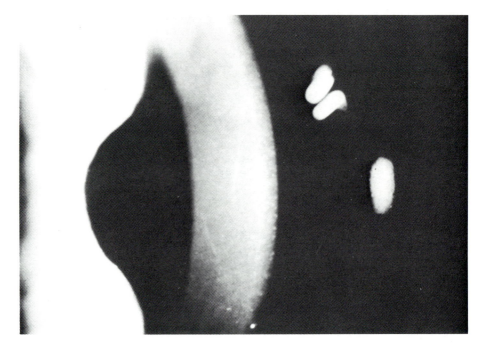

Fig 33-10 ■ Vertical striae are a frequent occurrence during first 2 weeks of extended wear. Patient should be observed to determine that condition does not worsen and disappears within that time. Recurrence after several months of extended wear signals the fitter that the lens has become soiled. (From Feldman GL: In Hartstein J, ed: Extended wear contact lenses for aphakia and myopia, St Louis, 1982, The CV Mosby Co.)

within the first 24 to 72 hours of wear. The cornea becomes edematous, with edema being present from endothelium to epithelium. Wrinkles may form in Descemet's membrane. The full diameter of the cornea is involved not just the corneal cap as seen with rigid-lens overwear reactions, this last being limited in depth as well as in diameter.

There is pronounced ciliary injection, extensive swelling of both upper and lower lids, and some flare and cells in the anterior chamber. The patient is often prostrate with pain, which is similar to a rigid-lens overwear reaction.

This type of reaction occurs in normal aphakic corneas with no vitreous touch or endothelial dystrophy. This reaction may occur in aphakia but is uncommon in myopia. It is also uncommon if suitable extended-wear lenses are used with high oxygen-permeability.

Diffuse corneal edema. Diffuse corneal edema is a reaction to the presence of a hydrogel lens without the acute congestive components. The cornea becomes edematous and steamy, there is some circumcorneal injection, vision is impaired, and the patient is uncomfortable. Under these conditions the lens cannot be tolerated, since visual performance is too poor, and in the milder forms corneal vascularization eventually develops. Again, this reaction is rare if lenses that are designed for extended wear are chosen. However, overzealous practitioners still experiment with lenses for extended wear that are not in the manufacturer's design for extended wear.

Milder forms of corneal edema are common. This may be manifest as:
1. an increase in myopia
2. corneal bedewings seen with retro-illumination
3. corneal epithelial erosions
4. an increase in the thickness of the cornea
5. polymegathism of the corneal endothelium
6. a dropout or loss of endothelial cells

In postcataract surgical cases in which we personally have attempted extended wear, we generally wait until the K readings are stabilized, the cornea is free of edema, there is no sign of post-operative inflammatory response, and the endothelium appears normal by slit-lamp assessment before insertion of the lenses. In the early years of extended-wear lenses we have at-

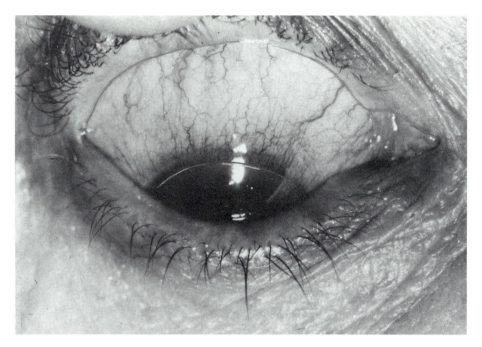

Fig 33-11 ■ Tightening of the lens. The lens dehydrated when the wearer was asleep, and it became immobile and caused limbal compression when he arose in the morning.

tempted large fenestrations of HEMA lenses. We also made a minihydrophilic aphakic lens with a diameter of 9.5 mm, but this lens centered poorly, was uncomfortable, and did not facilitate extended wear. Each attempt at modifying a conventional lens for extended wear was poorly received. Fortunately, with today's technology excellent oxygen-transmission lenses for extended wear have been developed.

Tightening of lens. The lens may become dehydrated during sleep, and this dehydration may lead to a tightening of the lens when the wearer arises in the morning. This tightening may cause limbal compression and a ciliary injection (Fig. 33-11). The incidence of contact lens adherence may be as high as 48% according to Kenyon, Polse, and Mandel but all lenses in their study began moving after 3 hours. A similar phenomenon may occur with RGP lenses. They may produce corneal and conjunctival indentation, SPK, and corneal indentation. This is more common with large-diameter lenses.

Dehydration may also affect the edge of the lens, causing it to evert. The turned-up edge may be displaced by the lid, which causes the lens to decenter and even eject from the eye.

Late complications

The following lens problems are frequently late complications of extended hydrophilic lens wear.

Protein and lipid buildup. Protein or lipid deposits on the surface of the lens occur anywhere from a few days to 1 year. Once protein is tenaciously deposited on the lenses, there is often hazy vision, an effective loss of clarity, and a change in the base curve of the lens (Fig. 33-12). Protein deposits may cover the lens even after one day of wear. They become a clinical problem if they create an uneven lens surface which in turn scatters light or presents a medium for the growth of micro-organisms.

Mineral deposits. Calcium deposits, seen as white discrete surface deposits on a lens, frquently grow in size. They may grow sufficiently in size to penetrate the pore structure of the lens so that when they are removed they leave large holes in the matrix. These holes in the matrix are often sufficiently large to permit bacteria to enter the substance of the lens.

Lens displacement. Lens displacement is a frequent complication in aphakia, since elderly patients often rub their eyes, especially when

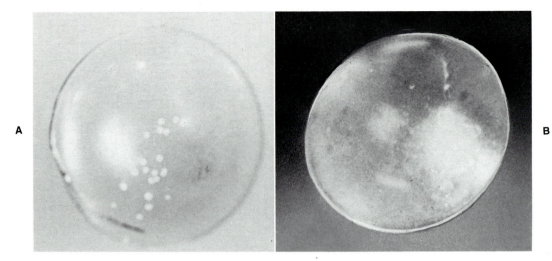

A

B

Fig 33-12 ■ A, Deposits on a soft lens. **B,** Protein buildup on a soft lens will vary with the duration of wear, the method of sterilization, and the tear composition and concentration of individual patients. (**A** from Stein HA, Slatt BJ, and Stein RM: The ophthalmic assistant, ed 5, St Louis, 1988, The CV Mosby Co.)

they wake up. The mechanical displacement of the lens often results in a lens that is wrinkled or folded, lying in the upper or lower fornix. Sometimes these lenses split when the eyes are rubbed, and occasionally they are lost. This problem is even more common in children. They require larger lenses (15 mm diameter) because they frequently rub their lenses out.

INFECTIONS

Infections are more common with extended-wear lenses than with daily-wear lenses. The susceptibility to infections is directly related to the length of time the lenses are worn. Extended wear for a month produces more frequent and serious infections than wearing the lenses for weeks straight. The risk of infection is so great that extended wear should be limited to one week or less. To reduce the incidence of infection:

1. Pre-select patients carefully, Reject those with chronic blepharitis, acne rosacea, dry eyes, poor hygiene habits, and recurrent chalazions.
2. Avoid contamination by water. Do not permit swimming with the lens in place in pools, lakes, rivers, or sea water. Lenses should not be worn while using hot tubs or jet spray baths. Do not allow the use of distilled water for the preparation of saline solution.

3. Restrict wearing time to a maximum of one week.
4. Patients who form adherent protein deposits to their lens quickly (in a matter of a month or two) should be placed on a disposable lens.
5. Check to see if the patient can fully close his eyes. An exposed eye with a lens resting on its surface is a hazard.

Vascularization of the cornea may occur even with the perfect patient wearing the perfect lens with a perfect fit. There is no method to predetermine who will develop this complication, so patients using extended-wear lenses have to be examined frequently, at least every six months, although every three months would be more desirable from the point of view of safety. Extensive vascularization of the cornea can occur in three months. Hypoxia is the cause of extensive vascularization. The cornea does not receive enough oxygen so the limbal vessels proliferate, penetrate the cornea, and bring more oxygen to the site. The growth of blood vessels may be uniform over the entire margin of the cornea or localized to one sector. It is more common superiorly where the lens is covered by the upper lid. It may be accompanied by an advancing nebula. It is essential that it be stopped.

What to do:
1. Inform the patient of the problem
2. Stop extended wear of lenses

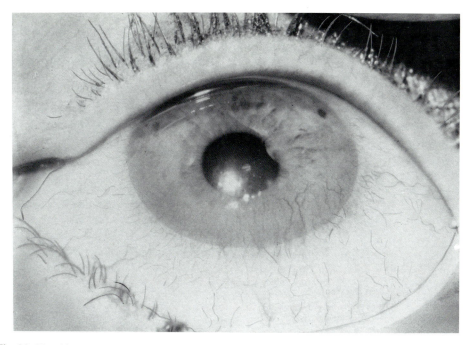

Fig 33-13 ■ Vascularization after use of low-water-content standard-thickness lens as an extended-wear lens.

3. Alternatives include
   a. Glasses
   b. Gas-permeable rigid lenses
   c. Thin soft daily-wear lenses

If lenses are chosen, the patient should be followed up every three months. Thin lenses provide more oxygen to the cornea than standard soft daily-wear lenses. The patient has to be seen routinely as this condition does not present with symptoms.

Corneal vascularization. Vascularization with today's lenses is very uncommon in our hands (Fig. 33-13). It occurs if one selects improper lenses that are not designed for extended wear or if the patient is not carefully fitted and the lenses are too tight. It may occur if there is excess deposit formation on the lens, which alters its parameters. When seen, the vascularization is usually confined to the limbal area but may extend either superficially into the cornea or deep into the stromal area.

Corneal vascularization is more apt to occur if:
1. The lenses are thick
2. Allergies are present
3. Extended wear is prolonged
4. Infection or inflammation is present

5. Chronic irritation exists in the form of a dry environment, chemical debris, cigarette smoke, or ultraviolet radiation from any source whatsoever

There are so many potential sources for corneal vascularization that it is no wonder that this is a common condition.

Marginal subepithelial infiltrates. Small round lesions occurring under the peripheral epithelium may occasionally be seen not only with daily-wear but also with extended-wear lenses. They may be small localized abcesses of *Staphylococcus aureus*. Alternatively they may be an allergic response of the cornea to antigen protein adherent to the contact lenses. Epithelial infiltrates have been reported by Josephson, Holden, and Zantos. Josephson has shown that lens-induced infiltrates may take up to 2½ months to resolve.

Many infiltrates are not infectious. They occur in quiet eyes. A clue to their presence is the inability of the eye to tolerate a lens for extended wear. For sterile infiltrates pain has been reported by one of us as a significant feature in identifying a bacterial infiltrate from a sterile infiltrate. Treatment may be simply to discontinue lens wear, which causes the infiltrates to fade away. Steroids may be useful; a short course of steroids for one or two weeks may be valid provided the intra-ocular pressure is checked regularly.

Minor corneal edema. Corneal edema is often undetected with the slitlamp microscope until there is at least an 8% increase in thickness as measured with the keratometer. Above this level early cases of corneal hypoxia can be detected by vertical striae.

Glued-on or "sucked-on" lens syndrome (tight-lens syndrome). The glued-on lens syndrome, reported by Wilson and associates, involves a tight, nonmovable lens that is associated with red eye (Fig. 33-14). Its cause is still controversial, but it may result from chemical or pH changes that alter the steepness of the lens. It may be relieved by the use of alkaline drops such as Balanced Salt Solution.

Wilson postulates a shift to an acid pH because of lactic acid buildup at night with consequent tightening of the lens and trapping of mucus and debris under the lens. The treatment is to culture the conjunctiva, remove the lens for a week, and treat the patient with antibiotics. After that insult, the patient should be placed on a morning and nighttime regimen of alkaline drops such as Blinks or Balanced Salt Solution. We have personally found this syndrome very uncommon in our practice.

Microcysts and vacuoles. With long-term use of extended-wear lenses, Zantos and others have reported vacuoles and microcysts present in the midperiphery of the cornea in at least 40% of patients. These may be clinically indistinguishable from Cogan's microcystic dystrophy. They may be a result of prolonged low-level anaerobic cell respiration and the resulting lactic acid buildup. There are thought to be inclusion areas of exfoliated desquamated cells. Less than 15 or 20 are probably a normal variant. They clear in time when the lens is removed.

Fungal infection. The classic fungal infection of a slow-growing infiltrate with small hypopyon and perhaps slight hemorrhage in the anterior chamber requires a rigid response in management. Usually the laboratory must be extra helpful in providing adequate fungal cultures.

FURTHER COMPLICATIONS AND WHY THEY OCCUR

1. At least 5% EOP (equivalent oxygen performance) is necessary for effective corneal oxygenation.

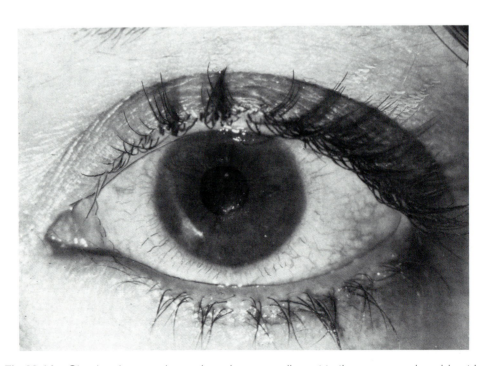

Fig 33-14 ■ Glued-on lens syndrome. Lens became adherent to the cornea and could not be dislodged causing corneal complications.

2. A large percentage of corneal cells lie at the outer peripheral ring, and consequently neovascularization occurs in this area if there is insufficient EOP for this portion of the cornea. This can be obstructed by the thickness of a myopic lens at the periphery.

3. Contamination of a lens and infection is more likely to occur with daily-wear lenses, when the patient does not follow the recommended manufacturer's method of cleaning and disinfection. Extended-wear lenses minimize the handling problem, and consequently, microbial contamination.

Despite decreased lens-handling, the actual frequency of infections is greater with extended-wear lenses. Moreover, these infections are apt to be more severe and are frequently associated with corneal ulcers. Infection is more apt to occur:

1. If there is water contamination of the lenses from hot tubs, lakes, etc.
2. If there are excessive deposits on the lenses
3. If there is a predisposition to infection — acne rosacea, dry eyes, chronic blepharitis, etc.
4. According to Allansmith, the deposits in extended-wear lenses are diffusely coated, whereas daily-wear lenses show peaks and valleys in the coating. The deposits in extended-wear lenses are flatter and result in a smooth refracting surface. Within 8 hours 95% of the lens is covered. These deposits can be up to 1 μm in depth. However, the oxygen permeability is not decreased.
5. Some authors (Binder, Allansmith) contend that deposit formation on lenses does not impair the oxygen transmission. However, Richard Hill believes that there is a progressive decrease in oxygen transmission as deposits form on lenses. Once the lenses are cleaned, there is an increase in oxygen transmission. Koetting has shown that the BUT (tear-film breakup time) is less than 15 seconds and a coating will develop on continuous-wear lenses and shorten the life of the lens.
6. Binder and Worthen have shown that prophylactic antibiotics are not necessary with continuous-wear hydrophilic lenses.
7. Hill has indicated that in areas of low humidity a lens loses 20% of its water content in 5 minutes. He has shown that if the water content is lower, there is a significant decrease in the EOP value and a reduction in oxygen flowing through the lens.

8. Farris and Gildar have developed a tear irregularity-determination test for dry eyes. In this a micropipette is used to collect a fine tear sample to be frozen and analyzed for its osmolarity content. He has shown that this is a more sensitive test for keratoconjunctivitis sicca than is rose bengal staining.

9. Because of the possibility of fungus infection causing microbial keratitis and ulcers, swimming with extended-wear lenses should not be condoned or approved even if swim goggles are used.

10. The initial cost for obtaining extended-wear lenses may be higher, but the maintenance cost is considerably less than that for daily-wear lenses even when one adds the cost of replacing lenses.

11. Because disinfection of extended-wear lenses is considerably reduced, there is less chance of chemical toxic or allergic corneal insult.

12. Patients with filtering blebs may displace lenses and create a problem. There is an additional risk of irritating the bleb and giving rise to bacterial infection.

13. Avoid fitting extended-wear lenses on patients who live in remote areas that are inaccessible to eye care.

14. In aphakia, large postoperative astigmatism may be a limiting factor unless the patient understands that an over-corrective spectacle lens will be worn.

15. All topical eye solutions and surfactants may be used with the content lens; ointments should be avoided because they blur vision.

THE DISPOSABLE SYSTEM

What are the advantages of the disposable contact-lens system? Firstly, there is a great deal of clinical evidence showing that bacteria adhere to contact-lens surface. This is more likely when the lens is coated and soiled. The work of many authors such as Mathea Allansmith shows that the coating continues on a progressive scale the longer the lens is worn. This coating is also aggravated by dietary habits: lipids may be more abundant in the tear secretions of some individuals.

Extended-wear lenses are a reality because there are a number of individual myopes who wish to become completely rid of spectacles. Radial keratotomy is popular with those who wish to rid themselves of spectacles completely. The disposable contact-lens system should be recommended to those individuals who are highly motivated and who take great pride in cleanliness and care and wish to wear extended-wear lenses. At this point in time the disposable lens seems to offer a valid solution to many of the problems associated with conventional extended-wear lenses. Disposable lenses are safer. The risk of infection is lower because protein build-up is cut off after one week of wear. The lens has minimal deposit formation because it is discarded on a weekly or twice weekly basis. In any six-week period, the protein that will deposit itself on a contact lens will be enough to create a risk situation for the patient. By weekly disposal this risk is eliminated.

Disposable lenses are less irritating. The patient is free from the effects of solutions and protein build-up. Also, the patient enjoys better vision. The optics are crisper because no debris accumulates and repeated dehydration of the lens surface does not occur.

Disposable lenses are more comfortable: a new lens is in place before the old lens, which has a life span of 7 days, has a chance to become spoiled. They also require less chair time. The lens fits in at least 70% to 80% of patients on a first fit basis. The parameter of one size fits all reduces chair time considerably for the individual practitioner.

No longer are patients burdened with the detailed instructions that are required for cleaning and disinfecting lenses in the other systems available. Patients fitted with disposable lenses have a much simpler regimen to follow.

Disposable lenses eliminate the possibility of toxic reactions to the ingredients in the care products that are required with conventional extended-wear lenses.

Disposable lenses also lower the likelihood of a patient developing GPC, which is said to be in part caused by an antigenic reaction to some of the protein that develops on the lens. Because there is minimal protein deposited on a disposable lens, the incidence of GPC is reduced. These lenses are also very useful for patients who have advanced GPC. Switching to a disposable lens minimizes the protein insult to the tarsal conjunctiva and so the GPC is gradually abated.

At this writing, only the Accuvue lens is available for use in powers from -0.50 to -6.00 D in 0.25 increments. It is a soft molded lens with a base curve of 8.8 mm and a diameter of 14.00 mm. It has a water content of 58% with an oxygen permeability of 28×10^{-11}. A minus 3 D lens has a center thickness of 0.07 mm with an oxygen transmissibility of $40 \times 10\ 19$ (DK/L). The Bausch & Lomb SeeQuence lens is a 38% hema spincast lens with a very thin 0.35 mm center, a 14.0 mm diameter, and a large 12.0 mm optical zone.

Each company offers its own form of manufacturing technology. What is most important is that mass producing these lenses is possible. Accuvue is manufactured by molding in the hydrated state unlike other soft lenses that are manufactured in the dry state and later hydrated. The pack lends itself to a simplified no-touch system in its manufacturing process.

Cost comparison

At first glance the disposable lens seems much more expensive than the regular lens system. However, the disposable lens user does not need solutions that can cost around $150 a year. There is no need for lens insurance.

Despite these factors, the cost of a disposable lens system is still higher than that of a regular lens. However, more than the cost of the lens has to be kept in mind. Disposable lenses are much safer than regular lenses. Drawbacks to the system are that there is only one base curve and diameter. Although one size is supposed to fit all, in reality one size fits most patients. There is also limitation of power correction. Only minus powers up to -6 correction are available. Plus lenses will soon be available. For the busy practitioner who has 104 lenses to dispense in a year per patient, a small room must be set aside to store the lenses. More time and personnel are required to handle the system. What is impressive is the technology that reproduces the lens with extreme reliability.

COMMENT. There is no doubt that the extended-wear lens of the future will be a disposable lens. Better fitting schemes and wider parameters no doubt will be introduced; we are impressed with the convenience that these will afford. We hope we will be impressed with their safety after long-term clinical studies have been conducted. The future of extended-wear lenses is bright because practitioners now are favorably disposed to extended-wear lenses.

Rigid gas-permeable lenses for extended wear

The newer gas-permeable rigid lenses enjoy the synergism of fluorine and silicone acrylate, which provides substantially increased oxygen-permeability and increased comfort due to enhanced in-the-eye wettability. The increase in oxygen delivery minimizes corneal swelling and its undesirable consequences such as epithelial microcysts, endothelial polymegathism, and endothelial pleomorphism. The better permability of these lenses makes them better able to eliminate hypoxic consequences than do soft lenses.

Moreover, with better dimensional stability, the rigid gas-permeable lens results in superior visual acuity. It does not dry out in arid environments and it has deposit-resistant features that ensure a clear optical surface. It is initially comfortable and after 1 or 2 weeks of wear, it is as comfortable as a soft lens. These lenses are quite durable and need not be replaced periodically. They delivery crisp optics if the person has moderate astigmatism of −2.00 D or less.

With hydrogel lenses patients feared damaging their lenses during removals. Because RGP lenses are more durable, patients are more likely to remove them regularly for cleaning. Thus a more flexible wear program can be followed.

Are there any special fitting techniques?

Extended RGP lenses are fitted in the same manner as daily-wear rigid lenses except that they are fitted flatter with the higher-DK material in order to prevent excess draping of the softer lens materials. In fact when first fit, it is desirable that the patient wear the lens as a daily-wear lens to ensure comfort and to eliminate fitting problems. If there is extensive 3 or 9 o'clock staining, the patient will have lateral and nasal episcleral injection and will not be comfortable or safe. Because the lens must roll with the eye during sleep it must be tight enough to stay on the eye during upward Bell's phenomenon (REM). If it is too tight, the trapped cellular debris under the lens will cause discomfort and lack of patient tolerance. If it is too loose, it will decenter off the cornea when the eye is opened. The threshold for fitting errors is low and only patients with the best fits should be allowed to graduate to extended wear.

The greater the power of the lens, the greater the chance of 3 and 9 o'clock staining, so high myopes should be evaluated carefully before going on to extended wear.

What about comfort?

Even the finest rigid lenses do not have the instant approval and acceptance that soft lenses enjoy. They are rigid and do not have the flexibility or the hydration of a soft lens, which can drape itself onto the entire surface of the cornea. This lack of draping can cause fitting problems if there is any deviation from normal in the peripheral cornea.

The patient requires some time to get used to the RGP lens. In that period, which normally may be to two weeks, the patient may experience sensitivity to light, tearing, and an awareness of the lens. Soft-lens patients in particular do not like the transfer to RGP lenses. They must be highly motivated to make the switch and should not work in a dusty or dirty environment. The soft lens protects the eye from debris whereas the smaller RGP lens permits dust particles to lodge between the lens and the cornea.

Sensitivity to light can be minimized by tinting of the lens and by using ultraviolet-light-absorbing lenses. At times, the patient's sensitivity to light is really caused by flare and can be remedied by increasing the size of the optical zone.

Patients with allergies should be warned not to rub their eyes. It is so easy to crack a lens while trying to rub away any mild early-morning itch.

Signs of marginal acceptance of the gas-permeable lens

1. Increasing myopia in the morning. Usually this is caused by corneal edema.
2. Corneal edema, from microcysts of the epithelium to vertical striae of Descemet's membrane.
3. Ptosis, which is usually caused by lid edema.
4. Persistent conjunctival hyperemia. This is largely caused by 3 or 9 o'clock staining.
5. Excessive mucous accumulation in the morning. This may be caused by allergies or even by early conjunctivitis from any cause whatsoever.

COMMENT Gas-permeable extended-wear lenses have far fewer complications than soft lenses used for the same purpose. However, they are less frequently prescribed because they

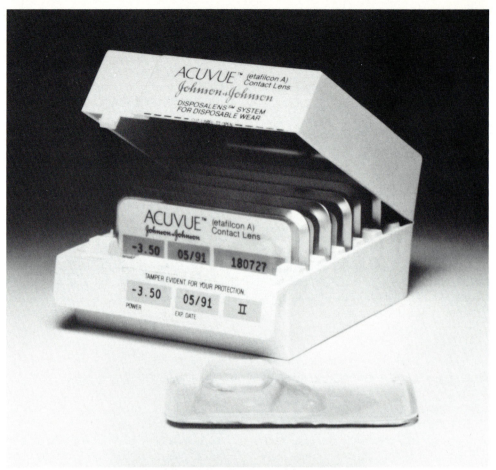

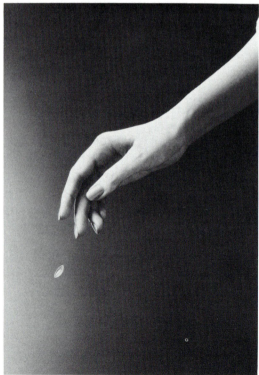

Fig 33-15 ■ The disposable contact lens. A revolutionary concept and method of packaging. (Courtesy Johnson and Johnson.)

require an adaptation period and patients and practitioners have not yet accepted a hard lens that rests on the eye for extended periods. However, the signs and symptoms of hypoxia are less with gas-permeable lenses and the frequency of infections is decreased with the rigid lenses. Also, rigid lenses have better durability, require less maintenance, offer clearer vision more consistently, and seldom cause vascularization of the cornea. However, soft lenses are preferred probably because of their promise of comfort—instant comfort, comfort at night without restriction, and the patient's freedom to work comfortably under dusty or brightly-lit conditions. We prefer the rigid gas-permeable lenses for extended wear although we probably prescribe more soft lenses because of patient request.

CONCLUSION

The thrust in this decade is toward the normalization of myopia. Radial keratotomy surgeons and orthokeratology specialists have created the large demand and have witnessed the technologic advance in a better and safer contact lens that can be worn on an extended basis. In addition, better care products for these lenses have improved to the point where extended-wear lenses are a feasible alternative to these other modalities for the correction of myopic and hyperopic refractive errors.

The prognosis for the young myopic person fitted with extended-wear lenses is much better than the prognosis for the aphakic person because of the thin lens centers, healthier corneas, and better tear film often found in myopic persons. Disposable lenses, now made sufficiently inexpensive so that they can be replaced weekly, have offered a new modality to the concept of extended wear (Fig. 33-15).

As lens technology advances, even more improved systems will undoubtedly be developed for visual restoration. Although careful monitoring of prolonged-wear aphakic patients is still the guideline of a careful and responsible fitter, the monitoring technique presently established may become more streamlined as confidence develops in newer extended-wear lenses.

34 ▪ *BANDAGE LENSES*

James V. Aquavella, Harold A. Stein, and Bernard J. Slatt

- ▪ *Therapeutic use of bandage lenses*
- ▪ *General principles of bandage lenses*
- ▪ *Other uses of therapeutic soft lenses*

THERAPEUTIC USE OF BANDAGE LENSES

The term *bandage lens* is used for a contact lens that is fitted primarily as a therapeutic modality, as opposed to it being fitted solely for the elimination of refractive error. In most instances the bandage lens will have plano (zero) power; however there are many situations when it is desirable to include refractive power though the lens is being used primarily for bandage purposes. Even if refractive power will ultimately be indicated, a thin plano lens should be tried first.

Although a wide variety of hydrophilic lenses is currently available, two basic manufacturing techniques are used—the spin-casting and the lathe-cutting techniques. The various hydrophilic lenses vary in design and polymeric constitution. For bandage purposes the primary concerns are the properties of flexibility and permeability, and the architectural configuration of the lens. These properties will vary with the observed thickness, diameter, and curvature of the finished bandage lens. Recently, collagen lenses or *shields* have been introduced and used both as bandage lenses and as drug delivery devices.

Indications for therapeutic lenses

Indications for therapeutic lenses may be divided into medical and surgical and are listed later in this chapter.

Fig. 34-1 represents an eye with severe painful bullous keratopathy after perforating injury with subsequent cataract extraction and glaucoma procedure. The eye is painful and there is no hope of visual rehabilitation. A hydrophilic bandage lens is a simple, nonsurgical option. A relatively tight fit with only 1 to 2 mm of motion will afford better pain relief. If unsuccessful, enucleation may be considered.

Fig. 34-2 is a case of Fuchs' dystrophy with secondary bullous keratopathy and a visual acuity limited to being able to counting fingers. In Fig. 34-3 we see the appearance of the eye with a hydrophilic bandage lens in place. Note the reduction in edema and the regularity of the surface. The acuity was only improved to 20/200, and penetrating keratoplasty was subsequently successfully performed. A therapeutic trial with hydrophilic lenses in such a case is often indicated because of its simplicity. In this particular instance there was no significant discomfort and the rationale for lens application was strictly related to an attempt to improve the acuity. A relatively flat fit will afford optimum acuity.

For intermediate and long-term use, hydrophilic lenses, as opposed to collagen lenses or shields, are indicated in bullous keratopathy. However, for short-term use in the event of an acute painful episode, one may consider the use of a 24-hour to 72-hour collagen lens that can be applied to the surface after fitting. The eye can be maintained with frequent instillations of artificial tear solution and daily application of a topical antibiotic (Fig. 34-4).

In Fig. 34-5 a case of aphakia with endothelial decompensation and epithelial edema can be seen. Fig. 34-6 shows the appearance of the eye with a thin hydrophilic bandage in place. The visual acuity in this instance was improved (with spectacle over-correction) from 20/200 to 20/60.

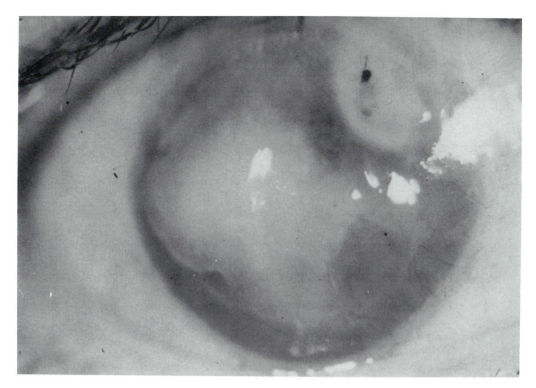

Fig 34-1

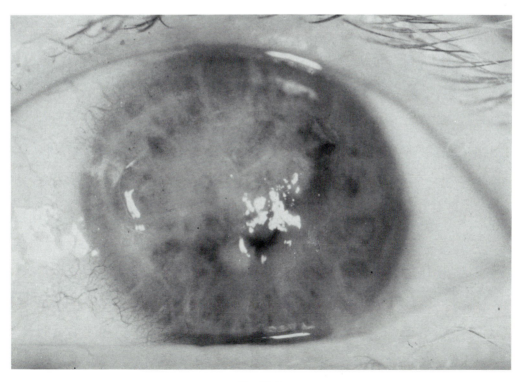

Fig 34-2

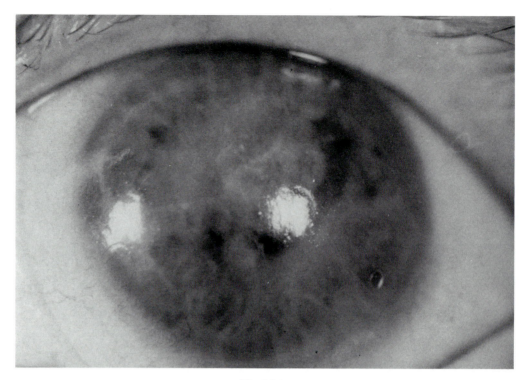

Fig 34-3

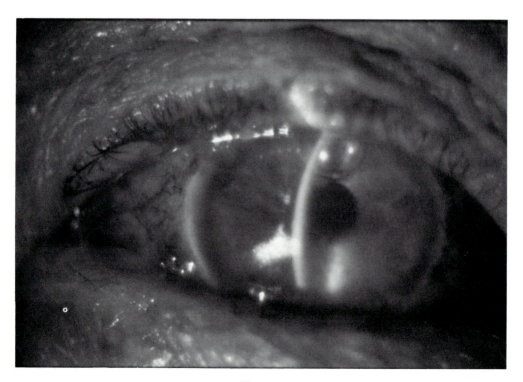

Fig 34-4

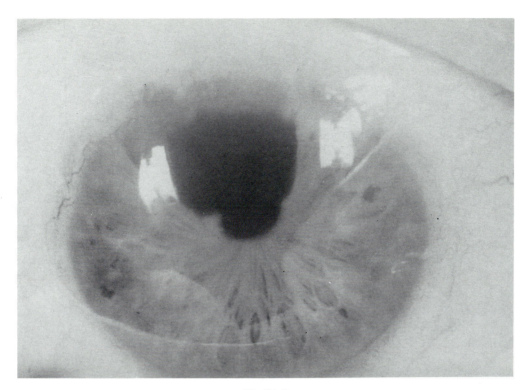

Fig 34-5

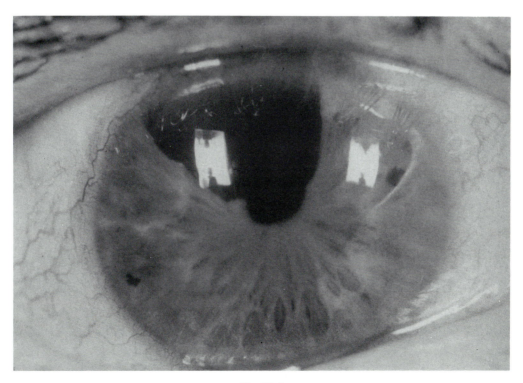

Fig 34-6

Our experience has shown that flat-fitting high-water-content lenses will provide best results in these cases.

Fig. 34-7 shows another case of aphakia with endothelial decompensation and secondary edema. In this particular instance the bandage lens was not efficacious in reducing corneal edema. Our preference in such a case is to begin treatment with frequent instillation of hypertonic saline solution alone. If the intra-ocular pressure is elevated, topical or systemic glaucoma medication is also used. Only when these conventional means have not resulted in improvement do we resort to a hydrophilic lens. We generally prefer the use of a thin, relatively high-fluid-content lathe-cut lens with plano power. The patient should be comfortable and, if able, may insert and remove the lens on a daily basis. Hypertonic saline solution is prescribed for use over the lens. Refitting and attempts at over-refraction are performed; if substantial improvement is to be obtained, it will usually occur in 4 to 6 weeks. At this point over-refraction using a K reading taken from the front surface of the hydrophilic lens is performed. The aphakic patient may then be fitted with a pair of aphakic spectacles. If an aphakic lens is used, the patient should be watched very closely. Because of the increased thickness of the aphakic lens and subsequently reduced oxygen-permeability, there are cases in which the eye will not support the use of the aphakic bandage lens but will do nicely with the thin plano lens system.

With current technology and the increased use of posterior chamber lenses in extracapsular surgery, a monocular aphakic eye is a rarity. Nevertheless, there are still some instances in which the anterior chamber is disorganized and the cornea is in a relative degree of decompensation. Some of these eyes can be rehabilitated with an epikeratophakia, others with an aphakic bandage contact lens. If there are signs of progressive decompensation, corneal transplantation may be unavoidable.

Fig. 34-8 reveals an eye with an old scarred cornea with the presence of a recurrent erosion. Note the irregularity of the epithelial surface indicated by the light reflexes. In fitting such a patient one should try not to use a local anesthetic so that the patient's comfort may be readily ascertained. One should have a variety of lenses available. We currently prefer the Per-

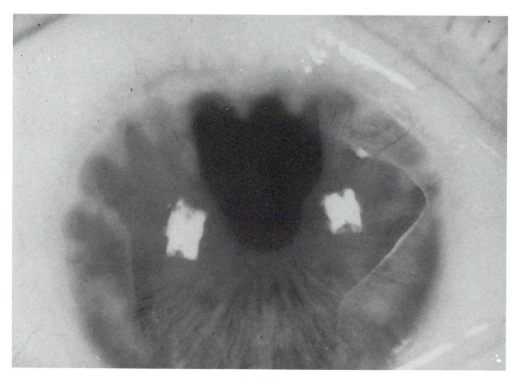

Fig 34-7

malens or Sauflon lenses. The CSI thin bandage lens is also highly desirable. On occasion a thin Softcon or Hydrocurve lens will work best. The principle in fitting the eye will depend on the specific location of the eroded area. Ideally, the lens should clear the eroded area, and a slightly steep fitting situation is indicated at least in the first few days. In addition one would hope to achieve a fit that would demonstrate only 1 or 2 mm of movement. Excess movement in erosion cases can sometimes result in increased discomfort. If the lens applied is very steep, 24 to 48 hours of increased stromal edema may result when one checks the appearance of the eye with the slit lamp. Consequently, a slightly flatter fit situation may be indicated. In most cases of erosions and abrasions the patient may be expected to have considerable discomfort periodically, even with the lens, for the first 48 to 72 hours. For this reason it is often wise to instill cycloplegics and to warn the patient that he or she will feel discomfort for the first few days.

If the lens has been used in a case of recurrent erosion, one should recall that 4 to 6 weeks are necessary for newly-formed epithelial cells to produce an adequate basement membrane. In many cases, if vision is adequate, the lens can be allowed to remain in place for 6 months to 1 year. We prefer to use topical instillation of artificial tear solution three or four times daily in such cases of long-term wear.

In cases of foreign-body removal, simple abrasion, or recurrent erosion, an alternative to patching the eye or using a hydrophilic bandage lens is to use a 24-hour or 72-hour collagen shield. This may be particularly useful if the patient does not know how to insert and remove a bandage lens and if it is difficult for the patient to return for follow-up. In such instances, the collagen lens can be hydrated and applied in the eye with a drop of topical anesthetic. An important consideration is that these lenses must be continuously hydrated in the eye with the use of artificial tear solutions, as well as with the application of a topical antibiotic, at least on a daily basis. With the biodegradation of the collagen lens, it is not necessary to instruct the patient on removal for there is a very small chance of complication during the time that the actual architectural configuration of a contact lens is in the eye.

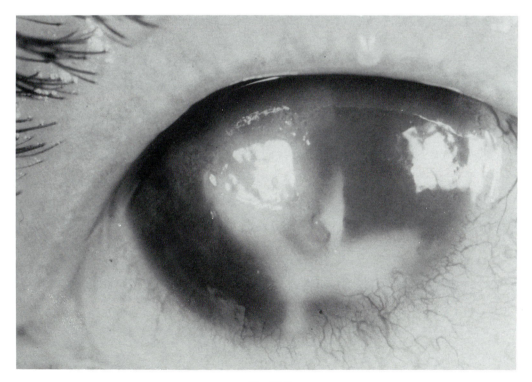

Fig 34-8

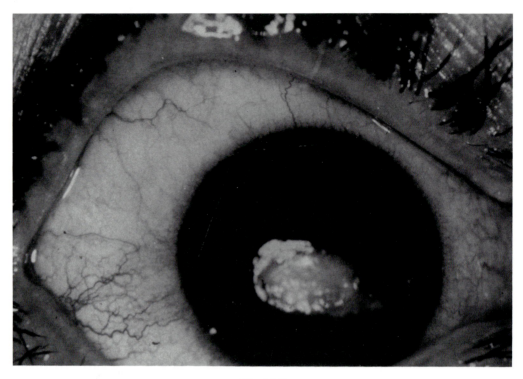

Fig 34-9

Fig. 34-9 represents the appearance of a 25-year-old patient with a combination of neurotrophic and neuroparalytic keratitis in a totally dry eye. She was fitted with a hydrophilic lens with parameters of plano power, 14.0 mm diameter, and 8.1 mm radius of curvature. There was no contact between the posterior surface of the lens and the ulcerated area. It was necessary for artificial tear solutions to be instilled every ½ to 1 hour. Prophylactic antibiotics should be used indefinitely. With this regimen visual acuity of 20/30 was achieved. One should realize that all of the dry-eye conditions are prone to secondary infection and inflammatory episodes. In addition, they are among the most difficult conditions to treat with or without hydrophilic lenses. Nevertheless in many cases the risks are relatively minor and the potential reward is great.

Fig. 34-10 shows the blepharitis that often accompanies keratitis sicca. In Fig. 34-11 we see the degree of corneal involvement in the same patient as seen in Fig. 34-10. With the use of a hydrophilic lens and frequent applications of artificial tear solution, accompanied by application of prophylactic antibiotics, the visual acuity as well as the physical appearance of the lesion improved within 2 weeks. Fig. 34-12 shows the eye after only 2 weeks of therapy. Lid scrubs, systemic antibiotics for severe blepharitis, topical antibiotics and steroids, and copious irrigation with artificial tear solutions are all necessary in these cases. Lenses used in patients with dry eyes should be disinfected and cleaned more frequently than when there is a normal tear flow. On occasion the dry-eye patients will develop deposits on their lenses in very short periods of time. This can be managed by the use of frequent friction cleaning, by the use of enzymatic hydrophilic lens cleaner, and often by the dispensing of two lenses for the patient. In some instances neovascularization will be a problem, and modified wearing schedules may very well be necessary. In all instances one should eliminate the environmental conditions that may result in further drying.

Punctum occlusion, moist chamber goggles or devices, and ocular inserts may also be indicated as part of a comprehensive therapeutic plan. More recently, ocular inserts composed of collagen have been advocated. These devices last for 24 to 72 hours, and slowly biodegrade re-

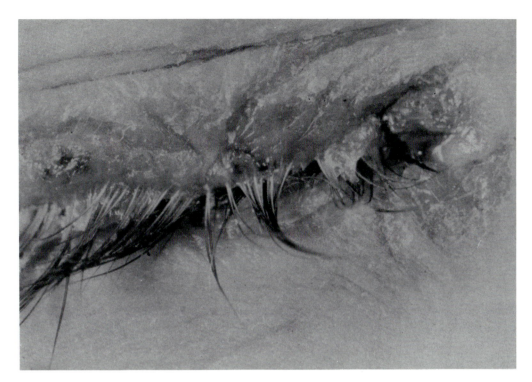

Fig 34-10

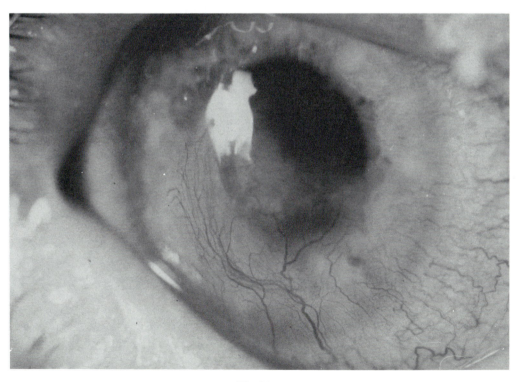

Fig 34-11

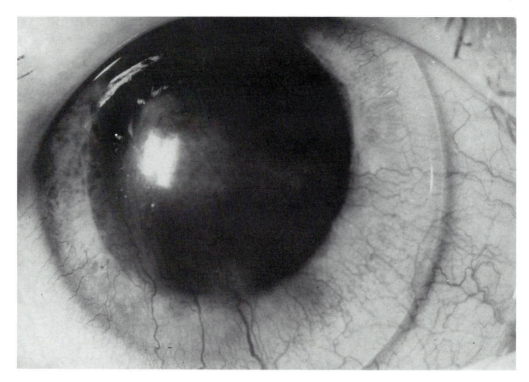

Fig 34-12

leasing a collagenous film over the entire ocular surface. In addition, the devices act as a reservoir for absorption of artificial tear solutions, which are instilled into the eye in conjunction with the collagen insert. Thus, a combined delivery system will often result in a significantly reduced need for artificial tear solution application. The introduction of low-cost ultrasound humidification has been a boon to the dry-eye population, particularly those who have been fitted with hydrophilic bandage lenses. Environmental humidification is an extremely important adjunct to the dry-eye therapy.

Fig. 34-13 shows an acutely inflamed eye with marginal ulceration. This lesion was very painful and was believed to be nonherpetic. The condition responded quickly to treatment with a hydrophilic bandage and topical instillation of both antibiotics and steroids. The ability of the hydrophilic lens to ensure all-over wetting in such irregular lesions is paramount in the therapeutic efficacy. A large-diameter lens to bridge the lesion will be comfortable.

Fig. 34-14 shows the appearance of an eye with severe marginal degeneration that is being treated with a thin lens. Note the serpiginous peripheral ulceration. Not all of these cases respond to hydrophilic lens therapy, but the use of the lens combined with other therapeutic modalities is often extremely helpful.

Fig. 34-15 shows an eye with exposure keratitis with the inferior lateral third of the cornea severely affected. The lesions responded rapidly to application of a hydrophilic lens and topical administration of antibiotics and steroids. A partial lateral tarsorrhapy was performed after the inflammation had subsided. Very often a partial lateral tarsorrhaphy will be helpful in maintaining seating and hydration of the hydrophilic lens. Without proper lid action it is difficult for the lens to be maintained in its proper position and there is a greater tendency for the lens to dry.

Fig. 34-16 shows a rather extensive recurrent erosion. In treating such lesions with hydrophilic bandage lenses, it is often wise to obtain cycloplegia to prevent the development of secondary ciliary spasm. Large, rather tight lenses to relieve pain are preferred.

In treating recurrent erosion, if traditional collagen shields and hydrophilic bandage lenses have failed, one may use 12-hour collagen

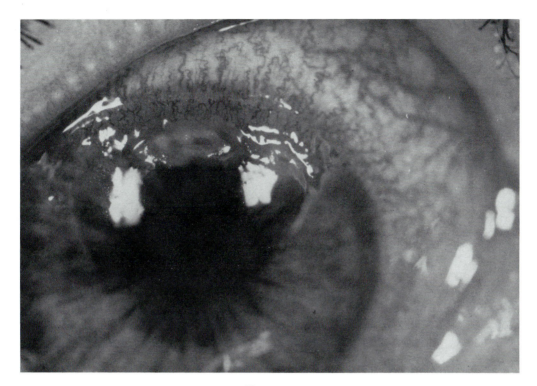

Fig 34-13

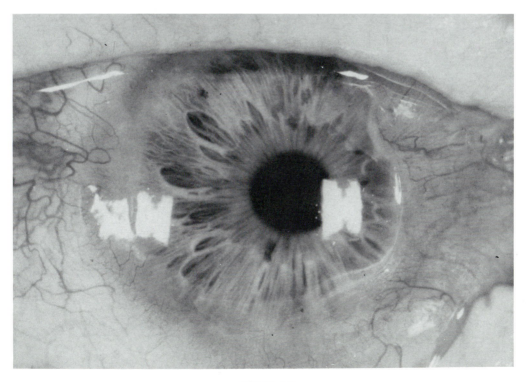

Fig 34-14

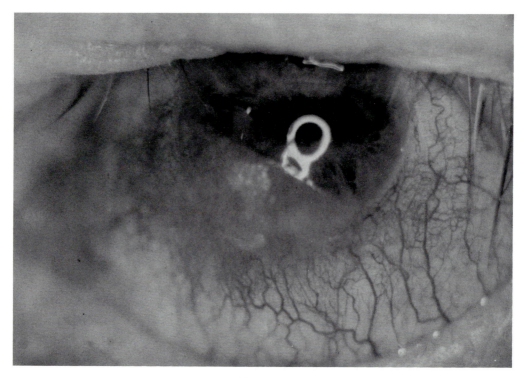

Fig 34-15

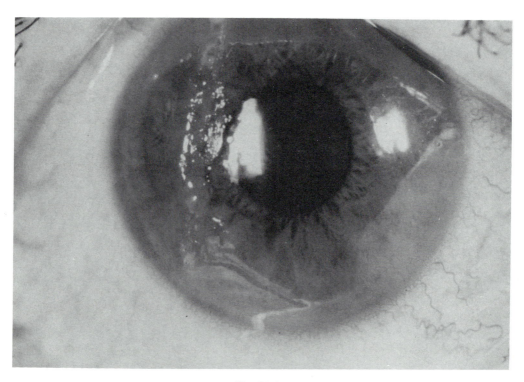

Fig 34-16

shields placed on the eye, and held in place by an overlying hydrophilic bandage lens. This will ensure that the collagenous material is in contact with the corneal epithelium for a longer period of time. When bandage lenses of all sorts have not proved efficacious, one may have to resort to micropuncture of Bowman's membrane, or superficial keratectomy in which the basement membrane is totally excised.

In Fig. 34-17 we see an almost totally opaque cornea as the result of an alkaline burn. However, the central corneal area is very thin and irregular and the application of the hydrophilic bandage lens improved the acuity from seeing hand motions to 20/80. Collagen shields have been very helpful in treatment of acute alkaline burns. Shields soaked in antibiotics and steroids can be applied to the corneal surface in the acute phase. Reapplication or the use of longer-acting shields will eliminate the need for very frequent topical medication with antibiotics, and steroids may be helpful in preventing opacification of the cornea.

Fig. 34-18 demonstrates the use of a hydrophilic bandage lens in a patient who had an excision of a hypertrophic filtering bleb. A partial peripheral keratectomy was necessary, and the application of a bandage lens resulted in a comfortable eye during the post-operative period. The lens can be applied on the operating table.

Fig. 34-19 demonstrates the use of a hydrophilic bandage lens in a case of spastic entropion with secondary corneal ulceration. Although surgical intervention is certainly indicated to restore the normal function of the lower lid, application of the hydrophilic bandage assists in obtainment of a comfortable eye until the surgery can be performed.

In cases in which a spastic entropion has been corrected surgically, the application of a collagen shield to the eye will restore epithelial integrity in a short period of time. This same concept indicates the use of collagen lenses or shields on the operating table following vitrectomy and retinal detachment procedures in which the corneal epithelium has been removed. The application of a 24-hour to 72-hour collagen shield will assist in the re-epithelialization process.

Fig. 34-20 illustrates the use of a hydrophilic bandage lens before keratoplasty. This patient, with a severe alkaline burn, had a very irregular calcified corneal surface with secondary inflammation and blepharospasm. The application of a hydrophilic lens combined with topical medi-

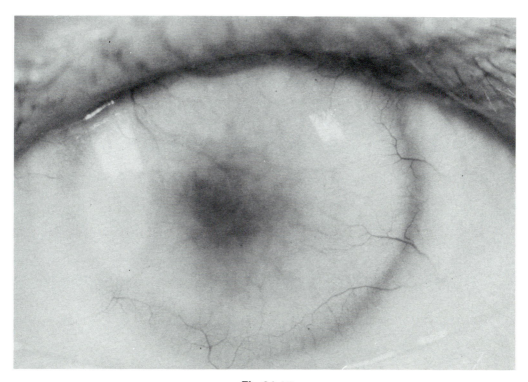

Fig 34-17

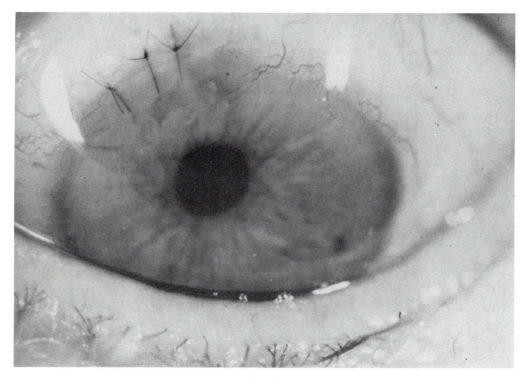

Fig 34-18

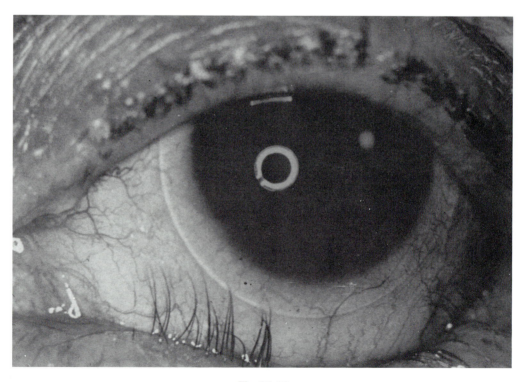

Fig 34-19

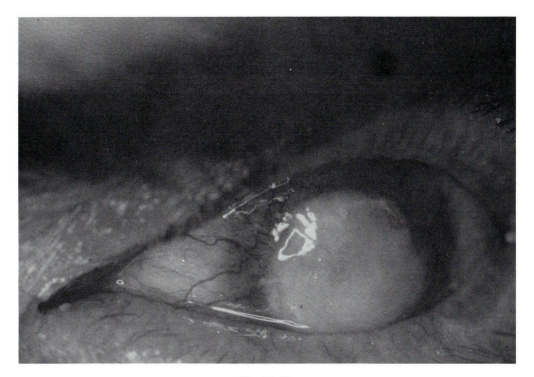

Fig 34-20

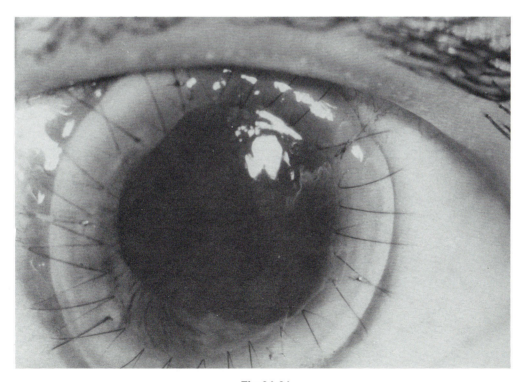

Fig 34-21

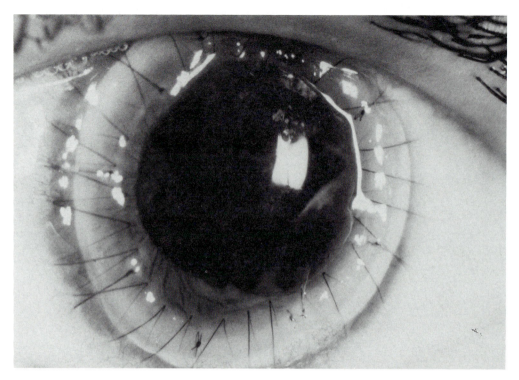

Fig 34-22

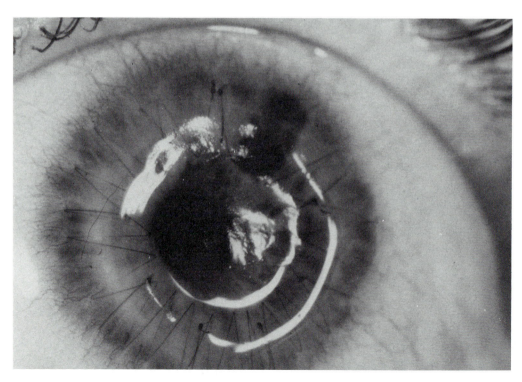

Fig 34-23

cation helped to quiet the eye before surgery.

Fig. 34-21 shows the post-operative appearance of a 10 mm graft in a case of keratoconus. Notice the paracentral area of corneal drying as a result of inadequate wetting of the surface associated with the plateau effect produced by the running monofilament nylon sutures.

In Fig. 34-22 we see the same case after application of a large lens ensuring the adequate wetting of the surface of the graft.

Fig. 34-23 shows another post-operative corneal graft in which the application of a hydrophilic lens has assisted in obtainment of proper wetting of the surface of the graft. The high-water-content, thin lenses are most useful in post-operative keratoplasty.

Twelve-hour and 24-hour collagen shields are now used routinely following penetrating keratoplasty to prevent desiccation of the remaining epithelial cells and to foster migration and mitosis of the cells to produce a more rapid re-epithelialization. The lenses are typically soaked in an antibiotic or antibiotic/steroid combination before they are applied on the operating table.

Fig. 34-24 shows the appearance of an eye after severe chemical injury with deep central ulceration and peripheral vascularization. The

hydrophilic lens was used both pre-operatively and post-operatively. In transplants performed on dry eyes and on eyes with chemical keratitis, the application of a hydrophilic bandage lens for the post-operative period assists in the preservation of the grafted epithelial cells.

There have been reports indicating higher incidence of secondary infection in corneal transplants treated with hydrophilic bandage lenses. Consequently, many corneal surgeons are advocating collagen lenses for use in the immediate post-operative phase. The use of topical prophylactic antibiotics with both collagen and hydrophilic bandage lenses is considered mandatory.

Fig. 34-25 shows a well-centered lens that has been fitted in a case of keratitis sicca. Generally speaking, in cases where it is important to preserve maximum visual acuity while the bandage lens is being worn, a well-centering lens with virtual contact between the posterior surface of the lens and the anterior corneal surface will usually afford maximum acuity.

Fig. 34-26 demonstrates a lens that is decentered inferiorly. Although such a lens may be perfectly adequate to control discomfort in bullous keratopathy, we should ensure that the lens

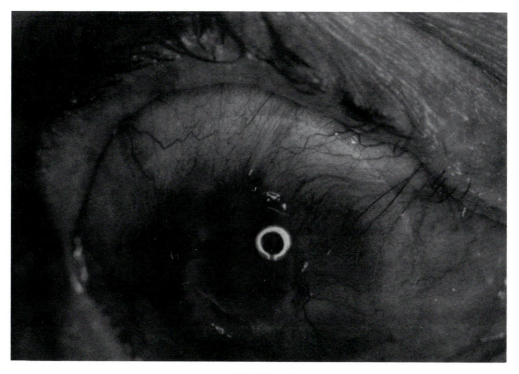

Fig 34-24

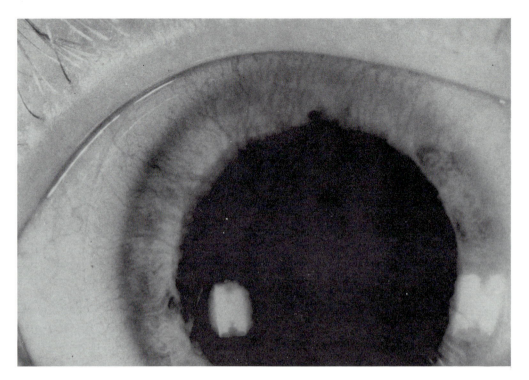

Fig 34-25

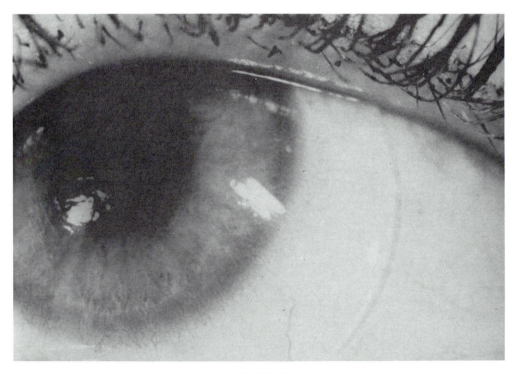

Fig 34-26

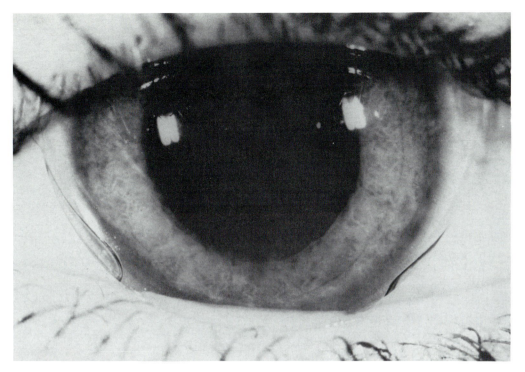

Fig 34-27

does not have a tendency to become displaced with a blink and with ocular rotations. However, in a case of recurrent erosion a lens that is loose may move excessively on the corneal surface and produce secondary irritation and occasionally blepharospasm.

Fig. 34-27 shows a lens that is so flat that its peripheral lip has become everted. If the edges of the bandage lens tend to flare, they can produce discomfort. It is important to inspect the periphery of the bandage lens with a slit lamp to determine that the lens is neither flaring nor gripping so tightly as to produce a suction-cup effect.

COMMENT. Another cause for an everted edge of a lens is that the lens was applied to the eye inside out.

Collagen lenses are available in only one lens size, having a 9 mm base curve with a 14.5 mm diameter. Although it may be easier to apply the lens in the dehydrated state, it is more comfortable for the patient to apply hydrated lenses only. Following a drop of topical anesthetic, a lens which has been hydrated either in antibiotic solution or in balanced salt solution for 15 minutes or more may be simply inverted on to the

ocular surface with the aid of a blunt forceps or with a spatula. These collagen lenses are extremely lightweight and are difficult to insert with a finger.

GENERAL PRINCIPLES OF BANDAGE LENSES

Bandage lenses are those contact lenses used for therapeutic purposes on a cornea to enhance epithelial regeneration and corneal healing. They should provide sufficient oxygenation to the cornea so as to minimally disturb corneal physiology. In addition, bandage lenses are used to provide ocular comfort and to act as a barrier to the cornea from the eyelids, lashes, and environmental conditions.

The corneal uses of therapeutic lenses are to:
1. Promote healing
2. Provide splinting over lacerations, perforations, and wound leaks
3. Provide comfort
4. Protect the eye
5. Improve the corneal rafters and improve vision
6. Act as a drug reservoir

Table 34-1 ■ Thickness of Bausch & Lomb lenses

	Plano T*	Plano U$_4$	Plano O$_4$	O$_4$ series (-2.00 D)
Thickness	0.10 mm	0.07 mm	0.06 mm	0.03 mm
Diameter	14.7 mm	14.5 mm	14.5 mm	14.5 mm

*Capital letters mean thickness; subscript numbers mean diameter.

Because the thickness affects the oxygen-permeability of a contact lens, the thinner the lens, the greater is its oxygen permeability. Since the 1960s and the pioneering days of Bausch & Lomb with the plano T series with a water content of 38% and the Softcon lens with a 55% water content, great strides continue to be made toward achieving a better contact lens with better oxygen-permeability and consequently providing a greater oxygen supply to the cornea. Commonly used lenses are shown in Table 34-1.

A comparison of the relative thickness of the Bausch & Lomb lenses is shown in Table 34-2. It is noteworthy that if a very thin lens is required the lenses of the plano O series have a center thickness of 0.06 mm. The standard O series are half this thickness, 0.03 mm, and are often used when an even greater amount of oxygen is required. They are however more flimsy with a greater tendency to wrinkling and edge rolling. If the standard O series of Bausch & Lomb is used, or the ultrathin series of other manufacturers, it is more practical to select a -2 or -3 D from an inventory set for better handling.

The CSI (Crofilicon) lens may be used as a bandage lens and has the advantage of uniform thickness throughout the lens body. It is available in a 14.0 mm diameter, three base curves (8.6, 8.9, and 9.35 mm), and in lower minus powers.

High-water-content lenses, usually 8.1, 14.0 plano, with 70% to 80% water, have an additional advantage in the therapeutic range by providing moisture to the cornea, and minimizing dehydration of the cornea in dry-eye syndromes. In addition, for every 10% increase in water content of a soft hydrogel lens, there is a 50% increase in the equivalent oxygen performance so that a 60%-water hydrogel lens, having 20% more water than a standard 40%-water lens, has

Table 34-2 ■ Commonly used therapeutic contact lenses

Lens	Content	Thickness	BC	Diameter	Polymer
Ultrathin:					
B & L-O	39%	.035	8.8	14.5	Hema
Syntex	39%	.035	8.6,8.9,9.35	14.8	Glycerol-methyl
CSI-T			8.0,8.3,8.6	13.8	methaceryate
Thin:					
CSI	38.5%	.06	8.0,8.3,8.6	13.8	Glycerol-methyl
			8.6,8.9,9.35	14.8	methacrylate
B & L U	39%	.07	(4) 8.5	12.5	Hema
			(63) 8.6	13.5/	
			(44)	14.5	
Hydrocurve II	55%	.06	8.8, 9.1	14.0-14.5	Hema/diacetone acrylamide
Hydron 04	38%	.04	8.6	13.8	Hema
Softcon	55%	.08	8.1,8.4,8.7	14.0-14.5	Poly (hema/vinyl pyrrolidone)
Higher water content:					
Cooper Therapeutic	71%	.24	9.0	15.0	Poly (hema/vinyl pyrrolidone)
Permalens	71%	.21	7.7,8.0,8.3	13.5	
			8.6	14.5	

2 times the equivalent oxygen performance at the same thickness. This factor may be extremely important in the selection of high-plus therapeutic lenses for bullous keratopathy of aphakia or marginal aphakic corneas in which the thickness cannot be sacrificed because of power requirements of the lens.

Collagen shields introduced by Bausch & Lomb are made of porcine scleral collagen (mostly type I although some type III collagen is present as well). The shields have been cross-linked so that varying biodegradation rates are available. The shields have an inherent oxygen-permeability of about twice that of a 55% water-content hydrophilic lens. But after an hour with the process of biodegradation as a result of exposure to proteolytic enzymes on the ocular surface, the oxygen-permeability of the shields increases exponentially. With the process of biodegradation, a fine collagenous biofilm forms to take the place of the contact lens configuration. The surface of this biofilm is covered with a tear film to protect the entire ocular surface. The therapeutic advantages of the collagen are thus protection and lubrication, both in the contact-lens format, as well as in the subsequent collagenous film stage.

Conditions that lend themselves to therapy with a bandage soft lens include corneas with broken epithelial surfaces (minimal movement lens) and corneas with intact epithelial surfaces.

Corneas with broken epithelial surfaces

Conditions in this category with which a minimal movement lens should be used include the following:
1. Recurrent corneal erosion
2. Painful bullous keratopathy with ruptured bullae (Fig. 34-28)
3. Corneal ulcerations (Figs. 34-29 to 34-32)
4. Thermal burns (Fig. 34-33)
5. Corneal lacerations with sharp, well-opposed margins
6. Severe forms of vernal conjunctivitis (Fig. 34-34)
7. Perforated cornea
8. Persistent epithelial defects

Therapeutic lenses may be left in place day and night for months. In particular, patients with painful bullous keratopathy are so relieved to have their lenses that often they are frightened to take them out. Such patients should return to the practitioner every 1 to 2 months for re-

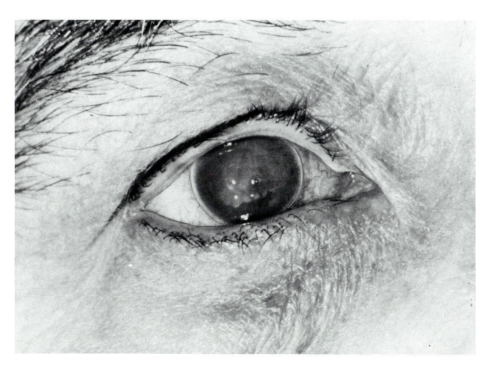

Fig 34-28 ■ Painful bullous keratopathy relieved by a soft bandage contact lens.

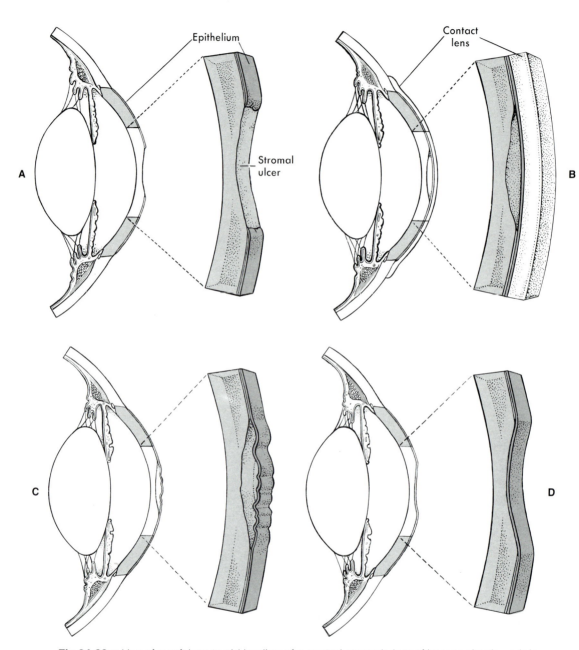

Fig 34-29 ■ Use of a soft lens to aid healing of a central stromal ulcer of herpes simplex origin, **A,** is depicted schematically. After the lens has been in place for some time, new epithelium bridges the ulcer site, **B.** When the lens is removed, **C,** the regenerated epithelium may initially appear as a flaccid bulla. Eventually regenerated tissue settles into the ulcer crater and adheres to the surface of the cornea, **D.** (**A** to **D** from Baum JL: Hosp Pract 8(8):89-95, Aug. 1973, and modified from Leibowitz HM and Rosenthal P: Arch Ophthalmol 85(2):165, 1971.)

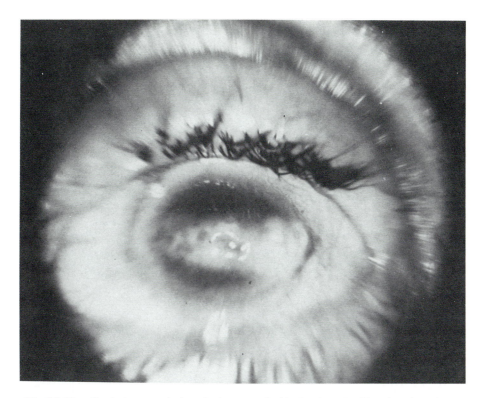

Fig 34-30 ■ Central corneal ulcer that responded to treatment with a bandage lens.

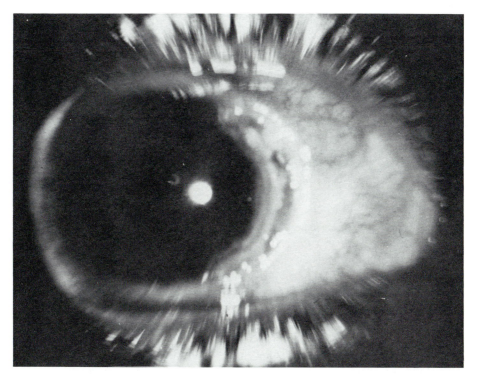

Fig 34-31 ■ Mooren's corneal ulcer. The soft lens may be employed temporarily until definitive therapy can be employed.

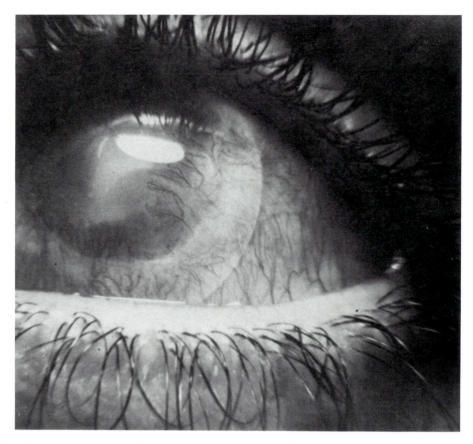

Fig 34-32 ■ Alkali burn of the eye. The soft lens provides a basis for the regeneration of epithelium to occur over the necrotic, ulcerated cornea.

moval, thorough cleaning, and disinfection or replacement of the lenses. Replacement is usually the most practical; otherwise the lenses become coated with mucous debris and mineral deposits, and may form a bacterial culture medium. In addition protein deposits can cause anoxia of the cornea or change the fitting characteristics of the lens by making it steeper. Thus, collagen lenses with a planned biodegradation time may be advantageous in some instances in that there is no necessity for the patient to return for removal of the lens by the physician.

A soft lens makes an excellent splint for small corneal lacerations and perforations until healing takes place. The corneal epithelium requires an intact basement membrane for tight adhesion of the new epithelium; the soft lens will aid in this formation. It is not uncommon for a collagen bandage lens to be used during the active phase of treatment of an epithelial erosion. If there are signs of distress from inadequate basement membrane formation, a hydrophilic bandage lens can then be fitted and worn for a period of 8 to 10 weeks.

Corneas with intact epithelial surfaces

A lens with normal movement should be used if the corneal epithelium is intact. Better vision is obtained and the movement of the lens aids in tear exchange.

Conditions that respond to a normal moving lens include the following:
1. Dry-eye syndrome (Fig. 34-35)
2. Keratoconus
3. Corneal dystrophies
4. Entropion, trichiasis, etc., to prevent lash irritation of the cornea
5. Neuroparalytic keratopathy
6. Ptosis with paralysis of superior rectus muscle (Fig. 34-36)
7. Aphakia with marginal corneas

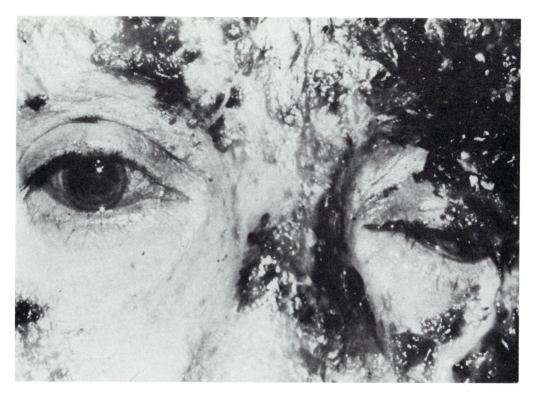

Fig 34-33 ■ Thermal burn around the eyes. The bandage lens can be used to heal the ulcerated cornea and prevent corneal exposure from lid retraction induced by scarring.

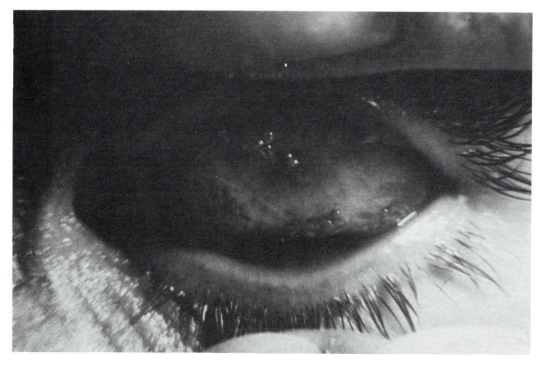

Fig 34-34 ■ Vernal conjunctivitis. Severe form with corneal ulceration requiring soft bandage lens for comfort and healing of the corneal ulcer.

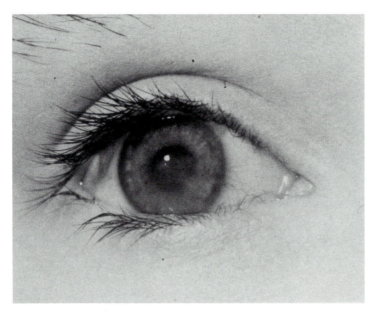

Fig 34-35 ■ Riley-Day syndrome. The soft lens protects the cornea from drying and erosion.

Ancillary medication must frequently be used with the soft lens in place. The medication must be water soluble; therefore substances that are soluble in oil, are in suspensions or in gels cannot be used. If steroids are to be used, it is important to use soluble steroids rather than those in suspensions, since the latter settle on the soft lens surface. Cycloplegics should be used for painful corneal disease, antibiotics for corneal ulcers of a bacterial origin, and tear supplements for dry-eye syndromes.

Standard drops containing preservatives are used. Freshly prepared solutions without pre-

servatives are easily contaminated. Preservative concentration in the presence of routine drop administration is not a clinical concern. All epinephrine and epinephrine-like drops should be avoided because they discolor the soft lens.

A plano lens is the most desirable bandage lens, since it is thin over the entire extent of its diameter whereas a lens with plus or minus power has a thicker center or periphery. In aphakics, however, with marginal corneas, or in cases of bullous keratopathy, where power requirements may be necessary, high-water-content lenses are more valuable in our hands.

Fitting the bandage lens

Bandage therapeutic lenses may be fitted with minimal or no movement as in the case of those corneas in which there is a broken epithelial surface. One may make these lenses steeper simply by increasing the diameter. The clinical appearance in the slitlamp is most usable in this determination because the flatness of a cornea with ulceration cannot be detected by keratometric reading. If there is lens movement in a denuded epithelial cornea with a conventional plano lens, a low-power lens with a known diameter and base curve should be selected. Antibiotic drops are often required.

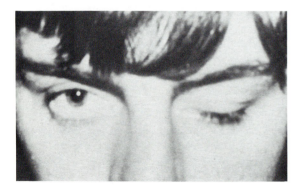

Fig 34-36 ■ The soft lens may be employed for corneal protection after surgery for ptosis where there is associated paralysis of the superior rectus muscle.

In those eyes in which the cornea has healed or the surface is intact so that there is a barrier

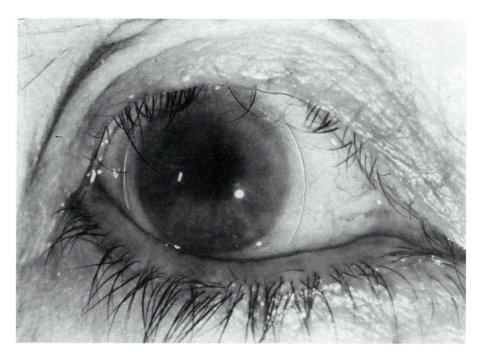

Fig 34-37 ■ Trichiasis of the upper lid after surgical removal of a carcinoma. The bandage lens protects the cornea from irritation.

protection from trichiasis or entropion (Fig. 34-37), the lenses should have some movement, (0.5 to 1 mm) to permit some tear exchange and transfer of metabolic products.

The fitting of collagen bandage lenses is relatively simple in that only one lens size and set of parameters is currently available. Since the collagen has a more acidic pH than do tears, insertion of the lens, even the hydrated form, will cause some stinging. It is advisable to use a topical anesthetic before inserting the lens. Lenses should also be hydrated in balanced salt solution with the addition of some topical antibiotics, or, for drug delivery purposes, they may be hydrated in the antibiotic alone.

OTHER USES OF THERAPEUTIC SOFT LENSES

1. Filling the plateau created by graft immediately after a corneal transplant.
2. Covering a disfigured eye (Fig. 34-38). Meschel has pioneered tinting of soft lenses as a shell and has produced irises on soft lenses. Several soft lens companies in Canada, Europe, and Japan manufacture colored soft lenses with black pupils that can cover a disfigured eye (Fig. 34-39). In ad-

dition a photographic process can be used to match the color of the soft lens with the iris of the fellow eye. These are referred to as iris-print lenses. Some practitioners have used epinephrine to turn a soft lens brown, but these lenses are not nearly as effective

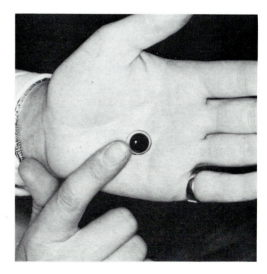

Fig 34-38 ■ Colored soft lens to cover cosmetically disfigured eyes. (From Stein HA and Slatt BJ: The ophthalmic assistant, ed 4, St Louis, 1983, The CV Mosby Co.)

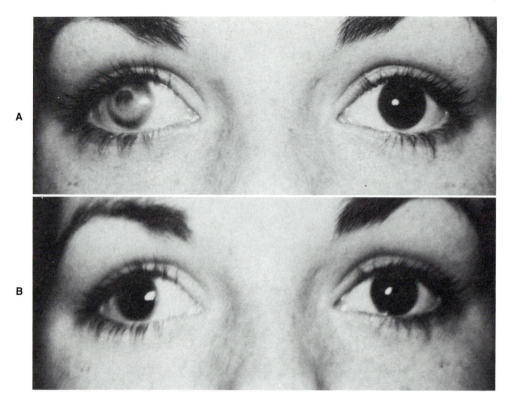

Fig 34-39 ■ Scarred, unsightly corneas, **A,** may be covered by a colored, therapeutic soft lens, **B.**

as lenses that are manufactured for this purpose.

3. Protecting the cornea during retinal and orbital surgery.

4. Used as cutaway pie for insertion of sutures in corneal transplants. Here a pie shape is cut away and used to splinter the corneal graft and maintain the anterior chamber while the cornea is sutured.

   COMMENT. A soft lens is not a panacea. Sometimes it does not work in conditions in which it is expected to work. Our best therapeutic use of the soft lens appears to be for indolent corneal ulcers and bullous keratopathy. The use of the soft lens is in many cases, a temporary solution to the problem of corneal disease and preserves future options of therapy.

5. The treatment of amblyopia in young children by soft lenses has been reported. A high-plus lenticular lens placed over the better seeing eye acts as a blurring lens and permits the amblyopic eye to develop its visual potential. The soft lens is used for daytime wear in children, and the parent is instructed in its insertion and removal.

6. Although soft lenses cannot usually seal a hole in a ruptured glaucomatous bleb, they may be used as an efficient mechanism to seal a leaking post-operative cataract wound and reform the anterior chamber.

7. Bandage lenses have only limited value in neurotrophic keratitis and mild cases of keratoconjunctivitis sicca. Usually they must be supplemented with artificial tears and antibiotics.

8. In keratoconus, a thin plano therapeutic lens may be used as part of a piggyback system in which a rigid lens is placed in front.

9. For drug delivery purposes, it has been demonstrated that high concentrations of Tobramicin and Gentamicin can be delivered to both the epithelial surface and to the anterior chamber by presoaking 12-hour and 24-hour collagen shields in the antibiotic solution for periods of 20 minutes. Concentrations achievable are higher than

those that can be obtained by the use of a hydrophilic contact lens or subconjunctival injection.

10. A bandage lens may be used over a perforated or ultra-thin cornea to which glue has been applied. The lens prevents the removal of the glue by the eyelid and provides comfort.

11. A delivery system for medication, using the collagen shield contact lens has been a major step forward. Its use in corneal ulcers and after cataract surgery indicates it is much more effective than infectious or topical medication. The medication is pulsed into the eye. The collagen shield is currently available in short duration (12 hours) and longer duration (24 and 72 hours) models.

35 ▪ *PRACTICAL PROBLEMS AND THEIR SOLUTION: CASE ANALYSIS*

Keith W. Harrison and Jean-Pierre Chartrand

The purpose of this chapter is to illustrate some common problems associated with contact lens wear. All cases cited here are patients who have been seen and treated in our office. It is our belief that one of the most important aspects of a successful practice is effective troubleshooting. The practitioner who is able to solve the patient's problems will not only keep that patient but also will receive word-of-mouth referrals. The unsuccessful trouble-shooter will not only lose the "problem patient" but also potential new patients.

PATIENT 1

22-year-old woman
Spin-cast soft lenses (Bausch & Lomb)
OD -2.75 U$_3$ K OD 45.00/44.62
OS -3.00 U$_3$ OS 45.00/44.75

Subjective complaint

Lens never looks clean, surface always smeary regardless of amount rinsed.
Enzyme cleaning of little help.
Visual acuity not as good as it should be.

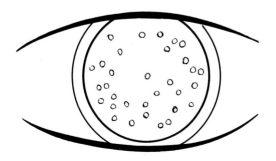

Fig 35-1 ▪ Fat lipids on lens surface. This type of "deposit" will move about during blinking and when the lens is rinsed.

Objective findings

Fit very good.
Lens has light-to-moderate accumulation of lipids.
Fig. 35-1.

Treatment

The patient had previously been using a cold disinfection system and, in our opinion, strict adherence was questionable.
The patient was put on a heat regimen using a daily surfactant cleaner (Pliagel) and the Barnes-Hind weekly cleaner.

Result

After 2 weeks of using this new system, the patient had no further complaints and the lenses appeared to be much cleaner. The patient also commented that the lenses "felt" cleaner than they had previously.

Comment

This case is important because it draws attention to the fact that all debris is not protein. Cleaners and enzymes that clear only protein will have no effect on this type of deposit.

PATIENT 2

76-year-old man with aphakia in right eye
Trans Canada Contact Lens Company, TC 75, extended-wear lenses
8.4 mm 14.0 + 13.75 K 43.50/42.50

Subjective complaint

The lens tends to coats over and becomes blurred and uncomfortable within 2 to 4 weeks, a process that necessitates removal and cleaning.

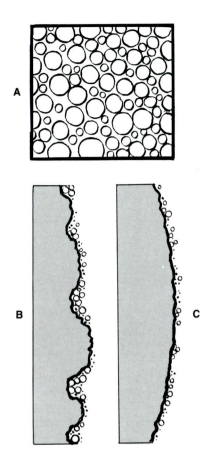

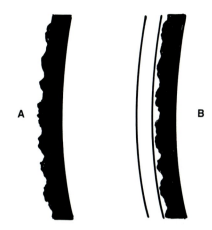

Fig 35-3 ■ **A,** Cross section of corneal epithelium denuded by keratitis. **B,** High-water-content bandage lens covering and protecting the epithelium.

Fig 35-2 ■ **A,** Pore structure of a soft lens (highly magnified). **B,** Cross section of the surface of a soft lens that holds debris because of its dehydrated state. **C,** Cross section of surface of a fully hydrated lens. The debris runs over the surface without binding.

time now. However, the effects of the drops are sometimes short lived. The eyecup used at night seems to be easier and more effective. Many of our patients use both. However, we now advise all extended-wear aphakes to wash with an eyecup nightly. We have also noticed that lubrication causes a reduction of tight lens reactions in our extended-wear patients.

PATIENT 3

27-year-old woman with severe keratitis in both eyes
Bausch & Lomb Plano T Bandage lenses
K OD 42.75/43.00
   OS 42.75/42.87

Subjective findings

Lenses feel dry and scratchy at end of day. Must wear fluid-filled goggles for sleeping.

Objective findings

Severe keratitis; dry eye.
Fig. 35-3.

Treatment

Refitting with high-water content lenses, TC 75 both eyes, 8.4 14.0 plano.

Lubricant drops twice a day onto lenses worn on an extended-wear basis, removed and cleaned weekly.

Result

Increased comfort. Virtually all drying problems were eliminated. There is no longer the need for fluid-filled goggles.

Objective findings

Moderately dry eye.
Tear-film breakup time 9 to 12 seconds, causing lens dehydration.
Fig. 35-2.

Treatment

Before retiring every night, he rinses for 30 to 60 seconds with an eyecup filled with normal saline solution.

Result

The period of time between cleanings increased from 2 to 4 weeks to 3 to 4 months.

Comment

We have advocated the use of lubricating drops for our extended-wear patient for some

Comment

Although generally it is not true that the drier the eye, the drier the lens required, the patient responded to a high-water-content lens as a bandage lens and was extremely pleased with the result.

The patient presented a hyperopic Rx of +1.00D over 2 years subsequent to this fitting and was given her Rx in the "bandage" lenses.

PATIENT 4

21-year-old woman
Bausch & Lomb
OD −2.75 U₄   *K* 43.00/43.75
OS −2.75 U₄   43.00/43.50

Subjective findings

Foreign-body sensation in both eyes, photophobia, and so on.

Objective findings

Foreign-body epithelial insult on both eyes. Many small fibers on and about the lenses.
Fig. 35-4.

Treatment

Lenses were removed for 48 hours, and the corneas were clear. Upon reinstructing the patient on care and handling, it was discovered that she was refilling her sample-size bottle of Boil n' Soak saline solution. The paper label was deteriorating, and the paper fibers from the bottle label were the root of the problem. This practice was discontinued and the problem was eliminated.

Comment

Inspection of the patient's care system, case, and so on can be of great value in problem solving.

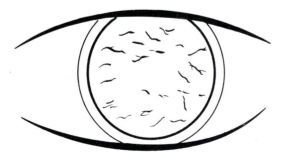

Fig 35-4 ■ Paper fibers on lens.

PATIENT 5

18-year-old woman
Rigid gas-permeable lenses, Boston material
Spectacle prescription
OD −3.00 −2.50 × 180   *K* 42.12/45.00
OS −3.25 −2.75 × 175   42.00/45.25
Lenses worn
OD 7.90 9.2 −3.75
OS 7.86 9.2 −4.00

Subjective complaint

Poor visual acuity.

Objective findings

Visual acuity with spectacles 20/20⁻ in both eyes.
Visual acuity with contact lens 20/30 in both eyes
Over-refraction of contact lenses was
plano −1.00 × 180 20/20⁻
     −0.25 −1.00 × 180 20/20⁻
The fit of the lenses appeared good and the corneas were clear.

K readings taken over the lenses indicated a 1.00 D flexing of the lenses on the eyes.

The center thickness of the lenses was measured and found to be 0.11 and 0.10 mm respectively.

Treatment

New lenses of the same specifications with a 0.14 mm center thickness were ordered.

Result

Visual acuity improved to 20/20 and 20/20⁻

The thicker lenses continue to hold their shape and do not mold to the corneal toricity.

Comment

The emphasis on these lenses in the rigid gas-permeable materials has brought with it an inherent soft lens problem: lens flexure. To fit moderate-to-high amounts of corneal astigmatism with gas-permeable lenses, slightly increased center thicknesses (0.03 to 0.05 mm) can be of considerable benefit. The effects of reduction of transmissibility caused by increased lens thickness appears to be negligible.

PATIENT 6

29-year-old woman
Bausch & Lomb
OD −7.00 U₃   *K* 43.50/43.62
OS −7.50 U₃   43.37/43.62

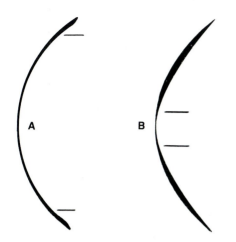

Fig 35-5 ■ **A,** Lathe-cut lens has a large usable optic zone. **B,** Spin-cast lens in the higher power range has a restricted usable optic zone.

Subjective complaint

Imbalance at near, blurring at the periphery.

Objective findings

Good fit, excellent centering large pupil 7.0 mm.

Treatment

U_4 lenses of the same power were tried and much the same problem persisted. Refitting with lathe-cut Hydron 0.06 lenses:

OD 8.4 14.0 −7.00
OS 8.4 14.0 −7.50

Result

Elimination of imbalance at near range and better general subjective response.

Comment

It would appear that the higher the correction with a spin-cast lens, the greater the peripheral distortion attributable to its asphericity. In this case the large pupil seemed to accentuate the problem, and therefore the larger, more defined optic performance of the lathe-cut lens was more satisfactory.

Fig. 35-5.

PATIENT 7

62-year-old man, monocular aphake
OD + 10.25 − 1.25 × 85 20/25 +2.75 add
OS − 6.25   20/50 +2.75 add
Cooper Permalens
OD 8.0 14.0 + 11.00   *K* 44.00/42.25

Subjective complaint

Patient wanted best acuity possible in both eyes, did not want the left eye to be fitted, and wanted to use present spectacles if possible.

Present spectacles
−6.50 sph +2.50 add
−6.25 sph +2.50 add

Objective findings

The fit of the Permalens was very good and need not be changed.

Treatment

A Permalens of the same fit but overcorrected to a +18.50 D was ordered.

Result

Visual acuity with the original minus spectacles over the lens gives 20/30 and reasonable binocularity. It seems to satisfy the patient and fit his needs.

Comment

Overcorrection and compensation of the monocular aphakic myope can save a great deal of work and aggravation. Upon the eventual extraction of the second cataract, the initial lens can be changed for optimum acuity.

PATIENT 8

24-year-old woman
Previously unsuccessful with Union lenses and Bausch & Lomb U_4 soft lenses, the latter being worn intermittently for 1 year.

Subjective complaint

All previous lenses caused irritation and inability to wear them more than 4 to 5 hours.

Objective findings

K OD 44.37/44.12
   OS 44.12/44.62
Spectacle prescription
−3.50 −0.50 × 5
−5.25 −0.50 × 180
Gutter dellen in both eyes
OD 11 to 7 o'clock
OS 1 to 5 o'clock
Tear-film breakup time 8 to 12 seconds

Treatment

High-water-content lenses (Permoflex) were fitted for daily wear.

Result

Initial results were good, but the lenses steepened excessively after 3 weeks of wear. Flatter lenses were subsequently fitted, and the patient now wears her lenses 10 to 14 hours daily with only the occasional dryness problems.

Comment

A high water content can compensate for the moderately dry eye and the transfer of enough oxygen to satisfy a moderately healthy cornea.

PATIENT 9

24-year-old woman
Wearing extended-wear Duragel 75
OD 8.8 14.0 −4.75 20/20   K 42.12/42.50
OS 8.8 14.0 −4.50 20/20   42.00/42.25

Subjective complaint

Excessive drying and lenses becoming "greased" over.

Objective findings

Some tightening late in the day because of dehydration; lenses coating heavily with oil and fat deposits.

Treatment

Refitting with ultrathin 38% H_2O lenses
Cibathin 0.035 center thickness
OD 8.9 13.8 −4.75 20/20
OS 8.9 13.8 −4.50 20/20

Result

Elimination of deposit formation and dryness complaints. Patient wears lenses for 1 week at a time before cleaning.

Comment

It is possible that in some instances for extended wear an ultrathin lens may be preferable to a high water-content lens. A large thin lens decreases the interaction between the lids and the lens.

PATIENT 10

58-year-old woman, monocular aphakic rigid lens, Boston II material
42.00 9.4 + 14.00 20/25 K 41.50/40.25

Subjective complaint

Constant irritation, gritty sensation

Objective findings

Recurrent keratitis
Lens low—inability to achieve lift even with flatter lens

Treatment

Refitting with a soft lens, heat-care regimen
Union Aquaflex
Vault II 13.8 + 14.00 20/25

Result

Increased comfort and wearability

Comment

Greater corneal coverage combined with the bandage effect of the soft lens can be of great benefit for the patient with a marginally dry cornea.

Gas-permeable lenses that fit low frequently cause severe 3 o'clock and 9 o'clock staining.

Note: This treatment was administered before the introduction of the Boston Equalens. It would be considered a possible solution now.

PATIENT 11

38-year-old woman
Spin-cast lenses, Bausch & Lomb
OD −4.50 O_3 K 43.00/43.25
OS −4.50 O_3 43.00/43.25
Lens age: 2¼ years

Subjective complaint

Injection in both eyes.
Six-hour maximum daily wear.

Objective findings

Mild injection in both eyes.
Visual acuity 20/30 OU fluctuating.
Lenses heavily coated, riding low.
Mild keratitis along lower edge of lens, arcuate stain.
Lids everted show early giant papillary conjunctivitis
Refracts −425 sphere OU 20/20

Treatment

Discontinue wearing lenses.
Steroid drops 3 times a day for 2 weeks.
Refit with AccuVue Disposable lenses
8.8 14.0 −4.50
8.8 14.0 −4.50
Daily-wear weekly replacement, AOsept disinfectant nightly.

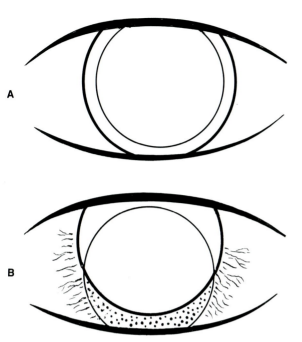

A

B

Fig 35-6 ■ **A,** Coated B₃ lens riding low causes inferior arcuate staining. **B,** New lens centering well provides good comfort, vision, and physiologic function.

Result

Visual acuity 20/20 OU.
Complete clearing of upper tarsus within 2 months.
Fourteen-hour daily wearing time
Fig. 35-6.

Comments

It is imperative when checking a contact-lens wearer that the lids be everted and observed. Some 50% of soft-lens wearers may exhibit papules of varying degrees on the upper tarsus. Old or coated lenses can trigger a reaction of this sort. These lenses (disposable) appear to reduce tarsal friction with the lens surface and lessen the recurrence of the giant papillary conjunctivitis through their frequent replacement.

In some instances, nothing will help because giant papillary conjunctivitis is believed to be an auto-immune response to the patient's own protein.

The most severe cases will always maintain a high level of muco-proteins in the tears. Other alternative therapy that can be tried is switching to gas-permeable lenses, preferably of a fluorosilicone-acrylate or fluorocarbon material.

PATIENT 12

32-year-old man
Lathe-cut soft lenses, Aquaflex II
OD Vault II 13.0 −4.50   K 41.00/41.75
OS Vault II 13.0 −5.00   41.12/41.75

Subjective complaints

Irritation.
Mild to moderate injection.

Objective findings

Keratitis.
Neovascularization from 9 o'clock to 12 o'clock position.
Good centering and movement.

Treatment

Refitting with high-water content lenses
TC 75
OD 8.4 13.5 −4.50
OS 8.4 13.5 −5.00
To be worn on a daily-wear basis

Result

Vessel regression.
Elimination.
Increased comfort.

Comment

Keratitis and neovascularization are signs of poor oxygen supply or a cornea with a high oxygen demand. Higher-water-content lenses are able to better supply the respiratory needs of this type of cornea. Close, long-term aftercare is required to maintain a patient of this nature. Extended-wear lenses can be excellent problem solvers when applied on a daily-wear basis.

PATIENT 13

31-year-old woman
Not presently wearing lenses
Spectacle prescription
OD −6.00 −1.50 × 90 20/20 K 43.00/41.25
OS −5.75 −2.00 × 90 20/20   43.50/41.50

Subjective complaints

Previously unsuccessful with both rigid and rigid gas-permeable lenses.
Very aware of the rigid lenses.

Objective findings

Ocular exam within normal limits.

Treatment

Fitting with large standard-thickness lenses
TC 50-S
OD 8.7 14.5 −6.25
OS 8.7 14.5 −6.25

Result

Visual acuity with the lenses is 20/25⁻ and 20/30
Binocular vision is 20/25.
All-day comfortable wear.

Comment

These lenses not mask significant astigmatism. But in higher refractive errors the presence of astigmatism is better tolerated. For this woman the loss of one or two lines of vision was acceptable. However, after wearing the spherical lenses for 3 years, the patient complained of VA more than at previous visits. Over-refraction of the lenses was $+0.75$ -1.00×90 20/20
                    $+0.50$ -1.50×90 20/200.

The patient was refitted with Ciba Torisoft lenses
8.6 14.5 −6.00 −1.00 × 90
                          VA 20/20 OU NVJ
8.6 14.5 −5.75 −1.75 × 90

Both distance and near vision are greatly improved and the patient is more satisfied. The older the patient, the less you can compromise visual acuity.

PATIENT 14

72-year-old man with aphakia in right eye
Rigid gas-permeable lenses, Boston material
43.00 9.2 + 12.25   K 44.00/42.75
Single-cut, center thickness 0.56 mm

Subjective complaints

Awareness of lens.
Some blurring of visual acuity when blinking.

Objective findings

Low-riding lens.
Visual acuity 20/25⁺ fluctuating.
Some greasing of lens.

Treatment

Refit with Boston Lens IV.
43.00 9.4 + 12.75
Lenticular minus carrier
Center thickness 0.40 mm

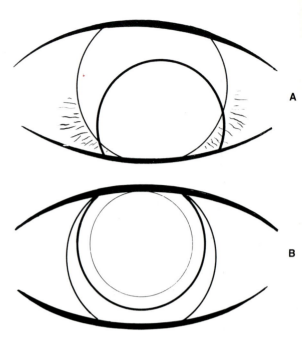

Fig 35-7 ■ **A,** Single-cut lens riding low causes irritation. **B,** Thinner, lighter lenticular lens centers well with the eyelid holding the lens. The lens also has a minus carrier to help the lifting action by the eyelid.

Result

Good centering.
Stable vision.
Better wetting.
Fig. 35-7.

Comment

In general, lenticulation of aphakic lenses is indicated to reduce lens thickness and weight. A minus carrier may help the upper lid to grasp the lens edge and promote better centering as well as lid sweep during blinking. A fluoronated monomer could be suggested where availability permits.

PATIENT 15

24-year-old woman
Hydron 0.06 soft lenses
OD 8.7 14.0 − 1.50 K 43.00/43.25
OS 8.7 14.0 − 1.75   43.00/43.37

Subjective complaints

Intermittent red eye for the past 8 months.
Some discharge in the morning.
Steroids used previously were of little help.

Objective findings

Fit of lens good, some coating because of discharge.

Cornea clear.

Some follicles on upper and lower tarsi.

Treatment

Culture and scraping taken.

Results

Cultures show inclusion conjunctivitis.
Tetracycline orally.
Sulfonamide II drops.
Replacement of lenses with same type.
All symptoms cleared within 3 weeks.

Comment

Red-eye problems are often not lens related. Herpes simplex infection is another offender of the cornea that may be mistaken for a lens abrasion.

PATIENT 16

39-year-old woman
Durasoft 2 lenses (Wesley-Jessen)
OD 8.6 14.0 −5.00
OS 8.6 14.0 −5.25

Subjective complaint

Poor visual acuity, especially for near vision.

Objective findings

Refraction −5.00 −0.75 × 180 20/20

                                              J-2

            −4.75 −1.25 × 180 20/20

K readings 41.75/43.75

            41.87/43.50

VA with present lenses OD 20/20

                    OS 20/30   NV J-4

Over-refraction OD −0.50 × 180 20/20

                                              J-3

            OS −1.00 × 180 20/25

Treatment

Refitting with Boston Equalens
OD 8.1 9.4 −4.75
OS 8.1 9.4 −4.50

Result

Distance VA 20/20 OU
Near VA J-1
All day comfortable wear in 10 days.

Comment

In many cases the astigmatic "pre-presbyope" will demand full correction for any residual astigmatism that may have been previously ignored. Correction of this cyl by using a RGP lens will usually improve both distance and near vision better than a toric soft lens will. Most patients will adjust from a soft lens to a rigid lens (especially a fluorinated material) within a couple of weeks and will not need reading glasses or bifocal lenses for two to five more years.

PATIENT 17

27-year-old male
Durasoft 3 on an extended-wear basis
OD 8.6 14.5 −2.75   K 43.50/43.75
OS 8.6 14.5 −3.00   43.50/44.00

Subjective complaint

Has no problems wearing on weekly extended-wear basis. Upon re-insertion after cleaning and disinfecting with papain enzyme, liquid surfactant, and AOsept, lenses feel extremely dry and eyes become injected.

Objective findings

When checked after 5 days wear, slit-lamp findings were good and patient was asymptomatic. When checked 7 hours subsequent to cleaning and disinfection, lenses appeared tight, corneas were slightly edematous, and moderate injection OU.

Treatment

Initially the type of enzyme cleaner used was changed, then soak time was reduced to as little as 10 minutes with no significant improvement. The enzyme was then discontinued completely at which time the *insertion reaction* disappeared. The lenses required replacement at 3 to 6-month intervals and the patient was subsequently fitted with disposable lenses.

Accuvue Johnson & Johnson 8.8 14.0 −2.75
                                   8.8 14.0 −3.00.

Result

The patient wears the disposable lenses on an extended-wear basis with weekly replacement. This eliminates solution preservative exposure, lessens the chance of reaction, and offsets protein build-up, which could trigger GPC.

Comment

A disposable lens can solve this problem because the patient is always wearing new lenses without exposure to enzymes or other chemicals.

PATIENT 18

33-year-old male
Keratoconus OU wearing Boston II material (4 years old)
OD 51.00 8.4 −8.75
OS 52.00 8.3 −7.50
Lenticular design McGuire type keratoconus PC2
K 48.00/56.00
    Slightly irregular, slightly oval cone
49.00/56.00

Subjective complaints

Wear time has dropped from 14 hours per day to 6 hours per day over past two months.

Objective findings

Moderately heavy touch indicating some progression of the cones. Some central eroding of the cornea as well as deposits on the lenses.

Treatment

Refitting with Boston Equalens in the same parameters as the Boston II lens.

Result

After one week of wear, all-day comfortable wear had been re-established.

Comment

The relatively high DK of the new material plus the fact that the lenses were new contributed to the success of the fit. This is also an excellent example of how lenses that contain a fluoronated monomer should exhibit flatter fitting characteristics than a silicone acrylate material. The "softer" material added to the comfort and the flat fit offset any tendency to on-eye flexure.

PATIENT 19

28-year-old female
Hydrocurve II 55% water soft lenses, extended-wear for 1 to 3 weeks at a time.
OD 8.5 14.0 −6.00   K 45.00/45.75
                     VA 20/25 OU
OS 8.5 14.0 −6.00   44.87/45.37

Subjective complaints

Eyes always look red. Has worn for 4 years. Present lenses 3 months old.

Objective findings

Lenses slightly tight, some circulimbal impression OU. Moderately injected neovascularization 1 - 2 mm OU. All vessels loop back out to the limbus. No active pannus.

Treatment

Refitting with extended-wear RGP lenses in an aspheric design—Bausch & Lomb Quantum
OD 7.45 9.6 −6.25
                     VA 20/20
OS 7.45 9.6 −6.25

Result

After one week of daily wear the patient began wearing the lenses on an extended-wear basis up to a maximum of one week at a time. The injection disappeared. After six months some of the neovascularization was observed as ghost vessels.

Comment

When faced with this type of problem, the most obvious treatment would be to refit with a flatter and perhaps a higher-permeability soft lens. It must always be remembered that a RGP lens provides greater oxygen-availability to the cornea than a soft lens of even equal DK because the RGP lens does not cover 100% of the cornea. The water content of the rigid lens is less than 0.5% and therefore is not dependent on tear quality or quantity in order to maintain its parameters. Patients presently wearing soft lenses usually have a faster adaptation time when refitted with rigid lenses than the average "virgin" contact-lens patient.

PATIENT 20

25-year-old female
Spincast soft lenses (Bausch & Lomb)
OD −3.75 04   K 45.00/45.25
OS −4.50 04   44.75/45.00

Subjective complaint

Patient must wear lenses constantly in order to maintain comfort. (History of extended wear for 30 days at a time for 3 years.) When lenses are removed for cleaning, eyes feel very dry and gritty.

Objective findings

Little movement or lag. Some microcysts OU. Keratitis (mild); staining when lenses removed.

Treatment

Lens-wear suspended for one month. Use of ocular lubricant drops *qid* and Lacrilube nightly. Weekly monitoring of corneas show keratitis and 90% of microcysts had cleared. Refitting with thin design Boston Equalens.

44.00 9.5 −2.75 .12 center thickness

44.00 9.5 −3.75 .7 heavy blended tri-curve PC

Result

After two weeks all-day wear had been established and the comfort was good. One year subsequent to refitting the patient wore the lenses on a daily-wear basis with occasional overnight wear. No microcysts are present and normal corneal integrity is maintained.

Comment

Some patients become dependent upon their soft extended-wear lenses as a result of extremely long wear periods (30 days or more). This is a result of the thinning of the mucoid

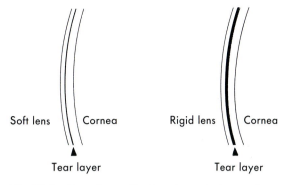

Fig 35-8 ■ Tear layer: the tear layer between the cornea and soft lens is 2 microns thick whereas the tear layer between the cornea and a rigid lens is 10-12 microns thick.

layer on the anterior surface of the corneal epithelium. The tear layer between the cornea and a soft lens is approximately one to two microns thick whereas the tear layer under a rigid lens is 10 to 12 microns thick. In addition to this, the total tear volume exchanged with each blink is approximately 2% to 4% for a soft lens compared to 10% to 15% in the case of a rigid gas-permeable lens (Fig. 35-8).

36 · PROBLEMS ASSOCIATED WITH CURRENT CARE SYSTEMS

John F. Morgan

- *Problems of compliance*
- *Problems associated with chemical care systems*
- *Problems associated with heat care systems*
- *Problems of incompatibility of care systems*
- *Problems of adverse reactions*
- *Problems of corneal infections related to care*
- *Problems of cleaning methods*
- *Diagnosis of "red eye" in patients wearing contact lenses*

The most significant complication that a contact-lens wearer can experience is an infection of the cornea. To reduce the chances of this happening, a contact lens must be as free from microbial contamination as possible when it is placed on the eye. The methods of disinfecting contact lenses, hard or soft, are numerous. There is no perfect system. The surface of contact lenses must be cleaned to maintain comfort and reduce the complications that coated lenses can produce. To effectively and safely monitor the course of the patient wearing the contact lenses, the fitter must know the possible and probable problems of the system of disinfection and cleaning that has been selected for the patient. Only by doing this can the fitter provide the patient with the safest and most comfortable contact-lens wearing course.

All the systems for disinfecting and cleaning contact lenses use chemicals. Chemicals that are strong enough to destroy bacteria, viruses, amoeba, and fungi have the potential to injure the cells of the anterior segment of the eye. This tendency to injure is called the *toxicity* of a compound. The body is equipped with elaborate systems to recognize nonself. When a chemical is identified as nonself the body tissues will react to it, producing unwanted changes. This process is called *sensitivity* or *hypersensitivity*. Some chemicals used in the care of contact lenses have a greater tendency to produce sensitivity than others.

The commercially available materials for the care of contact lenses are detailed elsewhere in this book (Chapters 8 and 14) and in other texts. This chapter will not primarily consider the commercially available care materials, but rather will present a discussion of the complications resulting from the methods and chemicals used in the care of PMMA, RGP, and soft contact lens. The problems associated with the care of contact lenses will be discussed in the hope that a fitter, on reviewing a patient's care system, will be able to arrive at a reasonable explanation for the patient's problem and solve it.

PROBLEMS OF COMPLIANCE
Factors affecting compliance

Choice of system. The fitter must know the strengths and shortcomings of different care systems to be able to provide the patient with the maximum possible protection against the serious complications of contact-lens wear. He must, for example, know that storing lenses, hard or soft, in an unpreserved saline solution will not protect the patient from significant contamination of the lenses. He must know that regular use of the system, even when the lenses are not being worn, is required to control the contamination of the lenses by micro-organisms.

The selection of a care system for a patient is a major factor in how well a patient complies with the system. In addition to the considerations for selection of the care system that are reviewed in Chapter 8, other circumstances must be given weight. For example, if the patient does not appear to be able to follow detailed instructions, it is unlikely that one of the hydrogen peroxide care systems, which require a "stop-watch" attention to details, will be complied with. A simpler system such as heat, if the lenses will tolerate it, may be a better choice. The ability of a patient to comply with a given system of care may not be accurately assessed at the initial visit. Continued follow-up and monitoring of the patient is required to determine how effectively the patient is using the method of care. A change in the care system may be required if compliance appears to be inadequate.

Vocational and avocational patient needs. The lifestyle of the patient must be considered in selecting a care system. The patient who travels extensively, without ready access to electricity, will not be a good candidate for a care system that is based on heat. The individual who works long or irregular shifts is not likely to able to comply with the needs of a hydrogen-peroxide care system.

Economic factors. The majority of patients wearing contact lenses are doing so for cosmetic reasons, which places contact lenses in the category of luxury items, so one would not expect the economics of care to be a factor. However, it is a significant one. Continuing ongoing expenses are a nuisance. Attempts to reduce the cost of care will be made by the average patient. In the long term the least expensive method of care will take advantage of bargains and so may end up with inappropriate care materials. Thus, regular monitoring of the care materials being used is required. The fitter of the contact lenses may well let economic considerations affect his judgment for the care recommended. To keep the initial costs of the lenses low, free samples of care materials supplied by the manufacturers may be dispensed and consequently recommended to the patient, although this may not be in the best interests of the patient.

Instruction and training

In any endeavor, time is money. It takes time to properly instruct and train a patient in the care of contact lenses. If the patient is not given this time, it is not hard to understand why compliance with contact lens care is as low as it is. The fitting office is ethically obligated to ensure that patients fully understand how to care for the lenses before they leave the office. Patients will seldom read the instruction brochures carefully. Training and instruction, in the care of the contact lenses, should be a hands-on session, where the patients can demonstrate their understanding of the system and their potential ability to use it.

Regular review of care

There is little doubt that the single most important cause of significant contact-lens complications is from failure to comply with the care system. Human beings are busy and will seek shortcuts to reduce the time spent performing a repetitive task such as lens care. Placing emphasis on the importance of compliance can best be achieved by regular follow-ups with a detailed review of the patient's care. Reinstruction in the proper methods of care is required for almost all contact-lens patients. A review of the care materials actually being used is necessary, as the patient may have made a substitution of materials that could have the potential for problems.

If a patient cannot or will not comply with the system selected for him, then the fitter must consider changing the care system to achieve a safe level of care.

Examples of failures of compliance

Two examples of failure to comply may serve to illustrate how involved this problem is. The first was common when patients were required to make their saline solution by mixing salt tablets with distilled water. Patients would have problems with the amount of water used, and would have either a hypotonic or hypertonic saline solution. The hypotonic solution would result in a soft lens that was "sticky" to handle. The lens would produce a mild discomfort on insertion that would rapidly improve as the tears adjusted the tonicity of the lens. A hypertonic saline solution would result in a lens that felt "stiff", with greater discomfort on insertion. In the more extreme cases of hypertonic saline solutions, the lens would have salt deposits evident on its surface (Fig. 36-1).

A more serious failure in compliance resulted in an *Acanthamoeba* corneal abscess that required two corneal grafts with long ongoing discomfort and visual loss. The tragedy of the situation was that the patient felt he was complying

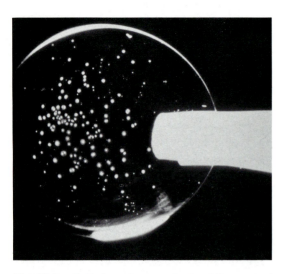

Fig 36-1 ■ Salt deposits on a hydrophilic contact lens from a hypertonic saline solution made from salt tablets and distilled water.

as best he could. The patient was instructed to use a hydrogen peroxide care system that used a tap-water rinse to remove the hydrogen peroxide. After he had cared for his lenses in this manner, he stored them for 5 days in a sterile nonpreserved saline solution. He failed to disinfect his lenses before he re-inserted them and the result was an *Acanthamoeba* infection of the left cornea (Figs. 36-2A and 2B).

PROBLEMS ASSOCIATED WITH CHEMICAL CARE SYSTEMS
Preservatives primarily for soft lenses

Hydrogen peroxide. Hydrogen peroxide disinfection is the oldest chemical care system for soft contact lenses. This care system was introduced in Canada in 1969. The original technique used, a powdered sodium bicarbonate neutralization method, was cumbersome. The present hydrogen peroxide care systems are simpler and more sophisticated. Hydrogen peroxide is very toxic to the anterior eye. It must be removed or neutralized before the lens is placed on the eye. The neutralizing materials used include platinum catalytic discs and solutions with catalase or pyruvate or thiosulfite. Simple dilution by repeated rinsing of the lenses is also used.

Hydrogen peroxide has enjoyed extreme popularity in recent years. It is the only system that can be used with many of the high water-content soft lenses that are commonly dispensed. It has an adjunct cleaning activity by means of its oxidative action. It is very effective in destroying bacteria within the times of exposure recommended by the manufacturers.

There are problems associated with its use as a care system that the fitter must be aware of to most efficiently monitor the patient in its use. The times of exposure to hydrogen peroxide re-

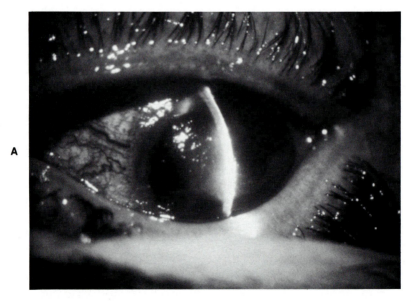

A

Fig 36-2 ■ **A,** Acanthamoeba corneal abscess in a patient who rinsed H_2O_2 from his hydrophilic contact lens with tap water.

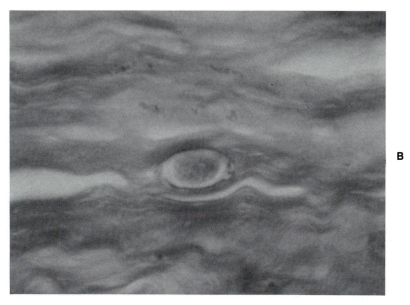

B

Fig 36-2, cont'd ■ **B,** Acanthamoeba cyst in the button taken for a corneal graft from the patient in Fig 36-2A.

quired to kill fungi is 45 minutes; the times recommended by the manufacturer are shorter than this. To kill *Acanthamoeba* requires 12 to 24 hours of exposure to hydrogen peroxide. This duration of time is impractical unless two sets of lenses are used. Leaving soft lenses in hydrogen peroxide for long periods will change

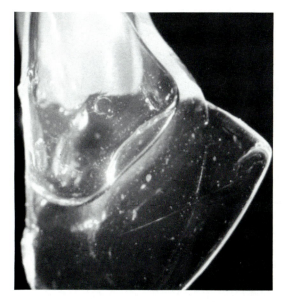

Fig 36-3 ■ Appearance of a hydrophilic lens after being left in H_2O_2 for several days.

their parameters (Fig. 36-3). It will require a long soak in the neutralizing solution to allow the lenses to return to their original parameters. Three sets of lenses might be required to achieve protection against *Acanthamoeba* with the hydrogen peroxide systems.

The method of neutralization of the hydrogen peroxide can be a source of problems. If the hydrogen peroxide is not neutralized, the residual hydrogen peroxide will produce marked discomfort when the lens is inserted. There will be variable degrees of punctate keratitis present (Figs. 36-4 *A* and *B*). This corneal epithelial insult heals well with no sequelae. The patient, however, may be reluctant to return to hydrogen peroxide care after experiencing this complication.

The neutralizing solution may be preserved with thimerosal. If the patient is sensitive to thimerosal, reactions of the eye will range from mild redness to severe corneal infiltrates or extensive epithelial loss. If the patient is not already sensitized to thimerosal, there is a 40% chance of developing a sensitivity to this mercury-based preservative. Toxic or sensitivity responses to the neutralizing chemicals (catalase, pyruvate or thiosulfite) are possible.

The neutralizing solution may be preserved with sorbic acid (sorbate). This preservative can do little more than maintain the sterile solution

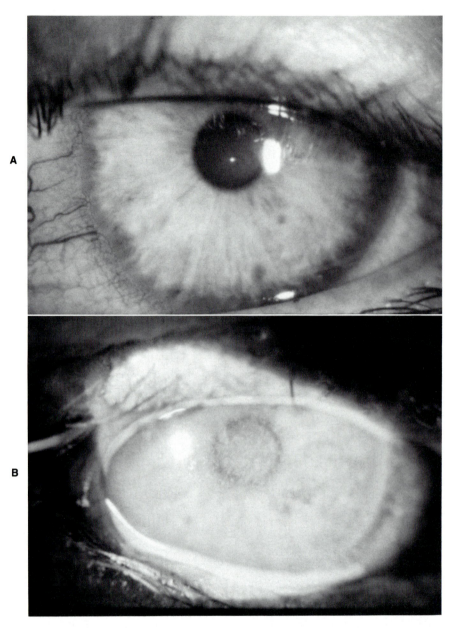

Fig 36-4 ■ **A,** Mild redness and punctate changes from residues of H_2O_2 on a hydrophilic contact lens. **B,** Severe redness and punctate changes from residues of H_2O_2 on a hydrophilic contact lens.

in the bottle free of major bacterial contamination. It cannot handle any load of micro-organisms placed in it, as will occur after the patient has handled the lenses. Lenses cannot be left in these sorbate preserved solutions with the confidence that microbial growth will not occur to potentially dangerous levels.

Acanthamoeba has become a serious threat to contact lens wearers. All tap water and distilled water may contain *Acanthamoeba*. As hydrogen peroxide is inefficient in destroying *Acanthamoeba*, tap water and distilled water should never be a part of a care system that relies on hydrogen peroxide for disinfection of the lenses. Systems that remove the hydrogen peroxide from the lenses by dilution with tap water or poorly preserved saline solutions increase the risks of *Acanthamoeba* infection (see Figs. 36-2A and B).

Sorbate (Sorbic acid). Sorbate (sorbic acid) has a minimal degree of activity against micro-organisms. It was introduced as a preservative for saline solutions when the problem of thimerosal sensitivity was becoming very evident. Sorbate cannot disinfect a contact lens; it can do little more than prevent the originally packaged sterile saline solution from contamination. A sorbate preserved saline is not adequate as a soaking solution for lenses. It must always be used in conjunction with a defined method for killing micro-organisms, such as heat or chemicals. Sorbate preserved salines may be used:

1. in the lens case for disinfection with heater units,
2. as a rinse after the lenses are removed from soaking solutions,
3. as a rinse after surface cleaning the lenses.

Toxic responses to sorbate preserved saline have not been found. However, sensitivity reactions do occur. They are usually mild, with a minimal degree of redness of the eyes and minimal punctate. If a sensitivity to sorbate is suspected, a sterile nonpreserved saline should be substituted for the sorbate preserved saline solution to see if the eye improves.

Sorbate preserved salines used in heater units will discolor hydrophilic lenses. The lenses turn a light brown color (Fig. 36-5). The lower the pH of the sorbate preserved saline, the faster the discoloring will take place. A commercially available sorbate preserved saline, with a pH of 6.07, discolored 38% HEMA lenses after only 22 cycles in a heater unit. Another brand of sorbate preserved saline, with a pH of 7.24, did not discolor the same type of 38% HEMA lenses after 50 cycles in the same type of heater unit.

Alkyl triethanolammonium chloride (TEAC.) Alkyl triethanolammonium chloride (TEAC) belongs to the family of quaternary ammonium compounds. It is relatively weak in its ability to kill gram-negative bacteria, yeasts, and fungi. To overcome these shortcomings TEAC is combined with thimerosal in the formulation for a soaking solution for hydrophilic lenses. This combination is effective as a disinfecting soaking solution for hydrophilic lenses.

TEAC is toxic to the epithelial cells of the cornea. 75% of patients in a study of a soaking solution with TEAC, in which the soaking solution was not rinsed off prior to the contact lens being placed on the eye, developed toxic epithelial corneal changes. The most common man-

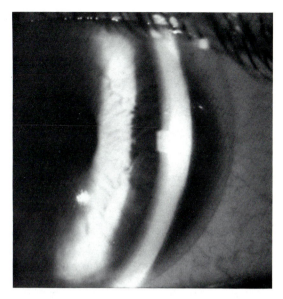

Fig 36-5 ■ Hydrophilic lens regularly disinfected with heat with brown discoloring from sorbate preserved saline solution.

ifestation of the toxic effect of TEAC was the appearance of intra-epithelial microcysts (Figs. 36-6A and B). When the soaking solution containing TEAC was rinsed off the lens, with a sterile nonpreserved saline solution prior to insertion, no toxic effects were found.

TEAC tends to be absorbed by high hydration hydrophilic lenses, particularly if the lens polymer contains methacrylic acid. Unless the manufacturer of a contact lens of hydration greater than 38% specifically recommends the use of TEAC containing soaking solutions, it is wise to avoid them. The level of adsorbed TEAC may produce toxic corneal changes because rinsing the lens before insertion may not remove the TEAC from the lens.

The need to combine TEAC with thimerosal to achieve a satisfactory disinfection effect exposes the patient to the risk of developing a sensitivity reaction to thimerosal.

Hypochlorite (sodium dichloroisocyanurate). This is a chlorine-based system which is available in Europe and has recently been introduced in Canada. The effervescent tablets dissolve rapidly in nonpreserved saline and release hypochlorite ions. The resulting solution contains 5 parts per million of free chlorine. Sodium bicarbonate formulated in the tablet transforms the hypochlorite into sodium chloride after 3 to

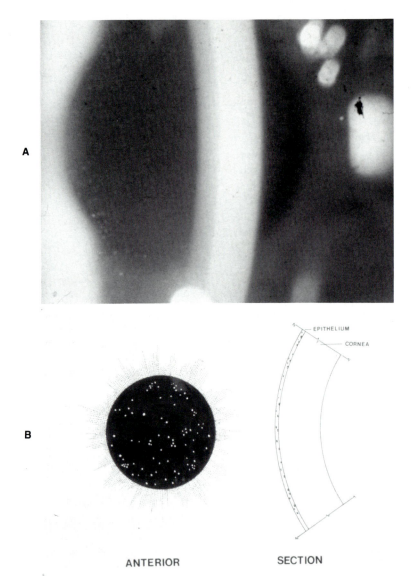

EPITHELIUM

CORNEA

ANTERIOR   SECTION

Fig 36-6 ■ **A,** Intra-epithelial microcysts produced by the toxic action of alkyl triethanolammonium chloride (TEAC). **B,** Artist's depiction of the intra-epithelial microcysts produced by the toxic action of alkyl triethanolammonium chloride (TEAC).

5 hours. The clinical results have been reported as good. Low- and high-water-content hydrophilic lenses and rigid gas permeable contact lenses, made from the siloxanyl acrylate materials, were used in the clinical trials.

The tablets cannot be used with preserved salines because the hypochlorite may bind with the preservative and reduce the available chlorine to below the levels required for disinfection. Chlorine is a highly reactive element and is readily bound by organic material. Lenses would have to be kept clean to maximize the disinfecting effectiveness of this system of care. A German study, over a 90-day period, indicated that there was a cleaning action with hydrophilic lenses as the hypochlorite is an oxidative agent.

The patients using this system of care should be strongly advised not to store their lenses in the solution, because it turns into an unpreserved saline solution. If the lenses are left in this solution for longer than a night, disinfecting them again prior to insertion would be the safest approach.

Polyquaternium 1 (Polyquad). Polyquaternium 1 (Polyquad) is a quaternary ammonium compound but it differs from TEAC in that Polyquad has a much higher molecular weight. Polyquad also has a wide spectrum of organisms against which it is effective. It is much less efficient against the Aspergillus fungus. It is formulated in a 0.001% concentration as a preserved saline solution.

The 0.001% preserved saline solution can be used with a heater unit. No toxic or sensitivity problems have been noted thus far. The solution does not have to be rinsed from the lens prior to insertion. Polyquad 0.001% has been used in clinical trials as a soaking solution with no evident clinical problems. If the patient who is using Polyquad preserved saline with the heater unit stores the lenses in the case for a number of days, there would appear to be added protection against microbial contamination. The acceptance of Polyquad preserved saline may be slow because of its relatively high cost compared to other preserved salines on the market.

The first formulations of the Polyquad preserved saline solutions that appeared on the market carried the caution not to use this saline solution with high-water-content lenses. The methacrylic acid in many high-water-contact lenses had the potential to adsorb the Polyquad to toxic levels. The more recent formulations appear to have overcome this problem; Polyquad may now be used with any hydrophilic lens and Polyquad preserved saline solutions are now being promoted in Canada as soaking solutions for all types of contact lenses.

Preservatives used for soft and hard (PMMA and RGP) lenses

Thimerosal. Thimerosal, a mercury-based preservative, has a bacteriostatic action against a wide range of micro-organisms. Its relative effectiveness as a preservative for solutions resulted in the widespread use of thimerosal in lens-care materials. It may be found in normal salines for hydrophilic lenses, soaking solutions for hydrophilic and hard contact lenses (PMMA, siloxanyl acetate, and fluorinated siloxanyl acetate lenses), surface-cleaning solutions for all lenses, and in eye wetters. Thimerosal is often present in lens care solutions in combination with other preservatives, such as Chlorhexidine and Alkyl triethanolammonium chloride, because of their inadequacies against groups of micro-organisms.

Unfortunately, thimerosal can induce a sensitivity (hypersensitivity) reaction in a high frequency of patients exposed to it. The frequency of sensitivity responses quoted in the literature varies considerably, from 15% to 40%. The 40% figure is more accurate according to our personal clinical observations. In a carefully monitored study conducted over a period of 2 years, 12 of 30 patients developed a sensitivity to thimerosal—a 40% frequency.

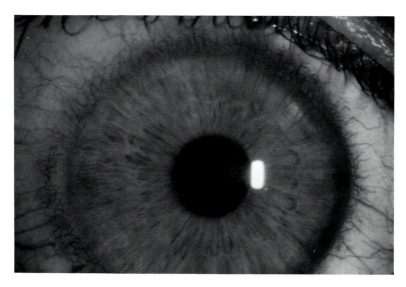

Fig 36-7 ■ Mild redness from a thimerosal sensitivity.

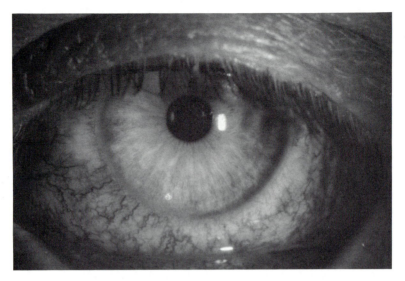

Fig 36-8 ■ Marked redness from a thimerosal sensitivity.

The diagnosis of a thimerosal sensitivity can present problems. The patient has typically used a thimerosal-containing solution for several months. A sensitivity is seldom seen until after 3 months of use, unless the patient has previously been sensitized to a mercury-containing compound. The most common presentation of a thimerosal sensitivity is a diffusely red eye with discomfort (Figs. 36-7 and 36-8). The reaction to thimerosal is a sensitivity response and can therefore mimic any eye disorder in which a sensitivity reaction is part of the clinical picture. A review in our clinic of the charts of patients wearing contact lenses who were exposed to thimerosal in their lens-care systems revealed that the thimerosal sensitivity response was mistaken for 15 other clinical entities (see list below).

CLINICAL DIAGNOSES MISTAKEN FOR THIMERO-SAL SENSITIVITY.

1. Hay-fever allergy
2. Contact allergy (cat dander)
3. Toxic keratitis
4. Bacterial conjunctivitis
5. Bacterial corneal abscess
6. Staphylococcal corneal infiltrates
7. Chlamydial conjunctivitis
8. Superior limbic keratopathy
9. Viral conjunctivitis
10. Herpes simplex keratitis (dendritic ulcer)
11. Adeno virus keratoconjunctivitis from APC Adeno virus
12. Adeno virus keratoconjunctivitis from epidemic adeno virus (see Fig. 36-19)
13. Anterior membrane dystrophy
14. Giant papillary conjunctivitis
15. Episcleritis (see Fig. 36-18)

Diagnosing a thimerosal sensitivity is often made more difficult because the patient does not know exactly what they are using for lens care. You cannot trust what the patient tells you. It is necessary to have the patient bring all the lens care materials and eye drops that they have used in the recent past to you for inspection. Only by doing this can the fitter be certain that thimerosal is not the culprit.

Thimerosal-sensitivity reactions are not restricted to the patients wearing hydrophilic contact lenses. It does occur in patients wearing rigid gas-permeable contact lenses or PMMA contact lenses (Fig. 36-18).

The high frequency of thimerosal sensitivity in hydrophilic lens wearers has resulted in reformulating many of the care products for hydrophilic contact lenses. However, thimerosal remains a preservative frequently found in care products for all types of contact lenses: hydrophilic, PMMA, and rigid gas-permeable. So called "fitting problems" of discomfort and redness in a patient wearing a contact lens made from a hard material may actually be the result of a thimerosal sensitivity.

Chlorhexidine. Chlorhexidine gluconate is bactericidal at levels greater than 100 mg/ml and bacteriostatic at lower levels, such as 60 mg/ml. Chlorhexidine is effective against the vegetative forms of gram-positive and gram-negative bacteria, with the important exception of the *Serratia* group. At the concentrations that chlorhexidine is used in hydrophilic care solutions it is less effective than desired against several of the yeasts and fungi. Chlorhexidine is, therefore, often formulated with thimerosal in hydrophilic contact-lens care solutions.

Chlorhexidine will accumulate in hydrophilic lenses to a concentration that may be considerably higher than that found in the solution in which the hydrophilic lens has been soaked. The concentration level of chlorhexidine in the lens reaches a stable level and does not increase.

Chlorhexidine is *not* noted for producing sensitivity responses. The literature where animal models are used indicates that chlorhexidine is relatively nontoxic; for the human eye, however, chlorhexidine *is* toxic. The variation of physiologic response may permit may patients to tolerate chlorhexidine-preserved care solutions without evident changes in the cornea. A reduced physiologic tolerance, exaggerated or produced by the hypoxia of the cornea that a contact lens can create, will result in toxic changes of the cornea. These changes appear as a superficial punctate keratitis with mild redness of the eye (Fig. 36-9). Soaking solutions for hydrophilic lenses that are preserved with chlorhexidine should be rinsed with a sterile nonpreserved saline solution, or a saline solution preserved with other than chlorhexidine, prior to being placed on the cornea.

Chlorhexidine is used as a preservative in the soaking or "conditioning" solutions for RGP contact lenses. Solutions for the disinfection of RGP lenses are difficult to formulate. These solutions, in which the RGP lenses are stored overnight, must also maintain and, ideally, enhance the wetting characteristics of the surface of the lens. The materials used to obtain good surface wetting properties of RGP lenses that contain siloxanyl are usually of high molecular weight and may impair the disinfecting action of chlorhexidine. These high molecular weight compounds may also serve as a substrate on which bacteria can "feed".

Serratia marcescens is a bacteria that is widely distributed in the environment in soil, food and

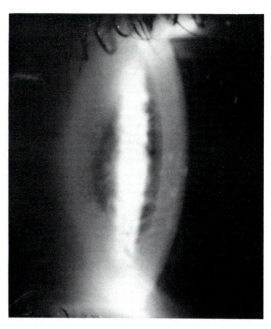

Fig 36-9 ■ Corneal punctate produced by the toxic action of chlorhexidine.

water. *Serratia marcescens* is a gram-negative, aerobic, nonspore-forming bacteria. Over a relatively short period of time, 12 patients wearing RGP contact lenses were treated for eye infections, 6 for conjunctivitis and 6 for keratitis (Fig. 36-10A). 5 of the 12 patients had *Serratia marcescens* recovered from swabs of the conjunctiva or corneal scrapings. The bottles of the Boston Conditioner that all 12 of these patients were using were found to be contamined with heavy growths of *Serratia marcescens* (Fig. 36-10B).

The observation that each of these 12 patients had *Serratia marcescens* growing in the chlorhexidine-preserved Boston Conditioner prompted us to culture the Boston Conditioner, or formulations identical to it marketed by Bausch & Lomb and CooperVision, of 73 patients. These 73 patients did not show any evidence of eye infections. They were all confirmed wearers of RGP lenses that contained siloxanyl. The 73 patients had 106 bottles of the Chlorhexidine preserved Boston Conditioner cultured. Of the 106 bottles 65 (61%) were contaminated with *Serratia marcescens*; 47 of the 73 patients (64%) had *Serratia marcescens* contamination of the Boston Conditioner in their bottles. It took as short a time as two days from the time a bottle of the chlorhexidine-preserved

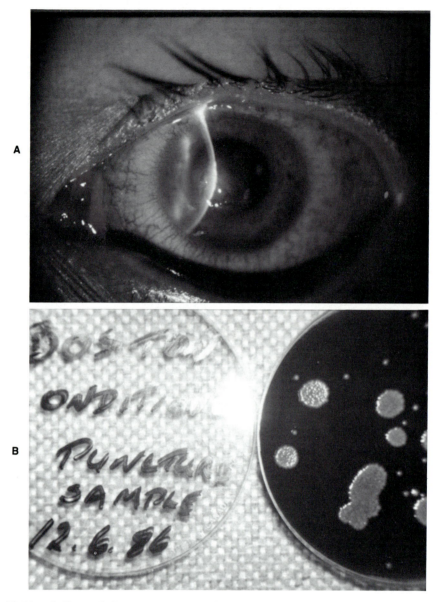

Fig 36-10 ■ **A,** Corneal abscess caused by *Serratia marcescens* that contaminated the RGP-conditioning solution. **B,** Colonies of *Serratia marcescens* growing on blood agar from a sample of Boston RGP conditioner that was obtained by a sterile needle puncture of the bottle.

conditioner was opened to when contamination by *Serratia marcescens* could be proven. Half of the bottles were found to be contaminated with *Serratia marcescens* within one week of being opened.

Polymer Technology, the manufacturer of the Boston Conditioner, reacted swiftly when this problem of *Serratia marcescens* contamination of the chlorhexidine-preserved Boston Conditioner formulation was brought to their attention. At the time of this writing clinical trials had

recently been completed for a Boston Conditioner formulation (Boston Advance Conditioner) with a new preservative Polyaminopropyl biguanide (PAPB). PAPB is discussed in the section that follows.

Polyaminopropyl biguanide (Dymed). Polyaminopropyl biguanide (Dymed) has been introduced as a preservative for hydrophilic contact-lens care materials in a saline solution and in a soaking solution within the past few years by Bausch & Lomb. Bausch & Lomb have elected to use the abbreviation *Dymed* for Polyamino-propyl biguanide.

Dymed is a cationic polymeric biguanide that is 5 to 10 times more effective against organisms than is chlorhexidine. It is very effective against *Serratia marcescens*. It is used in a concentration of 0.3 parts for million (0.0003 mgm per ml) in the preserved saline solution and 0.5 parts per million (0.0005 mgm per ml) in the hydrophilic lens-soaking solution.

No adverse responses to Dymed have yet been reported. It does not appear to be toxic to the cornea. It does not appear to produce sensitization of the external eye structures. The concentration of Dymed contained in the preserved saline solution and the soaking solution may be too low to achieve the best possible disinfection effects. Bausch & Lomb, the manufacturer of the Dymed preserved soaking solution and saline solution, feels that these concentrations are adequate. The low concentrations of Dymed in these hydrophilic contact-lens care solutions should permit their use with any type of hydrophilic lens.

Polyaminopropyl biguanide (PAPB). Polymer Technology Corporation considers that their method of using Polyaminopropyl biguanide as a preservative differs sufficiently from Bausch & Lomb's approach so that another synonym, PAPB, will be used for Polyaminopropyl biguanide in the labeling of the Polymer Technology solutions that contain it. Polymer Technology Corporation manufacturers the RGP contact lenses named Boston Lens and Equalens.

The major differences between Polymer Technology Corporation and Bausch and Lomb in the formulation of this chemical as a preservative for contact-lens care solutions, is the concentration used. Polymer Technology uses PAPB in concentrations of 15 parts per million (0.015 mgm per ml). This is 30 times the concentration that Bausch & Lomb uses in its soaking solution for hydrophilic contact lenses and 50 times the concentration of Bausch & Lomb's preserved saline solution.

The problems of *Serratia marcescens* contamination of the chlorhexidine preserved RGP contact lens conditioning solution have been discussed in the section on chlorhexidine. The new conditioning solution for RGP lenses produced by Polymer Technology are preserved with PAPB. The concentration of 15 parts per million of PAPB used in the Boston Advance Condi-

tioning Solution was dictated by several reasons that include:

1. Improved effectiveness against micro-organisms including *Acanthamoeba*
2. The presence in the formulation of the conditioning solution of high-molecular-weight "wetting" compounds that decrease the activity of preservatives,
3. The ability of gram-negative organisms, such as the *Serratia* species, to feed on high-molecular-weight wetting compounds.
4. The limited adsorption, by RGP contact lenses, of chemicals from soaking or conditioning solutions, compared to the adsorption by hydrophilic contact lenses.
5. The lack of toxicity of PAPB at the higher concentration.

The clinical study of the PAPB preserved conditioning solution for RGP lenses was completed in late 1988. The conditioner preserved with PAPB has been named *Boston Advance Conditioning Solution*. No confirmed cases of sensitivity or toxicity were found in the study. Patient acceptance of the conditioner in the study was excellent. Most important was the fact that numerous cultures of the new conditioner, preserved by PAPB, revealed no significant contamination by bacteria, especially *Serratia marcescens*. Only 3 bottles of the 460 (0.7%) submitted by the author for bacteriologic assessment, grew a *Serratia* species. The Boston Advance Conditioning Solution was placed on the market in Canada in May 1989. It should be available in the United States in late 1989.

During the bacteriology studies of PAPB as a preservative, Dr. DeCicco of the Catholic Universities of America in Washington DC, made an observation that will probably be of major importance in assessing preservative effectiveness. Dr. DeCicco observed that many of the preservatives used in lens-care products are effective against "standard" organisms obtained from commercial suppliers of bacteria for testing purposes. These preservatives, including chlorhexidine, thimerosal and benzalkonium chloride, were found to be inadequate against bacteria that had been cultured as contaminants in contact-lens soaking solutions. These organisms are termed *adapted* organisms. These adapted organisms are more representative of what the patient is likely to encounter. The testing of contact-lens care preservative formulations against adapted organisms is the best way to

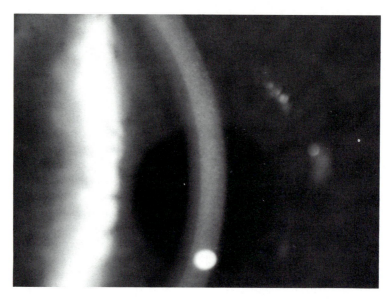

Fig 36-11 ■ Superficial punctate changes as a toxic reaction to the benzalkonium chloride preservative in the soaking solution.

determine their anti-microbial effectiveness (Table 36-2).

Preservatives primarily for PMMA lenses

Benzalkonium chloride. Benzalkonium chloride (BAK) is one of the oldest preservatives used in eye medications. It is a quaternary ammonium compound. It is not used in hydrophilic lens-care solutions because it is too toxic. BAK is toxic because it damages the material that holds the epithelial cells of the cornea to each other. This toxic effect is used to good advantage in an eye drop such as pilocarpine because it increases the penetration of the medication into the eye. Damaging the epithelium is not a desirable effect for contact-lens wearers. BAK is adsorbed by hydrophilic lenses to toxic levels very easily and epithelial damage will quickly result (Fig. 36-11). Epithelial damage has been seen after a soft lens was simply rinsed with Eye Stream™, a solution that is preserved by benzalkonium chloride.

BAK is found as a preservative in solutions meant for use with hard lenses. These solutions were formulated primarily for PMMA contact lenses. When BAK-preserved solutions are used with PMMA lenses, relatively few problems are seen unless the lens is coated, in which case the BAK may be retained in the debris on the lens

and may build up to toxic levels. BAK is not a suitable preservative for solutions to be used with hard lenses that are gas permeable. The benzalkonium chloride complex will cling firmly to the siloxanyl complexes that are present on

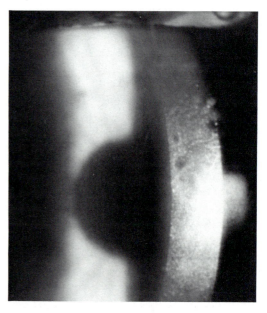

Fig 36-12 ■ Drying of the surface of a rigid gas-permeable contact lens that has siloxanyl in the polymer of the plastic, caused by the benzalkonium chloride in the soaking solution.

Table 36-1 ■ Effectiveness of preservatives against standard test bacteria and against adapted bacteria*†

RGP solution	Standard test *S. marcescens*		Adapted *S. marcescens*	
	Start	*6 hrs.*	*Start*	*16 hrs.*
.004 % Thimerosal (Alcon)	1.1×10^6	2.5×10^5	3.8×10^6	2.5×10^5
.004 % BAK (Allergan)	4.2×10^6	<10	5.4×10^6	8.5×10^5
.002 % Thimerosal	1.1×10^5	<10	6.0×10^6	4.0×10^1
.005 % Chlorhexidine (Titmus)				
.006 % Chlorhexidine (Boston)	4.2×10^6	<10	1.9×10^6	8.0×10^5
.0015% PAPB (Boston)	4.2×10^6	<10	1.2×10^6	<10

*Numbers in columns are colony-forming units per ml.
†Summarized from data provided by Dr DeCicco, Microbial Applications Laboratory, The Catholic University of America, Washington, DC

the surface of the lens. The hydrophobic part of the BAK complex will be the one that is exposed. The surface of the RGP lens will show an increasingly poor ability to wet. It may take 6 months of use of a BAK-preserved soaking solution to produce poor wetting of a RGP lens, but inevitably it will (Fig. 36-12). Also, RGP contact lenses tend to coat more readily than PMMA lenses. RGP lenses may retain the BAK in the debris on the lens at levels that will produce toxic changes in the corneal epithelium. BAK does not appear to be effective against adapted organisms (Table 36-1).

Chlorobutanol. Chlorobutanol is now rarely used as a preservative in soaking solutions for hard lenses; it is still commonly used as a preservative in eye drops. Chlorobutanol is not a fast-acting bacteriocide or fungicide. It is volatile and tends to change its concentration in solutions. Chlorobutanol is relatively toxic to the anterior eye structures.

PROBLEMS ASSOCIATED WITH HEAT CARE SYSTEMS

Disinfecting hydrophilic lenses has always been a major problem. The first hydrophilic contact lenses were introduced into the United States' market in 1969 were HEMA (polymacon) lenses of 38% hydration. These hydrophilic contact lenses could tolerate repeated heating without changing the structure of the polymer. The first hydrophilic contact lens available on the Canadian market, however briefly, was a lens made of a material that contained Poly-N-vinyl-pyrrolidone (PVP). The hydration of this material was close to 50%. Heat disinfection could not be used because repeated heating of the lens changed the polymer by modifying the PVP.

These lenses would lose their shape after repeated heating. Disinfection of these lenses was difficult to the point that the lenses were being shipped from the manufacturing laboratory heavily contaminated with *Pseudomonas aeruginosa*. This contamination of newly fabricated lenses led to the closing of this laboratory in Canada.

If the material of the contact lens is able to tolerate repeated heating without changing, moist heat is the most reliable disinfecting method available. Moist heat is an efficient method of killing micro-organisms. A temperature of 80° C maintained for 10 minutes will kill all the vegetative forms of organisms present, including the motile and cyst forms of *Acanthamoeba*. All of the commercially available heater units designed for the disinfection of hydrophilic contact lenses will achieve 80° C for at least 10 minutes. The heater unit is the only practical care method available on the market for the care of hydrophilic lenses that will reliably kill the motile and cyst forms of *Acanthamoeba*. Hydrogen peroxide will kill *Acanthamoeba*, but the time of exposure required to do so is 12 to 24 hours. This long exposure time does not make hydrogen peroxide disinfections practical for this purpose.

Lens problems

The single biggest drawback to recommending heat as a disinfection method for contact lenses is the number of hydrophilic and RGP contact lenses currently on the market that cannot tolerate repeated heating without changing their parameters (shape). The level of hydration of a hydrophilic contact lens can be a guide for the fitter. If the hydration of the contact lens is less than 40%, the lens will be made of HEMA material and will tolerate repeated heating. If the hydration is greater than 40%, then the polymer from which the contact lens is made may contain PVP or methacrylic acid and will not withstand repeated heating. There are lenses of high hydration, such as those made from lidofilcon, which can be disinfected with heat. The number of different materials that are available today may overwhelm the fitter of contact lenses. As a simple defense against this confusing situation, the fitter may avoid the use of heat disinfection because he knows that there are so many lenses on the market that will not tolerate heat. He will use a chemical-care method, particularly hydrogen peroxide, for hydrophilic contact lenses as it is compatible with all varieties of hydrophilic lens materials.

The contact-lens cases that had their contents cultured immediately after removal from a heater unit were the only ones that did not grow vegetative micro-organisms. Case cultures of all other care methods have yielded significant growth of bacteria or fungi. The fitter should be willing to offer the patient maximum protection from contamination of the contact lenses. Heat care will effect this better than any other disinfection method. A moment spent checking with the manufacturer of the particular hydrophilic contact lens chosen whether the lens can be cared for by repeated heating would allow the fitter to provide the patient with the most predictable disinfection method available.

Patients will have spells when they are not wearing their contact lenses regularly. They may leave their contact lenses in the lens case for days or weeks. It is vital to inform the patients that the lenses must be reheated regularly when not being worn each day. Although the temperatures achieved in the heater units will kill the vegetative forms of micro-organisms, the resting forms of bacteria and fungi will still be viable. With time, these resting forms will become vegetative and must be killed at this stage by reheating or the lens in the case may be invaded by fungal growth (Fig. 36-13 A and B).

The only RGP lens that will tolerate repeated heating is the Silcon™ lens, which is made from a thermosetting plastic, silicone resin. In the clinical trials of the lenses made from silicone resin, heat was used as the disinfection method. Most fitters who used this lens in their practices used chemical care for disinfection. Silicone

elastomer, from which the Silsoft™ lens is fabricated, can also withstand repeated heating. This was the method many fitters recommended for the care of the Silsoft™ lens when it was readily available. This lens is available now only in limited quantities, primarily for pediatric aphakic patients.

RGP lenses that contain siloxanyl cannot be disinfected by heat because the plastic is not thermosetting. It is also necessary to regularly "treat" the surface of hard lenses made from polymers that contain siloxanyl. This treatment is done with high-molecular-weight compounds that are in the soaking solutions. These act to maintain the wetting characteristics of the surface of the lenses because siloxanyl is hydrophobic.

CAB lenses imbibe water. Heating them in a saline solution is likely to change their parameters.

Saline solutions

Unpreserved nonsterile saline solutions. Unpreserved saline solutions would not pose any threat of infection if they were only to be used in the case when the lenses were being disinfected by heat. The heat cycle will kill any of the potentially pathogenic vegetative forms of organisms that may have contaminated the unpreserved saline solution. However, patients that make up their saline solution from distilled or de-ionated water and salt tablets will use this saline solution to rinse their lenses before insertion and after cleaning. They may even use this unpreserved saline solution to "moisten" the lens in the eye for greater comfort. Using unpreserved saline solutions for these purposes presents the very real and unacceptable risk of severe eye infection. The use of unpreserved nonsterile saline solutions is to be actively discouraged. Although the risk is statistically low and many patients may not have any problems, when a problem does occur, particularly an infection with *Acanthamoeba*, the consequences are severe and cannot be justified.

Distilled or de-ionated water is almost always the source of contamination. If tap water is used with the de-ionizing units, the risk of contamination is probably even greater. Distilled water is not sterile. *Pseudomonas species* organisms are often present in the distillation column of the water stills and will readily contaminate the distilled water.

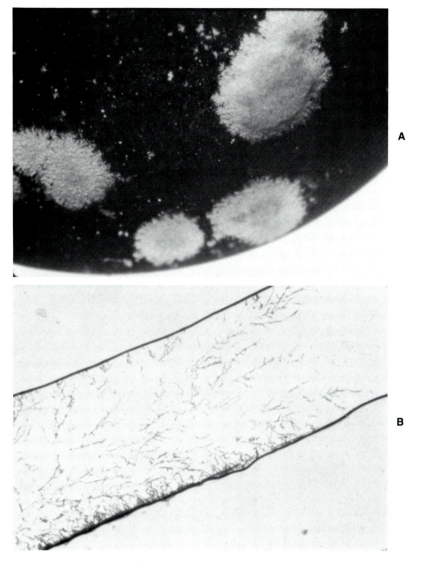

Fig 36-13 ■ **A,** Colonies of fungi growing on a hydrophilic contact lens. **B,** Fungi growing through the substance of a hydrophilic contact lens.

Distilling water does not remove inorganic materials that may act to discolor the hydrophilic contact lenses after repeated exposure. Also, the formulation of the salt tablets is not a simple matter. The buffers and stabilizers used in the preparation of the salt tablets may act to change or discolor the lenses.

The problems and risks that are inherent in making saline solutions from distilled water and salt tablets are compounded by failures in compliance by the patient. The original protocol for using distilled water with salt tablets required that the distilled water be brought to a boil im-

mediately before the salt tablet was added. Very few contact-lens fitters let alone patients remember that requirement. Patients will make several days' supply of saline solution rather than just the one-day supply originally called for. They will add too much or too little salt to the volume of distilled water. This produces a saline solution that gives discomfort on lens insertion because it is hypertonic or hypotonic.

The use of nonpreserved unsterile saline solutions is too great a risk to the patient to be tolerated and so it must be actively discouraged.

Preserved saline solutions. Preserved saline solutions are undoubtedly safer for the patient to use than are nonsterile unpreserved salines. But preserved saline solutions are not without their problems. The preservatives used in the preserved saline solutions, in historical order of use, include; chlorhexidine, thimerosal, sorbate (sorbic acid), Polyquad (polyquaternium 1) and Dymed (polyaminopropyl biguanide).

Chlorhexidine is toxic to the corneal epithelium and can produce a superficial punctate keratitis with resultant discomfort (see Fig. 36-9). It is relatively weak in its antimicrobial action against the *Serratia* species and other gram-negative bacteria. It tends to develop a higher concentration in the lens than is present in the care solutions. When a hydrophilic lens is coated, even higher levels of chlorhexidine will be retained by the lens to leach out onto the cornea to give a toxic change.

Thimerosal preserved saline solutions provide protection against a wide range of microorganisms from the bacteriostatic effect of this mercurial preservative. However, the use of thimerosal in any part of the care system exposes the patient to the risk of becoming sensitized to thimerosal (see Figs. 36-7, 36-8, 36-18 and 36-19). The frequency of sensitivity is as high as 40%. The large number of patients who developed thimerosal sensitivity helped to obtain early acceptance of an alternative preservative for saline solutions in the form of sorbic acid (sorbate).

Sorbic acid is used as a preservative only for saline solutions. It is an extremely weak preservative and cannot handle any degree of contamination. Sorbate saline solutions must always be used with some other method of disinfection, such as heat or chemicals. Sorbic acid preserved salines must never be relied upon as soaking agents with the expectation that they are providing the patient with protection from contamination of their contact lenses. The more acidic a sorbic-acid-preserved saline solution is, the more rapidly it will discolor hydrophilic lenses repeatedly heated in it (see Fig. 36-5). Sorbic acid will produce sensitization. Although this has not been a common event in contact-lens wearers using sorbic acid-preserved saline solutions, it must be watched for.

Polyquad-preserved saline solution currently provides one of the best disinfection options of all the preserved salines. It can even be used as a soaking solution with good patient safety and is now being promoted by its manufacturer, Alcon, as a soaking solution for hydrophilic lenses. However, a large volume of saline solution is used by contact-lens wearers. Consequently, the high cost of Polyquad preserved saline may make it unacceptable to patients. Toxic responses to Polyquad, which has a concentration level of 0.001%, have not been noted. Sensitivity reactions to Polyquad have rarely, if ever, been reported.

Dymed preserved saline solutions are the most recent to have been placed on the market. No evident toxic or sensitivity responses have been reported. The concentration of Dymed at 0.3 parts per million may be too low to allow much of a safety factor to control contamination of the lenses in the case. The lenses should be reheated regularly, if they are not being worn for some reason.

Sterile unpreserved saline solutions. Sterile unpreserved saline solutions were made available as an alternative saline solution for patients with toxic or sensitivity responses. Initially, sterile unpreserved saline solutions were available in unit dose packages. These were expensive and patients would try to minimize costs by making the volume of saline solution that was available last as long as possible. Once the unit dose was opened, contamination was inevitable. By using the opened container the next day, patients were asking for trouble.

Multiple-use containers of sterile unpreserved saline became practical with the introduction of aerosol type dispensers. With this system of packaging, the flow is only in an outward direction, with no back-drawing of contaminated materials. The saline solution in these containers is sterilized by high-dose radiation. There is only one case of these containers being contaminated and that was with *Pseudomonas maltophilia*. Some of the sterile unpreserved saline products in the multiple use aerosol cans is noted by a few patients to be uncomfortable to use as a rinse prior to lens insertion. This discomfort relates to the lack of a buffer in the saline solution. This minor shortcoming of the product has been rectified in most of the brands currently available. The greater cost of multiple-use sterile unpreserved saline solutions compared to preserved saline solutions has not been large enough to reduce patient acceptance of this product.

PROBLEMS OF INCOMPATIBILITY
OF CARE SYSTEMS

The contact-lens fitter must know what systems of care are compatible with the material from which the lens is fabricated. A hydrophilic lens material that contains PVP or methacrylic acid will not tolerate repeated heating. The presence of methacrylic acid in the polymer of a hydrophilic lens material will increase the likelihood of the lens adsorbing chemicals to toxic levels.

The most likely incompatibility in care systems is using a heater unit with hydrophilic contact lenses that have previously been disinfected with chemicals. The chemicals may be retained by the surface coating of the hydrophilic lenses or be adsorbed by the lenses. When the lenses are heated, the residual chemicals may react with the complex polymer plastic of the hydrophilic lens and damage it. The change produced may be evident to the patient, as the lens may become opaque. However, there may be changes in the parameters of the lens that will alter the manner in which it fits or functions, but patients may not be aware why they are having problems.

This problem may be less evident now in contact lens practices than it was 10 years ago. At that time Flexsol™ was popular as a soaking solution. It contained polyox, a high-molecular-weight polymer, and Adsorbobase. These compounds were present to help increase patient comfort on lens insertion. If a lens were heated in the presence of polyox and Adsorbobase, the lens would become opaque as the polyox and Adsorbobase reacted with the polymer of the hydrophilic contact lens (Fig. 36-14).

A patient heated his 38% hydration HEMA lenses in a Barnes-Hind soaking solution, then complained that the lenses no longer fit. The lenses had increased in diameter by 2 mm and the edge of the lens was fluted (Fig. 36-15). The specific chemical that caused this change in his lenses in the presence of heat was never discovered. Heating hydrophilic lenses with residual amounts of other soaking solutions changed the surface tension of the lenses.

Unfortunately, not all the materials contained in solutions for the care of contact lenses are listed on the labels. These lens-care products are patented and the companies are reluctant to list all the components in the formulation. Only "active" ingredients are listed.

Whenever possible, avoid interchanging chemical and heat care systems. If the patient wants to use heat with hydrophilic lenses that have been cared for by chemical or cold methods the lenses should be cleaned and rinsed thoroughly with sterile unpreserved saline. Allowing the lenses to soak overnight in sterile unpreserved saline and then replacing the saline prior to heating the lenses will further help in eluting any residual chemicals from the lenses.

Polyquad preserved saline can be used as a soaking solution. It was designed as a preserved saline for use in heater units with hydrophilic lenses. It may be the only product that can be used by a patient who is switching from cold care to heat care without having concerns that the lens will be changed in some way.

Hydrogen peroxide residues on a hydrophilic lens that is heated will damage the lens. However, this is unlikely to happen unless the patient takes the lens directly from the hydrogen peroxide and places it in the heater unit. Stranger things have happened. For example, an angry elderly aphakic patient complained bitterly about the short lifetime of his hydrophilic lens. The lens had changed color and caused significant eye discomfort and reaction on insertion (Fig. 36-16). The cause of these events was not

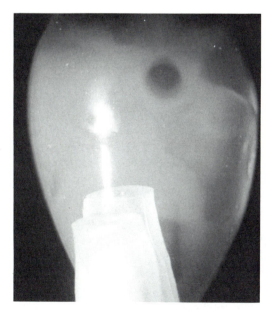

Fig 36-14 ■ Opaque appearance of a hydrophilic lens after it was heated in the soaking solution Flexsol™, which contained polyox and Adsorbobase.

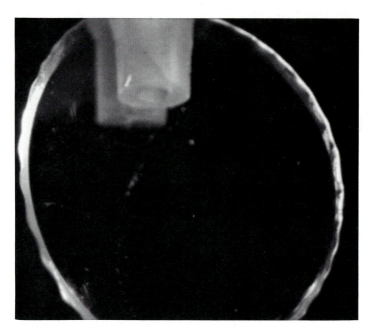

Fig 36-15 ■ Appearance of a hydrophilic lens that was heated in a Barnes Hind soaking solution. The lens became larger in diameter with fluted edges.

discovered until the patient was asked to bring all his care materials to the office for review. Then it was discovered that he had used a hair dye (Grecian Formula™) in his case when he heated the lenses rather than a saline solution!

All care materials and their methods of use should be reviewed by the fitter whenever a lens acts in a way that cannot be readily explained. The cause of the problem may be incompatible systems.

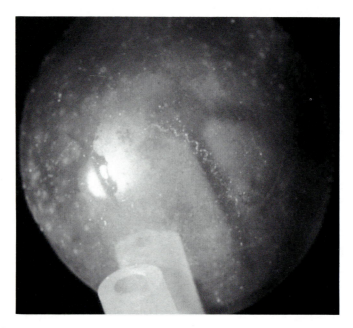

Fig 36-16 ■ Opaque appearance of a hydrophilic contact lens that was heated in a hair dye solution called Grecian Formula™.

There are numerous hydrogen peroxide care systems on the market. Not all the individual components of these care systems are interchangeable. The hydrogen peroxides that are sold specifically for the care of lenses should be the only ones used. 3% hydrogen peroxide for other uses is available in the stores, but it contains impurities that will change the color of the hydrophilic lens or damage it. Ultrazyme™ is an enzyme cleaner that is designed to be used in the hydrogen peroxide. If the patient is using a hydrogen peroxide system that has a platinum-coated disc as a neutralizing agent, the case must be vented to allow the use of Ultrazyme™. The patient may have been switched to a hydrogen peroxide care system by the fitter because of sensitization to chemicals. Such a patient can easily obtain another company's neutralizer or rinsing solution, which contains the chemical thimerosal, for example, that produced the sensitivity response.

Rigid gas-permeable contact lenses that contain siloxanyl are vulnerable to incompatible systems of care. These RGP lenses are damaged by the simple alcohols: ethyl, methyl, and isopropyl. Patients may have cleaned their PMMA lenses previously with alcohol without any evident problems. If they try cleaning their RGP lenses with a simple alcohol, the lenses will change shape and lose transparency (Fig. 36-17). Benzalkonium chloride (BAK) will, over a period of time, reduce the wetting characteris-

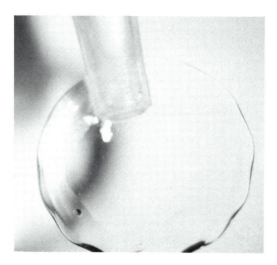

Fig 36-17 ■ Appearance of a RGP contact lens that has siloxanyl in the polymer after attempted cleaning with methyl alcohol.

tics of RGP lenses that contain siloxanyl (see Fig. 36-12). BAK should be avoided as a constituent of soaking solutions or cleaning solutions to be used with RGP lenses. A subtler incompatible situation for RGP lenses is the formulation of the soaking solution. If the soaking solution is not formulated to minimize the inherent hydrophobic character of siloxanyl, the lenses will not be comfortable to wear.

PROBLEMS OF ADVERSE REACTIONS

Adverse reactions to the chemicals used for the care of hydrophilic contact lenses or rigid gas-permeable contact lenses are either toxic or sensitivity responses.

Toxic reactions may be simply defined as poisonings. The degree of response to a given toxic insult is not the same from patient to patient. *LD 50* is a term used to define the dose of a poison or toxic substance that will kill 50% of the test animals to whom it is given; 50% of the animals survive. The analogy can be applied to patients. One patient may show significant corneal changes after exposure to a material and another may not have any evident change after the same exposure. However, if a large enough dose of a toxic material is administered, eventually all patients will show evidence of damage.

Sensitivity or hypersensitivity responses are much more individualized. The sensitivity response occurs only when the immune system of the patient "decides" that a substance to which it has been exposed is "nonself." A defense against the nonself material is then triggered when the patient next comes in contact with it. This defense reaction can produce significant symptoms and structural changes in the anterior segment of the eye.

Toxic reactions

Toxic responses do not require a period of use or exposure to a material to manifest themselves. Toxic reactions will occur soon after a patient begins to use a care system with a compound that is toxic to their eye. It is the toxic responses that are likely to be noted in the average clinical trial of a contact lens care solution as these clinical trials are seldom more than 90 days long. Sensitivity reactions usually require a period of exposure to the sensitizing material that is longer than 3 months. The history that the patient gives when he presents with eye discomfort can

Table 36-2 ■ Toxic responses in lens care systems

Chemical	Care component	Sequence	Clinical results
Hydrogen peroxide	Disinfecting solution	Failure to neutralize	Marked discomfort; redness; punctate
Enzymes	Cleaning solution	Residues in lenses	Moderate-to-severe redness on insertion
TEAC	Soaking solution	Failure to rinse lenses with saline	Mild redness; intra-epithelial microcysts
Chlorhexidine	Soaking solutions; surface cleaners; preserved salines	Failure to rinse lenses; coated lenses	Mild redness; superficial punctate
Benzalkonium chloride	PMMA and RGP lens solutions for soaking, cleaning	Used with soft Lenses or RGP lenses	Redness with mild-to-moderate punctate

therefore be very helpful. If the discomfort began within 3 months of use of a care system, then a toxic reaction is more probable than a sensitivity response. If the change did not occur until 3 months or more after starting use of the care system, a sensitivity response is more probable than a toxic reaction.

Toxic reactions are more likely to develop if the cornea is stressed. A lens that has very little oxygen flow or is providing poor tear circulation will weaken the cornea's ability to withstand any further insult. A cornea in this state is more vulnerable to a toxic injury than is a cornea that has adequate amounts of oxygen and fresh tears.

A toxic reaction will often appear as a redness of the eye, with diffuse punctate over the cornea. The patient may note varying degrees of a burning sensation. The degree of the redness and the severity of the punctate keratopathy can vary considerably.

The toxic reactions that are most likely to be seen by contact-lens fitters with the care systems that are popular today are shown in Table 36-2. Patients may also develop toxic changes of the cornea by failing to thoroughly rinse the cleaning solution from the lens prior to insertion. They may mistake the cleaning solution for the soaking solution and allow the lenses to remain in it overnight. They may work in an atmosphere of toxic vapors, such as formalin, which will damage the cornea (see Fig. 36-37). Foreign substances, such as perfumes, may be deposited on the lens from the patient's fingers and provoke a toxic corneal change.

If a toxic reaction is diagnosed, lens wear must be temporarily discontinued until the cornea has healed. Treatment often involves the use of topical steroids. The toxic material must be removed from the lens by thorough rinsing with a sterile unpreserved saline solution. Hydrophilic lenses should be soaked in the sterile unpreserved saline solutions for at least 24 hours and then disinfected. It may not be possible to remove some toxic materials from the contact lens and lens replacement may be necessary. The patient's care regime is then modified to avoid the offending chemical.

Sensitivity reactions

A sensitivity or hypersensitivity reaction does not occur when a patient is first exposed to a material. There must be previous exposure. Unless a patient has been exposed in the past to a chemical used in the care of contact lenses, no reaction to the offending substance will occur immediately. The patient will have been using the chemical in the care of their lenses for several months before the reaction occurs. Neither the patient nor the fitter may suspect that the problem is caused by a certain chemical because, as is often heard in the office, "I have been using that solution for months, so it could not be the cause of my problem."

An immune response is part of the reaction of the conjunctiva and cornea to many different things that act as sensitizers. The immune response is essentially the same, no matter what its etiology. The conjunctiva will show redness with edema. The cornea will show punctate and infiltrates. The fact that the sensitivity response is so similar regardless of the causes that trigger it, makes it easy to confuse a sensitivity to a chemical to one caused by something else. A review of the charts of patients wearing contact lenses who had red eyes with or without corneal involvement revealed that a chemical sensitivity had been confused with numerous other diagnoses.

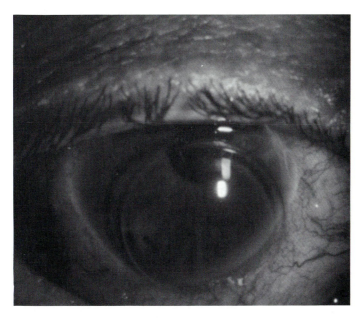

Fig 36-18 ■ Episcleritis as a manifestation of a sensitivity to the thimerosal preservative in a soaking solution for a RGP lens.

When it was recognized that thimerosal produced a sensitivity in 40% of patients, the accuracy of diagnosing sensitivity responses to chemicals used in the care of contact lenses improved significantly. All the care materials that the patient has used with the contact lenses should be looked at by the professional treating the patient. You cannot rely on what the patient tells you. Patients should bring everything they have been using with their contact lenses to the individual treating them to ensure an accurate assessment.

At the present time, thimerosal is the chemical that is most likely to be responsible for a sensitivity response. The degree of the severity of the reaction to thimerosal can vary widely. The response can be as mild as a decrease in the time a patient can wear the lenses comfortably or severe enough to produce episcleritis with pain (see Fig. 36-7, 36-8, and 36-18).

At the time of the initial examination, it is almost impossible to differentiate between a keratitis with infiltrates caused by an Adeno virus from a chemical sensitivity response (Fig. 36-19). Both these entities appear the same on examination. If the patient has had a flu-like illness, the cause of the corneal change is more likely to be an Adeno virus infection. But systemic symptoms of an Adeno virus infection may

be too mild to be noted in adults. If the corneal infiltrates clear quickly when lens-wear and the exposure to chemicals is discontinued, then the cause of the corneal change is more likely to have been a sensitivity response to chemicals.

Sorbic acid or sorbate is a preservative that can induce a sensitivity response. Its frequency

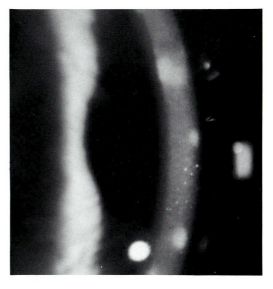

Fig 36-19 ■ Adenovirus-like infiltrates produced by a sensitivity to thimerosal.

is much lower than that produced by thimerosal. The severity of the sensitivity reaction is mild. The patient has mild symptoms of decreased wearing time associated with some discomfort. The eye shows a slight redness and the cornea may have a fine punctate present.

Any chemical used in the care of contact lenses is capable of producing a sensitivity reaction. This possible explanation for the patient's symptoms and eye changes must always be considered in the process of arriving at a diagnosis.

The diagnosis of a sensitivity reaction, as noted before, can be difficult to make. A detailed history, with very specific information on the care materials being used, must be obtained. Other causes that can produce the changes present will have to be ruled out with investigation. These investigations include swabs for cultures and scrapings for micro-organisms and the cell types present. If the removal of the contact lenses produces a rapid improvement in the eye changes, then a sensitivity response is the most likely diagnosis. If a bacterial, a chlamydial or a viral cause for the problem has been excluded, treatment of the eye with the use of topical steroids will result in rapid improvement.

When it has returned to normal, the eye can be challenged with drops of the suspected sensitizing agent to confirm the diagnosis. Changing the method of care to eliminate the suspected chemical is, of course, required when the patient returns to lens wear. A sensitivity response can be triggered by trace amounts of the guilty compound. Trace quantities may have been adsorbed by the lens or may be present in the surface coating on the lens. It may be necessary for the patient to obtain new lenses to avoid this possible source of continuing problems.

PROBLEMS OF CORNEAL INFECTIONS RELATED TO CARE

An infection of the cornea is a serious eye problem (Fig. 36-20). The stroma of the cornea lacks defenses against infection. An infection of the stroma will grow rapidly worse. If the infection is caused by *Streptococcus pneumonia* or *Pseudomonas aeruginosa*, the cornea may perforate within 24 hours and the eye may be lost. Dense scarring of the cornea can occur with infections. The vision of the eye may be significantly reduced. Rapid and accurate treatment of a suspected corneal infection is absolutely necessary to minimize the threat to vision that is present.

It must always be suspected that the source of an infection, in the eye of a patient wearing contact lenses, is from the care system. The case and solutions of a patient with an eye infection must be cultured. The method of use of the care system must be reviewed in detail with the patient to determine if he or she is complying with the care directions. The majority of corneal infections occur in patients who are not complying with the care system recommended. Unfortu-

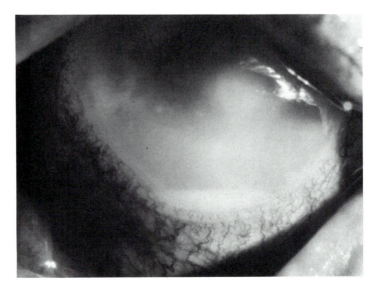

Fig 36-20 ■ Corneal infiltrate with hypopyon from an infection with a contact lens.

nately, there is also a group of patients who develops an infection because the individual who fitted the contact lenses is at fault. The fitter failed to recommend an adequate care system, failed to adequately train the patient in the care of the contact lenses, or failed to monitor the patient in the use of the care system. Compliance is not totally the responsibility of the patient. It is the obligation of the fitter to ensure that patient compliance is likely. If compliance is not occurring, then the patient should be advised to discontinue wearing the contact lenses.

A corneal infection is manifested by the presence of an infiltrate, which is an opaque area in the cornea of varying density and color (Figs. 36-21A and 21B). Infiltrates can also be produced by an immune response. The immune response may be to the infecting microorganism, the products of its metabolism, or the tissue destruction it produces. The immune response may also be part of a sensitivity reaction to a chemical in the care system, or to the coating on a lens (see Figs. 36-33A and B). An infiltrate from an infection will, in its early stages, look the same as an infiltrate that is a result of a chemical or lens-coating sensitivity reaction. If

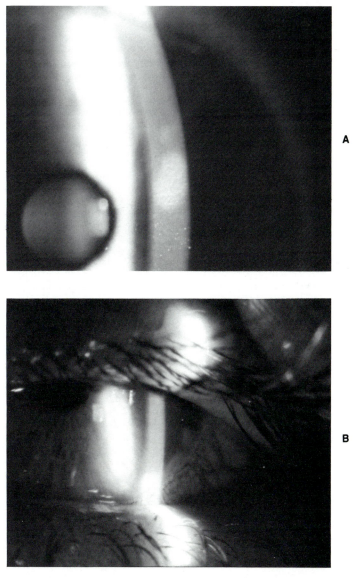

Fig 36-21 ■ **A,** Corneal infiltrate that could be from an infection but was caused by a thimerosal sensitivity. **B,** Marginal corneal infiltrates that could be from the toxins of a *Staphylococcus* infection but were caused by a thimerosal sensitivity.

the infiltrate is small in size and depth and the epithelium overlying the area of the infiltrate is intact, it is less likely that an infection is the cause. However, there is no guarantee of this. An irritable eye with a corneal infiltrate must always be treated as though it were infected until it is proved otherwise by the investigations done or by the clinical course. Time should not be wasted.

Swabs from the conjunctiva and scrapings from the infiltrate are taken for culture and for examination for micro-organisms after staining. It can be difficult to obtain enough of the causative organism, with the swabs and scrapings, to make an identification. For this reason, samples of the solution in the lens case and samples from all the bottles of the care solutions that the patient is using should be cultured. Cultures of the solution in the lens cases from patients who have no problems will almost inevitably yield growths of several bacteria. However, in the case of a suspected bacterial infiltrate, the recovery of a very pathogenic bacteria such as *Pseudomonas aeruginosa* from the lens case should lead the clinician to treat that organism, as it is probably the cause of the infection. Patients wearing RGP lenses have had corneal infiltrates and red uncomfortable eyes although no bacteria could be isolated from the swabs or scrapings taken from the eyes. When their chlorhexidine preserved conditioning solution was cultured, a heavy and pure growth of *Serratia marcescens* was discovered (See Figs. 36-10A and B). The patients were treated for this infection with good clinical results.

When it has been proved to the physician's satisfaction that an active infection is not present in the cornea, the infiltrates may be treated with topical steroids. Topical steroids should never be used initially in the treatment of the infiltrates because they will mask the symptoms and signs while the infecting element, bacteria, chlamydia or virus, continues its destructive activity. When the eye has been returned to normal, contact-lens wear may be resumed. It may be necessary to wait for months or even years before resuming contact-lens wear depending on the extent of the injury the eye has suffered. New lenses will be required and a different care system will probably be needed.

At present the most difficult corneal infection to treat is the one caused by *Acanthamoeba* (see Figs. 36-2 A and B). *Acanthamoeba* are present in all waters that are not rendered sterile. The best method of treating this disastrous corneal infection is to prevent it by instructing the patient not to use tap or distilled water in the care system of their contact lenses. The only care system for hydrophilic contact lenses that will kill *Acanthamoeba* reliably is a heater unit. Once *Acanthamoeba* infects the eye, it is hard to diagnose and its treatment is long and arduous.

PROBLEMS OF CLEANING METHODS
Lens surface coating

There are numerous materials available for cleaning contact lenses. Any contact lens that is placed on an eye will coat. The amount and type of coating that accumulates on the surface of a contact lens is primarily determined by the characteristics of the lens material. Information on the rapidity of coating of contact-lens materials in a given patient is provided in the box below.

The coating on the contact lens consists of a mixture of proteins, lipids, inorganic films, mucin, minerals, and material from the environment. The largest component of the protein coating is denatured lysozyme (Figs. 36-22A and B). Bacteria have been demonstrated to cling firmly to the surface of hydrophilic and RGP lenses.

Surface debris on a lens may be diffuse, mottled or concentrated in one area. The most common components of the surface debris are proteins and lipids. Proteins may show grossly on the lens surface with slit-lamp examination. Proteins can appear as a crazed layer on the surface of hydrophilic or RGP lenses. Allowing the lens to dry slightly while holding it in oblique illu-

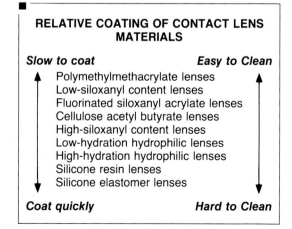

RELATIVE COATING OF CONTACT LENS MATERIALS

Slow to coat — *Easy to Clean*

Polymethylmethacrylate lenses
Low-siloxanyl content lenses
Fluorinated siloxanyl acrylate lenses
Cellulose acetyl butyrate lenses
High-siloxanyl content lenses
Low-hydration hydrophilic lenses
High-hydration hydrophilic lenses
Silicone resin lenses
Silicone elastomer lenses

Coat quickly — *Hard to Clean*

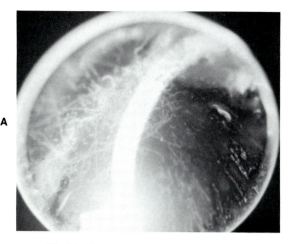
A

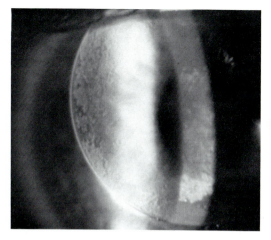
B

Fig 36-22 ■ **A,** Protein coating on a hydrophilic contact lens. **B,** Protein coating on a rigid gas-permeable contact lens.

mination will reveal less evident coating. Lipids may be more difficult to detect. A lens coated with lipids may look clean, but its surface tension has been significantly changed (Fig. 36-23). Calcium is the most common mineral found on the surface. This is most likely to occur in older patients with decreased tear production who are wearing high-water-content hydrophilic lenses (Figs. 36-24A and B).

In addition to the surface coating that will derive from the contents of the tears, there are many extrinsic elements from the environment of the patient that will contribute to spoiling the surface of any type of lens. Hands that are not washed well with a soap that is free of cream, perfume or oil additives may transfer grease, dirt, eye make-up, creams, lotions, and nicotine to the surface of the lens on insertion or removal.

Surface coating on contact lenses will produce numerous changes. The surface of the lens will not wet well. A hydrophilic lens will not hydrate properly. The layer of coating will obscure vision. The probability of developing giant papillary conjunctivitis is increased (Figs. 36-25A

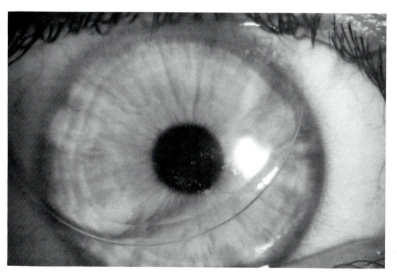

Fig 36-23 ■ A hydrophilic contact lens that appears clean but is coated with lipids and is displacing on the cornea.

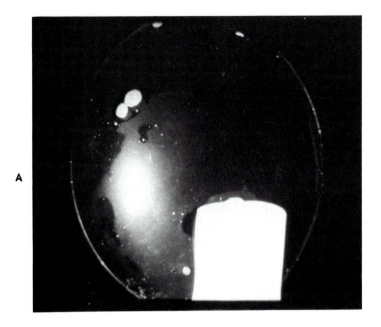

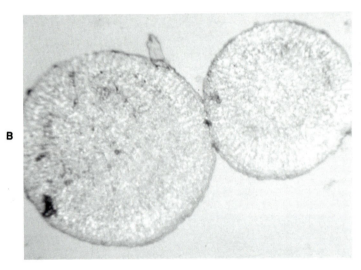

Fig 36-24 ■ A, Calcium deposits on a hydrophilic contact lens. **B,** High magnification of the calcium deposits on the hydrophilic contact lens shown in Fig 36-24A.

and B) and oxygen transmission is decreased.

Allansmith and Fowler have demonstrated that surface deposits extend over 50% of a hydrogel lens after 5 minutes and over 90% of the surface 8 hours after insertion. A cleaning system is required to remove the coating from the surface of the lenses. The cleaning system needed for hydrophilic lenses and RGP lenses consists, at the least, of a surfactant cleaner used

daily upon removal of the lenses and an enzyme cleaner used every 7 to 14 days.

The method of disinfecting hydrophilic contact lenses may contribute to the speed and amount of buildup of surface coating. Authors such as Kleist, Josephson, and Stein state that lens spoilage from surface coating will occur more rapidly when heat disinfection is used as compared to chemical disinfection. The infor-

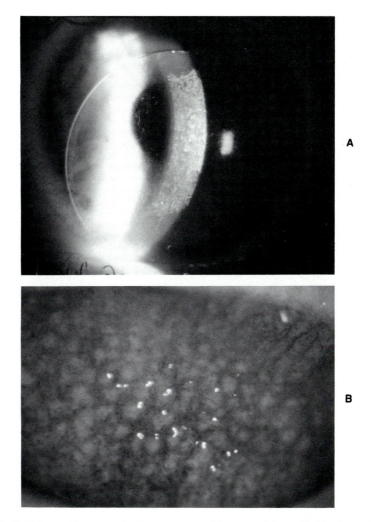

Fig 36-25 ■ **A,** Protein coating on a rigid gas-permeable contact lens. **B,** Giant papillary conjunctivitis present in a patient with evident protein coating on his or her rigid gas-permeable contact lens.

Table 36-3 ■ Incidence of common deposits on 370 lenses with deposits

| Type of deposit | Incidence | | |
	Overall (%)	Cold regimen (%)	Heat regimen (%)
Abrasions	25	28	22
Protein films	19	14	24
Pigment	25	9	38
Micro-organisms	10	4	28, unpreserved saline
			11, preserved saline
Inorganic films	10.5	5.9	14.4
Rust-colored spots	13	7	18
Lens calculi	13	13	13
Calcium carbonate	9.5	16	4
Calcium phosphate	4.6	9	1
Mercurial origin	10.5	5	21, preserved saline

From Kleist F: Deposits, International Contact Lens Clinics, May-June 1979.

mation from the study by Kleist is shown in Table 36-3.

My experience has been that there is little difference in how long low-water-content hydrophilic lenses last, no matter what the method of disinfection, heat or chemical, is used. The median useful lifetime for 38% hydration hydrophilic contact lenses has been 2 years for both heat and chemical care methods of disinfection. Cleaning these hydrophilic daily-wear lenses each day with a surfactant cleaner immediately after removal appears to allow the use of heat care without significantly reducing the useful lifetime of these lenses. The newer heater units do not heat the lenses to as high a temperature for long periods as the older heater units did. The lower temperature for shorter periods probably decreases the "baking-on" of the surface debris on the low-water content lenses.

Methods of cleaning and their problems

Cleaners for contact lenses include surfactants, enzymes, and oxidative compounds. Ultrasound maybe used as an in-office aid to clean lenses.

Surfactant cleaners. The surfactant cleaners used for hydrophilic, PMMA, and RGP contact lenses are either nonionic or amphoteric compounds in buffered isotonic preparations. Many of the brands can be used for the daily cleaning of any type of contact lenses. Daily surfactant cleaners are more efficient in removing loosely adherent surface debris than they are in cleaning the adherent denatured material on any lens surface. For this reason, daily surfactant cleaners should be used as soon as the lenses are removed from the eyes. The debris on the lens is more amenable to removal at that time than it is after being subjected to the heat or chemicals of the disinfection process. The problem is to convince patients to use a surfactant cleaner every day when they remove their lenses. Many patients have been instructed or have decided on their own that the surfactant cleaner should be used immediately before the lenses are to be inserted. Not only is this inefficient, it also exposes the patient to the toxic effects of the cleaners.

The efficiency of the different surfactant cleaners available is not significantly different. Slight advantages in cleaning may be obtained with polymeric beads for increasing the friction effect. The main factor in determining how well a surface cleaner performs is how it is used by the patient. There must be real friction applied to the lens when using the surface cleaner. The lens must be rinsed well to remove the mixture of surfactant cleaner and loosened debris or it will settle back on to the lens surface. Careful instruction of the patient in the use of surfactant surface cleaners is required.

Although many of the surfactant cleaners can be used on any type of lens material, there are certain combinations to avoid. A cleaner that is preserved with chlorhexidine or benzalkonium chloride should not be used with hydrophilic lenses because of the risk of toxicity. A cleaner that contains isopropyl alcohol is not suitable for RGP lenses that contain siloxanyl because simple alcohols act on the plastic of the lens, warping it or reducing its transparency (see Fig. 36-20).

Thimerosal is a preservative that is used in many of the daily surfactant cleaners. The ever-present risk of sensitivity to thimerosal must be kept in mind. Only a minute quantity of thimerosal can provoke the sensitivity response once it is established. Chronic exposure to small residues of thimerosal is as likely to induce a sensitivity to it as is exposure to larger amounts.

Surfactant cleaners may be formulated in a saline solution in the hope that its presence will keep the lenses cleaner. Friction is an essential part of the use of a surfactant cleaner, so these saline solutions add little to the cleaning of lenses.

Enzyme cleaners. The enzymes used for cleaning contact lenses are derived from three sources: plant, animal, and bacterial. The enzymes available for the care of contact lenses are summarized in Table 36-4.

The enzyme product that has been available the longest is papain, which is derived from a plant. It is efficient against protein residues. The molecule of papain is relatively small; it can be retained by hydrophilic lenses. As a general rule, the higher the hydration of the lens, the more papain it will retain. Papain enzyme residues were not a problem in practice when this valuable hydrophilic lens-cleaning substance was first introduced. At that time, the vast majority of soft lenses being used were 38% hydration lenses and the commonest method of disinfection was heat, which rapidly renders enzymes inactive. No residues of active papain were left on the lens to cause patient discomfort.

Table 36-4 ■ Enzyme cleaners for contact lenses

Enzyme	Source	Company	Active for	Method of use
Papain	Vegetable	Allergan	Protein	Effervescent tablet; dissolve in saline
Pancreatin	Animal	Alcon	Protein, lipids	Effervescent tablet; dissolve in saline
Subtilisin A	Bacterial	Allergan	Protein	Can be placed in H_2O_2
Subtilisin A	Bacterial	Bausch & Lomb	Protein	Effervescent tablet; dissolve in saline
Subtilisin A	Bacterial	Bausch & Lomb	Protein	Thermal formulation; use in case in heater

When cold or chemical disinfection methods were available, the problem of enzyme residues causing eye discomfort became evident. Patients continued to do what they had been told to do when using heat disinfection: they left their lense in the papain solution overnight and then they rinsed and inserted them with the papain residues present. The instructions for use of the papain where then modified. The patients soaked the lenses in the papain solution for a minimum of 3 hours, rinsed them well and placed them in the soaking solution overnight. Prior to inserting the lenses in the morning they were rinsed again. This technique alleviated the problem of enzyme residues with low-water-content lenses.

When high-water-content lenses came on the market, the problem of papain residues reappeared. These higher hydration lenses could not be cared for with heat disinfection, so enzyme residues could not be destroyed in this manner. In addition, the high-water-content lenses retained significantly more of the low-molecular-weight papain than did the 38%-hydration lenses. Leaving the highly hydrated lenses in the papain solution for at least 3 hours allowed them to accumulate more papain than the disinfection process could eliminate. Papain residues were present in the lens to cause a toxic reaction when it was inserted in the morning. The approach then was to shorten the time of exposure to the papain solution to 15 minutes. This solved the problem of papain residues on these lenses. However, the cleaning effect achieved by this short time of exposure to the papain was hardly worth the effort. Unfortunately for the patients who were using low hydration contact lenses the 15-minute time recommendation was included in the package insert instructions. This group of patients who read and

believed this information without consulting their fitter found that their lenses became coated rapidly despite the regular use of the papain enzyme 15 minutes at a time.

Pancreatin, which is derived from an animal source, was the second enzyme cleaning system made available. The pancreatin enzyme tablet contains protease, lipase, and amylase. This set of enzymes should be able to cope with all the major groups of materials that become firmly bound to the surface of a lens. The molecule size was larger. This made the problem of enzyme residues in higher hydrated soft lenses much less evident than when papain was used. In clinical practice pancreatin seems to be less efficient than papain in removing protein residues from hydrophilic contact lenses or RGP lenses with siloxanyl. The three enzyme types in pancreatin are not efficient enough in cleaning the lenses to obviate the need for the daily use of a surfactant cleaner.

Subtilisin A, which is derived from a bacterial source, is the most recent enzyme cleaner to appear on the market. The molecular size is much larger than papain. Enzyme residues are said not to be a problem because of the high molecular weight of this enzyme. Allergan has formulated Subtilisin A (Ultrazyme™) so that it may be placed directly in the hydrogen peroxide during disinfection. Bausch & Lomb has formulated Subtilisin A to permit the tablet, labeled "Thermal", to be placed in the saline solution in the case with the contact lens when the lens is being heat-disinfected. Bausch & Lomb also has a formulation of Subtilisin A in effervescent tablet form for dissolving in saline solutions. Barnes-Hind has recently introduced their Subtilisin A enzyme cleaner.

Cleaning hydrophilic lenses and RGP lenses with enzymes is needed for the average patient.

The correct use of enzyme cleaners will prolong the useful lifetime of both hydrophilic and RGP lenses. Lenses with clean surfaces are more comfortable. By reducing the amount of denatured protein on the surface of the lenses, the chances of developing GPC are decreased (see Figs. 36-22B, 36-25A and 36-25B).

The need to use an enzyme cleaner regularly is less evident to the practitioner and to the patient in the care of RGP lenses than it is with hydrophilic lenses. Without surface enzyme cleaning, hydrophilic lenses will show evidence of a surface coating that is impairing function or comfort within a few weeks of wear. RGP lenses that are not cleaned with an enzyme may not show evidence of the changes produced by the coating for 6 months or longer. Enzyme cleaning of both hydrophilic lenses and RGP lenses every 2 weeks is advised for the average patient in our practice. For patients with evidence of GPC an enzyme cleaner should be used once a week or even more often. Our clinical experience indicates the papain enzyme cleaner is the most efficient for use with RGP contact lenses. Exposing the RGP lens for at least 3 hours to the papain enzyme solution is recommended.

Oxidative cleaners. Hydrogen peroxide and hypochlorites are oxidative cleaners. The primary reason these compounds are used by patients is to disinfect the contact lenses. The cleaning action that hydrogen peroxide and hypochlorites produces through their oxidative action is a bonus. But is not sufficient to eliminate the need for surfactant and enzyme cleaning. Oxidative cleaners in general tend to produce degeneration of polymeric material. This degenerative effect is more evident with the stronger oxidative agents such as sodium perborate and sodium persulfate. Oxidative cleaners are seldom used with RGP lenses.

In-eye cleaners. In-eye cleaners, lubricators, rewetters or conditioners are designed with the hope that a few drops of them will solve problems of patient discomfort. The majority of times when these drops are recommended to a patient the reason for the problem is the poor blink pattern of the patient, that is, the blinking of the patient is inadequate in frequency or fullness or both. The drying or redness of the eyes that the patient notes when the blink is inadequate while wearing contact lenses will be relieved for such a very brief period of time by these "comfort" drops that they are hardly worth using for this complaint. The need for adequate blinking while wearing contact lenses must be taught to all patients. For many patients, the importance of blinking well must be re-emphasized frequently.

The "in-eye" drops may be preserved with thimerosal. Using them will not help the patient whose discomfort stems from a sensitivity to this chemical.

"In-eye" conditioners have been found to be a help for patients who wear their contact lenses overnight. The lenses often are reluctant to move when the patient wakes up. The "in-eye" drops and good blinking habit help the lenses to move, which improves vision and comfort. The use of "in-eye" lubricants may be a necessity in an environment with a very low humidity. Patients with a borderline volume of tear production who are wearing RGP lenses may find an "in-eye" wetting drop helpful if they are willing to use them frequently while wearing the lenses.

DIAGNOSIS OF "RED EYE" IN PATIENTS WEARING CONTACT LENSES
Introduction

The patient wearing contact lenses who presents with a red eye can be one of the more difficult clinical problems that an ophthalmologist has to diagnose. In the many years that I have taught residents in ophthalmology, the one clinical problem that seems to take them the longest to master is the patient with a red eye wearing contact lenses. One of the residents began his presentation on the red eye in contact lens patients with the phrase "Don't panic."

"Don't panic" neatly sums up the mental approach the clinician must adopt when a patient with a red eye, who wears contact lenses, sits opposite him. A logical detailed approach to the problem, coupled with an understanding of the factors that may be acting to produce the red eye, are essential.

Each of the three elements present: the lens, the care of the lens, and the patient, may be the reason for the red eye or all of them may be operative to varying degrees to produce the problem.

History from patient

A detailed history must be taken from the patient. The essential details that must be obtained from the patient are listed below.

PHYSICIAN ALERT

This patient may be wearing hard Contact Lenses.
Instructions for removal on back of this card.

NAME

	Power	B.C.	Diam.	Material
R				
L				

JOHN F. MORGAN, M.D., F.R.C.S.(C)
Eye Dept., Hotel Dieu Hospital
Kingston, Ontario — 544-4853

A

PHYSICIAN ALERT

This patient may be wearing Hydrophilic Contact Lenses
Instructions for removal on back of this card

NAME

	Power	B.C.	Diam.	Company
R				
L				

JOHN F. MORGAN, M.D., F.R.C.S.(C)
Eye Dept. Hotel Dieu Hospital
Kingston, Ontario - 544-4853

B

HYDROPHILIC LENSES

Instruction for Removal

1. Never probe about on the eye in search of a lens. Open eye lids. Find position of lens using a small beam of light **before** attempting to remove it.

2. Wash and rinse hands thoroughly before beginning the removal procedure. Retract the lower lid and place the index fingertip gently on the lower edge of the lens. Slide the lens down to the white part of the eye.

3. Compress the lens lightly between the thumb and index finger. Remove the lens from the eye.

4. If the carrying case is available, put the lens inside the cap of carrying case. If not, store in sterile normal saline as quickly as possible.
Caution: In case of severe trauma, shock or coma, the lens may adhere to the eye owing to insufficiency of tear flow. If the lens fails to move after gentle attempts to move it, flush the eye with sterile normal saline solution and wait for a few minutes before another attempt.

HARD LENSES

Instruction for Removal

1. Never probe about on the eye in search of a lens. Open eye lids. Find position of lens using a small beam of light **before** attempting to remove it.

2. Wash and rinse hands thoroughly before beginning the removal procedure.

3. Place fingertips of index fingers on upper and lower lids near margin. Open lids and then close lids with gentle pressure on cornea to "flip" lens out.

4. Place the lens in normal saline (in their own case if available).
Caution: In case of severe trauma, shock or coma, the lens may adhere to the eye owing to insufficiency of tear flow. If the lens fails to move after gentle attempts to remove it, flush the eye with sterile normal saline solution and wait for a few minutes before another attempt.

Fig 36-26 ■ Contact-lens identification card with instructions for removal, given to patients who have been fitted **A**, with hydrophilic contact lenses, and **B**, with rigid gas-permeable contact lenses.

Time of onset of the eye symptoms:
1. Was the lens in or out of the eye when the symptoms began?
2. Was the discomfort made worse with the lens in or out?
3. How soon after the lens was placed on the eye did the symptoms begin?
4. Has a similar problem occurred previously?

Details of lens wearing:
1. When were the contact lenses fitted?
2. Who fitted the contact lenses?
3. What type of lenses are they? Ideally, the specifications of the contact lenses should be obtained. Patients should be given a card (Fig. 36-26A, B, C, and D) with the specifications of the lenses to carry in their wallet. However, this is seldom done. You are lucky if the patient can tell you whether their contact lenses are soft, semi-soft, or hard.
4. How old are the present contact lenses?
5. How long does the patient wear the lenses on average each day?
6. Has the wearing time increased or decreased?

Details of the care of the lenses:
1. What method of care is being used?
2. What are the names of all the materials that are used in the care of the lenses? Patients are seldom able to give you this information accurately. If you know that you are to deal with a red eye in patients wearing contact lenses when they phone for an appointment, have them bring all their care materials with them. It is also usually necessary to request that the patient bring all their care materials for your inspection at their first follow-up visit. This is the only way to confirm exactly what the patient has been using.
3. How frequently are the lenses cleaned and disinfected? When was this last done?

Details of the patient:
1. General health, current or recent illness, medications.
2. Known allergies or sensitivities.
3. Recent exposure to others with "red eyes."
4. Topical eye medications or systemic medications used.
5. Environmental factors or change in the environment.

When the details of the history have been obtained, the examiner may know the reason for the red eye. The diagnostic process continues with a thorough examination of the physical state of the patient's eyes. The lenses must be examined for their type and physical condition. The parameters of the lenses, such as power, diameter, thickness, edge and blend appearance should be noted. The extent to which this can be done will depend on the equipment available and the type of lens.

The history and examination may determine that the red eye is not a result of wearing the

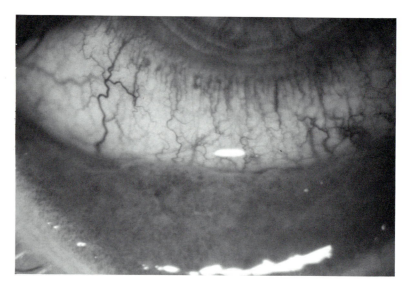

Fig 36-27 ■ Red eye caused by an inclusion conjunctivitis (TRIC) in a patient wearing contact lenses.

contact lenses (Fig. 36-27). The wearing of the contact lenses may have increased the discomfort, but the lenses or their care method were not the underlying cause of the red eye. A patient should never put a contact lens on a red irritable eye and a lens should always be removed immediately from a red irritable eye. Common sense is a difficult thing to teach.

Infection of the eye is the major concern when a patient wearing contact lenses presents with a red eye. In addition to redness, an infected eye will have a discharge that may be watery or purulent. If the redness is more marked in the conjunctiva on the inside of the lids than it is on the conjunctiva overlying the eye itself, then the patient has conjunctivitis. If the redness is more marked in the conjunctiva on the eye and there are infiltrates present in the cornea, the patient has a keratitis. Swabs from the conjunctiva and scrapings from the corneal infiltrate are taken to identify the causative bacteria. The case and the care materials should also be cultured. Treatment will be started with a broad-spectrum antibiotic. It must always be initially presumed that a red eye with corneal infiltrates has a bacterial infection until it is proved otherwise.

When an acute infection has been ruled out as the cause of the red eye, the examiner can assess the evidence for other causes of the red eye. Many of these causes relate to the lenses or their care. These are briefly discussed below.

Causes of red eye in lens wearers

Acute corneal hypoxia. This entity, historically and erroneously called the *overwearing syndrome* is seldom seen now as it resulted from the wearing of contact lenses made from materials that were not gas permeable. It used to be the most common cause of a red and uncomfortable eye in a contact-lens wearer. A foreign-body discomfort and redness of the eye would begin several hours after the lenses had been removed. The anoxic, dying epithelium would take a period of time to slough off the cornea and leave the nerves exposed to cause the pain (Fig. 36-28). The lens must be left off the eye and the eye firmly patched to achieve healing. This problem will recur if patients continue to wear lenses with poor gas permeability. When the cornea has healed, the patient should be refitted with a gas-permeable lens.

Chronic hypoxia. The gas-permeability of hydrophilic lenses and RGP lenses that are thick

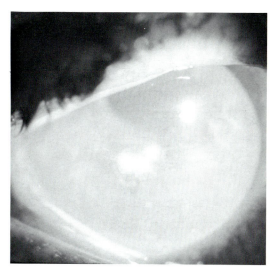

Fig 36-28 ■ Central epithelial erosion from acute corneal hypoxia in a patient wearing contact lenses that were not gas-permeable.

may be adequate enough to prevent acute corneal hypoxia but may leave a chronic shortage of oxygen. The lenses become more uncomfortable as the day goes on and as the eye becomes red. The cornea may show punctate, intraepithelial microcysts, and stromal edema. In the more severe and chronic cases there will be vessel invasion of the cornea (Fig. 36-29). To prevent these problems the patient should be refitted with lenses of higher gas permeability, if this is possible. If it is not possible to refit the patient, the daily wearing time must be restricted or lens wear should be discontinued.

Lens defects. The lens must be carefully examined for damage. An edge chip in a hard lens or a fissure in a soft lens will damage the corneal epithelium (Fig. 36-30A and B). The patient will note discomfort when the lens is inserted and relief when it is removed. The cornea will show an area of epithelial damage, loss or drying. The cornea should be allowed to heal, with patching if necessary, before the replacement lens is worn.

Mechanical effects. A hard or soft contact lens that has a poorly finished peripheral curve or edge area will be chronically irritating and produce redness of the eye. The lens is uncomfortable on insertion and the discomfort continues at the same level. A soft lens that has a poor peripheral area finish will produce a perilimbal

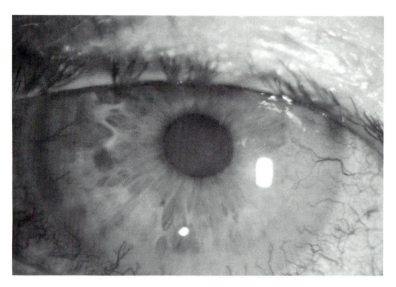

Fig 36-29 ■ Vessels invading the cornea caused by chronic corneal hypoxia from a contact lens that had inadequate gas permeability.

area of roughening. A hard lens with an inadequate peripheral area finish may produce an arcuate area of staining on the cornea. There may be no corneal changes in milder cases of this problem. Refinishing the periphery of the hard lens or changing the soft lens will be required.

Inadequate blinking. The failure to establish a blinking pattern that is adequate in frequency and fullness is the most common cause of redness of the eyes in contact lens wearers. The normal blink rate is 17 times a minute. A contact lens on an eye will invariably reduce the frequency and fullness of the blink. The contact lens wearer must reestablish the blink reflex when wearing contact lenses. To do this the fitter of the contact lens must inform the patient of the problem. The patient must be taught to "Think blink" to reestablish a good blink. The patient with poor tear distribution from the inadequate blink will note increasing redness of the eyes in the 3 and 9 o'clock positions with a burning discomfort as the wearing time increases (Fig. 36-31). The patient may also have punctate of the periphery of the cornea in the 3 and 9 o'clock positions. Six hours is usually the maximum time that a patient with this problem can tolerate this discomfort. If the patient gets over this hurdle, a good blink has been established. The patient can then proceed easily to all-day wear of his contact lenses. The problem of drying of the eye that a poor blink creates can

worsen if the lens design has a thick edge or if the lens diameter is inappropriate for the eye. The chronic drying can be severe enough to produce a dellen (Fig. 36-32). Redesigning the lens will be required.

Lens surface debris. If a contact lens made from any material accumulates surface debris, it will irritate the eye and make it become red. The debris on the surface of the lens may be evident with the lens on the eye when examined with the slit lamp. Not only should gross degrees of debris on the surface be specifically looked for, but the wetting characteristics of the lens surface should also be assessed when it is on the cornea. If the surface of the lens has areas that are drying rapidly, the lens will be a cause of irritation and redness. The lens may appear to be clear when on the eye, but it should also be examined, free of excess fluid, off the eye, using oblique illumination. Changes in the clearness and color of the lens will be more evident with the oblique illumination method of examination. A patient with lens-surface debris as a problem will usually give a history of gradually increasing discomfort when wearing the lens with vision that is less clear. The eye may be mildly red but the cornea is usually clear. However, occasionally surface debris on the lens can cause infiltrates of the cornea (Figs. 36-33A and B).

The tarsal conjunctiva of the upper lid should always be examined on a regular basis in every

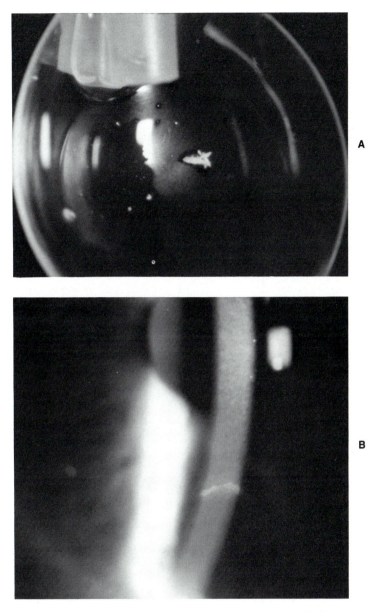

Fig 36-30 ■ **A,** Fissure in a hydrophilic lens that caused discomfort. **B,** Corneal roughening caused by the fissure in the hydrophilic lens shown in Fig 36-30A.

patient wearing contact lenses. It must always be done when the patient has a red eye. Surface debris on the lens is the cause of the immune response change, GPC, which occurs in the conjunctiva of the upper lid. It will not be diagnosed unless the upper lid is everted. Grossly coated contact lenses are the ones most likely to incite a GPC reaction (see Fig. 36-25B).

If a coated lens is determined to be the cause of the red eye, the lens will have to be replaced.

The patient's cleaning techniques will have to be improved. If coating continues to be the source of problems for the patient, then refitting the patient with a contact lens made from a material less prone to coating will be necessary.

Lens movement. If a contact lens does not move adequately, the tear layer between the lens and the cornea will not be frequently changed. The degree of lens movement required will vary with the type of material. Extended-

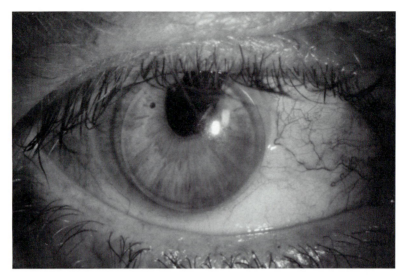

Fig 36-31 ■ 3 o'clock and 9 o'clock injection from inadequate blinking when wearing a contact lens.

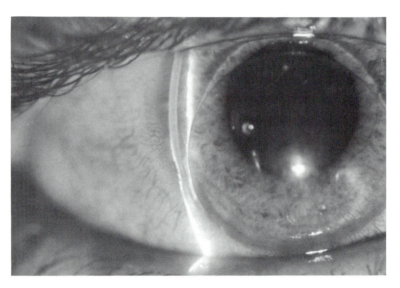

Fig 36-32 ■ A dellen at the edge of a RGP contact lens.

wear hydrophilic lenses, silicone elastomer lenses, and RGP lenses worn overnight are the ones most likely to lose all movement. Loss of movement can happen to any type of lens. The complete loss of movement of the lens produces stagnation of the tear layer. The epithelium is a rapidly growing cell layer and sheds old cells constantly into the tears, to be flushed away. If these dead cells are trapped behind the lens, the self-destruction enzymes that they release

will damage the living epithelial cells. The products of metabolism, such as lactic acid, are toxic and these are also retained. Various terms, such as *locked-on lens, stuck-on lens, tight lens syndrome* or *glued-on lens* have been used to describe this sequence of events.

The patient with the problem of loss of movement of the contact lens may have an eye that shows only mild redness and punctate. The non-moving lens may be evident. If the patient has

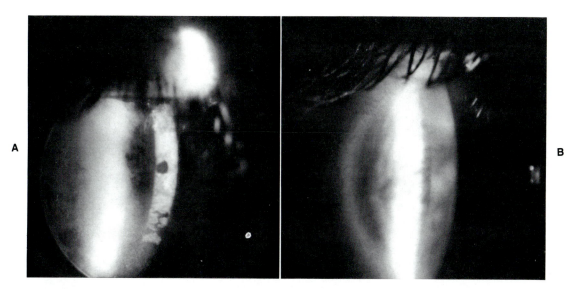

Fig 36-33 ■ **A,** Coating on a Fluorinated Siloxanyl Acetate (FSA) rigid gas-permeable contact lens. **B,** Corneal infiltrates seen in patient wearing the lens shown in Fig 36-33A.

managed to remove the RGP lens that has caused this problem, an indentation circle from the edge of the lens will be visible in the corneal epithelium (Fig. 36-34).

The patient with a non-moving lens may present with severe inflammation, corneal infiltrates, and iritis. This degree of reaction has been seen with all types of lenses for extended wear. A silicone elastomer (rubber) lens manufactured in Germany and used only in Europe caused very severe eye changes when it lost movement and became locked on (Fig. 36-35). With the silicone elastomer lens, the lens could be truly glued on as the tear layer would be completely lost. The corneal surface and the surface of the elastomer lens both become very hydrophobic and then stick to each to the extent that surgical removal of the lens may be required (Fig. 36-36). The patient who has had a tight lens syndrome must be refitted when the eye has returned to normal.

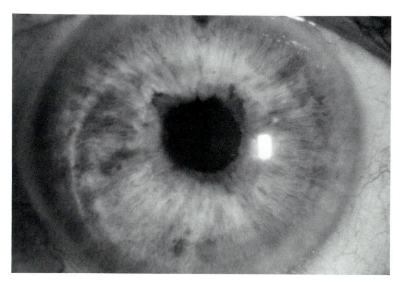

Fig 36-34 ■ Indentation ring on the cornea from a RGP contact lens that lost movement.

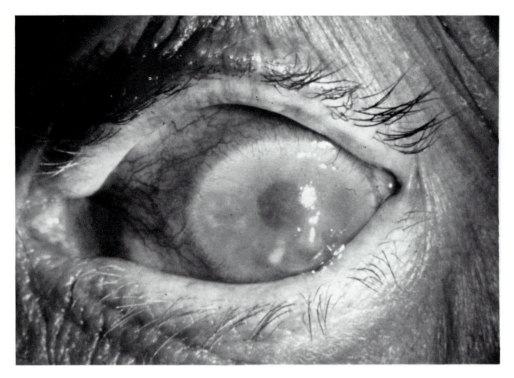

Fig 36-35 ■ Severe inflammation with corneal infiltrates and iritis from a "locked on" German silicone elastomer contact lens. (Courtesy of Dr H Roth, Ulm, West Germany.)

Lens care factors: toxic reactions. Toxic changes from the chemicals used for the care of the lenses can result in red, irritable eyes (see Table 36-2). Errors in the use of the surfactant daily cleaning solutions are common. The patient fails to adequately rinse the surfactant cleaner from the surface of the lens before inserting the lens on the cornea. The patient should have been instructed to use the daily cleaner immediately after removal of the lens and not immediately before inserting the lens. Daily surface cleaners for PMMA or RGP contact lenses are generally more toxic than the daily cleaners for hydrophilic lenses. The patient may inadvertently obtain a hard-lens cleaner and use it with hydrophilic lenses. The daily cleaner may be mistaken for a soaking solution. The results of this are painful when the lens is inserted. If a patient contaminates the lens with a material from his environment, such as perfume, suntan lotion, or solvents, the history of discomfort will be the same (Fig. 36-37). When the lens is inspected, it will often show evidence of the contamination. The patient with these problems will have discomfort and redness of the eyes as soon

as the lens is placed on the eye. A careful history and review of the care methods and materials should diagnose this problem. Topical steroids may be needed to treat the eye depending on the extent of the corneal damage present. A hydrophilic lens may have to be replaced as it tends to retain the chemical. A PMMA or RGP lens can usually be rinsed free of the residual chemical.

Hydrogen peroxide residues and enzyme residues will produce redness of the eyes from their toxic effects on the cornea. The symptoms are immediately present on lens insertion. The method the patient is using with these materials must be discerned to identify the reason for the problem. An understanding of the methods of hydrogen peroxide neutralization is required. The types of enzymes available (see Table 36-4) and their individual prediliction to be retained by high-water-content lenses must be known. The redness and corneal punctate changes are usually marked in these patients. The use of topical steroids for 4 to 5 days is often required to make the eye comfortable. The insult to the eye usually heals well. The patient's use of the

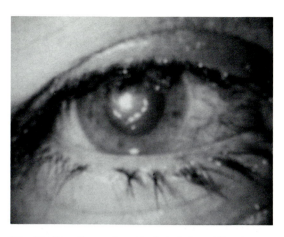

Fig 36-36 ■ Corneal epithelial defect left when a "glued on" German silicone elastomer lens had to be surgically removed. (Courtesy of Dr H Roth, Ulm, West Germany.)

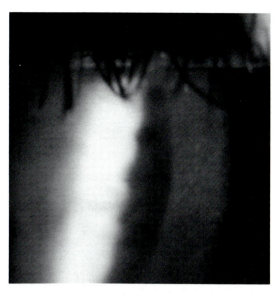

Fig 36-37 ■ Corneal punctate in a patient who was wearing a hydrophilic lens while working in an atmosphere of formalin vapors.

offending material must be modified to prevent a recurrence of the episode.

The toxic problems produced by care materials that are being used according to directions are less evident by obtaining a history. The materials actually being used must be inspected for the presence of chemicals known to produce a toxic effect. In the care of hydrophilic lenses, the chemicals to suspect for causing toxic changes are chlorhexidine and alkyl triethanolammonium chloride (TEAC). With RGP lenses, the potentially offending chemicals are benzylkonium chloride and chlorobutanol. The redness of the eyes will usually be most evident shortly after the lenses are inserted. The redness may actually decrease as the day goes on as the tears dilute the chemical residues. The problem may have dated from the time the patient began to use the chemicals. The cornea may show fine, diffuse punctate changes and intraepithelial microcysts. Another care system, with less toxic chemicals, will be required to solve the problem.

Lens-care factors: sensitivity reactions. It is possible to become hypersensitive to almost any compound in the systems for the care of contact lenses. However, the two chemicals most likely to be guilty are thimerosal, a mercury-based chemical, and sorbic acid (sorbate). Thimerosal, which has a 40% frequency of producing sensitization is by far the most common cause of a sensitivity reaction. The patients will have been using the solutions containing the chemical to

which they are sensitive for months. Sensitization requires a period of exposure to a complex. It does not occur immediately on first exposure. The eye with a thimerosal sensitivity reaction can show a wide range of changes that can be mistaken for many other causes as previously discussed. The care materials must be examined personally by the individual assessing the patient. Only in this manner can the presence of a sensitizing chemical in the care system or in eye drops being used by the patient be excluded as a cause of the difficulty. When the diagnosis of a sensitivity response is confirmed, treatment with topical steroids will rapidly improve the eye. The care method must be changed to eliminate the suspected chemical to which the patient is sensitive. Hydrophilic lenses will probably have to be replaced because they will retain minute amounts of the chemical and continue the sensitivity reaction. PMMA and RGP lenses should be thoroughly cleaned and rinsed.

Lens care factors: contaminated solutions. If the patient has the misfortune to have care solutions that have become contaminated with micro-organisms, serious eye infections may result. Solutions may become contaminated with bacteria, fungi, yeasts, amoeba, and viruses. Whenever an infection is suspected all the care solutions including the solution in the lens case should be cultured along with the swabs and scrapings from the eye. Unfortunately, viruses cannot be grown from these culture attempts. But if all the cultures are reported as negative, then it is more likely that a virus is the cause. *Acanthamoeba* infection is difficult to diagnose and to treat. It must always be suspected in a chronically inflamed eye with corneal changes.

Patient factors: allergies and sensitivties. The red eye that the patient presents with may have no relationship to the use of contact lenses except that wearing contact lenses when an eye is red for some reason will make it worse. A carefully taken history often reveals the presence of an allergy to spring pollens or ragweed as the cause of the red eye. The seasonal nature of the problem and the associated symptoms such as sneezing, nasal congestion, and possibly asthma, will explain the red eye. Sensitivities to materials in the environment as the reason for the red eye will require more investigation. The patient may have to keep a diary of what happens shortly before the eyes become red to discover the offending agent. The material that provokes the sensitivity reaction in the eye of the patient may be something as unlikely as carbonless duplicating paper or something as common as animal dander, particularly cat dander. The patient may only be able to wear the contact lenses for short periods of time if the material that the patient is sensitive to in the environment cannot be avoided. Topical steroids, as weak as possible, judiciously used, may be required. Sodium cromoglycate can be of value in treating these patients, but sodium cromoglycate should be used for 2 weeks before the time of exposure to the material that is provoking the allergic or sensitivity reaction.

Patient factors: medications. The patient may be taking systemic medications or using eye drops that may cause the eyes to be red. Again, a careful patient history should reveal these possibilities. Eye drops can produce the red eye because of a sensitivity to one of its components. Systemic medications can cause red eyes. It is often necessary to refer to a good Pharmaceutical Formulary to discover if the medication being used has been known to cause eye problems. Discontinuing the medication or discontinuing the wearing of lenses while the systemic medication is being used may be the treatment required. Some eye drops that are required on a regular basis to control a disorder of the eye, such as epinephrine for lowering pressure in the eye, cause redness of the eye in everyone who uses them. A degree of redness may have to be tolerated in such patients.

Patient factors: infection. The infection that a patient has may not have come from the lenses or care system. A history of exposure to someone with a red eye may indicate the reason for the problem. The patient with a chronic blepharitis or meibomitis is always at risk of a conjunctivitis or keratitis from the bacteria present in and on the lids. Even if the reason for the infection does not appear to be the lenses or care system, the lenses must not be worn until the infection is cured. The solutions being used may have become contaminated by the patient with the infecting agent. Replacing them is a safe approach.

Patient factors: multiple. Despite the best efforts made there is a small group of patients who will have red eyes when wearing contact lenses. These patients may lack the motivation to become adequate blinkers; they may work in a very dry environment; they may have a low-grade blepharitis, which they will not work to control. Their tear production or quality may be borderline in its adequacy. They may not be able to or wish to avoid environmental materials to which they are sensitive, such as cat dander. It is best that these patients not wear contact lenses at all; however, if they insist on wearing them they must be carefully monitored.

37 ▪ *ENDOTHELIAL RESPONSE TO CONTACT LENSES*

- Endothelial blebs
- Endothelial polymegathism and pleomorphism
- Conclusions

Contact lenses may induce short- and long-term corneal endothelial changes. These morphologic changes may be seen with daily-wear and extended-wear soft and rigid contact lenses. A brief review of the normal anatomy and physiology of the corneal endothelium (discussed in more detail in Chapter 1) will allow appreciation of the pathophysiology of these endothelial changes and of their potential significance.

The corneal endothelium is a single layer of cells and forms the most posterior layer of the cornea (Fig. 37-1). The integrity of this layer is crucial for maintenance of normal corneal transparency. Its main function is to keep the cornea in a relatively dehydrated state for optimum clarity. This is accomplished by means of an energy-dependent metabolic pump and a relative barrier to fluid flow between the endothelial cells. Loss of endothelial function results in prompt corneal swelling.

The endothelium appears to have limited regenerative potential. If the endothelial cells are damaged, the remaining cells in the area respond by enlarging and migrating to cover the

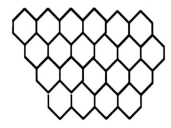

Fig 37-1 ▪ Corneal endothelium: normal mosaic.

defect. Mitotic activity is minimal. With increasing age there is a decrease in endothelial cell density and a concurrent increase in the variability of cell size. A variety of insults including trauma, infection, and intra-ocular surgery can damage and destroy endothelial cells and thereby hasten the aging process. Given their limited regnerative potential, as endothelial cell loss occurs a point may be reached where the remaining cells are not sufficient in number to enlarge and cover the entire posterior corneal surface which produces corneal decompensation with resultant edema and decreased vision.

ENDOTHELIAL BLEBS

The endothelial bleb response, which is the earliest endothelial cell change, develops within minutes after insertion of a thick soft or rigid contact lens. This endothelial change resolves slowly after 30 minutes of lens wear or rapidly after discontinuation of lens wear. This bleb response also occurs with atmospheric anoxia, lid closure, and exposure to carbon dioxide. The response is transient and does not seem to be associated with any lasting sequelae. This pathophysiologic endothelial change may be secondary to hypoxia, which results in a lowering in corneal stroma pH.

ENDOTHELIAL POLYMEGATHISM AND PLEOMORPHISM

Morphologic changes of the corneal endothelium can occur with daily-wear and extended-wear soft and rigid contact lenses. Although the mean cell size is normal, there is a wide variability in individual cell sizes. The cellular variability is similar to that seen in much older non-contact lens wearing populations. This gives the appearance of accelerated aging. These changes are thought to be secondary to hypoxia, which

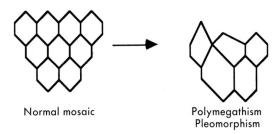

Normal mosaic   Polymegathism
                 Pleomorphism

Fig 37-2 ■ Corneal endothelium showing polymegathism and pleomorphism.

leads to lactate accumulation, elevated carbon dioxide levels, and pH changes. These changes lead to *polymegathism* (a variation in cell size) and *pleomorphism* (a variation in cell shape; Fig. 37-2). Polymegathism is a term used to describe an increase in the coefficient of variation in endothelial cell size (defined as the standard deviation of cell area divided by the mean cell area). The coefficient of variation in cell size in normal, non-contact lens wearers is usually below 0.32. Pleomorphism is defined as an increase in the proportion of non-six-sided (hexagonal) cells in the monolayer; hexagonality is normally above 60% in a non-contact lens wearing group.

Studies on polymethylmethacrylate (PMMA) hard contact lens wearers have demonstrated that the degree of ploymegathism is greater in patients who have worn their contact lenses for longer periods. The increase in polymegathism has ranged between 31% and 82% in these studies with a duration of contact lens wear that is between 9 and 23 years. A similar increase in polymegathism of 13% to 44% was noted in daily-wear soft contact lens wearers when compared to age-matched controls. Recent studies have also shown that these changes occur in patients who have worn RGP lenses and in former PMMA lens wearers who have switched to RGP contact lenses.

Polymegathism has been noted in cosmetic and aphakic extended-wear soft contact lens patients. These changes were noted by Holden et al. in 1985 in a study of patients wearing unilateral extended-wear soft contact lenses. With a mean duration of 5 years of wear they noted a 22% increase in polymegathism. Matsuda et al. published a study in 1988 in which they evaluated a group of contact lens-wearing aphakic individuals and an age-matched control group of non-contact lens-wearing aphakes who had uncomplicated intracapsular cataract extraction; they were evaluated approximately 2 years after cataract surgery. The extended-wear contact lens group had significantly increased coefficients of variation in cell size (51%) and a 28% reduction in the relative frequency of hexagonal cells, as compared to the control group.

MacRae et al. (1986) studied the reversibility of these endothelial changes in patients who had stopped wearing PMMA contact lenses for an average of 4.3 years after having worn them an average of 9.6 years. This study showed that the former hard contact lens wearers had persistent polymegathism and pleomorphism when compared to an age-matched control group. Additional studies by Holden's group (1985 and 1986) have demonstrated that although there is a slight trend toward reversal, there is no significant reduction in polymegathism 6 months after discontinuation of extended-wear contact lenses.

The majority of studies have noted no significant difference in endothelial cell density with the wearing of soft or rigid contact lenses. However, a study by Matsuda et al. (1989) showed a decrease in endothelial cell density in post-penetrating keratoplasty keratoconus patients who were fitted with PMMA hard contact lenses as compared to the donor-matched control group who did not wear contact lenses. The reduction in endothelial cell density in corneal transplant patients as compared to control groups may occur because transplanted corneas are more susceptible to stress. It remains unclear whether other contact-lens-wearing groups with polymegathism and pleomorphism will eventually develop a reduction in endothelial cell density. Further studies are necessary to clarify this important area of concern.

A long-term concern in contact-lens wearers with morphometric changes (polymegathism and pleomorphism) is that of corneal decompensation, especially when associated with stress such as that caused by ocular surgery. Rao et al. (1984) showed a relationship between abnormal endothelial cell morphology and corneal deturgescence; patients with a greater degree of pre-operative polymegathism were more likely to have irreversible corneal edema after cataract and intra-ocular lens implantation surgery. It is of interest that in the same study a reduced endothelial cell density was not associated with a greater corneal decompensation rate.

Since there is evidence that contact lenses may cause irreversible endothelial changes that may affect function especially under stressful conditions (e.g., intra-ocular surgery) it is wise to adopt a fitting policy that minimizes these morphometric changes. Some basic guidelines are as follows:

1. Since the highest risk group is made up of PMMA lens wearers who have worn their lenses for over 20 years, we recommend re-fitting these individuals with a highly oxygen-permeable rigid gas-permeable (RGP) lens.

2. For most soft or rigid contact lens wearers who are not wearing a relatively oxygen-permeable lens, we suggest switching to a more oxygen-permeable lens whether it be soft or rigid. This can be done at a convenient time such as when the patient needs a refitting or has lost a lens.

3. Although there are no recent guidelines for routine specular microscopy, it is not unreasonable to assess the endothelium after 20 years of lens wear. In patients with advanced polymegathism, pleomorphism, and endothelial cell counts of less than 1800 cells/mm^2, periodic specular microscopy may be indicated to monitor any progression. If there is progression, lens discontinuation should be considered.

CONCLUSIONS

Contact lens wear may be associated with morphometric abnormalities that indicate corneal endothelial stress. The clinical significance of contact lens-related polymegathism and pleomorphism is unknown. We know, however, that these morphometric changes in non-contact lens wearers are associated with an increased risk of corneal decompensation following intra-ocular surgery. In the future it will be important to further clarify the significance of contact lens-induced corneal endothelial changes and to develop strategies to minimize the potential risk of these changes in the contact lens wearer.

38 ▪ EPITHELIAL AND SUBEPITHELIAL COMPLICATIONS OF CONTACT LENSES

- Corneal abrasions
- Superficial punctate keratitis
- Arcuate defects
- 3 o'clock and 9 o'clock staining
- Epithelial microcysts
- Sterile infiltrates
- Superior limbic keratoconjunctivitis
- Dendritic keratitis
- Summary

The corneal complications of contact lenses may be mechanically induced (e.g., corneal abrasions, arcuate defects, etc.), may be secondary to chemical toxicity or an immunologic reaction, may be caused by an infective process, or may have a physiologic basis, through metabolic changes in the tear film and cornea. Several studies have shown that contact lens wear causes tear-film hypoxia, which leads to a reduction in corneal pH. Many of the documented changes in corneal morphology during contact lens wear (e.g., epithelial microcysts, endothelial blebs, and endothelial polymegathism) may be a direct result of hypoxia or indirectly caused by reduced pH.

The contact-lens fitter must be astute in the recognition of corneal complications in contact-lens wearers. Detection of these anatomic changes and the initiation of appropriate management can often prevent more serious sequelae. Although contact lenses are generally regarded as safe for optical use they are associated with a small risk of transient or permanent visual loss.

A review of the corneal complications of contact lenses will be presented. In this chapter, reversible epithelial and subepithelial compli-cations of contact lenses will be discussed. In Chapter 37 the endothelial response to contact lenses was reviewed. In Chapter 39 the more serious complications of corneal neovascularization and corneal ulcers will be presented.

CORNEAL ABRASIONS

Corneal abrasions in contact-lens wearers (Fig. 38-1) may be caused by a mechanical injury from the contact lens, sloughing of edematous epithelium, or a traumatic insertion or removal often caused by a fingernail injury. A mechanical abrasion is usually related to poor lens fit or to surface-edge defects. Occasionally, foreign bodies embedded in the lens substance can lead to surface breakdown with resultant abrasion. Hypoxia can lead to corneal edema, which can result in the sloughing of the epithelium especially with rigid contact lens wear. A chemical keratitis can result in loosely adherent epithelium, which can lead to corneal erosions.

Appropriate therapy in the past in the management of contact-lens-related abrasions has been to use a cycloplegic agent, an antibiotic

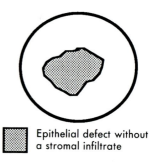

Epithelial defect without a stromal infiltrate

Fig 38-1 ▪ Corneal abrasion.

drop or ointment, and to apply a firm patch. Clemons et al. from the Cornea Service at the Wills Eye Hospital in Philadelphia suggest an alternative therapy. They reported five patients who developed *Pseudomonas* corneal ulcers after patching for what appeared to be a simple abrasion. It may be that some contact-lens patients who develop abrasions have a subclinical infection, so it is suggested that all contact-lens-related abrasions be considered as infected and treated with topical antibiotics. The use of the collagen shield soaked in an appropriate antibiotic solution (e.g., tobramycin) and placed on the eye will allow epithelial healing while also decreasing the chance of an infection.

SUPERFICIAL PUNCTATE KERATITIS

A superficial punctate keratitis (Fig. 38-2) in a contact-lens wearer may be mechanical, toxic-mediated, or related to an associated dry-eye condition. The same mechanical insults that can create a corneal abrasion can be responsible for a superficial keratitis. Chemical toxicity from contact-lens solutions can cause a diffuse punctate keratitis. This may be caused by the presence of preservatives in the saline solutions, from improper rinsing of the lenses after the use of surfactant or enzyme cleaners, or from failure to neutralize hydrogen peroxide disinfectants or elemental iodine disinfectants.

Probably the most common cause of a central punctate keratitis in a contact-lens wearer is the presence of a dry condition. Although fluorescein will detect changes in the corneal epithelium, it will not stain dry devitalized conjunctival epithelial cells as does the Rose-Bengal stain. The presence of interpalpebral Rose-Bengal staining suggests the existence of a dry eye condition. Schirmer strips may also be useful in confirming the presence of dry eyes. To test basic tear secretion, a drop of a topical anesthetic is placed on the eye and the conjunctival fornix is carefully wiped to remove excess moisture. The strips are then bent and placed over the lid margin so that tear production can be measured. After 5 minutes the amount of wetting can be easily quantified from the strips. Less than 5 millimeters of wetting is suggestive of a dry-eye condition.

Patients with a punctate keratitis should discontinue contact-lens wear until the epithelium heals. The use of lubricating drops or ointments can promote epithelial healing. When there is an absence of epithelial staining the patient can often return to contact-lens wear, but this depends on the etiology of the punctate changes. In cases of chemical keratitis the use of non-preserved saline solutions will decrease the chance of a punctate keratitis. The contact-lens fit should be re-evaluated and changes made if indicated. The frequent use of lubricating drops while wearing contact lenses should be encouraged in the mild dry-eye patient. The use of Freeman punctal plugs placed in the lower and, occasionally, in the upper puncta can be used to enhance the tear meniscus and provide improved comfort in patients with a moderate case of dry-eye. Patients with a severe case of dry-eye should refrain from contact-lens wear because of the high rate of corneal complications. These include superficial punctate keratitis, neovascularization, and corneal ulcers.

ARCUATE DEFECTS

Epithelial defects or punctate staining in an arcuate pattern (Fig. 38-3) often in the midperiphery or peripheral cornea may be seen in

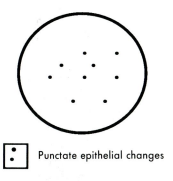

▪ Punctate epithelial changes

Fig 38-2 ■ Superficial punctate keratitis.

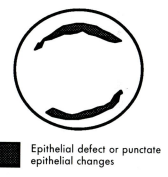

■ Epithelial defect or punctate epithelial changes

Fig 38-3 ■ Arcuate defects.

association with tight-fitting contact lenses. These may be caused by wearing soft or rigid contact lenses. Although the majority of reports in the literature attribute this staining pattern to tight-fitting contact lenses, one report documented this arcuate pattern in several patients who had tight lids and normal-fitting contact lenses. Management should include the use of topical prophylactic antibiotics and discontinuing contact-lens wear. When the epithelium heals these patients can be refitted with flatter contact lenses. If this recurs one should suspect the possibility of tight lids with compression of the contact lens against the cornea. Treatment may include changing the diameter of the contact lens.

3 O'CLOCK and 9 O'CLOCK STAINING

This is a common complication in rigid-contact-lens wearers. Abnormal tear flow dynamics because of the presence of a contact lens creates areas of poor wetting at the 3 o'clock and 9 o'clock positions of the peripheral cornea (Fig. 38-4). These superficial punctate epithelial changes stain with the use of fluorescein. By refitting patients with smaller or larger diameter contact lenses these changes can be minimized. In addition to observed wetting of the cornea, poor edge design can also be responsible for a punctate keratitis in the 3 o'clock and 9 o'clock positions.

EPITHELIAL MICROCYSTS

Epithelial microcysts (Fig. 38-5) occur frequently with soft contact lenses and most commonly with extended-wear lenses. They are associated with a depressed corneal epithelial me-

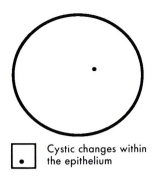

Cystic changes within the epithelium

Fig 38-5 ■ Epithelial microcysts.

tabolism sustained over a period of weeks to months. They appear as tiny dots of variable density in the corneal epithelium. They do not stain with fluorescein since the epithelial surface is intact. In advanced cases, the clinical appearance of microcysts is similar to Cogan's microcystic dystrophy that occurs in non-contact lens wearers. In this condition the cysts have been histologically identified as pockets of cellular debris that form when epithelial cells become trapped by an abnormal basement membrane that is secreted in excess and in an aberrant location.

STERILE INFILTRATES

Non-infected corneal infiltrates appear as whitish opacities of the subepithelial tissue, often with an overlying intact epithelium or limited to a superficial punctate keratitis. The infiltrates may be focal in nature, usually less than 1.5 mm in diameter, or multiple and peripheral (Fig. 38-6) often appearing as small subepithelial dots. These opacities are the result of an inflammatory

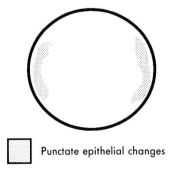

Punctate epithelial changes

Fig 38-4 ■ 3 and 9 o'clock staining.

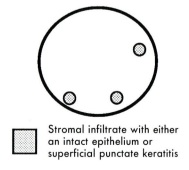

Stromal infiltrate with either an intact epithelium or superficial punctate keratitis

Fig 38-6 ■ Sterile infiltrates.

response to a specific antigen with resultant corneal infiltration of leukocytes. Because the cornea is avascular, the inflammatory cells must be derived from the limbal microvasculature or the tear film. The preservatives in contact-lens solutions have been identified as possible antigenic sources. The clinician must also be aware that subepithelial infiltrates can be unrelated to contact-lens wear as seen in hypersensitivity reactions to chlamydia or the staphylococcal organism.

The emergency management of contact-lens-related subepithelial infiltrates is to discontinue contact-lens wear. When the symptoms resolve the patient may return to contact-lens wear after switching to a nonpreserved saline solution. Although the use of topical steroids may hasten recovery, they are usually not necessary because the removal of the antigenic focus, i.e., the contact lens, will cause the inflammatory response to dissipate.

SUPERIOR LIMBIC KERATOCONJUNCTIVITIS

Superior limbic keratoconjunctivitis (SLK; Fig. 38-7) can occur in the hydrophilic lens wearer and resemble the idiopathic superior limbic keratoconjunctivitis described by Theodore. Patients may complain of a foreign-body sensation, dryness, redness, and contact-lens intolerance. On examination, findings may include injection of the superior bulbar conjunctiva that stains with Rose-Bengal, punctate staining and a micropannus of the superior cornea, and a fine papillary reaction of the superior tarsal conjunctiva. Larger papillae suggestive of giant papillary conjunctivitis do not occur.

This contact lens-induced superior limbic keratoconjunctivitis must be distinguished from the idiopathic form. In Theodore's SLK, the condition is usually bilateral and primarily affects middle-aged and older women. In 40% to 50% of cases there is a history of associated thyroid dysfunction, although therapy for the thyroid disease does not generally benefit the eye disease. Filaments of the superior cornea are common in the idiopathic SLK but rare in contact-lens-associated SLK.

The etiology of the condition in contact-lens wearers may be secondary to a hypersensitivity or toxic reaction to thimerosal or other preservatives in contact-lens solutions. An improper lens fit, such as a with a large-diameter lens, a loosely fitting lens, and/or a lens with an eccentric ride has also been implicated in contact-lens-associated SLK.

The treatment of choice for the lens-related condition is lens abstinence. The frequent use of lubricating drops may help to promote healing. Silver nitrate cautery, conjunctival recessions or resections, or thermo-cautery (which may be necessary in cases of idiopathic SLK) are generally not indicated in the lens-related condition. When the symptoms and signs abate the patient should be given replacement lenses with correction of any improper fit, changed to nonpreserved saline solution, and instructed to clean the lenses frequently.

DENDRITIC KERATITIS

Dendritic lesions of the cornea have been reported as a complication of soft contact lenses (Fig. 38-8). These dendrites are often associated with a conjunctivitis. The clinician must learn

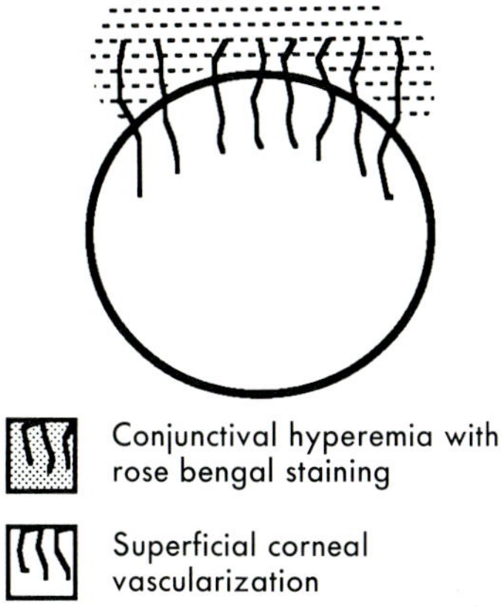

Conjunctival hyperemia with rose bengal staining

Superficial corneal vascularization

Fig 38-7 ■ Superior limbic keratoconjunctivitis.

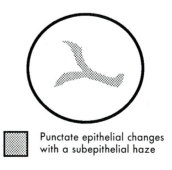

Punctate epithelial changes with a subepithelial haze

Fig 38-8 ■ Dendritic keratitis.

to differentiate the contact-lens-related dendrite from the infected dendrite of herpes simplex. The presence of bilateral disease suggests a non-herpetic etiology because herpes simplex keratitis is a uniocular condition except in primary or disseminated forms. The dendrites occurring as a complication of hydrophilic lenses are often multiple, are thinner than the herpes simplex dendrites, and are marked by an absence of swollen terminal knobs. Diminished corneal sensation can occur in herpes simplex keratitis and also from chronic contact-lens wear, and therefore is not a useful differentiating factor. Corneal cultures are negative in the contact lens-induced dendrites, and there is no response to antiviral medication.

These dendrites have been attributed to thimerosal hypersensitivity. Although contact-lens-related dendrites will improve spontaneously with lens abstinence, if topical steroids are used recovery may be hastened without the risk of progressive infection as can occur with herpes simplex.

SUMMARY

The reversible anterior corneal complications of contact lenses have been reviewed: corneal abrasions, superficial punctate keratitis, arcuate defects, 3 o'clock and 9 o'clock staining, epithelial microcysts, sterile infiltrates, and dendritic keratitis. The contact-lens fitter should have an understanding of the pathophysiologic mechanisms of disease involved, should be able to detect these clinical changes at the earliest stage, and should offer appropriate management solutions to ensure their reversibility.

39 ▪ SERIOUS CORNEAL COMPLICATIONS OF CONTACT LENSES AND THEIR MANAGEMENT

- ▪ *Corneal neovascularization*
- ▪ *Corneal ulcers*
- ▪ *Summary*

The most serious complications of contact lens use are corneal neovascularization and corneal ulcers, which can lead to a permanent loss of vision. The contact-lens fitter who has a practical understanding of the pathophysiologic mechanisms involved and follows his patients on a regular basis can provide important patient instruction and education to help reduce the risk of serious complications. Early recognition of the clinical symptoms and signs and the initiation of appropriate management steps may help to prevent progression of the disease process and consequent loss of vision.

CORNEAL NEOVASCULARIZATION

Corneal neovascularization (Fig. 39-1) may be superficial or deep, may be sectorial or may extend 360 degrees into the cornea. This is often the result of chronic hypoxia from a lens that is too thick or too tight.

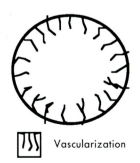

Vascularization

Fig 39-1 ▪ Corneal neovascularization.

The incidence of lens-induced corneal neovascularization is unknown. Small amounts (1 to 2 mm) of peripheral superficial vascularization are relatively common in extended- and therapeutic lens wear. Greater than 2 mm of progressive vascular ingrowth or ingrowth involving the middle or deep stroma is uncommon.

Stromal vascularization is a more serious complication of contact-lens wear and can lead to compromised vision via two mechanisms. Vascular ingrowth, if allowed to progress into the visual axis, can result in lipid exudation and scarring. A rarer cause of descreased vision is an intracorneal hemorrhage from the spontaneous rupture of a fragile new vessel. The hemorrhage is usually small and the blood usually clears spontaneously without a residual visual deficit.

The management of corneal neovascularization in contact-lens wearers depends on the degree of severity. As a general guideline, a patient with a mild degree of vascular ingrowth (less than 1.5 mm) can usually be refitted with a flatter or thinner soft contact lens or can be switched to a gas-permeable lens. This allows an increase in the amount of oxygen available to the cornea and therefore decreases the stimulus for neovascularization. At the other end of the spectrum, if the degree of vascular ingrowth is greater than 2.0 mm, the patient should discontinue contact-lens wear because progressive neovascularization could result in a loss of vision. If the neovascularization recedes significantly the patient can be refitted with gas-permeable contact lenses.

CORNEAL ULCERS

Infected corneal ulcers are the most serious complications associated with contact-lens wear.

Despite appropriate management corneal scarring may result with a resultant decrease in vision. The consequences of a delayed diagnosis and/or improper care may include severe scarring, corneal perforation, scleral extension, and loss of the eye. Corneal ulcers may occur in those who wear soft or rigid contact lenses but occur with greater frequency in wearers of soft contact lenses in general and extended-wear soft lenses in particular.

The most important organisms causing lens-related corneal infections include *Pseudomonas aeruginosa* and *Acanthamoeba*. *Pseudomonas* is the most common pathogen in bacterial ulcers among patients who use daily-wear and extended-wear lenses. *Acanthamoeba* is a parasite that is capable of causing a severe keratitis and whose diagnosis is easily confused with other causes of keratitis, especially in the early stages of the disease process. A variety of other bacteria may cause corneal ulcers associated with contact lenses less frequently. Fungi are not commonly seen in less-related corneal ulcers.

The pathogenesis of *Pseudomonas* lens-related corneal ulcers requires an epithelial defect in the corneal surface caused by a traumatic or hypoxic insult in the presence of a contaminated lens. A variety of factors may predispose to the development of a corneal ulcer. These may include incorrect or absent lens disinfection, lens removal and re-insertion without disinfection, lens overwear, continued lens wear despite the presence of a red eye, lack of hand-washing prior to lens manipulation, use of old lens-care solutions, use of homemade saline to store or to rinse lenses prior to insertion, and swimming while wearing contact lenses. All of these improper lens-care practices increase the risk of microbial infection.

Potential sources of infection that have been documented include the insides of bottle caps, the ribs of bottle tips, opened bottles of unpreserved saline solutions, and the use of homemade saline for lens storage and post-disinfection rinse. *Acanthamoeba*, a ubiquitous organism, has been identified in tap water, fresh water, saliva, and distilled water used in the preparation of homemade saline. Contamination of the contact lens can provide a continuous reservoir of the microbial agent for corneal infection. In addition the strong affinity of the *Pseudomonas* organism to the surface of the contact lens has been well documented.

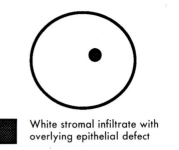

White stromal infiltrate with overlying epithelial defect

Fig 39-2 ■ Bacterial corneal ulcer—early stage.

The contact-lens fitter should recognize the symptoms and signs of an infected corneal ulcer. The patient may complain of increasing pain, redness, photophobia, tearing, and variably diminished vision. These symptoms may persist and worsen despite removal of the contact lens. Examination of the patient may reveal conjunctival injection, a ciliiary or limbal flush, a corneal infiltrate with an overlying epithelial defect (Fig. 39-2), granularity of the surrounding stroma, and an anterior chamber with a cell and flare reaction.

The presence of an inflammatory cell infiltrate in a contact-lens patient poses a diagnostic dilemma to the clinician who must decide whether it is infected or sterile. Non-infected infiltrates may be caused by a hypersensitivity reaction to preservatives in lens-care solutions. These infiltrates do not have to be cultured. On the contrary infected infiltrates should be cultured and treated aggresively with appropriate antibiotics. A clinical study by R. Stein et al., published in the American Journal of Ophthalmology in 1988 correlated symptoms and signs of contact-lens associated infiltrates with cultures of corneal scrapings. Clinical features that correlated with early infected infiltrates include significant pain, anterior chamber reaction, ocular discharge, and an overlying epithelial defect. When there was minimal pain and anterior chamber reaction, an absence of discharge, and the presence of an intact epithelium or one limited to a superficial punctate keratitis, these findings were more consistent with a sterile infiltrate. Large ulcers (greater than 2 mm) were always infected, but it was clinically significant that a third of the small ulcers were culture-positive. In general if confusion exists as to whether an infiltrate is infected or sterile it should be cultured and treated as infected until proven otherwise.

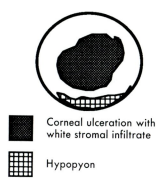

Corneal ulceration with white stromal infiltrate

Hypopyon

Fig 39-3 ■ Bacterial corneal ulcer—advanced stage.

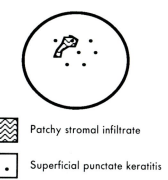

Patchy stromal infiltrate

Superficial punctate keratitis

Fig 39-4 ■ Acanthamoeba—early stage.

Pseudomonas aeruginosa is the most common organism encountered in contact-lens-related corneal ulcers. It should be suspected in any patient with an acute onset of severe pain regardless of the size of the infiltrate. Clinical findings may include an ulcer covered by thick adherent mucopurulent discharge, a wide area of surrounding stromal edema, the presence of a ring infiltrate around the ulcer referred to as a Wessely ring, and, in advanced cases, a hypopyon (Fig. 39-3). *Pseudomonas* corneal ulcers may progress rapidly if treatment is delayed or improper. This can lead to corneal scarring or loss of the eye. Although these features may be seen in *Pseudomonas* infections, they are not pathognomonic and can also be seen in other gram-negative rods.

Acanthamoeba keratitis is an uncommon but increasingly prevalent infection with the potential to cause severe ocular damage. The condition was first recognized in 1973. Twelve cases were reported between 1973 and 1983, and 36 between 1984 and 1986. More than 120 cases have now been reported in the literature. Many of the early cases were misdiagnosed as herpes simplex virus keratitis.

Acanthamoeba should be suspected in the contact-lens wearer, particularly in one who wears soft lenses and who uses homemade saline made from distilled water and salt tablets. Early in the course of the disease the pain is often greater than the clinical findings would lead one to predict. Early signs may consist of irregularity of the epithelium and a patchy stromal infiltrate (Fig. 39-4). At this stage the disease entity can be misdiagnosed as herpes simplex keratitis. With progression of the disease, a ring infiltrate is characteristically seen

(Fig. 39-5). Other clinical signs include infiltrates along corneal nerves, radial keratoneuritis, elevated nonbranching corneal epithelial lines, corneal stromal edema, iritis, and decreased corneal sensation. It is important for the clinician to be aware of this condition so that a diagnosis is made early in the disease course and treatment is initiated. If treatment is started at the ring infiltrate stage, prognosis for successful medical treatment is guarded.

All patients with a suspected infected infiltrate should have a corneal scraping for smears and culture prior to initiating treatment. The patient should be administered a topical anesthetic and a sterilized instrument such as a Kimura spatula can be used to scrape the corneal ulcer under slit-lamp visualization. The scrapings are smeared on a glass slide for Gram stain and Giemsa stain. The Gram stain is useful in detecting bacteria; the Giemsa stain is helpful in identifying fungi and *Acanthamoeba*. The Calcofluor stain can also be used to detect *Acanthamoeba* if a fluorescent microscope is avail-

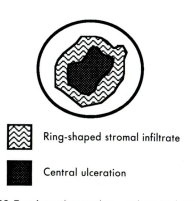

Ring-shaped stromal infiltrate

Central ulceration

Fig 39-5 ■ Acanthamoeba—advanced stage.

able. Cultures are performed by direct inoculation of the scraping onto multiple media, which include blood agar, chocolate agar, Sabouraud's media, and thioglycolate broth. *Acanthamoeba* is difficult to culture by standard means and is best done by applying the scraping to a non-nutrient agar with an overlay of *E. coli*.

Broad-spectrum fortified antibiotic therapy using tobramycin (15mg/ml) and cefazolinn (50 mg/ml) alternately every hour is started after the corneal scrapings are obtained. Small ulcers, especially if peripheral in location and associated with a modest degree of pain, can be managed on an outpatient basis with frequent follow-up visits. The indications for inpatient management of corneal ulcers include: when reliable antibiotic therapy cannot be ensured, in the case of large corneal ulcers, when there is significant pain or visual loss, and when the patient and clinician are separated by an inconvenient distance. In severe infections where *Pseudomonas* is suspected, fortified tobramycin may be given every 15 to 30 minutes for the first 24 hours in addition to hourly doses of cefazolin. Tobramycin is the antibiotic of choice for *Pseudomonas* because one third of the isolated strains are resistant to gentamicin.

Contact lenses made of collagen are being used increasingly in the management of corneal ulcers. The collagen shield can be soaked in an antibiotic solution and then placed on the eye to act as a delivery system of medication to the cornea. This provides the cornea with a steady and prolonged dose of the drug; it allows the frequency of topical drug administration to be reduced. The long-acting collagen shields (longer than 72 hours) are preferred for use in the management of corneal ulcers.

Subconjunctival injections of antibiotics are rare and generally are reserved for severe infections in which topical antibiotics are not available immediately. An injection of tobramycin (40 mg), cefazolin (50 mg), and 0.5 cc of 1% lidocaine can be administered in the subconjunctival space of the inferior cul-de-sac. Intravenous treatment is used only when there is scleral involvement of the infected process or when there is a corneal perforation. Adjunctive therapy includes a cycloplegic agent to relieve ciliary spasm and to prevent posterior synechiae of the iris to the lens. A relatively long-acting cycloplegic agent such as scopolamine, homatropine, or atropine can be used. If the intra-ocular pressure is elevated glaucoma therapy, which may include a topical beta-blocker and an oral carbonic anhydrase inhibitor, is initiated.

Topical antibiotic therapy can be modified after 24 to 48 hours depending on the clinical response and the culture results. For example, if *Pseudomonas* is isolated cefazolin can be discontinued. When antibiotic sensitivities are available, usually after 48 hours, further modifications can be made. Streptococcal ulcers may be treated with cefazolin exclusively. The frequency of topical antibiotic therapy is gradually reduced depending on the clinical response. Signs of improvement include diminished pain, decreased infiltrate size and epithelial defect, and less anterior chamber reaction.

The medical therapy for *Acanthamoeba* keratitis has not yet been clearly defined by controlled clinical studies. The organism often shows resistance to therapy because of its biphasic nature. The trophozites show a variable response to medical therapy while the cyst forms are more resistant. Topical drugs that appear to have some efficacy include propamidine isethionate (Brolene), neomycin, miconazole, clotrimazole, and oral ketoconazole. Current initial therapy may include topical Brolene, neosporin, and clotrimazole every 2 hours, and systemic ketoconazole. If *Acanthamoeba* keratitis is diagnosed in the early stages of the disease process, medical therapy can be effective in some cases. Penetrating keratoplasty is necessary in cases of progressive corneal involvement despite maximal medical therapy. Unfortunately, there is approximately a 25% recurrence rate of *Acanthamoeba* keratitis following corneal grafting.

In the prevention of contact-lens-related corneal ulcers the patient and the contact-lens provider have important roles to play. Lens-wearers must know the risk of infection that is associated with the use of contact lenses and understand the potential risk factors. Contact-lens wearers must know that they should remove a contact lens whenever the eye becomes red, irritated, or painful. If the symptoms worsen or persist despite lens removal, prompt ophthalmic care is warranted in order to rule out an early infection. The contact-lens provider should stress the importance of good hygiene and adherence to the recommended guidelines of the lens manufacturers. Homemade saline made from distilled water and salt tablets should not be used because of the high risk of contamination.

Asymptomatic patients should be evaluated twice a year. During these visits a careful history should be taken to make sure that proper hygiene and lens care is being practiced. The contact lenses should be re-evaluated with regard to their fitting characteristics and quality. Poorly fitting lenses or those with significant deposits should be replaced. The presence of a dry-eye condition or of blepharitis increases the risk of infection. If these conditions are mild patients can continue wearing their contact lenses but only with strict adherence to lid hygiene and to the guidelines on the use of lubricating drops. If the symptoms are moderate to severe in character it is usually best to have the patient refrain from contact-lens wear.

SUMMARY

The contact-lens fitter can help reduce the risk of serious corneal complications by:

1. Having a practical understanding of the pathophysiologic mechanisms of corneal disease;
2. Careful follow-up examinations on a regular basis;
3. Recognizing the early symptoms and signs of contact lens complications; and
4. Involvement in patient education and instruction. By these means the contact-lens fitter can decrease the patient's chances of developing corneal neovascularization and corneal ulcers and therefore prevent visual loss.

40 ▪ CONTACT LENS WEAR AND OCULAR ALLERGY

Mathea R. Allansmith
Robert N. Ross

- ▪ Hay fever conjunctivitis
- ▪ Vernal keratoconjunctivitis
- ▪ Atopic keratoconjunctivitis
- ▪ Solution intolerance
- ▪ Ocular anaphylaxis

Many conditions, allergic and non-allergic, can produce red, itchy, tearing, burning eyes. We will concentrate on the allergic conditions. Airborne allergens can readily adhere to the contact lens while it is in the eye. Moreover, the excursion of the lid across the worn contact lens can traumatize the tarsal conjunctiva, and each blink may introduce allergens into the lesion. If properties of the worn contact lenses are primarily responsible for the signs and symptoms of disease, treating the inflamed conjunctiva and finding the best tolerated contact lens material and design will be the most effective treatment. If, however, intrinsic ocular disease is the primary causative agent, adjusting the contact lens may be useless.

Our understanding of the etiology, pathophysiology, diagnosis, and treatment of allergic disease has advanced rapidly in recent years (Table 40-1). We are now in a position to recognize and treat the signs and symptoms of allergy, often without further compromising the patient's tolerance of the worn contact lens.

An estimated 20 to 40 million people suffer from hay fever, with seasonal or perennial rhinitis, sneezing, and conjunctivitis. In addition to hay fever, two other ocular conditions have major allergic components—vernal keratoconjunctivitis (VKC) and atopic keratoconjunctivitis (AKC). Hay fever conjunctivitis, VKC, and AKC

are not caused by wearing contact lenses. Although signs and symptoms of these diseases may be present independent of contact lens wear, the presence of ocular allergies may complicate contact lens wear for many patients. In addition, giant papillary conjunctivitis (GPC) and hypersensitivity reactions to the cleaning and disinfecting solutions are allergic conditions that result directly from wearing contact lenses.

HAY FEVER CONJUNCTIVITIS

Hay fever conjunctivitis (seasonal allergic conjunctivitis) (Fig. 40-1) is an inflammation of the conjunctiva that is usually but not always associated with allergic rhinitis (hay fever). Airborne allergens (for instance, pollen, molds, dust, and animal danders) can trigger an immediate allergic response in the nose (rhinitis) and conjunctiva (conjunctivitis). According to Kray, an estimated 15% to 21% of the population suffers from seasonal allergic conjunctivitis. The prevalence of perennial allergic conjunctivitis is much lower (3.5 per 10,000) but it is nonetheless a common and debilitating eye disorder as reported by Dart.

Hay fever conjunctivitis is probably caused by the solution of allergens in the tear film reacting with specific IgE receptors on conjunctival mast cells and basophils in susceptible individuals. The symptoms of hay fever conjunctivitis are mild-to-moderate itching, copious tearing, a burning sensation, photophobia, and the feeling of pressure behind the eyes. It is often impossible to detect any outward signs of disease despite the patient's report of bothersome symptoms. When signs are present, they are unmis-

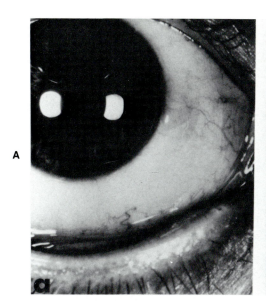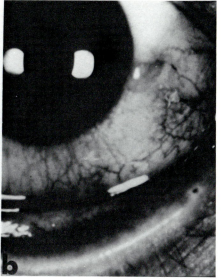

Fig 40-1 ■ Experimental hay fever conjunctivitis. **A,** White and quiet eye of patient allergic to grass pollen. **B,** Same eye 15 minutes after grass pollen extract applied topically. Note dilated vessels.

takable: conjunctival edema, dilation of conjunctival blood vessels, and swelling of the eyelids.

The treatment of hay fever conjunctivitis is not significantly complicated by the patient's wearing of contact lenses. Allergic patients can continue to wear their contact lenses and there is no reason to change the lens design or material. There is no need to treat the hay fever-associated conjunctivitis as if it were the more serious GPC. Hay fever conjunctivitis does not lead to GPC.

Treatment of hay fever conjunctivitis in patients who wear contact lenses is the same as in patients who do not wear contact lenses. Irrigating the eye with saline solution 2 to 4 times daily, cromolyn sodium applied topically to the eye 4 times daily, astringents, vasoconstrictors, and topical antihistamines are all effective measures. The use of corticosteroids is ordinarily not appropriate because of the undue risk of adverse reactions.

Mast cell stabilizers are becoming increasingly important in the treatment of hay fever conjunctivitis. The compound cromolyn sodium has been found effective in inhibiting mast cell degranulation in the treatment of asthma, allergic rhinitis, and a variety of allergic ocular disorders. Eye symptoms in scores of ragweed-

sensitive patients have been found to be reduced by topical application of cromolyn sodium 4% ophthalmic solution according to Greenbaum. Patients treated with cromolyn sodium were also found to use less antihistamine (chlorpheniramine maleate 4 mg) than patients in the comparison group. Cromolyn sodium is useful in combination with other medications as prophylactic treatment for patients with severe signs and symptoms of ocular allergy. Use of cromolyn sodium can reduce the use of corticosteroids in patients with severe hay fever conjunctivitis. Cromolyn sodium has also been found to be effective in the treatment of chronic allergic conjunctivitis according to van Bijsterveld.

Antihistamines are used extensively in the treatment of nasal and ocular symptoms of hay fever. Undesirable side effects of most antihistamines (notably drowsiness), however, have limited their effectiveness. In studies by Bende and Pecoud, levocabastine, astemizole, (studied by Vanden Bussche) and terfenidine (investigated by Kjellman) have all been found to reduce conjunctival hypersensitivity to airborne pollens.

In cases of hay fever conjunctivitis, consultation with an allergist is important to help identify offending allergens and, perhaps, to begin immunotherapy.

Table 40-1 ■ Contact lens (giant papillary) conjunctivitis

		Symptoms					
		Mucus or discharge in morning	Itching on removal of lens	Awareness of lens during wear	Vision with lens	Mucus while wearing lens	Lens wearing time
Stage 1 *Preclinical*		Minimal	Mild				
Stage 2 *Early clin-ical*		Moderate	In-creased	Begin to feel lens late in day	Mild blur-ring late in day		
Stage 3 *Moderate*		Moderate to severe	Moderate to se-vere, but variable	Increased awareness throughout day	Moderate blurring; requires in-creased blinking to see	Begins mu-cus accu-mulation on lens or eye	Begins to decrease but often little de-crease
Stage 4 *Severe or terminal*		Severe; eyelids stuck to-gether, must pry apart	Same as Stage 3	Distress on wearing lens, ap-proaching pain	Depends on mu-cus se-cretions, deposits on lens	Marked mu-cus secre-tion	Total loss of toler-ance; pain on insertion of lens depend-ing on condition

*UV indicates ultraviolet.

VERNAL KERATOCONJUNCTIVITIS

Vernal keratoconjunctivitis (Fig. 40-2) is a disease of youth, rarely appearing in children younger than 3 years or in people older than 25. Boys outnumber girls by an estimated 2:1. Vernal keratoconjunctivitis (VKC) accounts for 0.1% to 0.5% of all patients with ocular problems. It occurs more frequently in warm climates than in cooler climates.

VKC is a seasonal inflammation of the conjunctiva with giant papillae than run together giving the conjunctiva a characteristic cobblestone appearance. Signs and symptoms of VKC may occur throughout the year. They are often worse during the spring and summer months in the northern hemisphere, however, and may therefore be confused with hay fever conjunctivitis. Because VKC is severe and chronic, it significantly disrupts the lives of its victims. It may also involve the cornea and threaten vision. VKC usually appears on the tarsal conjunctiva; giant papillae may also appear on the limbal con-

Signs									
Itching while wearing lens	Lens movement	Lens condition (slit lamp)	Size and elevation of papillae	Morphology	Staining of tops of giant papillae with 2% fluorescein	Hyperemia and edema	Method of diagnosis	Mucus on conjunctiva	Corneal condition
			No change from baseline	Baseline			Symptoms only		
Mild by end of day, variable		Mild coating	Elevation of normal papillae and initial formation of giant papillae	Clover-like formations	Occasional staining of papillae	None or mild erythema	UV light,* 2% fluorescein, and high power on slit lamp	Usually mild, in sheets over papillae	Rare mild punctate staining superiorly
Mild to moderate, variable	Mild increase	Moderate to severe coating	Increased number, size, and elevation of papillae	Occasional mushroom forms	Staining during exacerbation	Variable erythema and edema	Slit lamp and sometimes naked eye	Heavy sheets, strands, and globs	Like Stage 2 but less rare
Mild to severe, variable	Lens moves to point where it may be pulled off cornea	Severe coating	Flattening of apex of elevation and progression of Stage 3	More of above	More papillae staining	Erythema more constant, edema variable	Naked eye	Severely increased	Occasional white arcuate infiltrate in superior cornea

Adapted from Allansmith et al.[1]

junctiva and trantas dots are sometimes seen in the limbal conjunctiva.

Intense itching that worsens late in the day is a constant feature of VKC. Physical exertion and exposure to dust, wind, and bright lights may also intensify the itching. Rubbing the eye also increases the itch. Patients also complain of irritation—an uncomfortable, hot, tight, sensitive feeling that is not like the foreign-body sensation. Tearing is profuse. Clear tears accumulate in the corners of the eyes. The constant presence of tears further irritates the skin of the lids and may lead to infection. Patients may pull thick strands of yellow or white material from the lids. This discharge may also accumulate while sleeping, but the lids are not stuck together on waking. Palpebral and limbal lesions, hard, elevated macro- and giant papillae, milky coating of conjunctiva, keratitis, and occasionally, ulceration of the conjunctiva may also appear.

The most serious features of VKC are those that affect the cornea. In one form of the disease,

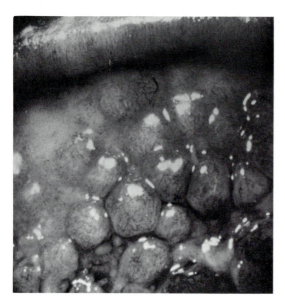

Fig 40-2 ■ Upper tarsal conjunctiva of eight-year old boy. Note giant papillae. Also note resemblance to giant papillary conjunctivitis.

the cornea develops tiny lesions that give it a stippled appearance. In another form of the disease, the corneal epithelium may begin to die, clouding the cornea. In severe cases, the entire cornea may be covered with gray patches that obscure vision.

Little is known about the pathophysiology of VKC. It clearly has an allergic component but no specific allergens have been identified. Almost all VKC patients (80%) also have a history of other allergic diseases, such as infantile eczema, allergic rhinitis, or asthma. The distribution of mast cells is abnormal in VKC. Normally no mast cells are found in the epithelium of the upper tarsal conjunctiva, but in VKC the number of mast cells may be as high as 16,000 cells per cubic millimeter of tissue. The normal density of mast cells in the substantia propria is 5000 cells per cubic millimeter of tissue, but in VKC patients, the density of mast cells is 9000 cells per cubic millimeter of tissue. Other inflammatory cells—lymphocytes, plasma cells, and eosinophils—may also migrate into the conjunctiva. Conjunctival scrapings reveal many eosinophils and eosinophilic granules. Tear histamine concentration and tear IgE levels are higher in vernal keratoconjunctivitis patients than in normal subjects.

The prognosis for eventual recovery from VKC is excellent, and when recovery comes, it is almost always complete. Nevertheless, patients need the benefit of treatment during the decade or so during which signs and symptoms of VKC are severe. Topical corticosteroids are used to treat VKC. Ophthalmic formulations of dexamethasone 0.1% or prednisolone 1% may be applied topically every 1 to 2 hours initially and then less often until signs and symptoms are brought under control. A mucolytic agent may be included in the treatment plan to help prevent accumulation of the mucus that is characteristic of VKC. Cromolyn sodium has also been shown to provide relief from itching, tearing, and photophobia in approximately two-thirds of VKC patients as reported by Jay.

ATOPIC KERATOCONJUNCTIVITIS

Atopic keratoconjunctivitis (AKC) resembles VKC but differs from it in several important ways (Fig. 40-3). AKC is a life-long disease, does not have the same sex distribution as VKC, and is usually not seasonal. AKC is an inflammatory skin disorder that affects the outer eye. Exacerbations of the skin disorders are accompanied by exacerbations of the AKC. It is seen in 25% of all atopic dermatitis patients. An estimated 3% of the population suffers from atopic dermatitis, which is allergic inflammation of the skin. Little is known about the etiology and pathophysiology of AKC. The disease typically appears in the late teen years and lasts until the fourth or fifth decade of life. The skin of the eyelids, the conjunctiva, and the cornea may be affected. The bulbar and tarsal conjunctiva may be thickened. Abnormal papillae appear on the conjunctiva. In severe cases, AKC may lead to scarring and vascularization of the cornea.

The symptoms of AKC are moderate-to-severe itching, burning, sensitivity to light, tearing, and discharge that may be watery or thick. These symptoms are perennial and do not seem to change with changes in the weather. Corneal changes may also occur. In addition, the following sequelae of AKC are serious because they can interfere with vision: pannus, ulceration, scarring, keratoconus, keratitis, and cataracts in 10% of cases (Fig. 40-4). AKC may also be complicated by secondary infection of the ulcers.

The prognosis for AKC is not good. Topical corticosteroids and brief courses of systemic corticosteroids are administered for the treatment of the most severe cases of AKC. Although this course of treatment may be somewhat effective

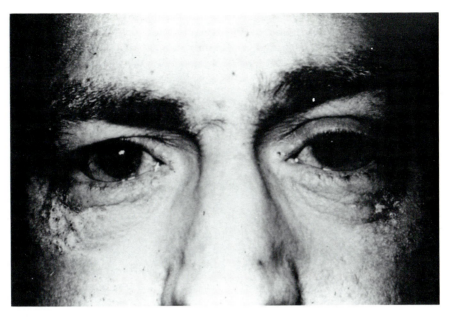

Fig 40-3 ■ Atopic keratoconjunctivitis. Note lichenified skin, thickened lids, and dilated conjunctival vessels. (Courtesy Phillips Thygeson, MD.)

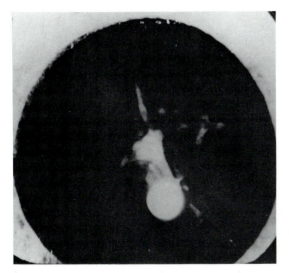

Fig 40-4 ■ Atopic cataract. Note "stretched bear rug" shape of opacity. (Courtesy David D. Donaldson, MD.)

in reducing its signs and symptoms, treatment with corticosteroids increases the risk of cataracts already associated with AKC. According to Simon-Licht, cromolyn sodium has not been found to be particularly effective in treating AKC.

SOLUTION INTOLERANCE

The incidence of intolerance to solutions used for cleaning and disinfecting soft contact lenses

has been estimated to be approximately 33% of those patients using chlorhexidine plus thimerosol and 5% to 8% of those using thimerosol alone as studied by Coward. Coward also found two disinfecting solutions to be particularly allergenic (Barnes-Hind and Alcon-Burton-Parsons). A family history of allergy was not a significant predictor of solution intolerance. In another study by Harrison, penicillin allergy, a family history of diabetes, and the use of birth control pills were all found to be significant predictors of sensitivity to solutions containing thimerosol. Approximately half the patients reporting hypersensitivity reactions to thimerosol-containing lens-disinfecting solutions also reported penicillin allergy or a family history of diabetes mellitus. The association of these conditions and thimerosol sensitivity has not been explained.

OCULAR ANAPHYLAXIS

Much remains to be learned about the pathophysiology of ocular allergy at the cellular and subcellular level according to Versura. When the basic mechanisms of these common ocular disorders are understood, treatment will be vastly enhanced. At present, however, treatment remains largely symptomatic.

The conjunctiva and other structures of the eye open to the external environment are normally well protected by lymphocytes, macrophages, plasma cells, neutrophils, and mast cells. The high concentration of mast cells in the conjunctiva and adnexa (an estimated 50 million cells in the tissue of each human eye) and the presence of basophils are especially important factors because of the role they play in ocular allergy. Eosinophils and basophils may also appear in disease.

The mast cell is responsible for both the immediate and the late-phase reaction. The rapid release of preformed mediators produces the familiar immediate allergic reaction. The production of longer acting and more powerful secondary, newly formed mediators from arachidonic acid creates the longer lasting inflammatory reaction.

Secretory granules in mast cells and basophils contain several preformed mediators (histamine, serotonin, heparin, neutral proteases, acid hydrolases, chemotactic factors for eosinophils, neutrophils, and lymphocytes) that have a profound effect on several tissues of the body, especially on venules. *Histamine* can contract bronchial smooth muscle, dilate the capillaries and arterioles, increase permeability of venules, and increase gastric secretion. *Serotonin* is a neurotransmitter that can constrict small blood vessels, reduce gastric secretion, and stimulate contraction of smooth muscle. *Heparin* is an anticoagulant. *Neutral proteases and hydrolases* may be responsible for tissue damage. *Chemotactic factors* for eosinophils, neutrophils, and lymphocytes are responsible for producing the signs and symptoms of inflammation.

Unlike the immediate reaction, the late-phase reaction is marked by the infiltration of inflammatory cells. Eosinophils, neutrophils, and basophils appear first (2 to 8 hours after challenge); followed by lymphocytes and monocytes/macrophages (24 hours after challenge). The late-phase reaction may be responsible for considerable tissue damage.

In addition to producing the observable inflammatory effects, the late-phase reaction may also "prime" tissue for the next immediate (and late-phase) reaction. Allergists have known for quite some time that a specific allergic reaction may make a person susceptible to a wide variety of nonspecific stimuli. The worn contact lens is an example of just such a nonspecific stimulus that can trigger or augment a specific allergic reaction in susceptible people.

41 ▪ *MANAGEMENT OF A CONTACT LENS PRACTICE*

DELEGATION

Many functions in the management of a lens practice may be delegated. Depending on the training, educational background, responsibility, and personality of the auxiliary personnel, several areas may be properly delegated so that the practitioner is free to spend time on the initial examination and fitting, with adequate time for the follow-up visits that are required.

COST

Lenses can be paid for in one of two ways. The first is an initial small cost outlay for the lenses, a fitting fee, and a visit fee for the practitioner, or a pay-as-you-go fee. In this way problem cases are charged proportionately, whereas "easy-fit" cases are charged less. The fitting fee may vary with the nature of the fit so that more difficult fittings, such as toric fitting or bifocal fitting, are charged a higher fee. Alternatively, one may use a total fee structure that can be broken down for the patient into the cost of the

material and the cost of professional fitting (Fig. 41-1). The same charge can be made for each standard fitting regardless of the number of visits required during the adaptation period. This all-inclusive coverage period may vary from up to 3 months, after which a fee per visit is charged. We favor the latter method, in which the patient is free to call on the practitioner without being concerned about the extra expense. It is important that the patient fully understand that the practitioner is not selling lenses but that the professional-fee component is added for professional time in evaluations to ensure a successful fit.

The contact lens area is extremely competitive and price-oriented. It is mandatory that the patient be fully aware of the fitting agreement, its cost, and the refund policy in the event of lack of satisfaction on the part of either the patient or practitioner. One must avoid misunderstanding and confusion and, above all, leaving the patient with the feeling that he was overcharged. Good public relations are important not only on the part of the fitter but also on the part of all personnel in contact with the patient (Fig. 41-2). One must be alert to exceptions to the rule, dissatisfied patients, and refunds. One must often customize the financial approach to patients.

HOW TO MAKE PATIENTS HAPPY

Making patients happy is not just good practice, it is also probably the best protection we have against lawsuits. The secret to making patients happy lies in developing good communication skills. Good communication skills start with an attitude of empathy and caring, and of letting patients know directly and indirectly that they are important. This attitude is reflected not only by what a doctor says and does, but what the office staff says and does and how psycho-

Our total fee is divided between the cost of material and a professional fee for fitting and service. This service is available for 3 months, after which a charge per visit will be made.
An inspection service will be provided at no charge at 6 months after initial visit.

Cost of lenses, case, and
initial supplies   _____
Fitting fee   _____
Warranty   _____
Miscellaneous   _____

         Total   _____

I have received lenses. _____
           Signature

         _____
           Date

Fig 41-1 ■ Sample of breakdown of fee structure that is provided to patient when lenses are received.

logically comfortable the patient is made to feel in the office environment. There are a number of ways in which one can create an impression that the office does in fact care.

1. Do not keep patients waiting for long periods of time. One of the key factors that go into a patient's overall rating of a practitioner is the time spent waiting in the reception area. Waiting time is a key factor in patient dissatisfaction and this dissatisfaction increases dramatically when waiting time exceeds 30 minutes. Office schedules cannot always be

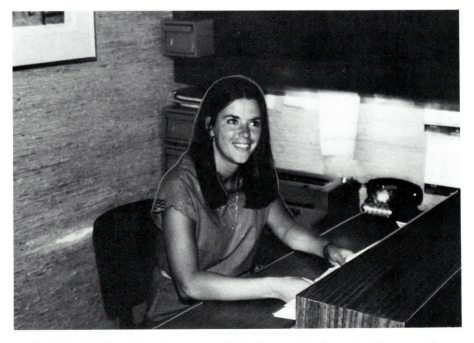

Fig 41-2 ■ Good public relations are vital to the growth of a contact lens practice.

controlled, especially if there are added emergencies to deal with. For those doctors who are chronically behind schedule one should take a close look at how bookings are made and try to prevent snarls in the schedule. If delays are unavoidable, patients should be told why they are waiting and how long the wait may be, to help minimize the aggravation. In addition, interesting time decoys should be available to help patients pass the time. These include topical magazines along with possible video information or even a television set in the waiting room.

2. Make patients feel important. The first contact the patient has with a doctor's office has to be courteous, respectful, and personalized. This can include little gestures of kindness, like the nurse asking after a recent baby, the receptionist asking for a preferred appointment time, or the doctor inquiring after an ailing family member or recalling some details of an earlier conversation.

   It is also appropriate for both male and female doctors to stand up and shake a patient's hand when first greeting a patient as well as touching patients in a neutral manner (on the arm, shoulder, or hand) during the course of a consultation. These are gestures that convey empathy, friendliness, and concern. It is critical to convey information in a tone that is neither patronizing nor too technical so that the patient understands what the basic problem is and what is going to be done to help correct it.

   The doctor should have eye contact with the patient being examined. It is often offensive to elder people if the doctor directs his advice to the younger person the patient may be accompanied by. Patients are often reluctant to ask questions and it is better to err on the side of too much information rather than insufficient information. Finally, doctors should not make patients feel they are too busy to listen to their problems because that patient may not only go elsewhere but may be thoroughly dissatisfied and litigious.

3. Create space for comfort. Surprisingly small details such as how the furniture is arranged can make a difference in overall patient response. In an eye practice a desk intervening between a patient and the doctor often serves as a barrier to communication. It is much better to have a direct, closer interaction with the patient. Both intimacy and empathy are given a head start by placing the chairs near each other to eliminate any broad expanse of space between the doctor and patient.

4. Respect a patient's right to privacy. Any discussions of fees both with the doctor or the receptionist should be conducted privately so that details of these conversations are not overheard by a room full of strangers.

5. Look the part. People do not respond well to individuals with long hair or those dressed in blue jeans, sport shirts, athletic shoes, and sports socks. In order to earn patient respect, the doctor and the staff should be dressed in conservative attire, the men wearing shirts and ties, and the women wearing suits, dresses, blazers, or dress pants.

6. Pay attention to detail. Unclean examining rooms make patients uneasy, especially when evidence from previous examinations is clearly visible. Interruptions during an exam can be particularly annoying. A loud intercom system undermines privacy and is unprofessional. Small conveniences such as a coat rack in the waiting room along with soothing decor, plants, and art prints all help create the impression of a pleasant, welcoming environment and a caring doctor.

7. Master communication skills. Conversation is an important factor in making or breaking the doctor-patient relationship. Here are a few tips:
   a. Be upfront. Give information right at the beginning of the visit and not at the end.
   b. Be creative. Use everyday language to explain what is wrong and how you are planning to correct it.
   c. Be personal. Ask questions about the patient's family and his or her social life so that they feel that they have not been forgotten from one visit to the next. Make notes on charts about a patient's interests and concerns for recall at future visits.
   d. Be caring. Put a hand on the patient's shoulder or arm to convey empathy.
   e. Be prepared. If you have something that needs to be shared with a patient's family, ask them to come in from the waiting room and share the information with them.
   f. Solicit patient feedback. Confirm that what you have told the patient has been understood by asking the patient to relay

back to you what he or she has understood. This is particularly important for educating patients on care systems for contact lenses. So often patients leave the office unable to manage their contact-lens care systems. Written information will make sure that the message gets across. Hand-outs are very important and are even more effective if they are personalized.

g. Be human. Patients want human beings looking after them. It is perfectly acceptable to tell patients that you also feel badly when the news you have for them is bad.

8. Be fair in all matters of finance. Charge fairly for your professional services but do not overcharge. Be fair in refunding patients who prove to be unsuited to contact lens-wear. Always look at the situation from the standpoint of the patient. Maintain good will at all costs.

OFFICE SPACE

Most ophthalmic practices gradually grow. Once the contact-lens practice is well established, three important areas are required in the office. First is a *fitting area*, which should be equipped with a variety of handy lens-storage trays that are easily accessible for use. Second, an *insertion and removal area* with a sink for patient and fitter to wash their hands is essential. This area permits the patient to practice insertion and removal until he or she is sufficiently comfortable with the procedure to take the contact lenses home. This area should also permit ancillary personnel to spend time with the patient. Third, an area for contact lens-evaluating equipment, storage, lens cleaning and sterilization and an area for making modifications to rigid lenses are also essential.

CHARTING

Careful documentation, including a careful history, slit-lamp examination, and recording of all pertinent factors should be made before fitting is begun. Important measurements and modifications must always be charted. It is often convenient to maintain separate lens records on each patient with cross-reference to standard clinical charts. A numeric system of charting with a cross-index containing patients' names arranged alphabetically is preferred.

WARRANTY OR INSURANCE

Patients are constantly worried about loss of or damage to their lenses. For most patients the initial expenditure of time and money represents a sizable investment and the fear of losing a lens can become an obsession with many patients. Their concern is justified, for insurance company profiles show a loss rate of 40% in the first year of wear, decreasing as the years go on. It is not surprising that private insurance floaters do not cover contact lenses.

Another argument in favor of insurance is that surveys of uninsured wearers show that 40% were no longer wearing their lenses because one or both lenses had been lost and they had not bothered to replace them. Lens insurance dramatically reduces the dropout rate among wearers. Without insurance there is a tragic waste of professional time and skill, to say nothing of the patient's time and money.

In those lens areas in which insurance is unavailable or the cost is excessive, we found that a simple warranty or guarantee of replacement by the practitioner at a fixed cost suffices, and encourages the patient to replace the lens when it becomes chipped, scratched, or coated. The warranty may be extended to include charges for fit and prescription changes as well as loss. A nominal replacement fee contributes greatly to the willingness of the patient to accept a new lens, particularly a soft lens, when the original lens shows the inevitable ravages of time.

We have found that most patients prefer to have a choice in the level of coverage that a warranty offers. The availability of a more comprehensive plan also prevents patients from feeling that they are being "nickled and dimed" every time they visit the office (Fig. 41-3). Our system includes a triplicate service agreement in which one copy is given to the patient, one is filed on the clinical chart, and one is filed alphabetically for quick reference and for notification of expiration date.

DUPLICATE LENSES

To reduce administrative inconvenience with rush orders for a replacement lens, every patient should have a duplicate pair of rigid lenses made up to the final prescription. This eliminates the weekend panic call before the annual school dance or speaking engagement. An extra pair of soft lenses may be ordered, but the autoclaved packed vial should not be opened because con-

CONTACT LENS SERVICE AGREEMENT

Prince Arthur Eye Associates hereby guarantees replacement of lost or damaged lenses for a period of one year.

Basic coverage: $30.00 per year

Charge per lens deductible varies according to lens material and design for loss or damage of lens will be _____ each.

Prescription change, check-ups, and lens adjustments are subject to a minimum $20.00 charge.

Comprehensive coverage: $45.00 per year

1. Loss or damage replacement as per basic coverage.

plus:

2. No charge replacement of any lens damaged within 60 days of purchase. (Damaged lens must be returned.)

3. No charge for regular check ups during the life of the warranty. (Limit two visits during 12 month warranty.)*

4. No extra charge for prescription change if the fit remains unchanged. Only the regular replacement deductible will apply.

5. Spare lenses for deductible fee only.

*Applies only to check ups by Prince Arthur Eye Associates. Regular examination rates apply to any examinations performed by doctors.

Fig 41-3 ■ Sample of service agreement for contact lens replacement.

tamination of the spare pair often results from neglect in maintenance.

When duplicate rigid lenses are not provided and a loss occurs, it may be several days before the replacement lens is received. When the replacement lens arrives, if the patient continues with the same wearing schedule there is a great risk of the overwear syndrome occurring, particularly with rigid-lens wearers.

The chief reason for replacing rigid lenses is loss. The chief reasons for replacement of soft lenses are deposit formation and clouding, tearing of the lens, yellowing, and roughening of the edges. There is generally a greater replacement rate for soft lenses than for rigid lenses, but the urgency factor is not so great for soft lenses because of the low loss rate.

REPLACEMENT LENSES

A systematic and efficient system should be developed to replace lost or damaged lenses. Many replacement lenses are often ordered by telephone, which is one way of minimizing the amount of traffic in an office. A duplicate telephone message system is invaluable as a way of minimizing errors and of rechecking the week's progress. Often patients will call repeatedly for lost lenses, and the ability to pinpoint the time the lenses were reordered and whether they have arrived is most helpful. A storage system that is alphabetized by surname when the lenses arrive effectively improves the efficiency of handling replacement lenses.

INVENTORY CONTROL AND RESTERILIZATION

The proper management of a lens practice necessitates the use of some measure of inventory control of lenses in addition to a list of names of patients awaiting special-order lenses. If the inventory is not controlled, one may easily expand one's own inventory of lens considerably beyond need and in addition have all the wrong powers on hand when a lens is required.

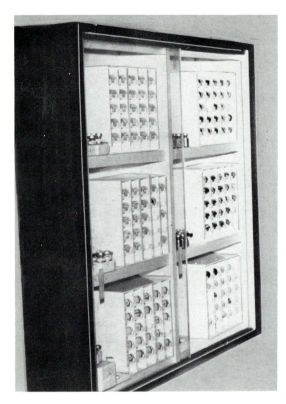

Fig 41-4 ■ Wall unit for storing soft lens wear.

Special lens-holding units may be used for inventory organization, enabling better control of both soft and rigid stock lenses (Fig. 41-4). It is important that all lenses that are used for trial fitting be properly cleaned and disinfected before being reused (Fig. 41-5).

At the beginning of a lens practice one should limit oneself to a select number of manufacturers in rigid and soft lenses whose reliability, quality control, and replacement service have been well established.

ORGANIZATION

Beside the fitter should be some lens wells in which contact lenses (from inventory lenses) can be placed during fitting. An organized system minimized the mix-up of lenses.

A special area should be set aside as the business area and for the verifying instruments in a proper lens practice. The orderly organization of this area is important. All lenses should be verified when received from the manufacturer. Proper drawers or boxes (Fig. 41-6) for lenses, clearly labeled with power and base curve, should be maintained. A disorganized system

leads to repeated confusion and loss of time in rechecking the parameters of a lens to identify the stock of trial or inventory lenses. Ledger books and adequate recording of lenses and payments should be maintained.

REFUNDS

This is a difficult area in which to have any hard-and-fast rules. In the first 6 weeks some persons will reject their lenses for justifiable reasons. It is important that practitioners listen with sympathy and understanding and put themselves in the patient's position. In those cases in which the lenses have been used only for a few days and are still adequate for replacement into the inventory after sterilization, it is usually appropriate to consider the amount of professional time and professional visits and charge accordingly, refunding the balance of the payment. This maintains the goodwill of the patient. In some of our patients a trial charge may be levied and the rest of the balance deferred for the lenses until the patients conclude that they are satisfied and wish to continue using the lenses. Most patients, once they have been shown the benefits of the lenses and their ability to manage them more easily, will usually prefer contact lenses to spectacles. This is particularly true in the case of patients who have aphakia and keratoconus. One should have a consistent and fair fee policy. Some practitioners provide this in writing at the time of the initial visit.

It is important that starter supplies of cleaners, disinfecting solutions, enzyme tablets, and so on, are provided, along with a detailed description of the usage. So often patients are given purchasing slips for their local drugstore and the selected supplies are unavailable and substitutions are made. This can adversely affect the success of the lenses.

INSTRUMENTATION

Many sophisticated instruments are available today for the evaluation of the patient and the lenses. In the establishing of a lens practice it is important that the practitioner have reliable and efficient diagnostic instruments for patient evaluation on both the initial and follow-up visits. As a lens practice grows, further equipment for evaluation of lenses received from the laboratory should be added and the practitioner should become less dependent on the laboratory for quality control. As the practice increases fur-

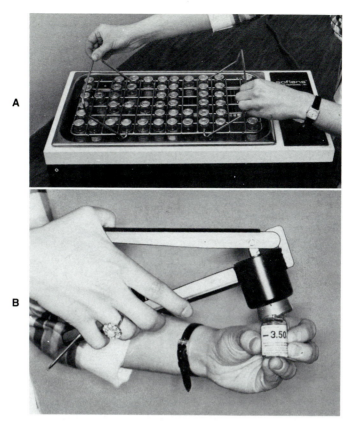

Fig 41-5 ■ **A,** Practitioner resterilizing Bausch & Lomb lenses in large carrying case. **B,** Recapping Soflens in vial for sterilization. (From Stein, HA and Slatt BJ: The ophthalmic assistant, ed 4, St Louis, 1983, The CV Mosby Co.)

ther, modifying and grinding facilities may be added to complete the picture and provide added services (Fig. 41-7).

LENS SERVICING

If a lens practice is sufficiently large, certain lens services should be provided. Such services as buffing and polishing a hard lens can be easily performed by an experienced technician with an inexpensive modification unit. A small charge may be levied to pay for the time involved.

Modifications are an important added feature to a contact lens practice. One can achieve instant success by slight increases in the power of a rigid lens, blending the junctional curves, flattening the peripheral curve, or making the lens diameter smaller. With the increased use of gas-permeable rigid lenses in the last few years, in-office modifications of gas-permeable lenses can be a great time-saver as well as a practice-builder for achievement of rapid success.

Perhaps the most problematic area for the lens practitioner is that of replacement lenses. The patient must be made fully aware at the time of fitting that the lens has a limited life expectancy and will require replacement every year or two.

Both soft and rigid lenses may from time to time require professional cleaning, and the patient should be encouraged to return for this service. Extended-wear lenses invariably build up protein and deposits that interfere with oxygen exchange and may embarrass the integrity of the cornea. The patient should return at regular intervals and should have the lenses removed and either professionally cleaned or replaced. This is most important for the elderly aphakic patient with poor tear function.

A SUCCESSFUL PRACTICE

Most professional offices cannot and do not advertise or retail lenses at a discount price. Therefore, they are not widely known or chosen

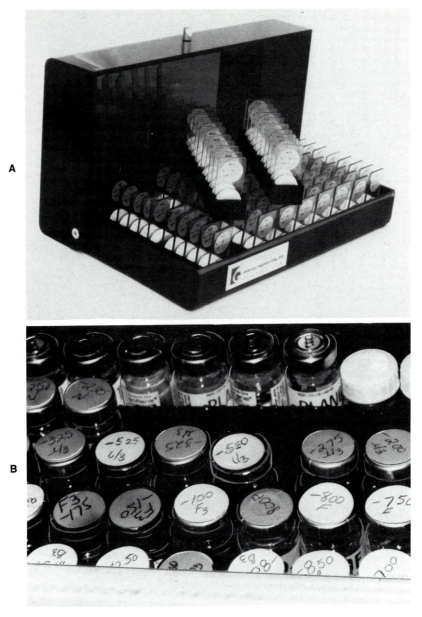

Fig 41-6 ∎ **A,** Orderly lens control case. **B,** For tidiness, a drawer system may be used for storage of contact lenses.

because they are not the cheapest purveyors of lenses. The only advantages of going to the doctor are his superior skills and his willingness to take a personal interest in the patient's welfare.

How to achieve these aims:

1. Be thorough. Check tear film and lids and examine every facet of lens fitting so as to maximize your success rate.

2. Be selective. Choose patients carefully. The happy patient is your only source of advertisement.

3. Inform your patient. Pamphlets, letters, etc., tell the patient about possible problems and complications and how to prevent them.

4. Emphasize safety. Many patients think contact lenses are products like shoes or socks. A lens is a prosthetic device that requires expert supervision.

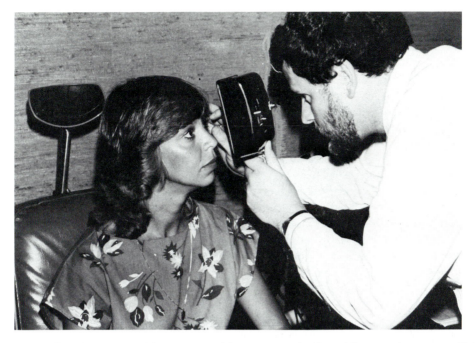

Fig 41-7 ■ The Burton ultraviolet lamp provides gross evaluation of fluorescein patterns. This gross assessment may be superior as an overview of the fitting pattern to the slitlamp, which may be too detailed.

5. A follow-up service is essential. Many contact-lens-induced problems are quite asymptomatic. The patient should be monitored carefully. The commercial way is to sell the lenses to the patient and then say good-bye.
6. Offer personal services. Do special things for the patients such as providing free starter kits, loaner lenses, loaner autoclaves, etc.
7. Be current. Attend lectures, seminars, and read journals in order to stay up to date on developments in the field.

ORDERING LENSES

In the initial stages of lens practice one may wish to order lenses on a per-case basis in which the laboratory makes new lenses and modifications without charge to the fitter. As the practice develops, fitting and ordering from trial sets is a far better and quicker method of arriving at the final lens, and it minimizes the number of repeat office visits for the patient. As the practice grows still further, an inventory set of common powers and sizes in both rigid and soft lenses should be obtained. This further minimizes the number of office visits required, creates instant success with patients while their enthusiasm is high, and identifies the problems very easily in repeat visits, providing on-site correction.

FOLLOW-UP OF PATIENTS

It is most important that lens patients be adequately followed up. A number of satisfied lens-wearers will simply forget to return for regular examination. However, lens patients require ongoing care. The rigid lens may warp, thus altering the corneal curvature, and the soft lens may become coated with protein, causing chronic anoxia of the cornea with vascular invasion.

One may ask patients to return at regular intervals, but it is the responsibility of the practitioner to see that they actually do return. In a busy practice it is all too easy to overlook the dropouts who do not return. Thus an effective recall system, either by phone or mail, is most important. Addresses and phone numbers of patients may change, but a little detective work on the part of ancillary personnel may greatly aid in the locating of patients if for no other reason than to ensure that they obtain follow-up care either by the initial fitter or by another practitioner. We suggest that a patient-agreement form be used, outlining the minimum follow-up requirements.

One may gear the recall system to a set time of the year when all contact files are reviewed and those patients who have not returned are duly notified. Some practices use the birthday cross-reference or date of initial fit system by reviewing each chart during the month of the patient's birthday or date of initial fit, thus spreading the load over the year.

Disposable contact lenses permit a system of follow-up that is based on the patient returning for his or her supply of additional lenses. It is important with disposable lenses that the patients adhere to the throw-away system and not use the same lenses for too long in an attempt to save money.

CONTACT LENS INFORMATION

The general information that a new patient has about contact lenses is often confusing and incorrect. The initial consultation should set some of this information straight and put all the questions in the proper perspective. However, sensible handouts reinforce the question's answer and often answer other questions overlooked in the initial interview. Some of these pamphlets are available from manufacturers and from contact-lens societies. They can however be customized for your own practice. Handouts are great practice builders and should be encouraged. In addition, video has significantly changed the communication system. Good video-tapes on the care of contact lenses are available and they reinforce the spoken and written word.

42 ■ COMPUTERS IN A CONTACT LENS PRACTICE

Alan Mandelberg

- ■ *Inventory*
- ■ *Patient tracking, recalls, and service agreements*
- ■ *Chart information*
- ■ *Data reports*
- ■ *Labels*
- ■ *Getting started*
- ■ *Equipment*
- ■ *Summary*

As the contact-lens industry approaches the twenty-first century, contact-lens fitters are faced with a unique new challenge: competition is reducing profits, while the vast number of lenses available requires larger inventories than ever before. To keep up with these changing times and their challenges, contact-lens practitioners are using computer systems because of the significant advantages that they offer.

Primarily what the right software program offers today's lens-fitters are fast and effective ways to track inventory, gather patient data, automate recalls, reconcile vendor bills, keep up-to-date mailing lists, and measure profitability. All this can be done with a few simple key strokes.

The following discussion describes exactly how a computer system assists in these functions. The specific software system used for this purpose—and as far as we know the *only* software system designed exclusively for the comprehensive management of a contact lens practice—is Contact Tracker.*

---

*Contact Tracker is available from CL Tracker Company, Burbank, California 91505, telephone number (818) 841-4727. At the time of printing, the program was being sold for $1695.

INVENTORY

Fitters who take advantage of a computer system for contact lens management can say goodbye to labor-intensive manual tracking methods. No longer is every pair of lenses recorded by hand in a log as the lenses are ordered, received, and dispensed. In a modern office, a computer does the tracking (Fig. 42-1).

In the days when a practitioner fitted only hard lenses and kept only a small trial-fitting sets of lenses on hand, inventory control was not as complicated as it is today. With the advent of soft contact lenses and their many variables however, a large stock of lenses is necessary to better ensure that a patient is fitted successfully on the first visit.

Ideally, one would like the patient to leave with a pair of lenses in hand. A customer-oriented practice, then, needs to have available all the latest lenses, including those with differing water contents and varied parameters. As new lenses evolve and others become less popular, a practitioner may find himself with a surplus of older, less frequently used lenses. Even on a consignment agreement, these lenses take up storage space and are a considerable investment.

A computer system that tracks and reports lens inventory daily can readily tell practitioners which lenses are moving, which are sitting idly, and which need to be re-ordered. The computer can also identify patients who are wearing lenses that you wish to eliminate from your inventory. One way to get rid of your surplus of these lenses is to offer them to these patients as spares.

Besides knowing at any time which lenses are in stock and which need to be ordered, practitioners can also track performance records of

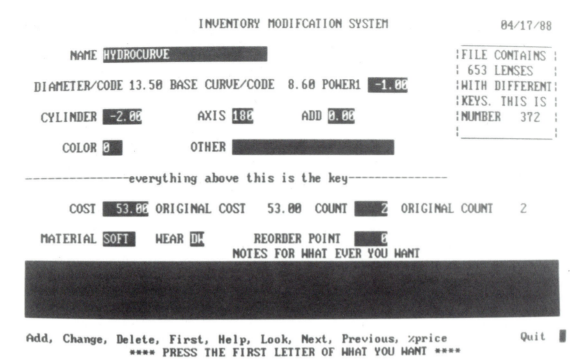

Fig 42-1 ■ Inventory modification. This screen shows how many lenses are in stock and accepts the user's instructions to change inventory with additions, corrections or deletions. Users can enter 100 or so lenses in an hour, since only new information needs to be entered for each lens stocked. Other parameters remain constant until changed.

individual lens types based on parameter, type, and company. If a practitioner wants to keep, for example, a one-month supply of each lens on hand, he or she can now easily know how many to stock. A daily report can signal when a particular lens has fallen below its minimum supply.

Entering inventory information is easy with a good data base program. Such a program allows quick entry of large numbers of lenses without the need to re-enter information on each parameter. For example, if you order 20 lenses with the same base curve, diameter, and cost that vary only in power, then you should change only the power and the number of lenses of that power. Each time you enter lens information and press "A" for "add," that order is transferred to inventory, and the same lens information appears on the screen for the user to modify for the next order. Thus, much re-keying of information is avoided and inventory orders can be entered in batches rather than singly.

The best designed system would allow the lens to be automatically subtracted from inventory as it is dispensed (Fig. 42-2). After a pair of lenses is selected, the technician should only have to type in a few letters into the computer. "CI," for example, might call up all Ciba lenses. The screen would display the Ciba lenses in inventory by base curve and power. By moving the cursor around, the dispenser could select the exact lens he or she is dispensing. When the lens is chosen, "I" is typed, thereby subtracting the lens from inventory and adding it to the patient's record. If the lens is not in inventory, the key "O" is pressed for "order." The time and date of the transaction is automatically logged. Now all the dispenser has to do is to type in whether the lens is new, a refit or a replacement, and bill the patient.

Such tracking methods are not unusual in any business that maintains inventories, and contact-lens practices should be no exception. In short, by maintaining a more selective and consumer-responsive inventory, the practitioner can improve patient service, inventory control, and profits.

```
Screen ID: CL_LK      CL TRACKER IS LOOKING AT PATIENT            Date 04/17/88
                         A CENTER FOR VISION CARE
    ID          NAME SMITH           THOMAS                     TITLE  MR
                     RIGHT LENS( 04/16/88)        LEFT LENS(04/16/88)
LENS NAME             QUALIPERM II                QUALIPERM II
VENDOR               QUALITY                      QUALITY
BASE CURVE            8.15   DIAMETER   9.20       8.15   DIAMETER    9.20
POWER-1              -6.00                        -6.00
CYLINDER x AXIS       0.00 X   0 ADD   0.00        0.00 X   0 ADD   0.00
OTHER-1              OPEN 2 DGR THING APPX .2     OPEN 2 DGR THING APPX .2
MATERIAL             GP            COLOR   GY     GP            COLOR   GY
WEAR(DW/EW)          DW                           DW
OTHER-2
ORDER/INVENTORY      0        DATE    04/04/88    0        DATE    04/04/88
FIT TYPE             NF       REP REASONFIT       NF       REP REASONFIT
COST                 22.50    FEE     150.00      22.50    FEE     150.00
FITTER               G                            G

        TO GO TO THE PATIENT'S PREVIOUS LENS PRESS G OTHERWISE PRESS M ▮
```

Fig 42-2 ■ Contact lens screen. Here the screen is showing data pertaining to a particular set of patient hard lenses. Every parameter is available for detail, plus two "Other" fields can be used for miscellaneous or unique patient or lens data. When a lens is pulled from inventory, it appears here.

PATIENT TRACKING, RECALLS, AND SERVICE AGREEMENTS

If a computer was to do nothing but handle recalls and service agreements, it would pay for itself many times over. As most practitioners know, simply sending notice cards does not guarantee return visits. Although many of these patients have moved or have chosen other fitters, a great many others simply forget to call. This latter group may include patients who are wearing old extended-wear lenses and are running the risk of developing corneal problems. Whatever the case, if a patient problem arises because of lack of follow-up, the practitioner is partly to blame. To prevent this, practitioners should keep not only a list of no-shows, but also one of people who did not respond to their reminder card.

Outside service agreements help skirt the issue somewhat; however, they still do not guarantee follow-up visits and are expensive to maintain. By tying yearly recalls to an in-office service agreement, practitioners can maintain patient control, receive payment for the agreement, and track patients via personal letters requesting appointments and agreement renewals. Ideally, you should combine the yearly recall and the service agreement visit so that patients only receive one recall mailing a year.

The month after letters are sent, the computer can generate a list of names and phone numbers of those patients who have not responded. Then follow-up calls can be made. Most patients realize the importance of the annual visit and appreciate the personal concern and the convenience of being able to make an appointment at the time of the call.

CHART INFORMATION

Basically, all pertinent patient information can be stored in the computer and printed out in reports and onto sticker labels for the outsides of patient charts (Fig. 42-3). Patient data includes name, address, home and work phone numbers, age, sex, the types of lenses currently being worn and length of time they have been worn, date of last visit, whether the patient has a service agreement, and a complete contact-lens history. When reviewing a hard-copy report, the doctor can confirm this information and can correct any data that has been entered incorrectly or that is not current.

The patient history should cover all the lenses the patient has worn, any associated problems,

```
Screen ID:CL_LK      CL TRACKER IS LOOKING AT PATIENT          Date 04/17/88
                          A CENTER FOR VISION CARE

   ID           NAME SMITH           THOMAS                   TITLE  MR
   SOCIAL SECURITY 123-00-0000  DATE OF FIRST VISIT 04/14/86
 C/O                              ADDR 4418 VINELAND AVE. #106

 CITY NO HOLLYWOOD  STATE CA ZIP 91602+0000

 TELEPHONES:HOME 818-762-0653  WORK 818-762-0647
 BIRTHDAY 04/01/52 LAST EXAM 04/04/88 NEXT EXAM 04/04/89
 DOCTOR    M           INSURANC BLU CROS  PAT TYPE  0        CL PAT     G
 GLAUCOMA  *           CATARACT  *        KORNEA   KG        RETINA     *
 VITREOUS  *           FLORANG   *        PHOTOS-K  *        CATSURG    *
 KORSURG   *           SURGERY   *        LASER     *        LATER SU   *
 SPECIAL   *           REFERRAL  *        FIELD19   *        FIELD20    *
 FIELD21   *           FIELD22   *        FIELD23   *        FIELD24    *
 Press any key to continue..._
```

Fig 42-3 ■ All-purpose screen. The program comes with 24 blank code fields for the user to name. Help fields are also user defined. In this example, cornea is spelled with a "K", so the "K" command can differentiate from "C" for cataract. Fields can be labeled for diagnoses, therapies, referrals, or whatever other information is pertinent to the practice.

reasons for changing, and cost to the doctor, fees, and profit. Additional information could include the patient's refractive error, i.e., whether they have keratoconus or high myopia, and whether they were referred, and if so, by whom.

Besides providing a concise and thorough record, this data has other advantages. For example, the flow sheet helps the fitter decide which lenses to try based on previous experience. Having access to previous patient costs and fees may help the fitter solve problems without consulting the front office. Finally, it may persuade him to give a valued patient a free replacement lens, or convince him not to give away a lens to a patient who has received numerous free lenses in the past. In addition, tracking referral patients helps you know who are key referral sources. All this data is difficult and time-consuming to track without a computer.

DATA REPORTS

More important than what you put into the computer is what you get out of it. Depending on the user's request, the computer can create lists and reports containing selective or general information. Patient reports, inventory, and office information are all literally at the user's fingertips. Any information can be included or excluded in any particular search; this is a helpful research tool.

For example, one can follow only those patients who have been fitted with certain lenses, patients of a certain age, or those who have a certain condition, or one can follow the patients who have been successfully fitted with gas-permeable lenses. Changing trends in lens popularity and shifts in practice demographics can also be tracked.

When tracking inventory, the practitioner can generate a daily list of lenses dispensed and ordered. The same report can tabulate gross receipts and costs of those lenses, and whether they were new, refitted or replaced lenses.

Also, when the bill comes from a contact-lens vendor, it can be easily reconciled against a report of the lenses ordered from that vendor. Often these vendor bills are sizable and many contain errors. For example, some vendors charge for lenses that should be under warranty. Because of limited staff time, office managers cannot always sort through these bills as they should. The computer, however, makes such checking easy.

Similarly, there is virtually no limit on the number of reports available to assess practice growth, and office and fitting efficiency. For example, it is easy to measure how many lenses one fitter uses on an average per patient as compared to another fitter. Program users unanimously report increased efficiency as well as few complaints and problems. Having access to more information more easily means practitioners can spend less time managing their practice and more time with patients, thus enjoying the rewards of a more competitively run, streamlined practice.

LABELS

The quick, easy production of patient labels is another singular advantage of computers and one that allows most systems to pay for themselves (Fig. 42-4). Labels both for charts and for mailings go a long way toward improving office management and marketing efforts.

All health-care professionals are realizing the relationship between marketing and survival in today's competitive climate, and ophthalmologists are no exception. Therefore, the benefits of computer-generated selective and mass mailing lists are a tremendous asset to practitioners.

The virtue of selective lists is that you can target a unique population of patients; for example, soft-lens patients can receive mailings on tinted lenses; high-astigmatic patients can receive information about new toric lenses. You can mail your over-40 population information on bifocal lenses, and so on. Demonstrating your personal interest in such a way enhances the practice's image and growth.

Similarly, mass mailings with more general yet pertinent information also create a positive exposure. Information on new services and products, new equipment, plans for office expansion, and Medicare updates can be provided in an office newsletter. Computerized sorting by zip codes allows you to save costs by bulk-mailing, and the computer-printed labels or envelopes save office time. Since the Contact Tracker program is compatible with several more popular word-processing programs including WordStar and New Word, specific data, such as names, can be included in form letters for bulk mailings.

Besides simple name-and-address labels however, more detailed labels can go on the cover

```
Screen ID: CL_LBL        CL TRACKER PATIENT LABELS          Date 04/17/88
                           A CENTER FOR VISION CARE
Place a P next to a label to print it now or an F to write it to a file to be
   printed later. Press G to go on.

■ NAME & ADDRESS LABEL                ANNUAL SERVICE AGREEMENT LABEL

 ┌──────────────────────────┐          ┌──────────────────────────┐
 :MR THOMAS SMITH          :          :SMITH, MR THOMAS          :
 :4418 VINELAND AVE. #106  :          :EXP.04/04/89 OD   45.00   :
 :NO HOLLYWOOD, CA 91602+0000          :OFF.04/04/88 OS   45.00   :
 :                         :          :REF.   /  /               :
 :                         :          :                          :
 :                         :          :                          :
 └──────────────────────────┘          └──────────────────────────┘

 CHART LABEL                          LENS Rx LABEL

 ┌──────────────────────────┐          ┌──────────────────────────┐
 :        MB0G**K***** 04/04/88:       :SMITH, MR THOMAS          :
 :04/01/52 ************ 04/04/89:      :QUALIPERM II      04/04/88:
 :MR THOMAS SMITH          :          : 9.20  8.15  -6.00  0.00X  0:
 :4418 VINELAND AVE. #106  :          :QUALIPERM II      04/04/88:
 :NO HOLLYWOOD, CA 91602+0000          : 9.20  8.15  -6.00  0.00X  0:
 └──────────────────────────┘          └──────────────────────────┘
```

Fig 42-4 ■ Labels. Basically, the computer generates four types of labels: 1) Name and address labels for mailing; 2) Annual service agreement labels for patient charts or other files. These carry expiration dates and lens cost; 3) Chart labels contain key data, such as birth date, last visit, next visit, patient diagnostic codes, etc. These are placed on the chart cover for easy scanning; 4) Lens prescription labels indicate the current lenses the patient is wearing. These can go right on the chart, or, if lenses are on order, may go to the front office for the "Lenses Ordered" box or file. All labels can be easily printed in any quantity.

of patient charts. The practitioner can obtain key identifying information without opening the chart.

Another helpful label can be generated when ordering contact lenses. This label can go in a front-office file until the order is received. Because the label contains the exact parameters of the lens, checking accuracy upon arrival is simple. The front-office person can verify that the lens is correct and call the patient, thus avoiding the embarrassment of calling a patient in for the wrong lenses.

If a patient calls to inquire about an order, the front office staff does not need to look up the chart or call the back-office technician; they just look in the box of "lenses ordered" labels. Because the date of order is on the label, the front office person can call the vendor if the lenses are late.

Labels identifying patients who have service agreements also help staff to quote accurate costs of replacement lenses. A label can be placed on the ledger as well as on the chart, so that the chart does not have to be pulled each time.

GETTING STARTED

No doubt, there are 3 major factors that account for the resistance practitioners express when considering a computer system: initial work load, training, and cost. Practitioners who have adopted the system will testify that it is indeed easy to enter old patient data and that the technology is not that difficult to use. While the Contact Tracker system was designed specifically for technicians, even part-time temporary help can learn it quickly.

The two most recommended approaches for getting patients into the new system are the *month-to-month method* and the *all-at-once method*. Probably the easiest way is to enter only those patients who are due to come in for office visits the following month, plus new patients or those calling for other than annual visits. All that needs to be entered are the names, addresses, phone numbers, and the type of lenses that they are currently wearing. However, the practitioner may decide that entering more complete data at this time would be beneficial.

If only ten patients were added an hour, an office that sees 80 patients a month could have a month's patient load entered in a day. If only one day a month were dedicated to data entry, by the year end the practice would have more than 1000 names on the computer.

The all-at-once method has the obvious benefit of more complete access to information sooner, but it disrupts the office more. Those who used this approach reported that the transition took about two weeks. Of course, this varied widely depending on the size of the practice.

Once the system is in place, practitioners notice the cost efficiency immediately. The system pays for itself time and time again thanks to its speed, ease of storage and retrieval of information, inventory control, and accuracy.

EQUIPMENT

The Contact Tracker system can be used on both single-user and multi-user systems. If an office has an IBM PC, it should be upgraded to an XT, which means that the computer will add a hard disk of memory. The hard disk will contain the Contact Tracker program and its memory. On a multi-user system, the XT can still tie in with the rest of the office's system. When getting a computer, a practitioner should get one with 20 megabytes of memory, which will be more than sufficient. A computer with a clock and a dedicated printer will also be necessary.

IBM or IBM clones (which are cheaper) both serve the purpose. If you're new to computers, however, buy from a retail computer store, where the salespeople will be patient in answering questions. The support is worth the few extra retail dollars.

Above all, an office needs computer hardware and software that is easy to use and fits smoothly into the work flow.

SUMMARY

Clearly, a computer system as described here is essential to any sophisticated contact-lens practice that wants to be competitive now and in the future. Such a system allows the practitioner to better control his practice and to make key decisions. Being able to track the amount of cash generated, the ebb and flow of inventory, enhanced marketing options to select and general patient groups, cost controls, proper charging and payment of bills, complete patient information, and clerical accuracy are all advantages that are now available to the practitioner—with less expense and less effort. When these factors can all be combined in one easy, interconnected network, then the practitioner is in a much better position to manage his practice effectively and to remain competitive.

43 ▪ COSMETICS AND CONTACT LENS WEAR

- Mascara
- Face powder
- Eyeliner
- Eye shadow
- Hair spray
- Removal of cosmetics
- Helpful hints

It may be beneath the dignity of contact-lens fitters to deal with cosmetic problems, but unfortunately it is not beneath the dignity of patients to present them. For this reason an appreciation of the most suitable types of cosmetics for lens wearers is as important as the correct type of solution to be used with their lenses.

In our opinion cosmetics should be applied after the lenses have been inserted. This prevents both contamination of the lens by makeup and, from the patient's point of view, disruption of her artwork by the occasional dropped tear. Also it is easier to apply a lens to a naked eye.

Skin care products are used by both sexes. Products such as hair-grooming agents, acne medications, aftershave lotions, perfumes, deodorants, and perfumed soaps can all have an adverse effect on a contact-lens wearer. Even such hand and face cream residues, nicotine products, and newspaper ink may contaminate both soft and rigid contact lenses.

MASCARA

Used for lash augmentation, mascara should be used sparingly, and only on the outer half of the lashes. The type of mascara that is enriched with small, hairlike fibers to produce extra lash length should be avoided because the fibers often dry and fall into the eye (Fig. 43-1). Water-

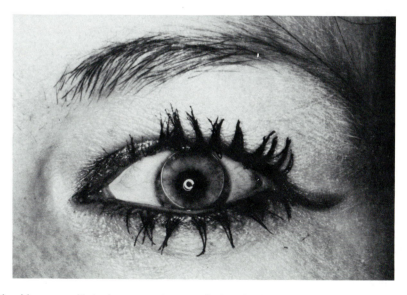

Fig 43-1 ▪ Mascara with lash augmentors applied to the base of the eyelashes. Some of the pigment has fallen off and is deposited at 8 o'clock on the cornea.

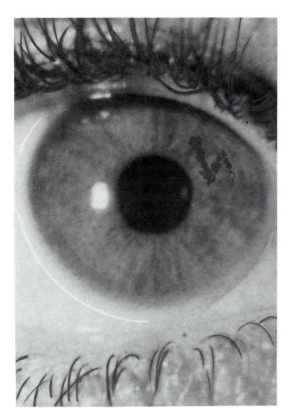

Fig 43-2 ■ Water-soluble mascara avoids the deposition of pigment deposits on the surface of lenses as noted in this illustration.

INGREDIENTS OF EYE MAKE-UP

Mascara
Beeswax, carnauba wax, stearic acid, tryethenolamine, cocoa butter, petroleum jelly, paraffin wax, cellulose ether, polyvidone, phenoxyethanol, polyolesters, alcohol.

Eye shadow
Petroleum jelly, lanolin cream, isopropyl myristate, talc, fatty esters, p-hydroxybenzoates.

Eye shadow powder
Talc, titanium oxide, magnesium myristate pigment, polyglycol, kaolin, cellulose ether, polyol stearates, fish scales, metallic dust, pearl shell.

Eye liner
Glycerine, lanolin, polyvinyl pyrolidine, diethylene glycol monostearate, sodium lauryl sulphate, pigments, polyvinyl alcohols, propylene glycol, p-hydroxybenzoates.

Face powder
Ingredients are many and varied, including colloidal kaolin, talc, precipitated chalk, rice starch, powdered silica and silicates, powdered silk, fatty esters, zinc stearate, kohl, lead.

---

soluble brands are preferred because they do not act as a foreign body if some of the pigment accidentally falls behind a lens (Fig. 43-2).

Besides being a potential irritant, contaminated mascara is frequently a source of blepharoconjunctivitis in women. The product itself is free of contamination when sold; it is after it is used that it becomes contaminated with bacteria and fungi. The most common contaminant is *Staphylococcus epidermidis*, whereas the most dangerous is *Pseudomonas aeruginosa*, which grows in a liquid mascara medium and can invade a small corneal erosion or abrasion.

It is prudent to culture the cosmetics, especially the mascara and its applicator, in any serious ocular infection in women who wear cosmetics. Also it is best if women discard their cosmetics after 3 months of use because of the likelihood of contamination.

FACE POWDER

Face powder comes in either a loose powder or a pressed, compact form. It contains fatty acids and magnesium silicate, which leaves residues on the fingers and are thus transferred to the lens (see box above). Care should be exercised in handling face powder to avoid this problem.

EYELINER

This substance, which comes in a liquid form or as a solid to be mixed with water, should be applied on the lid margin beyond the lash line. A soft pencil is ideal. The "Cleopatra look" achieved by the application of heavy deposits of eyeliner over the entire margin of the lid should be deplored because it may cause blepharitis, styes, and chalazions (Fig. 43-3). Again, water-soluble brands are the only type that should be used and should be replaced every 3 to 4 oz.

Recently the procedure of blepharopigmentation has become available in which a fine dye is tattooed permanently as eyeliner. This elim-

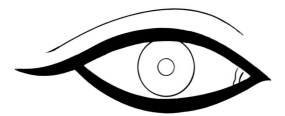

Fig 43-3 ■ The Cleopatra look. The eyeliner covers the lid margin, Moll's glands, and the glands of Zeis as well as the meibomian glands, which may lead to blepharitis, styes, and chalazions.

inates the chances of eyeliner pigment getting into the tear film.

EYE SHADOW

Iridescent types of eye shadow should be avoided. These contain such things as ground glass and oyster shells (Fig. 43-4). Greasy smudge pots and pomades should be another sacrifice for the lens wearer. The creamy-stick eye shadow or the compressed cream powder and brush-on type can be used.

HAIR SPRAY

Hair spray, used widely by both men and women, can cause severe keratitis, erosions of the cornea, and surface opacities of contact lenses (Fig. 43-5), which manifests itself as a salt-and-pepper spotting of the lens. Hair spray

comes most commonly in an aerosol form, which frequently contains lacquer. Normally persons are gazing in the mirror while applying hair spray, therefore their eyes are open. This practice should be discouraged (Fig. 43-6). The eyes should be closed and kept closed for several minutes, since the spray tends to linger. It is simplest to leave the room if a spray has just been released. Even plastic spray guards or a hand, which is of some help in protecting the eyes, cannot stop a vapor. Probably the best routine is not to apply hair spray while lenses are being worn; hair spray should only be used before the lenses are inserted.

REMOVAL OF COSMETICS

At the end of the day cosmetics should be removed after the lenses are removed because the fingers are less likely to be contaminated by the pigments, creams, and oils comprising the make-up complex. It is important to encourage women to use noncreamy or nongreasy cleansing lotions to remove their cosmetics. The greatest harm is often caused by eye make-up remover, probably because copious amounts are used and it often spills into the eye. It must be used carefully.

HELPFUL HINTS

1. Patients should be told never to swap, borrow, or lend eye make-up or applicator brushes. Trachoma and staphylococcal kera-

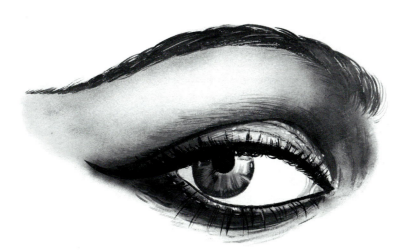

Fig 43-4 ■ Eye shadow with organic additives such as oyster shells frequently acts as an irritant and sensitizer.

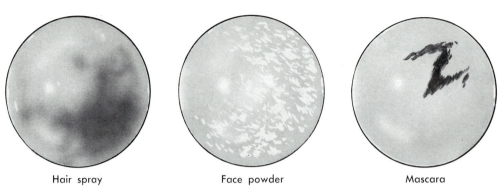

Hair spray   Face powder   Mascara

Fig 43-5 ■ Lenses spoiled by poor handling of facial cosmetics.

titis have been spread in this manner. Brushes should be washed frequently or, preferably, replaced by new ones.

2. Lenses should not be worn in beauty salons. The sprays and fumes in the air can damage the lenses and cause a chemical keratitis. The heat and warm air from hair dryers can cause visual hazing, discomfort, and inability to tolerate the lenses.

3. False eyelashes should not be used. Blepharitis frequently ensues on the basis of an allergic reaction to the adhesive or lash. The adhesive may also be a direct irritant (Fig. 43-7). When the lashes are removed, they frequently take with them some of the real ones; this adds further insult to the lid margin.

   If the patient requires false eyelashes for some valid reason (singers, performers, or entertainers often require them as part of their costume), they should be encouraged to use human lashes tacked on above their own lashes (Fig. 43-8). A waterproof adhesive that has been allowed to dry slightly to a tacky stage should be used.

4. The use of brands made by well-known cosmetic firms should be encouraged. Chances are that the quality control of the product will be better. Federal regulations regarding cosmetics are not nearly as stringent as those regarding food and drugs.

5. Hypoallergenic compounds should be used. Avoid all oily and creamy items. Approximately one woman in 10 has either a respiratory or skin allergy to perfume. Some of

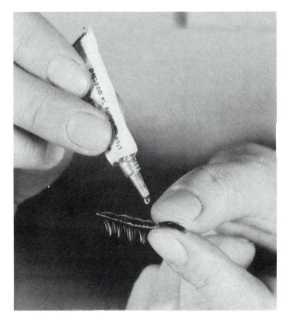

Fig 43-6 ■ Hair spray on a lens inadvertently exposed to an aerosol vapor.

Fig 43-7 ■ The adhesive of false eyelashes may be an irritant and source of sensitization with repeated applications.

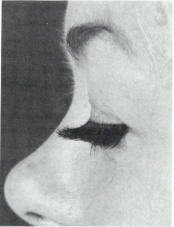

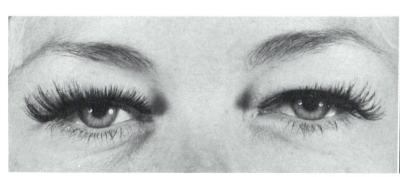

Fig 43-8 ■ False eyelashes should be worn above the real lashes.

the oils in perfumes such as oil of lemon, oil of orange, and oil of bergamot are derived from citrus fruits, so people allergic to citrus fruits may also be allergic to perfumes containing such oils.

Hypoallergenic brands are designed to eliminate from their preparation obvious sensitizers such as perfumes and lanolin (Fig. 43-9). Lanolin is used regularly in cosmetics and soaps and is one of the most common allergens, causing severe redness, itching, and blotchy skin spots.

6. Beauty soaps should be avoided as they are made up of oils, emulsions, and perfumes. There are soaps specially designed for contact-lens wearers such as AOSoap, Optisoap, Neutrogena or glycerin soaps.

Unfortunately trial and error must be employed to discover which hypoallergenic brand is most suitable. Cosmetic firms are not required to label the ingredients of their products; therefore the physician cannot assess a given compound on the basis of its ingredients. Some fitters provide handouts on the dos and don'ts of cosmetics.

7. Do *not:* apply cosmetics to red swollen eyes; share make-up products; use saliva or tap water with the make-up; apply make-up in a moving vehicle; and apply eyeliner to the inner eyelid margin as it may block the pores and result in chalazions and styes.

■
PROBLEMS THAT MAY ARISE FROM COSMETICS

Lids
Blepharitis
Allergic response
Foreign particulate matter. Blocking of ducts from oily cleaners.

Lashes
Overloaded with mascara. Distorted lash roots.

Cornea
Minute abrasions from free talc and organic materials, titanium oxide, precipitated chalk, powdered silica, powdered silk, powdered shell, powdered fish scales.

Pre-corneal tear film
Imbalance due to oily suspension and particulate matter in the tear film

Fornices
Accumulated debris, mascara, etc.

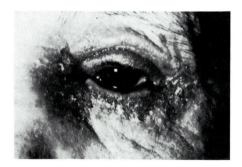

Fig 43-9 ■ Contact dermatitis. Reaction to face powder on eyelids.

8. If facial make-up (foundation) and blush (rouge) are used, the patient should be advised to wash her hands thoroughly as pigment particles can be transferred to the lenses.

9. There are a number of cosmetic removers such as I-Scrub that are non-irritating even if they do enter the eye. These scrubs are important in the care of extended-wear lenses. Clinical problems caused by cosmetics are listed in the box on p. 509.

44 ▪ *HOW TO START A CONTACT-LENS PRACTICE*

James E. Key
Carole L. Mobley

- ▪ *Why fit contact lenses*
- ▪ *Strategy for starting the practice*
- ▪ *Assessing your resources*
- ▪ *Forms and office policies*
- ▪ *Promoting the new practice*

WHY FIT CONTACT LENSES

Before deciding to start a contact-lens practice, which is probably the most commercially exploited and competitive branch of eye-care services, the practitioner must decide if this is an area to which he wants to commit his resources. The primary purpose for starting a contact-lens practice is that it will enhance the array of services the practitioner can offer patients. Contact lenses give the practitioner another treatment option, enabling the office to provide better, more comprehensive care than the competition. Practitioners who do not dispense contact lenses often lose patients once a surgical or medical treatment is completed.

Contact-lens patients, moreover, need routine follow-up care and at least yearly return visits. This repeat business from an established base is much more likely to attract new patients than is marketing. Numerous surveys have shown that the satisfied contact-lens patient will come back for other eye care needs and is the best source of referral for new patients with other needs and problems.

From a purely economic point of view, contact lenses provide a hedge against changes in Medicare reimbursement and other third-party encroachments upon payment for services. The contact-lens branch of the practice also helps keep all facilities and personnel fully productive, which distributes the overhead cost. The contact-lens aspect of the practice can also be very profitable on its own if professional expertise, image, and reputation raise the practitioner above the price-cutting level, and if the proper strategy is used to begin a practice.

STRATEGY FOR STARTING THE PRACTICE

The most important step in establishing or expanding a contact-lens practice is to survey the needs of your community or practice area. Determine what contact-lens products and services are available, and at what prices. There may be unsatisfied needs if the commercial chains are only interested in the high-volume, simple spherical lenses. In addition, if most professional fitters have given up contact-lens work because of price discounting, there may now be a need for a professional who can handle problem fits for patients who require or want premium lenses and personalized care. It is also helpful to talk to the other eye-care professionals in the area. If any of them do not do contact-lens work, they may be an untapped source of referrals within the community.

A second important step in getting started is to establish goals for the contact-lens practice. You need to decide how much time and effort you will actually devote to the contact-lens area. For example, if you decide that you will only fit spherical designs in soft and gas-permeable lenses, you will still be able to fit 80% of the target population. You can do this without an inventory base that is too varied, and you can be somewhat price-competitive with discounters. On the other hand, if you decide to also fit specialized lens designs, you can provide full-service contact-lens fitting. This will build a referral practice, but does require large and varied fitting sets, and will need more of your personal direction and staff resources.

ASSESSING YOUR RESOURCES

As you decide to fit contact lenses, you must assess what resources you will devote to this aspect of the practice. These resources not only includes your own time, but also the skills and time of your staff. Contact-lens work also requires some specialized equipment and materials, as well as consideration as to office space and layout. Lastly, inventory and its effect on cash flow are very important considerations.

Staffing

Staff is probaby the most important resource and it is also the most expensive resource that you will have in a contact-lens practice. By their personality and training, the staff must always present an image of competence, quality, and willingness to help. Finding the right people is the most difficult aspect of starting a lens practice. The screening process starts when you or your office manager gives the applicant an application to fill out. You need to judge right away the prospective technician's manner and to decide if he or she is polite and courteous and whether he or she is likely to make a good first impression. Assess whether the applicant is neat and clean and can speak clearly because clear communication is very important in patient education.

References should always be checked if at all possible. You are mainly looking for dependability, honesty, and courtesy, and if any letter of recommendation or previous employer sounds the least bit hesitant, this usually indicates a deficiency. While interviewing the applicant, you must present your own expectations for the job of contact-lens technician. Not only must the applicant have the necessary skills or be willing to learn them, but he or she must understand exactly the job you wish them to do. Lastly, an assessment of the applicant's educational level is very important. Determine whether the applicant has ever attended regional contact-lens courses or annual professional meetings such as those of the CLAO. Has the applicant pursued a source of home education? If not, we believe the applicant should

certainly be willing to do so and to obtain certification within a reasonable length of time. If you are fortunate enough to find an applicant who is already certified by the National Contact Lens Examiners, American Board of Opticians or Joint Commission on Allied Health Personnel in Ophthalmology (JCAHPO), that person has already indicated a level of commitment and expertise.

Potential applicants might be found by contacting a Fellow of the Contact Lens Society of America because these recognized fitters do much training and teaching through regional and national courses.

Inventory

After obtaining the proper staff, inventory selection and control is the next most important area as it involves the expenditure of a fairly significant amount of money. If the inventory is poorly chosen and becomes quickly obsolete, it is of no use and that part of the entire investment must be written off.

Inventory control harkens back to the nature of your contact-lens practice. If your practice is built around a high volume of fairly easy, mostly spherical contact-lens fits, you only need to choose one or two manufacturers' most popular products and learn to fit them well. Many patients can be fitted from stock with dispensing done at the time of the visit if practicable.

If your practice is more specialized, less inventory is required for dispensing purposes. Although your trial sets may be more varied, patients fitted with soft bifocal or soft toric lenses are usually willing to wait while lenses are being ordered. In this specialty practice, it is important to choose lens' types carefully. You should use a manufacturer who has a good return and warranty policy and one who will be cooperative about lens exchanges.

In determining how many lenses of each lens type to stock, you must decide what level of patient service you wish to provide. It has been estimated by management experts that 80% of patients can be fitted with 20% of the lenses stocked by a specialized fitter. It follows, therefore, that 80% of the specialized fitter's inventory is required to fit only the remaining 20% of patients. However, in a full-service contact-lens practice, the remaining 20% is the "market niche" that the practice hopes to capture and use to build its reputation. The best advice for launching a practice is to choose only one or two manufacturers who have a good line of soft toric and spherical lenses available both with or without tints. In addition, choosing the highest quality RGP-lens manufacturing laboratory will definitely pay off in terms of well-made and well-finished lens edges with minimal central thicknesses and less need for in-office modification.

Office space and equipment

In assessing resources for starting a contact-lens practice, evaluate your office space. This is particularly important because space for a contact-lens practice is often just adapted from existing space without a great deal of thought. Ideally, the room for fitting contact lenses should be larger than the standard examining room. There should be numerous shelves for the storage of lens-fitting sets and contact-lens accessories and solutions. A locked closet within the room for the storage of lens inventory is mandatory. The area for teaching the patient how to insert and remove the contact lenses should be separate from the fitting room because the time required for this procedure cannot always be adequately determined. Since the patient must be allowed to practice insertion and removal until he is comfortable with the procedure, it is important not to tie up the fitting area. The contact-lens fitting room should also be large enough for the installation of a sink and a counter top where lens modification as well as lens-cleaning and lens-polishing can take place.

Equipment needed for a contact lens practice

Equipment costs will be affected by the decision to offer patients contact lenses. The following pieces of equipment are absolutely necessary for basic contact-lens fitting:
1. Keratometer
2. Radiuscope
3. Lensometer
4. Profile analyzer
5. Hand magnifier with measuring grid
6. Millimeter ruler
7. Lens thickness gauge
8. Modification unit for polishing with various tools for redefining edges.

These capital costs must be taken into account when starting a contact-lens practice. The room for fitting will, of course, have to be equipped with a slitlamp and a phoropter, but the room can also double as a refracting lane when not needed for contact lenses.

FORMS AND OFFICE POLICIES

Starting a contact-lens practice will require the use of various forms and hand-outs necessary to solicit and to impart information. Patients appreciate receiving these packets of printed information about contact-lens care when they are considering the purchase of new contact lenses. These hand-outs can be prepared by the office, but they can usually be obtained from individual manufacturers, describing the particular lens types each offers. You can ask for literature from the manufacturer for those lenses you are choosing to fit, and display them in the contact-lens area or even in the reception area if you do not consider this too commercial. Many prospective patients are likely to take these brochures and hand-outs home to show them to other prospective lens-wearing candidates.

There are other forms that the office will need for contact-lens work that must be adapted from the experience of previous fitters. Many of these forms have been detailed in contact-lens publications or are available from various contact-lens buying groups. Examples of these forms follow:

1. A contact-lens information form, which is to be sent to the previous fitter in order to obtain information such as original keratometry, which will be needed in the evaluation of the patient's refitting.
2. A contact-lens service agreement, which describes the exact services the office will provide the patient and specifically states the cost of replacing the lenses. It is also wise to tie this contact lens service agreement into the annual examination so that the office has an easy yearly recall method.
3. A contact-lens prescription form, which would authorize the patient to obtain fitting from a registered contact-lens fitter only, and to return to the practice within a specified period of time for evaluation of that fit.
4. Numerous completed forms on the care and handling of the various types of lenses. These would include instructions for extended-wear soft contact lenses, extended-wear RGP lenses, and daily-wear lenses of all varieties. It is best to have separate forms for each of these and to write in, at the time of dispensing, instructions on the specific care reg-

imen for that particular lens. Having an adequate supply of all these forms at the time of the initial establishment of a contact-lens practice will save a great deal of time as well as avoid confusion on the part of the staff. Such written reminders are also greatly appreciated by patients and are taken as a sign of the care and professionalism of the office.

Office policies regarding contact-lens fees must also be decided upon before the first patient is fitted. In general, the best policy is to collect one-half of the contact-lens fee at the time of initial fitting and one-half when the patient returns to pick up the contact lenses. As contact lenses are rarely an emergency, this policy must be applied consistently to everyone. Patients do better with contact lenses when they have already made a significant financial investment in them. A new contact-lens practitioner cannot afford to order lenses without having at least one-half of the fee pre-paid. An office policy should also be established concerning the return of contact-lens patients. A quality practice will be built through service, and part of that service is to be sure the lenses are performing well on the patient's eyes. The fact that a patient does not return should not be taken to mean that the patient is completely satisfied. If a patient misses one of his important follow-up visits, particularly the three-month visit, he should be notified and told to return. Again, most patients appreciate being reminded if they have simply forgotten their appointment.

PROMOTING THE NEW PRACTICE

Professional promotion of your contact-lens practice is the practitioner's only hope against the aggressive retail promotion and competition. Indeed, good marketing has the potential to protect your practice from the "cheap lens" price wars. This is the reason that the most successful practitioners market their contact-lens' skill and expertise to the exclusion of any particular brand or type of contact lens. Always stress that your contact lens service provides individualized care and solutions to particular problems and is not simply "selling lenses." This also gives the practitioner the opportunity to upgrade the existing contact-lens patients to premium products with greater performance that also have greater profit margins. There are several important steps in the marketing of a new contact-lens practice. The first of these is to establish yourself as a

source of up-to-date information on all types of contact lenses and contact-lens care products. The advertising done by discounters has created a great deal of confusion and the practitioner has a marvelous opportunity to build patient confidence by clearing up this confusion.

Even though you may be most familiar with the lenses from only two or three manufacturers and know them to be of high quality, in your marketing you must avoid brand identification. Stress that you have knowledge of all of the eye-care options and that patients are free to select the one that will be best for them. Never forget that you are selling service with a professional, caring approach. Remember that the telephone is your link with new patients. All calls should be treated seriously and without interruption, if possible. For those callers who need a more prolonged conversation regarding lens services or prices, a number where they can be contacted should be taken and the call returned as soon as possible. All calls about price should be turned into conversations about quality. The advantages of contact lenses should be stressed with the use of open-ended questions in order to maintain a dialogue with the patient. This gives the prospective patient the opportunity to know that your office puts his eye health and vision above selling contact lenses. It is often helpful to obtain the names and addresses of all callers so that an introductory booklet concerning contact lenses can be mailed to them even if they do fail to make an appointment.

Once the patient is in the office, professionalism should be reinforced. Here the office staff is part of the upgrade process and should try to emphasize the advantages of new contact lenses or care systems. The staff should be careful not to criticize "cheap" lenses, but should always offer a better-quality real option if one exists. Fortunately, the new soft contact lens designs, as well as the gas-permeable polymers now provide lenses that will fit almost any refractive error and yet satisfy the oxygen demands of the cornea. Visual aids and lens performance brochures are very helpful in explaining to the patient why a change in their contact lenses might need to be made, or why contact lenses might be a better alternative for visual correction for them than spectacles.

Lastly, effective marketing means keeping the lines of communication open with both past and present patients. Continuing communication with those patients presents the best opportunity for increased patient loyalty and referrals. The annual warranty letter not only reminds patients to renew their contact-lens warranty, but also reinforces your continued interest in their eyes and reminds them of their yearly visit. Even prior to that annual letter, special postcards reminding patients about recent advances in areas that are of interest to them would be helpful. For example, a postcard about the availability of new gas-permeable bifocal lenses might be very interesting for those patients who are wearing reading glasses over their present contact lenses.

If you decide to use newsletters, they should carry informative articles on advances in contact-lens technology. These newsletters can be written by you or adapted from those that are now offered by marketing companies as well as professional societies such as the American Academies of Ophthalmology and Optometry. Direct-mail pieces to existing patients can be useful if these mailings are credible and informative. They should continue to promote your office as a knowledgeable source of objective information on eye health. Patients are interested in whether the doctor or his office staff has attended a recent contact-lens meeting or taught a course or presented a paper on some new lens or care product.

Marketing does not require a heavy expenditure of dollars nor would this even be advisable for the early contact-lens practice. The best marketing continues to be through an existing and growing patient base who needs to know that you do have an interest in contact lenses, and needs to be reminded that contact lenses might be appropriate for them. In starting this practice, simply remember to offer more than competitive prices to the patients by marketing the quality of your practice as well as the fact that you are striving for good corneal health and better vision for your patients. By doing so, the contact lens part of your practice will be both profitable and enjoyable.

45 ▪ *PHOTOGRAPHY OF THE ANTERIOR SEGMENT**

Csaba L. Martonyi

- ▪ Photographic terms
- ▪ Film size
- ▪ Film speed and types
- ▪ Exposure
- ▪ Setting
- ▪ External photography
- ▪ Photo slit-lamp biomicrography
- ▪ Goniography
- ▪ Endothelial specular photomicrography
- ▪ Cinematography and video recording
- ▪ Processing
- ▪ Cataloging slides
- ▪ Slides for presentation
- ▪ Summary

In 1960, Novotny and Alvis performed the first successful fluorescein angiogram on a human. That event marked the advent of modern ophthalmic photography. Subsequent development of sophisticated instrumentation has made it possible to consistently produce precise documentation of subtle changes within the eye. Intravenous fluorescence angiography has contributed greatly to a better understanding of the posterior segment of the eye and continues to be of particular importance in the diagnosis and treatment of many of the diverse disease processes that affect it. Since 1976, endothelial specular photomicrography has made possible the documentation of the cell density of the posterior layer of the cornea of the living eye. Moreover, photography plays an indispensable role in many areas of research and teaching. With the techniques of external photography, photo

slit-lamp biomicrography, fundus photography, fluorescein angiophotography of both the posterior and anterior segments, motion picture and video recording, and endothelial specular photomicrography, ophthalmic photography is today a vital, well-established specialty area.

Although this chapter cannot treat the full scope of ophthalmic photography, it provides an overview and an introduction to its most practical applications.

PHOTOGRAPHIC TERMS

Standard, hand-held 35 mm cameras are of two basic types: single-lens reflex, and those using a rangefinder or a viewfinder. (The latter type is not recommended unless specifically designed for eye photography.) Numerous lenses are available, and their important characteristics include focal length, lens speed, depth of field, and resolution. Exposure is determined with an exposure meter and regulated by means of an adjustable diaphragm, or "f" stops, and shutter speeds.

Focal length

The focal length of a lens is the distance between the lens and the film plane in the camera (actually measured from the principal plane of the lens when focused at infinity). The focal length, expressed in millimeters, is engraved on most lens systems along with the serial number and trade name. The normal, or standard, camera lens is that which will produce an image of a scene in the same perspective as seen by the unaided eye. The normal focal length for a camera is roughly equivalent to the diagonal measurement of the film size used. For a 35 mm (film size) camera, the standard lens is 50 mm

---

*Modified from Stein HA, Slatt BJ, and Stein RM: Ophthalmic assistant, ed 5, St. Louis, 1988, The CV Mosby Co.

in focal length and has approximately a 45- to 55-degree angle of view. A wide-angle lens, such as a 35 mm (focal length), has a short focal length with an angle of view of about 62 degrees; a telephoto lens, such as a 135 mm, has a long focal length and is restricted to an angle of 18 degrees.

Lens speed

Lens "speed," or widest aperture, refers to the maximum light-gathering power of the lens. It is expressed in the form of an "f number," which represents the ratio of the diameter of the lens to the focal length. Engraved on the lens system, it may appear as f2.5 or f1 : 2.5 (or merely 1 : 2.5). The diameter of an f1 lens is equal to its focal length and is termed a *fast* lens because it permits a great amount of light to reach the film. Such a lens would be well suited for photography in available light. Most lenses have adjustable f stops, operated by a diaphragm between lens elements.

Depth of field

The distance within which all objects closer to and farther from the camera are acceptably sharp is called the *depth of field*. As a general rule, one third of the total depth of field will fall in front of the point at which the camera is focused and two thirds beyond that point. For instance, if the depth of field covers a distance of 3 feet when the camera is focused at 15 feet, all objects that are between 14 and 17 feet from the camera will appear sharp on the photograph. (Depth of focus is the same phenomenon occurring at the film plane.)

Depth of field is a function of focal length and f number. It increases with the use of larger f numbers (smaller apertures) and decreases with smaller f numbers (larger apertures). Depth of field is also greater for a wide-angle lens (short focal length) and less for a telephoto lens (long focal length) when both are set at the same f number. Depth of field is further affected by the camera-to-subject distance. The effective distance covered by the depth of field when a lens is focused at or near infinity is far greater than that of the same lens focused on a very near object. The closer a lens is focused, the more "shallow" becomes the depth of field. Since most photography in ophthalmology is done at high magnifications with a short distance between the camera and the subject, natural limitations in

depth of field must be compensated for by using the highest possible f number (referred to as *stopping down*) and by using a light source that is sufficiently bright to provide the necessary exposure.

Resolution

Resolution, or resolving power, is the ability of a lens, film, or the eye to distinguish fine detail. This resolving ability of films and lenses is measured by the highest number of lines per millimeter that they are able to define clearly without blurring together.

Shutter speed

Shutter speed is measured by fractions of a second, indicated by numbers such as 30, 60, and 125, which stand for 1/30, 1/60, or 1/125 of a second. These numbers represent the length of time the shutter is open when the shutter release is activated—the interval during which the light passes through the lens and strikes the film.

Shutters may also have a "B" or "T" setting for time exposures. These are impractical for patient photography since a blurred image will result. Time exposures are useful when photographing nonmoving objects in dim light, when the camera is mounted on a tripod.

FILM SIZE

Although film comes in many sizes, the one most commonly used in eye photography is the full-frame 35 mm, which yields transparencies with the dimensions of 24 mm × 35 mm (⅞″ × 1⅜″). These are mounted in 2″ × 2″ cardboard mounts, from which their name *two-by-two slide* is derived.

FILM SPEED AND TYPES

The *speed* of a film refers to its sensitivity to light, expressed in International Standards Organization (ISO) numbers (formerly American Standards Association [ASA] numbers). The higher the number, the more sensitive, or "faster," the film. Standard color films range from 25 to 400 ISO, or greater, and black and white films for general use range from 32 to 400 ISO, or greater. Films having low ISO numbers will have fine-grained patterns on the film emulsion and higher resolution. The sharp detail offered by slower films (color or black-and-white) makes them valuable to scientific or diagnostic study, particularly when large prints are to be made from the slides or negatives.

There are two types of color film: positive transparency and negative. The name of each film indicates its type. Names ending in "-chrome" (for example, Kodachrome, Ektachrome, Anscochrome) signify positive transparency films that produce color slides. Names ending in the word "color" (for example, Kodacolor, Ektacolor, Fujicolor) refer to films that produce negatives from which prints are made. When desired, the preparation of *internegatives* will permit prints to be made from slides. Black-and-white negatives and subsequent prints can also be made from color slides for publication purposes.

Color films are also designated *daylight* or *tungsten*, which refers to the lighting conditions under which the film must be used. All lighting sources have a *color temperature*, which is expressed in degrees Kelvin. Normal daylight, around midday, has a color temperature of approximately 5,400° K. The light produced by an electronic flash, blue flashbulbs, or a blue filter over white bulbs has the same color temperature and requires the use of daylight film. Photo floods and other sources of tungsten illumination have a much lower color temperature and require the use of tungsten film. Tungsten films were designed to be used with lamps that produce 3200° Kelvin.

The use of daylight film under tungsten illumination will result in pictures having a yellow-orange or "warm" cast; the use of tungsten film outdoors, or with electronic flash or blue bulbs, will result in a decidedly blue, or "cold"-appearing picture, inappropriate for patient photography. If a single type of film must be used under both lighting conditions, conversion filters can be placed over the lens, but an increase in exposure is required.

In general, daylight films have a higher ISO rating than comparable tungsten films. The exception is some high-speed motion picture films that are currently manufactured in tungsten only.

EXPOSURE

Exposure is the total volume of light that strikes the film. It is the *sum* of light *intensity* and *duration* of exposure. Correct exposure is achieved through the balanced interaction of film sensitivity, brightness of illumination, f stop, and shutter speed.

When using available light, the shutter speed is used to control the duration of the exposure and the f stop is used to regulate the intensity of the light striking the film. Each full f stop setting (f8, f11, f16, and so on) and each shutter speed setting (30, 60, 125, and so forth) affects the total exposure by a factor of two. For example, if the camera were set at a correct exposure of $\frac{1}{60}$ of a second at f11, and then the lens were opened to f8, twice as much light would reach the film and the image would be overexposed. Conversely, if the lens aperture were closed down to f16, only half the needed light would reach the film, and the image would be underexposed. Likewise, if the f stop remained constant and the shutter speed varied, the same alteration in total exposure would result. By decreasing the shutter speed from $\frac{1}{60}$ to $\frac{1}{30}$ of a second, the exposure would be doubled; by increasing the shutter speed from $\frac{1}{60}$ of a second to $\frac{1}{125}$ of a second, the exposure would be halved. Correct settings, therefore, are vital to correct exposure. If either f stop or shutter speed is off by just one setting, a serious overexposure or underexposure may result on the film.

Exposure meters

Whenever a light source other than a flash is used, the correct exposure must be determined with a light meter. All modern light meters are marked in ISO numbers that correspond with the ISO ratings of available films. Before taking a reading, the light meter must be set to the ISO of the film being used. When using a hand-held exposure meter, care should be taken to read the average intensity of light reflected from the subject. If the light meter is allowed to respond to an area that is either much brighter or much darker than the average, a proportionate underexposure or overexposure will result. Also, to prevent underexposure, the sensing element of the meter should be shielded from sources of light that do not strike the subject itself. Another manner of determining exposure is to take an incident reading. Rather than measuring the light being reflected by the subject, a special filter is placed over the sensor of the light meter, and the light source itself is measured from the position of the subject to be photographed.

The newest single-lens reflex cameras have built-in exposure meters that offer automated exposure control when set to correspond to the ISO rating of the film being used.

Flash illumination

When using electronic flash, the *duration of the exposure* is usually determined by the *duration of the flash*. Since most modern electronic flash units have a duration of approximately $\frac{1}{1,000}$ of a second, the length of the exposure will be $\frac{1}{1,000}$ of a second. This very short, motion-stopping duration makes the electronic flash ideally suited for eye photography. Since the duration of the exposure is now essentially beyond our control, correct exposure is achieved by regulating the *intensity* of the light, either at its source or when it passes through the lens, or both. In most cases, the intensity of the flash source itself need not be altered. In fact, it is desirable to have ample light to guarantee a good exposure at very high f stops, thereby ensuring the greatest possible depth of field at close working distances, especially when using slower, fine-grained film. Should it be impossible to stop down sufficiently to compensate for flash intensity, a diffuser can be used over the flash source itself.

All flash sources (electronic or flashbulb) are assigned a *guide number*, which is a numeric representation of the intensity of that particular flash source when used with a specific sensitivity (ISO) of film. The correct exposure is determined by dividing the guide number by the number of feet between the camera and subject. For instance, a guide number of 40 used with 25 ISO film, at a camera-to-subject distance of 5 feet, requires a lens aperture of f8, or at 10 feet, a lens aperture of f4. That same light source would have a guide number of 55 when used with a film rated at 50 ISO, requiring an aperture of f11 at 5 feet and of f8 at 10 feet. As one can see, doubling the ISO rating influences the exposure again by a factor of two. Using a film with an ISO rating twice as great, under the same lighting conditions, requires a reduction of exposure by one half.

Although no longer a variable when using electronic flash illumination, the shutter speed *must* be set at the speed prescribed by the manufacturer to provide proper *synchronization* (maximum light output coincident with a fully open shutter). In addition the synchronization cord of the flash unit must always be connected to the *X* outlet on the camera. Incorrect shutter speed settings, or using the wrong synchronization connector, can result in the loss of part or all of the picture. For electronic flash, *only* the X outlet may be used.

When using flashbulbs, the synchronization selector (when available) is set to *M* and the synchronization cord is attached to the M outlet. When using flash bulbs with a camera equipped with a focal plane shutter, the synchronization cord must be attached to the *FP* outlet, and only FP type flashbulbs are used.

SETTING

A specific area should be set aside for ophthalmic photography if possible. The photographic environment, including background and room lighting, can thus be better controlled, providing more consistent results. A degree of privacy, an important courtesy to the patient, will also be ensured.

EXTERNAL PHOTOGRAPHY

A 35-mm single-lens reflex camera with interchangeable lenses is recommended for external eye photography. The single-lens reflex feature permits viewing and photography through the same lens system. Composition and sharp focus are thus made easy since the image being photographed is seen in the viewfinder exactly as it will appear on film. To achieve the necessary magnification, a macro lens (specially designed to permit focusing on very near objects) is recommended. Macro lenses for 35 mm cameras are available from approximately 50 mm to 120 mm in focal length. The advantage of a longer (100 mm and over) focal length macro lens is that it permits a greater working distance between camera and subject and will produce less perspective distortion. (An extreme example of perspective distortion is that which results from the use of a very wide lens, such as a "fish-eye" lens.) Photography of an intra-operative procedure, for example, would dictate the use of a longer focal length lens to provide a suitable working distance-to-magnification ratio.

The close focus range capabilities of a macro lens can be further extended with the use of an *extension ring* or *tube*, which merely extends the lens further from the camera, enabling one to focus on an even closer object. Similarly, lenses designed for normal photographic use can also be extended for close focus applications. Varying lengths of rigid extension tubes may be

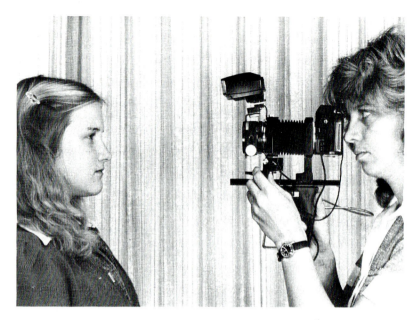

Fig 45-1 ■ Contax RTS Camera, Contax Auto Bellows, 100 mm Yashica Bellow Lens, and pistol grip.

used on the same camera interchangeably to provide an extended range of magnifications. Another method of extending lenses is the use of a bellows-focusing device between the camera body and the lens. Effectively a variable extension tube, it allows for continuous adjustment over a wide range when used with the appropriate focal length of lens (Fig. 45-1). A good, practical magnification-to-working distance ratio can be achieved with the use of a 100 mm or 135 mm lens.

If only a fixed (noninterchangeable) lens camera is available, an add-on portrait lens can be used; however, whereas it is seemingly simple and inexpensive, it may provide limited magnification and resolution. Whenever its use is elected, it must be with a single-lens reflex camera to ensure proper framing and focus.

Illumination

For illuminating external photographs, an electronic flash device is recommended. Problems created by rapid eye movements or blinking are eliminated by the extremely short duration of the flash. Many inexpensive flash units are available today, some with automatic exposure control, eliminating the need to change f stops while being able to alter the distance be-

tween camera and subject over a given range. If such a flash is being contemplated, its ability to function in the automatic mode at such close distances must be ensured. Not all have that capability.

A flash source should always be positioned to provide even, diffuse illumination over the area being photographed. The bridge of the nose, prominent brows, and so forth should never be allowed to cast a shadow onto the area of interest. When making photographs of a single eye area, the light should be positioned on the patient's temporal side. When taking a two-eye view or full-face photograph, the light should be positioned directly above the lens. The resulting photograph will show uniform illumination over the subject area, with shadows falling directly behind and below the patient. Using a lens of 100 mm or more in focal length will considerably lessen the problems attendant upon the use of the sharply oblique illumination, which results from working at too close a range to the subject.

A suitable background should be provided. A simple solution is to obtain several large (30″ × 40″) matte boards available in a variety of pleasing colors. Fairly light, warm colors, such as yellow or light orange, are best. Greens and especially blues are seldom complimentary to

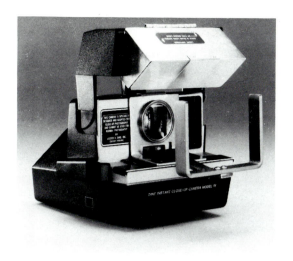

Fig 45-2 ■ Dine Instant (Polaroid) camera with closeup lens and built-in flash. (Courtesy Lester Dine Co.)

flesh tones. As a general rule, the lighter the subject, the darker should be the background, and vice versa. Patients with oculocutaneous albinism, for instance, might be best photographed in front of a dark background, whereas a lighter background must be used for darkly pigmented individuals. Another point to keep in mind is that when photographing extremely dark subjects, it is advisable to make additional, lighter exposures by "opening up" half an f stop (half the distance to the next smaller f number).

For persons not familiar with photography, the Lester A. Dine system (Fig. 45-2), which incorporates a Polaroid camera, is most useful. It is supplied wth a color-coded series of lenses and frames to establish framing and camera-to-subject distance, and a flash source preset to provide correct exposure.

Whenever flashbulbs are used for patient photography, a clear protective shield must be placed over the bulb; this will prevent the possibility of injury should a bulb explode during the photographic session.

PHOTO SLIT-LAMP BIOMICROGRAPHY

Many conditions affecting the anterior segment of the eye, especially the transparent cornea, anterior chamber, and lens, are of such a subtle nature that they defy detection by any means other than *slit-lamp biomicroscopy*. Since the adverse conditions occurring in these trans-

parent or translucent structures are themselves commonly transparent, conventional, diffuse illumination in unsuitable for their visualization. Only the specialized "optical sectioning" ability of the slit-beam illumination and high magnification of the slit-lamp biomicroscope provide an adequate view of the subtle changes that are of interest to the ophthalmologist.

Fundamental to producing consistently useful photo slit-lamp documentation is a thorough knowledge of (1) the structures of the eye, (2) the location and general appearance of the diverse conditions affecting the eye, and (3) the basic forms of illumination and their application to these conditions. Basic illumination techniques include direct focal, tangential, direct and indirect retro-illumination from the iris; retro-illumination from the fundus; transillumination; sclerotic scatter; proximal illumination; and Tyndall's phenomenon for aqueous cells and flare.

A slit-lamp biomicroscopic examination is a dynamic process. With the use of a narrow slit beam to provide optical sectioning, transparent structures like the cornea can be examined in minute detail, a small section at a time. The result is, in essence, a mental composite image of the entire cornea. In slit-lamp photography, however, each photograph is restricted to a single moment in that examination. To overcome this limitation, some slit lamps are equipped with a diffuse illuminator as well. When used in conjunction with the slit illuminator, the result can be a pleasingly subdued image of the overall eye with a superimposed narrow slit beam to provide specific information about that section of the structure that it isolates (Fig. 45-3). Although diffuse illumination will cause some fine detail to become obscured through the scattering of light, it is useful to provide general, introductory photographs. With these as a basis, additional photographs can illuminate areas of more precise interest, further isolated through increased magnification. The result then will be a series of slides that lead the viewer through a logical progression from an overview to the most subtle detail. Fig. 45-4, *A* through *L*, shows some of the forms of illumination, along with recommended exposures as used on the Zeiss photo slitlamp. For other photo slitlamps, exposures should be established by exposing test films using the manufacturer's recommendations.

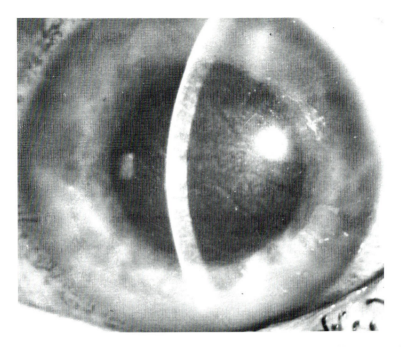

Fig 45-3 ■ Slit-lamp photograph showing diffuse, overall illumination with a superimposed narrow slit beam.

Fig 45-4 ■ **A,** Optical sectioning with fill illumination. Overall, diffuse illumination (fill light) provides a view of the entire eye, and the superimposed, direct focal illumination of the narrow slit beam provides specific information about the area that it isolates. Direct focal illumination in the form of a very narrow slit beam, without overall, diffuse illumination, is the most selective, direct method of examining the structures of the eye.

Fig 45-4 ■ **B,** Tangential illumination. A moderate to wide slit beam is projected onto the area of interest at a sharply oblique angle to produce clearly defined highlights and shadow areas, greatly enhancing topographic detail.

Fig 45-4 ■ **C,** Pinpoint illumination, based on Tyndall's Phenomenon, is used to visualize and photograph aqueous cells and flare. The smallest circle beam is directed through the anterior chamber at an oblique angle. If the aqueous is turbid with cells and protein the small cone of light will be visible to a variable degree depending on the amount of abnormal material it contains, demonstrating anywhere from "one" to "four-plus" aqueous cells and/or flare.

Fig 45-4 ■ **D,** Specular reflection. A moderate slit beam is projected onto the surface of interest (the corneal endothelial surface in this example) and viewed at an angle from the perpendicular that is equal to the angle of incidence. An area of nonreflectance from normally flat, reflective surfaces, indicates an abnormality.

All exposures listed assume the use of $2\times$ magnifiers on the side arms. When $2\times$ magnifiers are not used, increase magnification or f-stop.

ISO 200
Diffuse illum. open $10\times$
Slit 9
Side arm f16

ISO 200
No diffuse illum. $16\times$
Slit 9
Side arm f32-44

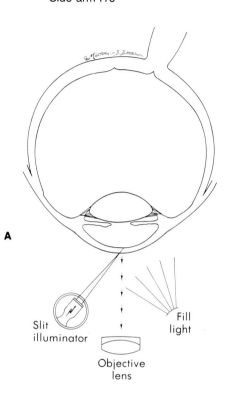

A

Slit
illuminator

Fill
light

Objective
lens

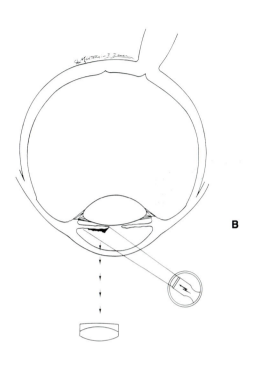

B

ISO 800 or greater
No diffuse illum. $16\times$
Slit 9
Side arm f16

ISO 200
No diffuse illum. $16\times$
Slit 9
Side arm f44

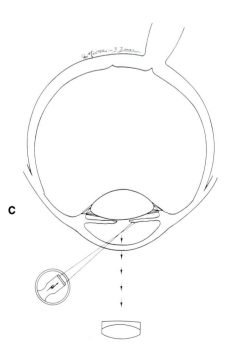

C

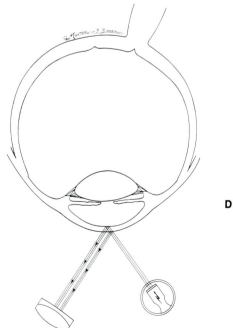

D

ISO 200
No diffuse illum.
Slit 9   16-25×
Side arm f16-22

ISO 400
No diffuse illum.
Slit 9   16×
Side arm f16

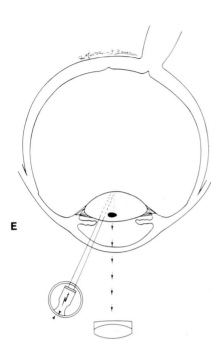

E

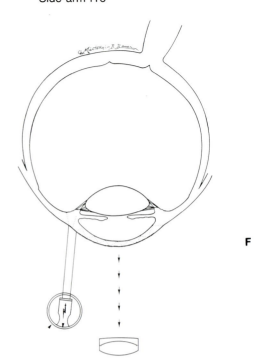

F

Fig 45-4 ■ E, Proximal illumination. A moderately narrow slit of light is directed to strike an area just adjacent to the area of interest. The light is absorbed by the surrounding tissue and scattered behind the abnormality, outlining it in relief against a now lighter background. This is an especially useful technique for delineating the general size and shape of an opaque object obscured by overlying soft tissue (such as an imbedded foreign body).

Fig 45-4 ■ F, Sclerotic scatter. A wide slit beam is directed to strike the limbal area where the light is absorbed and "piped" throughout the cornea. When corneal changes are present, they become visible by reflecting a small portion of the light passing through the cornea.

Fig 45-4 ■ G, Direct retro-illumination from the iris. A moderate slit beam is directed onto the iris surface behind the corneal abnormality. (The slit beam must not strike the corneal changes directly.) The corneal abnormality is then examined or photographed in silhouette against the light background of the illuminated iris. The slit illuminator is rotated from its normally isocentric position to permit centration of the principal subject area in the final photograph.

Fig 45-4 ■ H, Indirect retro-illumination from the iris. A moderate slit beam is directed to strike the iris just adjacent to the area which lies directly behind the corneal abnormality. The light striking the iris will be reflected in all directions and the subtle corneal changes can be seen, diffusely retroillumi-nated, against the dark background of the unilluminated iris and even darker pupil. The most useful zone of information will often be at the interface of light and dark backgrounds at the pupillary margin. The slit illuminator is rotated from its normally isocentric position to permit centration of the principal subject area.

Fig 45-4 ■ I, Retro-illumination from the fundus. A moderate slit beam is projected through the dilated pupil to strike the fundus in an area behind the abnormality to be examined or photographed. The slit illuminator must be brought into a nearly coaxial position with the biomicroscope and the slit beam decentered to enter at the pupillary margin. Through careful positioning of the slit illuminator and the slit beam in the pupillary area, the red reflex will be seen, against which subtle corneal and lenticular changes will be outlined. Considerably greater levels of illumination may be achieved by rotating the subject eye to position the optic nerve head to provide a much brighter background. This is an especially useful technique when photographing patients with dark fundi.

Fig 45-4 ■ J, Iris trans-illumination. Photographs should be taken with the pupil only partly dilated (3 to 4 mm when light stimulated). With the slit illuminator in a coaxial position with the biomicroscope, a small, full circle beam of light is projected through the pupil into the eye. Defects in the iris will be visible by transmission of the orange light reflected from the fundus.

ISO 200
No diffuse illum.
Slit 9
16-25 ×
Side arm f22-32

ISO 200 to 400
No diffuse illum.
Slit 9
16-25 ×
Side arm f16

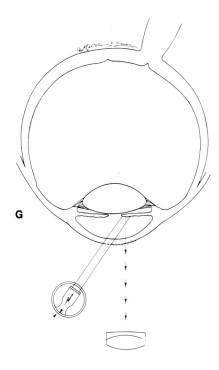

G

H

ISO 200
No diffuse illum.
Slit 9
10-16 ×
Side arm f32

ISO 200
No diffuse illum.
Slit 9
16 ×
Side arm f14

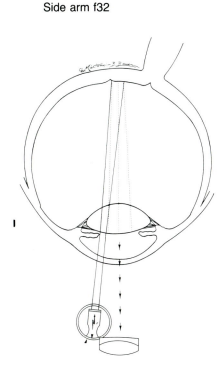

I

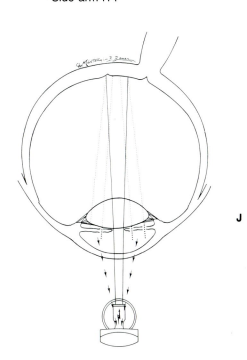

J

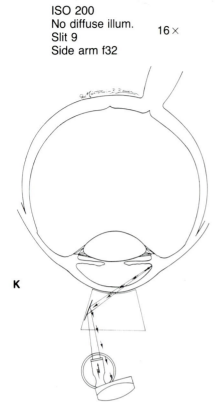

ISO 200
No diffuse illum.
Slit 9   16×
Side arm f32

K

ISO 400
No diffuse illum.
Slit 9   16-25×
Side arm f16

L

Fig 45-4 ■ K, Goniography. After placement on the eye, the goniolens is rotated to bring the desired mirror into position opposite the area to be examined or photographed. A slit beam of moderate width, made parallel with the angle, is usually used. The same basic technique is used for the study and documentation of peripheral vitreal and retinal conditions, through a well-dilated pupil.

Fig. 45-4 ■ L, Photography of the posterior pole through a fundus lens. A contact lens is placed on the eye, which permits a view of the fundus with the biomicroscope. With a narrow or moderate slit beam, the structures of the posterior fundus can be examined in minute detail. The slit illuminator must be placed in a relatively coaxial position with the biomicroscope; the larger the pupil, the better the opportunity for oblique sectioning.

Several photo slitlamps are available today. Desirable features include coaxial viewing (viewing and photography through the same lens system) and a flash source for both the slit and diffuse illuminators. Slitlamps not designed for photography may, on occasion, produce satisfactory photographs with the appropriate attachments. Of these attachments, electronic flash illumination is the most essential to provide the short exposures necessary to "freeze" eye movements and provide the correct color temperature of light for daylight film. Most tungsten bulbs used in slit-lamp biomicroscopes do not produce the exact color temperature required by available films. Another important attachment for a nonphotographic slitlamp is a diffuse illuminator to provide the overviews mentioned earlier.

Beyond the mastery of the mechanics of a photo slitlamp, the diligent practice of slit-lamp biomicroscopy is important to gain experience in disease entity recognition and light source manipulation to achieve maximum detail enhancement.

GONIOGRAPHY

Certain important structures of the anterior segment of the eye, such as the filtration angle, cannot be seen directly. To obtain a view of the angle, a gonioscopic lens (contact lens, some containing mirrors) is placed on the eye. Using

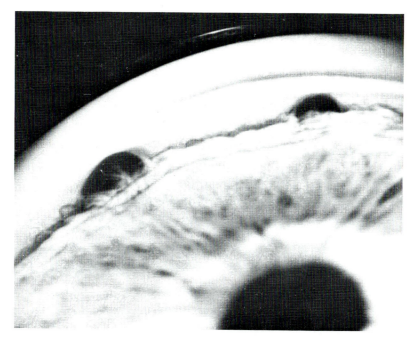

Fig 45-5 ■ A goniograph showing pigmented cysts in the angle.

a moderate beam from the slit-lamp illuminator and the standard exposure for that slit width, excellent photographs are obtainable (Fig. 45-5). Diffuse illumination is not used in goniography because of the increase in light scatter within the gonioscopic lens.

Before the placement of the lens on the eye, a topical application of proparacaine hydrochloride, 0.5%, is used to anesthetize the corneal surface. The concave, contact end of the lens is filled with a viscous solution of methyl cellulose to provide the necessary optical medium and a cushion between the lens and the eye. Once on the eye, the lens is rotated to place the desired mirror *opposite* the area to be viewed and photographed (see Fig. 45-4). (Goldmann and Haag-Streit lenses are available with three mirrors set at varying angles to facilitate a view of the angle, anterior vitreous, and retina.) Care should be taken to position the lens to eliminate reflections from its flat, rear surface. A three-mirror Haag-Streit lens with a special anti-reflection coating (similar to coatings on photographic lenses) is available from Ocular Instruments, Inc., Redmond, Washington. This coating, as on photographic lenses, permits a more efficient passage of light and contributes to the quality of the photographs. Another type of goniolens, the

Koeppe, not containing mirrors, is ideal when examining or photographing patients in the supine position or children under anesthesia. In this case, a hand-held fundus camera, such as a Kowa, is used instead of the slitlamp and produces excellent results.

When desired, slit-lamp photographs of the fundus can be obtained through the center of the Goldmann-type contact lenses (Figs. 45-6 and 45-7). The slit-lamp illuminator must be placed in a fairly coaxial position with the microscope to provide adequate illumination through the relatively small aperture of the pupil.

All contact lenses, especially those used for photography, must be carefully maintained. By rinsing with running warm water immediately after each use, the methyl cellulose is easily removed and will prevent the formation of a crusty residue, which can easily scratch the surface of the lens if one attempts to wipe it away. At this point, the lens should be placed in an appropriate solution for sterilization. After it is rinsed, the lens should be carefully dried with a soft cloth or tissue to remove droplets (which may leave precipitates behind), and stored in a sturdy, dust-free container.

To ensure the quality of goniographs, new

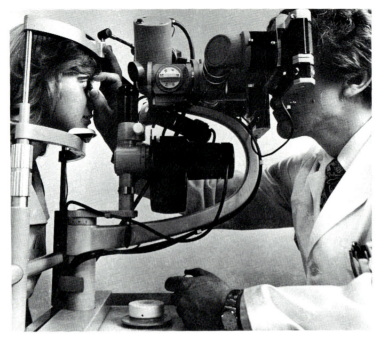

Fig 45-6 ■ The Zeiss Photo Slit Lamp in use with a contact lens to obtain the slit fundus photograph shown in Fig 45-7.

lenses should be purchased and their use restricted to photographic purposes only.

Goniography, like all slit-lamp biomicroscopy, should be practiced as often as possible under the direction of the ophthalmologist.

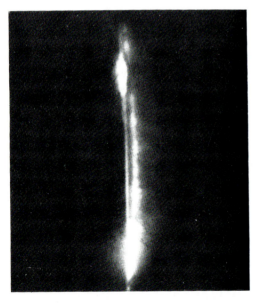

Fig 45-7 ■ The double slit indicates a shallow, serous detachment of the neurosensory retina.

ENDOTHELIAL SPECULAR PHOTOMICROGRAPHY

Specular micrography is a method of photographing and evaluating the endothelial surface of the cornea. As its name implies, specular micrography is based on a system of projecting a light onto the endothelial surface and photographing the information contained within the *specular reflection* of that light source. *Specular,* from the Latin *specularis,* means "mirrorlike." A specular reflection can be obtained from any relatively smooth surface. To be visible, however, it must be viewed at an angle from the perpendicular directly proportionate to the angle of incidence. The glossy surface of the endothelial cells will reflect a considerable amount of light, whereas their borders, not being smooth and flat, will absorb some of the light, providing a discrete "negative" outline for the cells (Fig. 45-8).

Though endothelial cells play a critical role in maintaining corneal clarity, they are of a finite number and do not regenerate. Several conditions, including age, can contribute to their compromise, and an assessment of their density and general health can be of significant value when considering such procedures as cataract extraction or intra-ocular lens implantation.

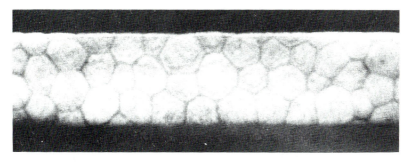

Fig 45-8 ■ Mosaic pattern of corneal endothelial cells.

Two types of endothelial microscopes, contact and noncontact, are available. The former requires direct contact with the patient's cornea. Before use of the contact microscope, the patient's cornea must be anesthetized, and extreme care should be taken during the procedure to avoid inadvertent, excessive pressure on the eye. To this end, the patient must be positioned in the head rest assembly so as to be able to maintain steady, gentle pressure against the chin rest and, most importantly, the forehead stabilizing bar. If the patient's forehead is allowed to move away from the camera, there is the risk of the patient moving abruptly forward and applying excessive pressure to the eye. The slight amount of pressure required for photography is no more than that needed to slightly flatten the cornea against the applanator surface. Contact microscopes help minimize the normal movements of the eye. Noncontact types may have variable magnification and may be extremely useful when direct contact with the patient's cornea is contraindicated.

CINEMATOGRAPHY AND VIDEO RECORDING

Both forms of motion recording have advantages and disadvantages. The foremost advantage of cinematography over video recording is its ability to produce finer detail, crucial if duplication for wide distribution is anticipated. The "original" film can be completely edited, then reproduced many times, either onto film or video cassettes, without an excessive loss of information and without a striking increase in contrast. Among the disadvantages of cinematography however, are the high cost of film and processing, the time required for processing,

and the time lost reshooting because of poor exposure or other technical problems.

Major advantages of video recording are the relatively low cost of tape and our ability to monitor and make immediate adjustments when necessary. Sound may be recorded simultaneously or narrated after the video portion has been recorded. Playback is instantaneous and duplication is simple and relatively inexpensive. Video's major disadvantage is its relatively poor resolution. An *edited master* is in fact a copy of the original, and subsequent copies tend to further increase in contrast with a proportionate degradation of image quality.

Requests for motion recording may be made for patient eye movements and intra-operative procedures. Extra-ocular motility studies are most easily recorded on videotape but can, of course, be recorded on motion picture film as well. Macro lenses are available for both television cameras and motion picture cameras, but standard lenses may be extended for close-up applications in the manner described under External Photography. The television camera should always be used with a monitor (built-in or accessory), and the motion picture camera should be of the reflex type to ensure correct framing and focus. When television is used to document a patient's eye movements, instructions to the patient can be recorded simultaneously with the video to positively identify the direction of gaze being attempted. If desired, the sound portion can be eliminated or recorded over at another time. Videotapes may be completely erased and reused.

For much of the intra-operative recording of surgical procedures today, both motion picture film and television cameras are mounted on the

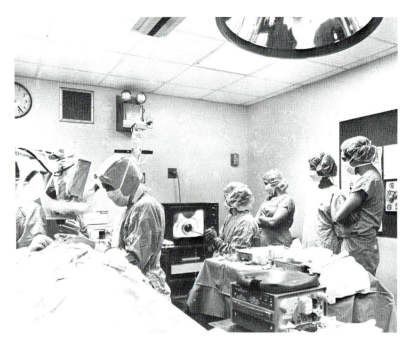

Fig 45-9 ■ Operating room personnel observe a surgical procedure on closed circuit television.

operating microscope and may be coaxial with the surgeon's view (necessary for documenting intra-ocular procedures such as vitrectomies, and so on).

A video system is generally left on for an entire procedure. When using a motion picture camera, however, the surgeon usually activates the system to document selected portions of the operation. A major limitation of microscope-mounted motion picture cameras is their limited film capacity. A video system can record almost indefinitely, and even while a completed tape is being replaced with a fresh one, monitor display of the procedure can usually continue. A major, obvious benefit is the teaching value of such a system, which allows a number of observers to benefit from the view normally seen only through the microscope oculars (Fig. 45-9).

For documenting procedures not requiring an operating microscope, a system as described for ocular motility may be used. A long focal length macro lens is recommended to provide a suitable magnification-to-working distance ratio. Regular lenses may also be used by extending with extension rings or spacers. The camera must be placed on a sturdy tripod of sufficient height to provide the desired angle of view. The photographer may have to be positioned on a short

stepladder to provide a comfortable stance.

Whereas the color temperature of light sources, such as the operating field lights, is of importance to both video and motion picture photography, it is much more important for the latter. The operating lights may be used with tungsten-type film, and the slight shift to the warm tones can be corrected, when desired, with the use of color correction filters.

In cinematography, titles may be superimposed over scenes by

1. shooting the scene
2. rewinding the film in the camera, and
3. re-exposing that section of film by photographing titles made of white or colored letters on a pure, nonreflective black background.

Only the letters are thus recorded, and the result will be letters superimposed over the scene previously photographed. Titles may be faded in by initially stopping the lens down completely, and as the camera is running, slowly (over a 1- to 2-second period) opening the lens to the f number required for correct exposure. The process is reversed to fade off the titles. Titles for videotapes are most easily done with the use of two cameras, one recording the scene and the other recording the title simultaneously onto the same tape. Titles can be prepared and faded on and off as with cinematography. Some video cameras have character generations built in, which can create titles electronically.

PROCESSING

Kodachrome film must be returned to a major processing plant for developing, but some films, such as Ektachrome, can be processed by local photofinishers with little delay. If local services are unavailable, special mailers may be purchased and the film may be sent for processing elsewhere.

Black-and-white processing, though much simpler, should be carried out in a suitably equipped darkroom. Fluorescein angiograms can be made into positive transparencies by "proof" printing onto 8″ × 10″ graphic arts film. After processing, the angiogram can be studied on a light table with a suitable magnifier. When desired, individual frames can be cut from the sheet, mounted into 2″ × 2″ mounts, and projected. Enlargements, or paper prints, can also be made from selected frames.

CATALOGING SLIDES

It is essential to establish an editing and filing system that will guarantee positive identification and ready retrieval of all patient photographs.

We have already mentioned the maintenance of the photographic log to include patient name, date of photography, medical identification number (when used), eye being photographed (OD/OS), types of photographs requested (stereo, slit-lamp, external, and so on), and provisional diagnosis. A separate log should be kept for each camera to avoid confusion. If a photograph is taken of the patient's data first, all photographs following the identification slide will belong to that patient. When processed slides are kept in order and consecutively numbered (as they are when processed by Kodak), they are simple to identify even when several rolls of film are involved.

Upon receipt from the processor, slides should be grouped by patient, sorted for quality, properly labeled with the patient's name and number and date of photography, and identified as a right or left eye. The inclusion of the patient's age and diagnosis is also recommended, since this will facilitate its use for future lecture or research purposes.

Stereo pairs may be mounted either in stereo glass mounts or simple aluminum frames covered by a protective plastic shield. Correct orientation of stereo pairs can easily be determined by using a light table and a stereo map viewer. When right and left sides are interposed, a reverse stereo effect will be seen. When mounting is not desired, the slides should be marked as being a stereo pair, left and right sides identified, and placed side by side into plastic loose-leaf sheets for filing.

Photographic records can be filed either alphabetically or by patient registration number. Perhaps the simplest method is to place 2″ × 2″ slides into readily available plastic loose-leaf pages accommodating 20 slides each. Specular micrography negatives should always be stored in sleeves designed for that purpose. Both the negatives and the prints may then be placed into an 8½″ × 11″ envelope and filed along with the slides, Polaroid prints, and so on in a letter-size drawer file. Pendaflex folders may be used in conjunction with Steelcase-type files.

Since most photographic files are eventually used for teaching or lecturing, it is wise to initiate at the onset a cross-indexing system to permit retrieval by disease entity. Although several methods have been tried and are in use across the United States, it is difficult to establish a card file system that is both complete and manageable. Whenever the resources are available, a computer program,* with its inherent ability to handle considerable data with speed and accuracy, should be established. At the minimum, the photographer should maintain a list of those patients and cases that the photographer or the ophthalmologist find to be of special interest or teaching value.

Whenever a photographic procedure is carried out, a notation indicating date, type and extent of photography, and signature or initials of the photographer should be entered into the patient's records.

SLIDES FOR PRESENTATION

Projection slides in the most commonly used 2″ × 2″ format can be made easily with a minimum of equipment.

*Montague PR, Weingeist TA, and Eichmann DA: Iowa data retrieval system: computers in ophthalmology, New York, IEEE, 1979. Also: University of Iowa Press, 1983.

A 35 mm single-lens reflex camera equipped with a close focusing lens (macro lens or normal lens extended with bellows or extension rings) can be mounted on an inexpensive copy device consisting of a platform, a movable (up and down) stand for the camera, and four lights for illumination. Printed materials can then be copied from a book or manuscript, or the desired information can be typed onto white paper with a carbon-ribbon typewriter. Capital letters and adequate spacing are helpful, and the number of lines should be restricted to 12 or less. To liven up the presentation, this information can be typed onto colored paper, or a color filter should be placed over the lens and exposed on color film. A new film from Polaroid (PolaBlue) is now available that will produce white (clear) letters on a blue background, and can be processed in 6 minutes in a desk-top processor.

Today, a number of programs are available for generating slides on a computer. They can be quite flexible and are fairly easy to learn. The actual slide of the computer-generated image is produced at a central station to which one is linked by a modem (a device that makes it possible for computers to communicate with each other over telephone lines). When a direct link is not possible, the electronic information can be stored on a disk and mailed to a central station for conversion into slides.

For projection, slides must be placed in the projector upside down. To simplify loading, the standard marking system should be used: the slide should be placed on a light table in its correct position and the lower left-hand corner of each slide should be marked with a red dot. (Self-adhering labels are not recommended since they may separate from the mount and cause the slide to jam.) The slides should be loaded with the red dot in the upper right-hand corner.

SUMMARY

In ophthalmology, a picture can truly be "worth a thousand words," and ophthalmic photography has indeed become an indispensable adjunct to the eye care profession.

To provide this vital service, the ophthalmic photographer must learn proven methods and stay abreast of new developments in technique and instrumentation. The success of each individual hinges primarily on his or her interest in photography, as well as in ophthalmology, along with a keen desire to excel in this challenging specialty.

SUPPLEMENTARY READINGS

Allansmith, MR: The eye and immunology, St Louis, 1982, The CV Mosby Co.

Allansmith, MR and Ross, RN: Immunology of the tear film. In Holly, FJ, editor: The preocular tear film in health, disease, and contact lens wear, Lubbock, Tex, 1986, Dry Eye Institute.

Allansmith, MR and Ross, RN: Ocular allergy and mast cell stabilizers, Surv Ophthalmol 30-229, 1986.

Allansmith, MR et al: Giant papillary conjunctivitis in contact lens wearers, Am J Ophthalmol 83:697-708, 1977.

Aquavella, JV: Hydrophilic bandages in chronic corneal edema, Medcom Special Studies, New York, 1973, Medcome Press.

Aquavella, JV and Rao, GN: Which lens: contact lenses currently available for extended wear in aphasia, Ophthalmology 87(2):151-154, 1980.

Aquavella, JV and Rao, GN: Contact lenses, JB Lippincott Co, Philadelphia, 1987.

Aquavella, JV et al: The effect of collagen bandage lens on corneal wound healing: a preliminary report, Ophthalmic Surgery, 18:8, 1987.

Bailey, NJ: The examination and verification of a contact lens, JAOA 30(8):557-560, 1959.

Bailey, NJ: Residual astigmatism with contact lenses. I. Incidence, Optom J Rev Optom 98(1):30-31, 1961.

Bailey, NJ: Residual astigmatism with contact lenses. II. Predictability, Optom J Rev Optom 98(2):40-45, 1961.

Bailey, NJ: Residual astigmatism with contact lenses. III. Possible sites, Optom J Rev Optom 98(3):31-32, 1961.

Bailey, NJ: Residual astigmatism with contact lenses. IV. Corrective techniques, Optom J Rev Optom 98(4):43-44, 1961.

Bailey, WR: Preservatives for contact lens solutions, Contact Lens Soc Am J 6(3):33-39, Oct 1972.

Baldone, J: Contact lenses in the aphakic child, Contact Lens Med Bull 3(2):25-27, April 1970.

Baum, JL: Therapeutic uses of soft contact lenses, Hosp Pract 8(8):89-95, Aug 1973.

Baum, J and Boruchoff, SA: Extended wear contact lenses and pseudomonal corneal ulcers, Am J Ophthalmol, 101:372-373, 1985.

Bayshore, CA: Astigmatic soft contact lenses: a report of 140 patients, Int Contact Lens Clin 4(1):56-59, Jan-Feb 1977.

Beier, CG: A review of the literature pertaining to monovision contact lens fitting of presbyopic patients: clinical considerations, Int Contact Lens Clin 4(2):49-56, March-April 1977.

Bier, N: The contour lens: a new form of corneal lens, JAOA 28(7):394-397, 1957.

Bier, N and Lowther, G: Contact lens correction, Sevenoaks, Kent, 1977, Butterworth & Co, Publishers.

Benjamin, WJ and Hill, RM: Ultra-thins and oxygen update, Contact Lens Forum, pp. 43-45, Jan 1979.

Bende, M and Pipkorn, U: Topical levocabastine, a selective H1 antagonist, in seasonal allergic rhinoconjunctivitis, Allergy 42:512-515, 1987.

Berger, RO and Streeten, B: Fungal growth in aphakic soft contact lenses, Am J Ophthalmol 91:630-633, 1981.

Bergmanson, JP and Chu, LW: Contact lens-induced corneal epithelial injury, Am J Optom Physiol Opt 59(6):500-506, June 1982.

Binder, PS and Worthen, DM: Clinical evaluation of continuous wear hydrophilic lenses, Am J Ophthalmol 83(4):549-553, April 1977.

Binder, PS: The physiological effects of extended wear soft contact lenses, Ophthalmology 87(8): Aug 1980.

Blanco, M: A method for detection of dissolved materials in hydrophilic lenses, Contacto 20(2):11-14, March 1976.

Boeder, P: Power and magnification properties of contact lenses, Arch Ophthalmol 19(1):54-67, 1938.

Bonnet, R and Cochet, P: New method of topographical ophthalmometry: its theoretical and clinical application, Am J Optom Arch Am Acad Optom 39(5):227-251, 1962.

Bowman, RW, Dougherty, JM, and McCulley, JP: Chronic blepharitis and dry eyes, Into Ophthalmol Clin 27:27, 1987.

Boyd, H: Analysis of 1000 consecutive contact lens cases, First Scientific Congress of the European Contact Lens Society of Ophthalmologists, London, June 1971.

Boyd, H: Complications of contact lens fitting, Contact Lens Med Bull 4:6-8, April-June 1971.

Boyd, H: The red eye syndrome, Contact Intraocular Lens Med J 1(1-2):198-199, Jan-June 1975.

Boyd, H, Gould, HL, and Sampson, WG: Enlightened concepts in contact lens medical practice, Highlights Ophthalmol 12(3):139-163, 1969.

Bronstein, L: Accuracy of fluorescein for determining corneal curvature, Contacto 3(6):170-171, 1959.

Brucker, D: The Hydrocurve lens, Contact Intraocular Lens Med J 1(3):13, July-Sept 1975.

Brungardt, TF: The optics of fluorescein patterns, JAOA 53(4):305-306, April 1982.

Burns, RP, Roberts, H, and Rich, LF: Effect of silicone contact lenses on corneal epithelium metabolism, Am J Ophthalmol 71(2):486, Feb 1971.

Buxton, JN and Locke, CR: A therapeutic evaluation of hydrophilic contact lenses, Am J Ophthalmol 12:532, 1971.

Caldwell, DR, Kastl, PR, Dabezies, OH, Miller, KR, and Hawk, TJ: The effect of long-term hard lens wear on corneal endothelium, Contact Intraocular Lens Med J 8(2):87-91, April-June 1982.

Callender, M and Egan, DJ: A clinical evaluation of the Weicon-T and Durasoft-TT toric soft contact lenses, Int Contact Lens Clin 5(5):209-221, Sept-Oct 1978.

Carmichael, C: Safety and efficacy of a new enzyme cleaner, Int Contact Lens Clin 10(5):286, 1983.

Carney, LG and Hill RM: Human tear pH diurnal variations, Arch Ophthalmol 94:821, 1976.

Carter, DB and Brucker, D: Hydrophilic contact lenses for aphakia, Am J Optom Physiol Opt 50(4):316-319, 1973.

Cavanagh, HD, Bodner, BI, and Wilson, LA: Extended wear hydrogel lenses, Ophthalmology 87(9):871, Sept 1980.

Cedarstaff, TH and Tomlinson, A: Human tear volume, quality, and evaporation as a comparison of Schirmer, tear break-up time, and resistance hygrometry techniques. Ophthal Physiol Opt 3:239, 1983.

Chaston, J and Fatt, L: Corneal oxygen uptake under a soft contact lens in phakic and aphakic eyes, Invest Ophthalmol Vis Sci 23(2):234-239, Aug 1982.

Clinch, TE, Benedetto, DA, Felberg, NT, and Laibson, PR: Schirmer's test: a closer look. Arch Ophthalmol 101:1383, 1983.

Collins, M and Carney, LG: Patient compliance and its influence on contact lens wearing problems, Am J Optom Physiol Opt 63:952-956, 1986.

Cope, C, Dilly, PN, Kaura, R, and Tiffany, JM: Wettability of the corneal epithelium: a reappraisal, Curr Eye Res 5:777, 1986.

Cotter, J: Soft contact lens testing on fresh water scuba divers, Contact Intraocular Lens Med J 7(4):323-326, Oct-Dec 1981.

Coward, BD, Neumann, R, and Callender, M: Solution intolerance among users of four chemical soft lens care regimens, Am J Optom Physiol Opt 61:523-527, 1984.

Couzi, J: Ocular hypertension with contact lenses, Contactologia 3(3):120-124, Aug 1981.

Cureton, GL: Clinical experience with soft lens solutions, Contacto 20(2):25-29, March 1976.

Dabezies, OH: Accessory contact lens solutions. In New Orleans Academy of Ophthalmology: Symposium on contact lenses, St Louis, 1973, The CV Mosby Co.

Dabezies, OH: Soft contact lens hygiene, Contact Intraocular Lens Med J 1(1-2):103-108, Jan-June 1975.

Dabezies, OH: Contact lenses: CLAO guide to basic sciences, San Diego, 1984, Grune & Stratton.

Dart, JK, et al: Perennial allergic conjunctivitis: definition, clinical characteristics, and prevalence. A comparison with seasonal allergic conjunctivitis, Trans Ophthalmol Soc UK 105:513-520, 1986.

Davis, HE: Technique in the fitting of bifocal contact lenses, Contacto 3:70, 1959.

De la Iglesia, FA, et al: Evaluation of hydrophilic contact lens effects on rabbit eyes, Contacto 20(2):18-24, March 1976.

DeCarle, J: Further developments of bifocal contact lenses, Contacto 3:5, 1959.

DeCarle, J: Further developments of bifocal contact lenses, Contacto 4:185, 1960.

DeDonato, LM: Changes in the hydration of hydrogel contact lenses with wear, Am J Optom Physiol Opt 59(3):213-214, March 1982.

D'Halnens, J: Soft lenses, Contact Lens Med Bull 7(1-2):10, Jan-June 1976.

Dilly, PN: Contributions of the epithelium to the stability of the tear film. Tran Ophthalmol Soc UK 104:381, 1985.

Dixon, JM: Emotional symptoms in contact lens patients, Contact Intraocular Lens Med J 7(4):327-330, Oct-Dec 1981.

Dixon, JM: Ocular changes due to contact lenses, Am J Ophthalmol 58(3):424-441, 1964.

Dixon, JM et al: Complications associated with the wearing of contact lenses, JAMA 195:901, 1966.

Dixon, JM and Lawaczeck, E: Corneal dimples and bubbles under corneal contact lenses, Am J Ophthalmol 54(5):827-831, 1962.

Dixon, JM and Lawaczeck, E: A mechanism of glare due to corneal lenses, Am J Ophthalmol 54(6):1135-1137, 1962.

Dixon, WS, and others: Unilateral aphakia and corneal contact lenses, Can J Ophthalmol 8:97-105, 1973.

Doane, MG: Tear spreading, turnover, and drainage. In Holly, FJ (ed): The preocular tear film in health, disease and contact lens wear. Lubbock, Texas, Dry Eye Institute, 1986.

Dohlman, CH: Complications in therapeutic soft lens

wear, Trans Am Acad Ophthalmol Otolaryngol 78:399, 1974.

Donshik, P, et al: Treatment of contact lens-induced giant papillary conjunctivitis, CLAO J 10:346, 1984.

Donshik, P, et al: Disposable hydrogel contact lenses for extended wear, CLAO J 14:4, 1988.

Doughman, DJ, et al: The nature of "spots" on soft lenses, Ann Ophthalmol 7:345, 1975.

Dyer, JA: A practical nomogram for fitting corneal contact lenses, Contact Lens Med Bull 1(4):8-11, 1968.

Dyer, JA: XIIIth Conrad Berens memorial lecture: corneal contact lenses in perspective: 1948-1981, Contact Intraocular Lens Med J 8(1):3-8, Jan-March 1982.

Dyer, JA and Ogle, EW: Correction of unilateral aphakia with contact lenses, Am J Ophthalmol 50(1):11-17, 1960.

Editorial: The adjustment to aphakia, Am J Ophthalmol 35:118, 1955.

Ehrich, W and Epstein, D: Colour atlas of contact lenses, New York, 1983, Thyme Medical Publishers Inc.

Elmstrom, GP: The legal aspects of contact lens practice, JAOA 35(9):775-777, 1964.

Enriquez, AS and Korb, DR: Meibomian glands and contact lens wear, Br J Ophthalmol 65:108, 1981.

Fatt, I and Chaston, J: Measurement of oxygen transmissibility and permeability of hydrogel lenses and materials, Int Contact Lens Clin 9(2):76-88, March-April 1982.

Fatt, I and Chaston, J: Relation of oxygen transmissibility to oxygen tension or EOP under the lens, Int Contact Lens Clin 9(2):119-120, March-April 1982.

Feldman, GL, et al: Fitting characteristics and gas permeability of thin hydrogel lenses, Contact Lens J 10(3):13-20, Dec 1976.

Feldman, F, and Wood, MM: Evaluation of the Schirmer tear test, Can J Ophthalmol 14:257, 1979.

Fowler, SA and Allansmith, MR: Evolution of soft contact lens coating, Arch Ophthalmol 98:95-99, Jan 1980.

Fowler, S and Allansmith, M: The effect of cleaning soft contact lenses: a scanning electron microscopic study, Arch Ophthalmol 99:1382, 1984.

Fowler, S and Allansmith, M: Removal of soft contact lens deposits with surfactant-polymeric bead cleaner, CLAO J 10:229, 1984.

Fowler, S, et al: Surface deposits on worn hard contact lenses, Arc Ophthalmol 102:757, 1984.

Fraunfelder, F: Which type of saline solution for soft contact lenses is best? Am J Ophthalmol 91:540, 1981.

Garcia, GE: Continuous wear of gas permeable contact lens in aphakia, Contact Intraocular Lens Med J 2(1):29-34, Jan-March 1976.

Gasset, AR and Kaufman, HE: Bandage lenses in the treatment of bullous keratopathy, Am J Ophthalmol 72:36, 1971.

Gasset, AR and Kaufman HE: Soft contact lens, St Louis, 1972, The CV Mosby Co.

Ghormley, R: Hydrogen peroxide: the hydrogel disinfection system of the future? I. Int Contact Lens Clin 11(11):714, 1984.

Girard, LJ, Soper, JW, and Sampson, WG: Corneal contact lens, St Louis, 1970, The CV Mosby Co.

Goldberg, JB: Must the gas go through? Optom Weekly 66(34):15, Oct 2, 1975.

Goldberg, JB: The conventional corneal lens: safety and efficiency, Optom Weekly 67(6):135-138, Feb 5, 1976.

Gordon, S: An evaluation of small, thin contact lenses, Optom Weekly 55(5):21-25, 1964.

Gordon, S: Designing a minimum-thickness hard contact lens, Contact Lens Forum, pp. 41-53, June 1976.

Grant, SC and May, CH: Orthokeratology—the control of refractive errors through contact lenses, Optician 163:8-11, 1972.

Grayson, M: Diseases of the cornea, ed 2, St Louis, 1983, The CV Mosby Co.

Green, WR: An embedded ("lost") contact lens, Arch Ophthalmol 69(1):23-24, 1963.

Greenbaum, J, et al: Sodium cromoglycate in ragweed-allergic conjunctivitis, J Allergy Clin Immunol 59:437-439, 1977.

Gregg, BR: Aspheric contact lenses: development and doubt, Contact Lens 2(5):20-24, 31, 1969.

Grosvenor, T: Clinical use of the keratometer in evaluating corneal contour, JAOA 38(5):237-246, 1961.

Grosvenor, T: Optical principles of soft contact lenses, Optom Weekly 67(3):29-31 Jan 15, 1976.

Gruber, E: Six years experience with Soflens, Contact Intraocular Lens Med J 1(2):70-82, Jan-June 1975.

Gruber, E: An unusual case of keratitis, Contact Lens Forum 9(10):68, 1984.

Gruber, E: The disposable contact lens: a new concept in extended wear, CLAO J Oct 14:4, 195-198, 1988.

Guillon, JP and Guillon, M: Tear film examination with a contact lens patient, Contax May:14, 1988.

Gundel, RE: Determining appropriate cylinder correction with soft toric lenses, J Am Optom Assoc 59:3, March 1988.

Hall, KC: A special contact lens for complete ptosis, JAOA 30(2):121-123, 1958.

Hall, NC and Krezanoski, JZ: Antimicrobial synergism in a contact lens soaking solution, N Engl J Optom 13(9):229-233, 1963.

Hamano, H: The change of precorneal tear film by the application of contact lenses, Contact Intraocular Lens Med J 7(3):205-209, July-Sept 1981.

Hamano, H, et al: A new method of measuring tears, Contact Lens Assoc Ophthalmol J 9:281, 1983.

Hamano, H and Kaufman, HE: The physiology of the cornea and contact lens application, New York, 1987, Churchill Livingstone.

Hamano, H and Kaufman, HE: Physiology of the cornea and contact lens applications, New York, 1987, Churchill Livingstone.

Hamano, H and Kawabe, H: Standardization of soft contact lenses, Contacto 20(4):14-19, July 1976.

Hamano, H and Kawabe, H: Variation of base curve of soft lens during wearing, Contacto 22:10-14, Jan 1978.

Hamano, H, et al: Statistical trends of wearers of contact lenses, Contact Intraocular Lens Med J 8(1):29-37, Jan-March 1982.

Harris, MG, Harris, KL, and Ruddell, D: Rotation of lathe-cut hydrogel lenses on the eye, Am J Optom Physiol Opt 53(1):20-26, Jan 1976.

Harris, MJ, et al: Flexure and residual astigmatism with Paraperm 02 and Boston II lenses on toric cornea, Am J Optom Physiol Opt, April 1987, 64:4, 269-273.

Harrison, DP: Contact lens wear problems: implications of penicillin allergy, diabetic relatives, and use of birth control pills, Am J Optom Physiol Opt 61:674-678, 1984.

Harrison, K and Stein, HA: Nomogram for fitting fluorosilicone acrylate contact lenses, CLAO J 14:3, July 1988.

Hart DE, et al: Spoilage of hydrogel contact lenses by lipid deposits, Ophthalmology 94:13-15, 1987.

Hartstein, J: Astigmatism induced by corneal contact lenses. In Becker, B and Drews, RC: Current concepts in ophthalmology, vol 1, St Louis, 1967, The CV Mosby Co.

Hartstein, J: Practical points in contact lens fitting, Eye Ear Nose Throat Mon 46(8):1004-1005, 1967.

Hartstein, J: Basics of contact lenses, ed 3, 1979, American Academy of Ophthalmology.

Hartstein, J: Extended wear contact lenses for aphakia and myopia, St Louis, The CV Mosby Co, 1982.

Helers, N: The precorneal tear film. Biomicroscopical, histological, and chemical investigations, Acta Ophthalmol Suppl 81:5, 1965.

Highman, VN: High water content soft contact lenses for continuous wear, Contact Lens J 5(5):1976.

Hill, JF: Variation in refractive error and corneal curvature after wearing hydrophilic contact lenses, JAOA 3(46):290-294, 1975.

Hill, RM: Extended wear: closing the gap. Contact Lens Forum 4(12):67-69, Dec 1979.

Hill, RM and Carney, LG: Extended wear systems, Contact Lens Forum 1(6):29-31, Oct 1976.

Hind, HW and Szekely, IJ: Wetting and hydration of contact lenses, Contacto 3(3):65-68, 1959.

Holden, BA: The principles and practice of correcting astigmatism with soft contact lenses, Aust J Optom 58:279-299, 1975.

Holly, FJ: Formation and rupture of the tear film, Exp Eye Res 15:515, 1973.

Holly, FJ: Tear film physiology and contact lens wear. II. Contact lens-tear film interaction, Am J Optom Physiol Opt 58:331, 1981.

Holly, FJ: Tear film formation and rupture: an update. In Holly, FJ, editor: The preocular tear film in health, disease and contact lens wear. Lubbock, Texas, 1986, Dry Eye Institute.

Holly, FJ and Lemp, MA: Tear physiology and dry eyes, Surv Ophthalmol 22(2):69-87 Sept-Oct, 1977.

Holly, FJ and Refojo, MF: Oxygen permeability of hydrogel contact lenses, JAOA 43:1173-1178, 1972.

Holly, FJ and Refojo, MF: Wettability of hydrogels, J Biomed Mater Res 9:315-326, 1975.

Houde, WL and Rubin ML: Extended wear lenses: an update, Surv Ophthalmol 26(2):103-105, Sept-Oct 1981.

Clinics of North America, Problems with contact lenses, Philadelphia, 1988, WB Saunders Co.

Jay, JL: Clinical features and diagnosis of adult atopic keratoconjunctivitis and the effect of treatment with sodium cromoglycate, Br J Ophthalmol 65:335-340, 1981.

Johnson, DG: Soft hydrophilic contact lenses, Can J Ophthalmol 6:342, 1971.

Johnson, DG: Keratoconjunctivitis associated with wearing hydrophilic contact lenses, Can J Ophthalmol 8:92,1973.

Josephson, JE: Hydrogen lens wearer utilizing preserved solutions, J Am Optom Assoc 49:280, 1978.

Josephson, JE: Appearance of the preocular tear film lipid layer, Am J Optom Physiol Opt 60(11):883, Nov 1983.

Josephson, JE and Caffery, BE: Hydrogel lens solutions, Int Ophthalmol Clin 21:163, 1981.

Josephson, JE, Caffery, BE, and Pope, CA: Clinical experience with tinted hydrogel lenses, Can J Optom 44(3):21, 1983.

Josephson, JE and Caffery, BE: Corneal staining after instillation of topical anesthetic (SSII). Invest Opthahlmol Vis Sci 29:1096, 1987.

Josephson, JE, et al: Hydrocurve II bifocal contact lenses: a clinical perspective, CLAO J 14:2, 1988.

Josephson, JE: Appearance of the preocular tear film, Am J Optom Physiol Opt 60:883, 1983.

Junzo, A and Manabu, A, editors: Menicon hard and soft contact lenses, Tokyo, 1977, Tokyo Contact Lens Co.

Kaetting, RA and Boyd, WS: Surface artifacts found on unboiled hydrophilic lenses, Int Contact Lens Clin 3(4):37-41, Dec 1976.

Kamiki, T and Kikkawa, Y: Ozone sterilization technique of hydrophilic contact lenses, Contacto 20(3):16-18, May 1976.

Kaufman, HE: Problems associated with prolonged

wear soft contact lenses, Ophthalmology 86:411-417, March 1979.

Keates, RH and Falkenstein, S: Keratoplasty in keratoconus, Am J Ophthalmol 74(3):442-444, 1972.

Kenyon, E, Polse, KA, and Mandell, RB: Rigid contact lens adherence: incidence, severity and recovery, J Am Optom Assoc 59:168-74, 1988.

Kenyon, E, Polse, KA, and O'Neil, M: Ocular response to extended-wear hard gas-permeable lenses, CLAO J 11:2, April 1985.

Kerns, RL: Contact lens control of myopia, Am J Optom Physiol Opt 58(7):541-545, July 1981.

Kersley, HJ: Soft contact lenses in aphakia, Contact Lens J 5(8):29-30, 1977.

Kimura, SJ: Fluorescein paper, Am J Ophthalmol 34(3):446-447, 1951.

Kjellman, NI and Anderson, B: Terfenadine reduces skin and conjunctival reactivity in grass pollen allergic children, Clin Allergy 16:441-449, 1986.

Kline, M: The lacrimal strip and the preocular tear film in cases of Sjogren's syndrome, Br J Ophthalmol 33:387, 1949.

Kleist, F: Appearance and nature of hydrophilic contact lens deposits, Int Contact Lens Clin 6(3):120-130, May-June 1979.

Koetting, RA, Castellano, CF, and Wartman, R: Patient compliance with new instructions, Contact Lens Spectrum, 23-30, Nov 1986.

Koliopoulos, J and Tragakis, M: Visual correction of keratoconus with soft contact lenses, Ann Ophthalmol 13(7):835-837, July 1981.

Korb, DR: Edematous corneal formation, JAOA 44(3):March 1973.

Korb, DR and Korb, JE: A new concept in contact lens design. I and II, JAOA 41(12):1023-1032, 1970.

Korb, DR, Finnemore, VM, and Herman, JP: Apical changes and scarring in keratoconus as related to contact lens fitting techniques, JAOA 53(3):199-205, March 1982.

Korb, DR and Herman, JP: Corneal staining subsequent to sequential fluorescein instillations, J Am Optom Assoc 50:361, 1979.

Kray ST, et al: Cromolyn sodium in seasonal allergic conjunctivitis, J Allergy Clin Immunol 76:623-627, 1985.

Krezanoski, J: The significance of cleaning hydrophilic contact lenses, JAOA 43:305, 1972.

Krezanoski, J: Where are we in the developments of pharmaceutical products for soft (hydrophilic) lenses? Contacto 20(1):12-16, Jan 1976.

Kurihashi, K: Fine cotton thread method of lacrimation. Am J Ophthalmol 83:151, 1977.

Lambert, SR and Klyce, SD: The origins of soft contact lens fit, Ophthalmology 91(1):51-56, Jan 1981.

Lamp, M, Goldberg, M, and Roddy, M: The effect of tear substitutes on tear film break up time, Invest Med 14(3):255, March 1975.

Lebow, KA: The clinical evaluation of the Boston Equalens for cosmetic extended wear, Contact Lens spectrum, August 1987.

Lee, R: Contact lens handbook, Philadelphia, 1986, WB Saunders Co.

Leibowitz, HM and Rosenthal, P: Hydrophilic contact lenses in corneal diseases, Arch Ophthalmol 85:163, 1971.

Leibowitz, H and Kapino, D: Experiences with a new detergent lid scrub in the management of chronic blepharitis, Arch Ophth 106:719, June 1988.

Leibowitz, HM: Continuous wear of hydrophilic contact lenses, Arch Ophthalmol 89:306, 1973.

Lembach, RG, McLaughlin, R, and Barr, JT: Crazing in a rigid gas-permeable contact lens, CLAO J 14:1, Jan 1988.

Lemp, MA, Dohlman, CH, and Holly, FT: Corneal desiccation despite normal tear volume, Ann Ophthalmol 2:258, 1970.

Lemp, MA, Holly, FJ, and Dohlman, CH: Corneal desiccation despite normal tear volume, Ann Ophthalmol 2(3):258-261, 1970.

Lemp, MA, et al: The precorneal tear film. I. Factors in spreading and maintaining a continuous tear film over the corneal surface, Arch Ophthalmol 83:89, 1970.

Lemp, MA, et al: The preocular tear film. I. Factors in spreading and maintaining a continuous tear film over the corneal surface. Arch Ophthalmol 2:258, 1970.

Lenz, MA and Hammil, RH: Factors affecting tear film breakup in normal eyes, Arch Ophthalmol 89:103, 1973.

Lester, RW: Fluorescein and contact lenses, Contacto 2(4):91, 1958.

Levinson, A and Weissman, B: An analysis of the general fitting of hydrophilic contact lenses in Israel, Int Contact Lens Clin 3(4):64-70, Nov-Dec 1976.

Levy, B: Rigid gas-permeable lenses for extended wear: a 1-year clinical evaluation, Am J Optom Physiol Opt 62:889-94, 1985.

Lippman, JI: Gas-permeable contact lenses: an overview, Contact Intraocular Med J 7(1):15, Jan-March 1981.

Lowther, G: Caring for hard GP lenses, Int Contact Lens Clin 11(2):75, 1984.

Lowther, G: Disinfection of extended-wear lenses, Int Contact Lens Clin 11(1):14, 1984.

Mandell, R: Is there an angle to wetting? Contact Lens Forum 9(8):45, 1984.

Marcus, W, et al: Safe disinfection of contact lenses after contamination with HTLV-III, Ophthalmology 93:771-774, 1986.

Mackie, IA: Localised corneal drying in association with dellen, pterygia, and related lesions, Trans Ophthalmol Soc UK 91:129, 1972.

Mackie, IA and Seal DV: The questionably dry eye, Br J Ophthalmol 65:2 1981.

Mandell, RB: Corneal oxygen need and gas permeable contact lenses, JAOA 53(3):211-214, March 1982.

Mandell, RB: Keratopography, Encyclopedia Contact Lens Pract 3:12-51, 1962.

Mandell, RB, editor: International Contact Lens Clinics, Chicago, 1974, Professional Press.

Mandell, RB: Contact lens practice, ed 3, Springfield, Ill, 1981, Charles C Thomas, Publisher.

Mandell, RB and Kang, L: Rigid contact lens area and corneal oxygenation, Am J Optom Physiol Opt, 65:5 387-394, 1988.

McDonald, JE: Surface phenomena of tear films. Trans Am Ophthalmol Soc 6:905, 1968.

McGill, J, et al: Tear film changes in health and dry eye conditions, Trans Opthalmol Soc UK 103:313, 1983.

McMonnies, CW and Hoe, A: Marginal dry eye diagnosis: history versus biomicroscopy. In Holly, FJ (ed): The preocular tear film in health, disease and contact lens wear, Lubbock, Texas, Dry Eye Institute, 1986.

Meisler, DM, et al: Cromoly treatment of giant papillary conjunctivitis, Arch Ophthalmology, 100:1608-1610, 1987.

Mengher, LS, et al: Effective fluorescein instillation on the pre-corneal tear film stability, Curr Eye Res 4:9, 1985.

Mengher, LS, et al: Non-invasive assessment of tear film stability. In Holly, FJ (ed): The preocular tear film in health, disease and contact lens wear, Lubbock, Texas, Dry Eye Institute, 1986.

Meschel, LG: Second generation soft contact lenses, Contact Intraocular Lens Med J 2(3):26-39, July-Sept 1976.

Miller, D: An analysis of the physical forces applied to a corneal contact lens, Arch Ophthalmol 70(6):823-829, 1963.

Mitra, S and Lamberts, DW: Contact sensitivity in soft lens wearers, Contact Intraocular Lens Med J 7(4):315-322, Oct-Dec 1981.

Mishima, S and Maurice, DM: Oily layer of the tear film: an evaporation from corneal surface, Exp Eye Res 1:39, 1961.

Mobilia, EF, Yamamoto, GK, and Dohlman, CH: Cornea wrinkling induced by ultra-thin soft contact lenses, Ann Ophthalmol 12(4):371-375, April 1980.

Molinari, JF: The clinical assessment of giant papillary conjunctivitis, Am J Optom Physiol Opt 58(10):886-891, Oct 1981.

Mondino, BJ, Salamon, SM, and Zaidman, GW: Allergic and toxic reactions in soft contact lens wearers, Surv Ophthalmol 26(6):337-343, May-June 1982.

Morgan, JF: Induced corneal astigmatism with hydrophilic contact lenses, Can J Ophthalmol 10:207-213, 1975.

Morrison, R: Small thin contact lens use, Optom Weekly 54(18):853-855, 1963.

Norn, MS: Lacrimal apparatus test, ACTA Ophthalmol 43:557, 1965.

Norn, MS: Desiccation of the precorneal film, Acta Ophthalmol 47:865, 1968.

Norn, MS: Vital staining of the cornea and conjunctiva, Acta Ophthalmol Suppl 113:66, 1972.

Norn, MS: Studies of surface phenomenon in external eye: methods of examination, ed 2, Copenhagen, 1983, Scriptor.

Norn, MS: The tear film break-up time: a review. In Holly, FJ, editor: The preocular tear film in health, disease and contact lens wear. Lubbock, Tex, 1986, Dry Eye Institute.

Obean, MF and Winter, FC: Contact lens storage, Am J Ophthalmol 57(3):441-443, 1964.

Occhipindi, JR, et al: Fluorophotometric measurement of human tear turn-over rate, Curr Eye Res 7(1):995, 1988.

Patel, S, et al: Effects of fluorescein on tear break-up time and on tear fitting time, Am J Optom Physiol Opt 62:188, 1985.

Pecoud, A, Zuber, P, and Kolly, M: Effect of a new selective H_1 receptor antagonist (levocabastine) in a nasal and conjunctival provocation test, Int Arch Allergy Appl Immunol 82:541-543, 1987.

Penley, C, et al: Efficacy of hydrogen peroxide disinfection systems for soft contact lenses contaminated with fungi, CLAO J 11:65, 1985.

Pinkers, A, et al: Contact-lens-induced pseudodystrophy of the cornea, Documenta Ophthalmologica 65:433-437, 1987.

Polse, HA, Sarver, MD, and Harris, MG: Corneal effects of high plus hydrogel lenses, Am J Optom Physiol Opt 55:234-237, 1978.

Poster, MG; Hydro-dynamics of corneal contact lenses, Am J Optom Arch Am Acad Optom 41(7):422-425, 1964.

Price, MJ, et al: Tarsal conjunctival appearance in contact lens wearers, Contact Intraocular Lens Med J 8(1):1-22, Jan-March 1982.

Refojo, MF: A critical review of properties and applications of soft hydrogel contact lenses, Surv Ophthalmol 16:233,1972.

Refojo, MF: Materials in bandage lenses, Contact Intraocular Med J 5(1):34-44, Jan-March 1979.

Refojo, MF and Holly, FJ: Tear protein adsorption on hydrogels: a possible cause of contact lens allergy, Contact Intraocular Lens Med J 3(1):23-35, Jan-March 1977.

Rietschel, RL and Wilson, LA: Ocular inflammation in patients using soft contact lenses, Arch Dermatol 118(3):147-149, March 1982.

Rocher, P and Francois, J: Choice of total diameter of a contact lens, Contacto 12(2):30-35,1968.

Rosenthal, JW: Clinical pathology in contact lenses. In Raiford, M editor: Contact lens management, Boston, 1962, Little, Brown & Co.

Rosenthal, P: Corneal contact lenses: large or small, Arch Ophthalmol 76:631-632, 1966.

Ruben, M: The fitting of corneal contact lenses, Trans Ophthalmol Soc UK 87:661, 1967.

Ruben, M, editor: Soft contact lenses: clinical and applied technology, London, 1978, Bailliere Tindall Pubs. (New York, Wiley Medical Publications).

Ruben, R, Tripathi, C, and Winder, AF: Calcium deposits as a cause of spoilation of hydrophilic contact lenses, Br J Ophthalmol 59:141-148, 1975.

Sampson, WG: The properties of ophthalmic prisms and their application in corneal contact lenses. Presented at First Annual Ophthalmology Alumni Meeting, Houston, Texas, April 1964.

Sampson, WG: Contact lenses and the AC/A ratio: applications in accommodative esotropia, Contact Lens Med Bull 2(3):9-15, 1969.

Sampson, WG: Curvature irregularity and its dioptric effect on corneal contact lenses, Contact Lens Med Bull 1(1-2):4-7, Jan-March 1968.

Sampson, WG: Correction of refractive errors: effect on accommodation and convergence, Trans Am Acad Ophthalmol Otolaryngol 75(1):124-132, 1971.

Sampson, WG, Soper, JW, and Girard, LJ: Topographical keratometer and contact lenses, Trans Am Ophthalmol Otolaryngol 69:959-969, 1965.

Santos, S: Cystic formation in the corneal epithelium during extended-wear contact lenses, Int Contact Lens Clin, 10(3):128-146, 1983.

Schuller, WO, Young, WH, and Hill, RM: Clinical measurements of the tears: viscosity, J Am Optom Assoc 43:135,1972.

Sclossman, A: The ophthalmological advanced fitting contact lens symposium. Part 2, Eye Ear Nose Throat Mon 45(1):94, 118, 1966.

Seal, DV and Macie, IA: The questionably dry eye as a clinical and biochemical entity. In Holly, FJ (ed): The preocular tear film in health, disease, contact lens wear, Lubbock, Texas, Dry Eye Institute, 1986.

Shaw, EL: Diagrams and pathophysiology of keratoconus, Contact Lens Med Bull 7(3):56, July-Sept 1974.

Shivitz, IA: Optical correction of postoperative radial keratotomy patients with contact lenses, CLAO J 12(1):59-62, 1986.

Sibley, MJ: Tailoring solutions for new lens material, Contacto 20(5):32-33, Sept 1976.

Simon-Licht, IF and Dieges, PH: A double-blind clinical trial with cromoglycate eye drops in patients with atopic conjunctivitis, Ann Allergy 49:220-224, 1982.

Slatt, BJ and Stein, HA: Why wear glasses if you want contacts? Richmond Hill, Ontario, 1972, Simon & Schuster of Canada Ltd.

Sloan, DP: A report on continuous contact lens wearing, Contacto 4(4):117-122, 1960.

Smelser, GK: Relation of factors involved in maintenance of optical properties of cornea to contact lens wear, Arch Ophthalmol 47:32, 1952.

Smelser, GK and Chen, DK: Physiological changes in cornea induced by contact lenses, Arch Ophthalmol 53(5):676-679, 1955.

Snyder DA, Litinsky, SM, and Gelender, H: Hypopyon iridocyclitis associated wth extended wear soft contact lenses, Am J Ophthalmol 93(4):519-520, April 1982.

Soft lens care: scientific and clinical aspects (Roundtable discussion), PanAmerican Congress of Ophthalmology, April 23, 1975.

Soper, JW: A new lens for keratoconus. Presented to the annual convention of the Contact Lens Society of America, Las Vegas, 1969.

Soper, JW, editor: Contact lenses: advances in design, fitting, application, New York, 1974, Stratton Intercontinental Medical Book Corp.

Soper, JW: Fitting keratoconus with piggy-back and Saturn II lenses, Contact Lens Forum, 11:25-30, 1986.

Stehr-Green, JK, et al: Acanthamoeba keratitis in soft contact lens wearers: a case-control study, JAMA 258(1):57-60, 1987.

Spring, T: Corneal endothelium: the effects of contact lenses and keratoconus, Contact Intraocular Lens Med J 8(1):9-11, Jan-March 1982.

Stark, WJ and Martin, NF: Extended-wear contact lenses for myopic correction, Arch Ophthalmol 99(11):1963-1966, Nov 1981.

Stark, WJ, et al: Extended-wear contact lens and intraocular lenses for aphakic correction, Am J Ophthalmol 88(3 Pt 2):535-542, 1979.

Steele, E: The fitting of aspheric corneal contact lenses, Contacto 13(4):5-57, 1969.

Stein, HA: Therapeutic uses of soft lenses, Contact Lens J 10(3):25-28, Dec 1976.

Stein, HA: Aphakia—selection of patients for contact lenses, intraocular lenses or spectacles: review of 1,000 cataract operations, Contact Intraocular Lens Med J 7(3):210-218, July-Sept 1981.

Stein, HA: Gas-permeable hard lenses, CLAO J, 10:3, July 1984; 10:7, April 1985.

Stein, HA: Correction of presbyopia with contact lenses, CLAO J, 11:3, July 1985.

Stein, HA: Where have contact lenses gone? Cataract, Int J of Cataract Surg, Oct, 1985.

Stein, HA: Canadian experience with soft and hard extended-wear contact lenses, Contactologia, Vol 1:8, 1986.

Stein, HA: Innovations in rigid gas-permeable and soft contact lenses, Highlights of Ophthalmol, 14:9, 1986.

Stein, HA: Specialty Contact Lenses, Conrad Berens Memorial Lecture, CLAO J, 13:5, Sept 1987.

Stein, HA: Basic Sciences 2, American Academy of Ophthalmology, Optics Refraction & Contact Lenses, January 1987.

Stein, HA, et al: Multicentre comparative clinical evaluation of daily care solutions for rigid gas permeable contact lenses, Can J Ophthalmol 19:4, 1984.

Stein, H and Harrison, K: The safety and effectiveness of Polyclens: an all-purpose cleaner for hydrophilic soft contact lenses, CLAO J 9:39, 1983.

Stein, H and Meltzer, D: Current management of presbyopia, Am Acad Ophthalmol, 6:2, 1987.

Stein, HA and Slatt, BJ: Clinical impressions of hydrophilic lenses, Can J Ophthalmol 8:83, 1973.

Stein, HA and Slatt, BJ: Contact lenses after cataract surgery, Can J Ophthalmol 9(1):79-80, 1974.

Stein, HA and Slatt, BJ: The ophthalmic assistant, ed 5, St Louis, 1988, The CV Mosby Co.

Stein, HA and Slatt, BJ: Swimming and contact lenses, Contact Intraocular Lens Med J 3(3):24-26, July-Sept 1977.

Stein, HA and Slatt, BS: Assessment of soft toric lenses, Curr Can Ophthal Pract 3:3, 1985.

Stein, HA and Slatt BS: Correcting astigmatism with rigid contact lenses, Curr Can Ophthal Pract 3:3, 1985.

Stein, HA, et al: Duane's clinical textbook of ophthalmology: fitting soft contact lenses, vol 1, Philadelphia, JP Lippincott, 1988.

Stone, J: Comments on orthokeratology and extended wear contact lenses, Can J Ophthalmol 40(1):4, March 1978.

Stone, J and Phillips, AJ, editors: Contact lenses: a textbook for practitioner and student, ed 2, Sevenoaks, Kent, Butterworth & Co Ltd, 1981.

Stuchell, RN, Farris, RL, and Mandel, ID: Methods of studying proteins in the tear fluid. In Holly, FJ, editor: The preocular tear film in health, disease and contact lens wear, Lubbock, Tex, Dry Eye Institute, 1986.

Swanson, K; Dispensing contact lenses, St Louis, 1975, Mo-Con Laboratories, Inc.

Szekely, IJ and Hind, HW: Treated polyvinyl alcohol for contact lens solution, United States Patent 3, 183, 152, 1965.

Szekely, IJ, Hind, HW, and Krezanoski, JZ: Accessory contact lens solutions, Encyclopedia Contact Lens Pract 4(20):13-26, 1963.

Tajiri, A: Impression technique to determine edge contour of contact lenses, Contacto 4(9):391-397, 1960.

Tannehill, JC and Sampson, WG: Extended use of the Radiuscope in contact lens inspection, Am J Ophthalmol 62:538, 1966.

Temprano, J: Therapeutic use of soft contact lenses, Contact Intraocular Lens Med J 2(3):60-67, July-Sept 1976.

Tiffany, JM: The role of meibomian secretion in the tears, Trans Ophthalmol Soc UK 104:396, 1985.

Tiffany, JM: Tear film stability and contact lens wear. Trans Br Cont Lens Assoc 19:35, 1988.

Tripathi, RC and Tripathi, BJ: The role of the lids in soft lens spoilage, Contact Intraocular Lens Med J 7(3):234-241, July-Sept 1981.

Tripathi, RC, Tripathi, BJ, and Ruben, M: The pathology of soft contact lens spoilage, J Ophthalmol 87(5):365-380, May 1980.

Tsuda, S, et al: Corneal physiology and oxygen permeability of contact lenses, Int Contact Lens Clin 8(3):11-22 May-June 1981.

Ullen, RL: Legal implications in fitting contact lenses, JAOA 38(4):288-291, 1961.

van Bijsterveld, OP: A double-blind crossover study comparing cromolyn sodium eye drops with placebo in the treatment of chronic conjunctivitis, Acta Ophthalmol 62:479-484, 1984.

Vanden Bussche, G, Emanuel, MB, and Rombaut, N: Clinical profile of astemizole. A survey of 50 double-blind trials, Ann Allergy 58:184-188, 1987.

Van Haeringen, NJ: Clinical biochemistry of tears, Surv Ophthalmol 26:84, 1981.

Vaughan, DG: The contamination of fluorescein solutions, Am J Ophthalmol 39(1):55-61, 1955.

Versura, P, et al: Scanning electron microscopy study of human cornea and conjunctiva in normal and various pathological conditions, Scan Electron Microsc 4:1695-1708, 1985.

Vidal, FL: Medical complications of contact lenses, Int Ophthalmol Clin 1(2):495-504, 1961.

Vinita, H, Bennett, ES, and Forrest, J: Clinical investigation of the paraperm EW rigid gas-permeable contact lens, Am J Optom Physiol Opt 64:5, 1987.

Wechsler, S and Wilson, G: Changes in hydrogel contact lens power due to flexure, Am J Optom Physiol Opt 55:78-83, 1978.

Weidt, AR and Cunin, BM: The bifocal alternative, Contact Intraocular Lens Med J 7(3):250-251, July-Sept 1981.

Weinberg, RJ: Corneal vascularization in aphakia, Am J Ophthalmol 83(1):121, Jan 1977.

Weinstock, FJ: Contact lens fitting, Philadelphia, JB Lippincott, 1989.

Weis, DR: Contact lenses for athletes, Int Ophthalmol Clin 21(4):139-148, Winter 1981.

Weissman, BA: Contact lens primer, Philadelphia, 1984, Lea & Febiger.

Weissman, BA: Results of the extended-wear contact lens survey of the Contact Lens section of the American Optometric Association, JAOA, 58:159, 1987.

Weissman, BA, Fatt, I, and Rasson, J: Diffusion of oxygen in human corneas in vivo, Invest Ophthalmol Vis Sci 20(1):123-125, Jan 1981.

Welsh, RC: Contact lenses in aphakia, Int Ophthalmol Clin 1(2):401-440, 1961.

Wilson, LA, Schlitzer, RL, and Ahearn, DG: *Pseudomonas* corneal ulcers associated with soft contact lens wear, Am J Ophthalmol 92(4):546-554, Oct 1981.

Wilson, LA, et al: Delayed hypersensitivity to thimerosal and soft contact lens-wearers, Ophthalmology 88:8, Aug 1981.

Winkler, CH and Dixon, JM: Bacteriology of the eye. III. A. Effect of contact lenses on the normal flora. B. Flora of the contact lens, Arch Ophthalmol 72(6):817-819, 1964.

Wolf, E: The muco-cutaneous junction of the lid-margin and the distribution of the tear fluid, Trans Ophthalmol Soc UK 66:291, 1946.

Zekman, TN and Krimmer, BM: The treatment of conical cornea: introduction of a new multicurve fluidless corneal contact lens, Arch Ophthalmol 54(2):481-488, 1955.

Zekman, TN and Sarnat, LA: Clinical evaluation of the silicone corneal contact lens, Am J Ophthalmol 74(3):534, Sept 1972.

Zantos, SG and Holden, BA: Research techniques and materials for continuous wear of contact lenses, Aust J Optom 60:86-95, March 1977.

APPENDIXES

APPENDIX A

THICKNESS
CONVERSION TABLE

Inches	mm	Inches	mm
0.001	0.025	0.021	0.525
0.002	0.050	0.022	0.550
0.003	0.075	0.023	0.575
0.004	0.100	0.024	0.600
0.005	0.125	0.025	0.625
0.006	0.150	0.026	0.650
0.007	0.175	0.027	0.675
0.008	0.200	0.028	0.700
0.009	0.225	0.029	0.725
0.010	0.250	0.030	0.750
0.011	0.275	0.031	0.775
0.012	0.300	0.032	0.800
0.013	0.325	0.033	0.825
0.014	0.350	0.034	0.850
0.015	0.375	0.035	0.875
0.016	0.400	0.036	0.900
0.017	0.425	0.037	0.925
0.018	0.450	0.038	0.950
0.019	0.475	0.039	0.975
0.020	0.500	0.040	1.000

From Hartstein, J.: Questions and answers on contact lens practice, ed. 2, St. Louis, 1973, The C.V. Mosby Co.

CONVERSION TABLES FOR DIOPTERS TO MILLIMETERS OF RADIUS

Diopter conversion table

Diopters	mm	Diopters	mm	Diopters	mm	Diopters	mm
20.00	16.875	36.00	9.375	39.00	8.653	42.00	8.035
22.00	15.340	36.12	9.343	39.12	8.627	42.12	8.012
24.00	14.062	36.25	9.310	39.25	8.598	42.25	7.988
26.00	12.980	36.37	9.279	39.37	8.572	42.37	7.965
27.00	12.500	36.50	9.246	39.50	8.544	42.50	7.941
28.00	12.053	36.62	9.216	39.62	8.518	42.62	7.918
29.00	11.638	36.75	9.183	39.75	8.490	42.75	7.894
29.50	11.441	36.87	9.153	39.87	8.465	42.87	7.872
30.00	11.250	37.00	9.121	40.00	8.437	43.00	7.848
30.50	11.065	37.12	9.092	40.12	8.412	43.12	7.826
31.00	10.887	37.25	9.060	40.25	8.385	43.25	7.803
31.50	10.714	37.37	9.031	40.37	8.360	43.37	7.781
32.00	10.547	37.50	9.000	40.50	8.333	43.50	7.758
32.50	10.385	37.62	8.971	40.62	8.308	43.62	7.737
33.00	10.227	37.75	8.940	40.75	8.282	43.75	7.714
33.50	10.075	37.87	8.912	40.87	8.257	43.87	7.693
34.00	9.926	38.00	8.881	41.00	8.231	44.00	7.670
34.25	9.854	38.12	8.853	41.12	8.207	44.12	7.649
34.50	9.783	38.25	8.823	41.25	8.181	44.25	7.627
34.75	9.712	38.37	8.795	41.37	8.158	44.37	7.606
35.00	9.643	38.50	8.766	41.50	8.132	44.50	7.584
35.25	9.574	38.62	8.738	41.62	8.109	44.62	7.563
35.50	9.507	38.75	8.708	41.75	8.083	44.75	7.541
35.75	9.440	38.87	8.682	41.87	8.060	44.87	7.521

From Stein, H.A., and Slatt, B.J.: The ophthalmic assistant, ed. 4, St. Louis, 1982, The C.V. Mosby Co.

Diopters	mm	Diopters	mm	Diopters	mm	Diopters	mm
45.00	7.500	48.00	7.031	51.00	6.617	54.00	6.250
45.12	7.480	48.12	7.013	51.12	6.602	54.12	6.236
45.25	7.458	48.25	6.994	51.25	6.585	54.25	6.221
45.37	7.438	48.37	6.977	51.37	6.569	54.37	6.207
45.50	7.417	48.50	6.958	51.50	6.553	54.50	6.192
45.62	7.398	48.62	6.941	51.62	6.538	54.62	6.179
45.75	7.377	48.75	6.923	51.75	6.521	54.75	6.164
45.87	7.357	48.87	6.906	51.87	6.506	54.87	6.150
46.00	7.336	49.00	6.887	52.00	6.490	55.00	6.136
46.12	7.317	49.12	6.870	52.12	6.475	55.12	6.123
46.25	7.297	49.25	6.852	52.25	6.459	55.25	6.108
46.37	7.278	49.37	6.836	52.37	6.444	55.37	6.095
46.50	7.258	49.50	6.818	52.50	6.428	55.50	6.081
46.62	7.239	49.62	6.801	52.62	6.413	55.62	6.068
46.75	7.219	49.75	6.783	52.75	6.398	55.75	6.054
46.87	7.200	49.87	6.767	52.87	6.383	55.87	6.041
47.00	7.180	50.00	6.750	53.00	6.367	56.00	6.027
47.12	7.162	50.12	6.733	53.12	6.353	56.50	5.973
47.25	7.142	50.25	6.716	53.25	6.338	57.00	5.921
47.37	7.124	50.37	6.700	53.37	6.323	57.50	5.869
47.50	7.105	50.50	6.683	53.50	6.308	58.00	5.819
47.62	7.087	50.62	6.667	53.62	6.294	58.50	5.769
47.75	7.068	50.75	6.650	53.75	6.279	59.00	5.720
47.87	7.050	50.87	6.634	53.87	6.265	60.00	5.625

SPECTACLE LENS POWER WORN AT VARIOUS DISTANCES TO EQUIVALENT CONTACT LENS POWER

Vertex conversion table

Spectacle lens power	Effective power at corneal plane of spectacles at designated distance from cornea (vertex distance/millimeters) Plus lenses							
	8 mm	9 mm	10 mm	11 mm	12 mm	13 mm	14 mm	15 mm
4.00	4.12	4.12	4.12	4.12	4.25	4.25	4.25	4.25
4.50	4.62	4.75	4.75	4.75	4.75	4.75	4.75	4.87
5.00	5.25	5.25	5.25	5.25	5.25	5.37	5.37	5.37
5.50	5.75	5.75	5.75	5.87	5.87	5.87	6.00	6.00
6.00	6.25	6.37	6.37	6.37	6.50	6.50	6.50	6.62
6.50	6.87	6.87	7.00	7.00	7.00	7.12	7.12	7.25
7.00	7.37	7.50	7.50	7.62	7.62	7.75	7.75	7.75
7.50	8.00	8.00	8.12	8.12	8.25	8.25	8.37	8.50
8.00	8.50	8.62	8.75	8.75	8.87	8.87	9.00	9.12
8.50	9.12	9.25	9.25	9.37	9.50	9.50	9.62	9.75
9.00	9.75	9.75	9.87	10.00	10.12	10.25	10.37	10.37
9.50	10.25	10.37	10.50	10.62	10.75	10.87	11.00	11.12
10.00	10.87	11.00	11.12	11.25	11.37	11.50	11.62	11.75
10.50	11.50	11.62	11.75	11.87	12.00	12.12	12.25	12.50
11.00	12.00	12.25	12.37	12.50	12.75	12.87	13.00	13.12
11.50	12.62	12.87	13.00	13.12	13.37	13.50	13.75	13.87
12.00	13.25	13.50	13.62	13.87	14.00	14.25	14.50	14.62
12.50	13.87	14.12	14.25	14.50	14.75	15.00	15.25	15.37
13.00	14.50	14.75	15.00	15.25	15.50	15.62	16.00	16.12
13.50	15.12	15.37	15.62	15.87	16.12	16.37	16.62	16.87
14.00	15.75	16.00	16.25	16.50	16.75	17.12	17.50	17.75
14.50	16.50	16.75	17.00	17.25	17.50	17.87	18.25	18.50
15.00	17.00	17.37	17.75	18.00	18.25	18.62	19.00	19.37
15.50	17.75	18.00	18.25	18.75	19.00	19.37	19.75	20.25
16.00	18.25	18.75	19.00	19.37	19.75	20.25	20.50	21.00
16.50	19.00	19.37	19.75	20.25	20.50	21.00	21.50	21.87
17.00	19.75	20.25	20.50	21.00	21.00	22.00	22.25	22.87
17.50	20.50	20.75	21.25	21.75	22.25	22.75	23.25	23.75
18.00	21.00	21.50	22.00	22.50	23.00	23.50	24.00	24.62
18.50	21.75	22.25	22.75	23.25	23.75	24.50	25.00	25.62
19.00	22.50	23.00	23.50	24.00	24.75	25.25	26.00	26.50

From Stein, H.A., and Slatt, B.J.: The ophthalmic assistant, ed. 4, St. Louis, 1982, The C.V. Mosby Co.

Effective power at corneal plane of spectacles at designated distance from cornea
(vertex distance/millimeters)

Minus lenses

8 mm	9 mm	10 mm	11 mm	12 mm	13 mm	14 mm	15 mm
3.87	3.87	3.87	3.87	3.87	3.75	3.75	3.75
4.37	4.37	4.25	4.25	4.25	4.25	4.25	4.25
4.75	4.75	4.75	4.75	4.75	4.75	4.62	4.62
5.25	5.25	5.25	5.12	5.12	5.12	5.12	5.12
5.75	5.62	5.62	5.62	5.62	5.50	5.50	5.50
6.12	6.12	6.12	6.00	6.00	6.00	6.00	5.87
6.62	6.62	6.50	6.50	6.50	6.37	6.37	6.37
7.12	7.00	7.00	6.87	6.87	6.87	6.75	6.75
7.50	7.50	7.37	7.37	7.25	7.25	7.25	7.25
8.00	7.87	7.87	7.75	7.75	7.62	7.62	7.50
8.37	8.37	8.25	8.25	8.12	8.00	8.00	8.00
8.87	8.75	8.62	8.62	8.50	8.50	8.37	8.37
9.25	9.12	9.12	9.00	8.87	8.87	8.75	8.75
9.62	9.62	9.50	9.37	9.37	9.25	9.12	9.12
10.12	10.00	9.87	9.75	9.75	9.62	9.50	9.50
10.50	10.37	10.37	10.25	10.12	10.00	9.87	9.87
11.00	10.87	10.75	10.62	10.50	10.37	10.25	10.12
11.37	11.25	11.12	11.00	10.87	10.75	10.62	10.50
11.75	11.62	11.50	11.37	11.25	11.12	11.00	10.87
12.25	12.00	11.87	11.75	11.62	11.50	11.37	11.25
12.62	12.50	12.25	12.12	12.00	11.87	11.75	11.50
13.00	12.75	12.62	12.50	12.37	12.25	12.00	11.87
13.37	13.25	13.00	12.87	12.75	12.50	12.37	12.25
13.75	13.62	13.50	13.25	13.00	12.87	12.75	12.62
14.25	14.00	13.75	13.62	13.50	13.25	13.00	12.87
14.50	14.37	14.12	14.00	13.75	13.62	13.50	13.25
15.00	14.75	14.50	14.25	14.12	14.00	13.75	13.50
15.37	15.12	14.87	14.75	14.50	14.25	14.00	13.87
15.75	15.50	15.25	15.00	14.75	14.62	14.37	14.12
16.12	15.87	15.62	15.37	15.12	14.87	14.75	14.50
16.50	16.25	16.00	15.75	15.50	15.25	15.00	14.75

TABLE OF SAGITTAL VALUES

Diameter of CPC (mm)	Radius of curvature of central posterior curve (CPC) (mm)								
	8.44 mm 40.00 D	8.33 mm 40.50 D	8.23 mm 41.00 D	813. mm 41.50 D	8.04 mm 42.00 D	7.94 mm 42.50 D	7.85 mm 43.00 D	7.76 mm 43.50 D	7.67 mm 44.00 D
5.4	0.444	0.450	0.455	0.461	0.467	0.473	0.479	0.485	0.491
5.6	0.478	0.485	0.491	0.497	0.503	0.510	0.516	0.523	0.529
5.8	0.514	0.521	0.528	0.535	0.541	0.549	0.555	0.562	0.569
6.0	0.554	0.559	0.566	0.574	0.581	0.589	0.596	0.603	0.611
6.2	0.590	0.598	0.606	0.614	0.622	0.630	0.638	0.646	0.654
6.4	0.630	0.639	0.648	0.656	0.664	0.673	0.682	0.691	0.699
6.6	0.672	0.682	0.691	0.700	0.708	0.718	0.727	0.737	0.746
6.8	0.715	0.725	0.735	0.745	0.754	0.765	0.775	0.785	0.795
7.0	0.760	0.771	0.781	0.792	0.802	0.813	0.823	0.834	0.845
7.2	0.806	0.818	0.829	0.840	0.851	0.863	0.874	0.886	0.897
7.4	0.854	0.867	0.879	0.891	0.902	0.915	0.927	0.939	0.951
7.6	0.904	0.917	0.930	0.943	0.955	0.968	0.981	0.994	1.008
7.8	0.955	0.969	0.983	0.996	1.009	1.024	1.037	1.051	1.066
8.0	1.098	1.023	1.037	1.052	1.066	1.081	1.096	1.110	1.126
8.2	1.063	1.079	1.094	1.110	1.124	1.140	1.156	1.172	1.188
8.4	1.119	1.136	1.152	1.169	1.184	1.202	1.218	1.235	1.252
8.6	1.178	1.196	1.213	1.230	1.247	1.265	1.282	1.300	1.319
8.8	1.238	1.257	1.275	1.294	1.311	1.331	1.349	1.368	1.388
9.0	1.300	1.320	1.339	1.359	1.377	1.398	1.418	1.438	1.459
9.2	1.364	1.385	1.406	1.427	1.446	1.468	1.489	1.510	1.533
9.4	1.430	1.453	1.474	1.496	1.517	1.541	1.563	1.585	1.609
9.6	1.498	1.522	1.545	1.568	1.590	1.615	1.639	1.663	1.669

From Creighton, C.P.: Contact lens fabrication tables, Tonawanda, New York, 1964, Creighton Publishers.

Diameter of CPC-POZ* (mm)	Radius of curvature of central posterior curve (CPC) (mm)							
	7.59 mm 44.50 D	7.50 mm 45.00 D	7.42 mm 45.50 D	7.34 mm 46.00 D	7.26 mm 46.50 D	7.18 mm 47.00 D	7.11 mm 47.50 D	7.03 mm 48.00 D
5.4	0.496	0.503	0.509	0.515	0.521	0.527	0.533	0.539
5.6	0.535	0.542	0.549	0.555	0.562	0.568	0.575	0.582
5.8	0.576	0.583	0.590	0.597	0.604	0.612	0.618	0.626
6.0	0.618	0.626	0.634	0.641	0.649	0.657	0.664	0.672
6.2	0.662	0.671	0.679	0.687	0.695	0.704	0.711	0.720
6.4	0.708	0.717	0.725	0.734	0.743	0.753	0.761	0.771
6.6	0.755	0.765	0.774	0.784	0.793	0.803	0.812	0.823
6.8	0.804	0.815	0.825	0.835	0.845	0.856	0.866	0.877
7.0	0.855	0.867	0.877	0.888	0.899	0.911	0.921	0.933
7.2	0.908	0.920	0.932	0.943	0.955	0.968	0.979	0.992
7.4	0.963	0.976	0.988	1.001	1.014	1.027	1.039	1.052
7.6	1.020	1.034	1.047	1.060	1.074	1.088	1.101	1.116
7.8	1.079	1.094	1.108	1.122	1.136	1.152	1.165	1.188
8.0	1.140	1.156	1.170	1.186	1.201	1.217	1.232	1.249
8.2	1.203	1.220	1.236	1.252	1.269	1.286	1.301	1.319
8.4	1.268	1.286	1.303	1.320	1.338	1.357	1.373	1.393
8.6	1.336	1.355	1.373	1.391	1.410	1.430	1.448	1.468
8.8	1.405	1.426	1.445	1.465	1.485	1.506	1.525	1.547
9.0	1.478	1.500	1.520	1.541	1.563	1.585	1.605	1.629
9.2	1.553	1.576	1.598	1.620	1.643	1.667	1.689	1.714
9.4	1.630	1.655	1.678	1.702	1.727	1.752	1.775	1.802
9.6	1.711	1.737	1.762	1.787	1.813	1.840	1.865	1.894

*POZ, Peripheral optic zone.

CONVERSION TABLE RELATING DIOPTERS OF CORNEAL REFRACTING POWER TO MILLIMETERS OF RADIUS OF CURVATURE

Diopters	Radius (mm)	
	Curvature	
Drum reading	Convex	Concave
52.00	6.49	6.51
51.87	6.50	6.53
51.75	6.52	6.54
51.62	6.54	6.56
51.50	6.55	6.57
51.37	6.57	6.59
51.25	6.58	6.61
51.12	6.60	6.62
51.00	6.62	6.64
50.87	6.63	6.66
50.75	6.65	6.67
50.62	6.66	6.69
50.50	6.68	6.71
50.37	6.70	6.72
50.25	6.73	6.75
50.12	6.73	6.75
50.00	6.75	6.77
49.87	6.76	6.79
49.75	6.80	6.82
49.62	6.80	6.82
49.50	6.82	6.84
49.37	6.83	6.85
49.25	6.85	6.87
49.12	6.87	6.89
49.00	6.89	6.91
48.87	6.90	6.93
48.75	6.92	6.95
48.62	6.94	6.96
48.50	6.96	6.98
48.37	6.97	7.00
48.25	6.99	7.02
48.12	7.01	7.03
48.00	7.03	7.05

Conversion table relating diopters of corneal refracting power to millimeters of radius of curvature for an assumed index of refraction of 1.3375. The column under convex curvature should be used when the keratometer is used to measure the cornea, and the third column is used to measure concave surfaces such as the CPC of a corneal contact lens in terms of its equivalent corneal refracting power in diopters.

Diopters	Radius (mm)		Diopters	Radius (mm)		Diopters	Radius (mm)	
	Curvature			Curvature			Curvature	
Drum reading	Convex	Concave	Drum reading	Convex	Concave	Drum reading	Convex	Concave
47.87	7.05	7.07	43.87	7.67	7.72	39.87	8.47	8.50
47.75	7.07	7.09	43.75	7.72	7.74	39.75	8.49	8.52
47.62	7.08	7.11	43.62	7.74	7.77	39.62	8.52	8.55
47.50	7.10	7.13	43.50	7.76	7.79	39.50	8.54	8.58
47.37	7.12	7.15	43.37	7.78	7.81	39.37	8.57	8.61
47.25	7.14	7.17	43.25	7.80	7.84	39.25	8.60	8.63
47.12	7.16	7.19	43.12	7.83	7.86	39.12	8.63	8.66
47.00	7.18	7.21	43.00	7.85	7.88	39.00	8.65	8.69
46.87	7.20	7.23	42.87	7.88	7.90	38.87	8.68	8.72
46.75	7.22	7.25	42.75	7.90	7.92	38.75	8.71	8.75
46.62	7.24	7.27	42.62	7.92	7.95	38.62	8.74	8.78
46.50	7.26	7.29	42.50	7.95	7.97	38.50	8.77	8.80
46.27	7.28	7.31	42.37	7.97	8.00	38.37	8.80	8.84
46.25	7.30	7.33	42.25	8.00	8.02	38.25	8.82	8.86
46.12	7.32	7.35	42.12	8.01	8.05	38.12	8.85	8.89
46.00	7.34	7.37	42.00	8.04	8.07	38.00	8.88	8.92
45.87	7.36	7.39	41.87	8.06	8.10	37.87	8.91	8.95
45.75	7.38	7.41	41.75	8.09	8.12	37.75	8.94	8.98
45.62	7.40	7.43	41.62	8.11	8.15	37.62	8.97	9.01
45.50	7.42	7.45	41.50	8.13	8.17	37.50	9.00	9.04
45.37	7.44	7.47	41.37	8.16	8.19	37.37	9.03	9.07
45.25	7.46	7.49	41.25	8.18	8.22	37.25	9.06	9.10
45.12	7.48	7.51	41.12	8.20	8.24	37.12	9.09	9.13
45.00	7.50	7.53	41.00	8.23	8.27	37.00	9.12	9.16
44.87	7.52	7.55	40.87	8.26	8.29	36.87	9.14	9.19
44.75	7.55	7.57	40.75	8.28	8.32	36.75	9.19	9.23
44.62	7.57	7.58	40.62	8.31	8.34	36.62	9.22	9.26
44.50	7.59	7.60	40.50	8.34	8.37	36.50	9.25	9.29
44.37	7.61	7.62	40.37	8.36	8.39	36.37	9.28	9.32
44.25	7.63	7.65	40.25	8.39	8.42	36.25	9.31	9.35
44.12	7.65	7.67	40.12	8.41	8.44	36.12	9.35	9.38
44.00	7.67	7.70	40.00	8.44	8.47	36.00	9.38	9.42
						34.00	9.93	9.97

COMPENSATION FOR EFFECT OF VERTEX DISTANCES (USED WHEN PLUS LENS IS MOVED FROM THE EYE)

℞ power (D)	Distance moved (mm)									
	1	2	3	4	5	6	7	8	9	10
7.00	6.95	6.90	6.86	6.81	6.76	6.72	6.67	6.63	6.59	6.54
7.25	7.20	7.15	7.10	7.05	7.00	6.95	6.90	6.85	6.81	6.76
7.50	7.44	7.39	7.33	7.28	7.23	7.18	7.13	7.08	7.03	6.98
7.75	7.69	7.63	7.57	7.52	7.46	7.41	7.35	7.30	7.24	7.19
8.00	7.94	7.87	7.81	7.75	7.69	7.63	7.58	7.52	7.46	7.41
8.25	8.18	8.12	8.05	7.99	7.92	7.86	7.80	7.74	7.68	7.62
8.50	8.43	8.36	8.29	8.22	8.15	8.09	8.02	7.96	7.90	7.83
8.75	8.67	8.60	8.53	8.45	8.38	8.31	8.24	8.18	8.11	8.05
9.00	8.92	8.84	8.76	8.69	8.61	8.54	8.47	8.40	8.33	8.26
9.25	9.17	9.08	9.00	8.92	8.84	8.76	8.69	8.61	8.54	8.47
9.50	9.41	9.32	9.24	9.15	9.07	8.99	8.91	8.83	8.75	8.68
9.75	9.66	9.56	9.47	9.38	9.30	9.21	9.13	9.04	8.96	8.88
10.00	9.90	9.80	9.71	9.62	9.52	9.43	9.35	9.26	9.17	9.09
10.25	10.15	10.04	9.94	9.85	9.75	9.66	9.56	9.47	9.38	9.30
10.50	10.39	10.28	10.18	10.08	9.98	9.88	9.78	9.69	9.59	9.50
10.75	10.64	10.52	10.41	10.31	10.20	10.10	10.00	9.90	9.80	9.71
11.00	10.88	10.76	10.65	10.54	10.43	10.32	10.21	10.11	10.01	9.91
11.25	11.12	11.00	10.88	10.77	10.65	10.54	10.43	10.32	10.22	10.11
11.50	11.37	11.24	11.12	10.99	10.87	10.76	10.64	10.53	10.42	10.31
11.75	11.61	11.48	11.35	11.22	11.10	10.98	10.86	10.74	10.63	10.51
12.00	11.86	11.72	11.58	11.45	11.32	11.19	11.07	10.95	10.83	10.71
12.25	12.10	11.96	11.82	11.68	11.54	11.41	11.28	11.16	11.03	10.91
12.50	12.35	12.20	12.05	11.90	11.76	11.63	11.49	11.36	11.24	11.11
12.75	12.59	12.43	12.28	12.13	11.99	11.84	11.71	11.57	11.44	11.31
13.00	12.83	12.67	12.51	12.36	12.21	12.06	11.92	11.78	11.64	11.50
13.25	13.08	12.91	12.74	12.58	12.43	12.27	12.13	11.98	11.84	11.70
13.50	13.32	13.15	12.97	12.81	12.65	12.49	12.33	12.18	12.04	11.89
13.75	13.56	13.38	13.21	13.03	12.87	12.70	12.54	12.39	12.24	12.09
14.00	13.81	13.62	13.44	13.26	13.08	12.92	12.75	12.59	12.43	12.28
14.25	14.05	13.86	13.67	13.48	13.30	13.13	12.96	12.79	12.63	12.47

R power (D)	Distance moved (mm)									
	1	2	3	4	5	6	7	8	9	10
14.50	14.29	14.09	13.90	13.70	13.52	13.34	13.16	12.99	12.83	12.66
14.75	14.54	14.33	14.12	13.93	13.74	13.55	13.37	13.19	13.02	12.85
15.00	14.78	14.56	14.35	14.15	13.95	13.76	13.57	13.39	13.22	13.04
15.25	15.02	14.80	14.58	14.37	14.17	13.97	13.78	13.59	13.41	13.23
15.50	15.26	15.03	14.81	14.60	14.39	14.18	13.98	13.79	13.60	13.42
15.75	15.51	15.27	15.04	14.82	14.60	14.39	14.19	13.99	13.79	13.61
16.00	15.75	15.50	15.27	15.04	14.81	14.60	13.39	14.18	13.99	13.79
16.25	15.99	15.74	15.49	15.25	15.03	14.81	14.59	14.38	14.18	13.98
16.50	16.23	15.97	15.72	15.48	15.24	15.01	14.79	14.57	14.37	14.16
16.75	16.47	16.21	15.95	15.70	15.45	15.22	14.99	14.77	14.56	14.35
17.00	16.72	16.44	16.18	15.92	15.67	15.43	15.19	14.96	14.74	14.53
17.25	16.96	16.67	16.40	16.44	15.88	15.63	15.39	15.16	14.93	14.71
17.50	17.20	16.91	16.63	16.36	16.09	15.84	15.59	15.35	15.12	14.89
17.75	17.44	17.14	16.85	16.57	16.30	16.04	15.79	15.54	15.31	15.07
18.00	17.68	17.37	17.08	16.79	16.51	16.25	15.99	15.73	15.49	15.25
18.25	17.92	17.61	17.30	17.01	16.72	16.45	16.18	15.92	15.68	15.43
18.50	18.16	17.84	17.53	17.23	16.93	16.65	16.38	16.11	15.86	15.61
18.75	18.40	18.07	17.75	17.44	17.14	16.85	16.57	16.30	16.04	15.79
19.00	18.65	18.30	17.98	17.66	17.35	17.06	16.77	16.49	16.23	15.97
19.25	18.89	18.54	18.20	17.87	17.56	17.26	16.96	16.68	16.41	16.14
19.50	19.13	18.77	18.42	18.09	17.77	17.46	17.16	16.87	16.59	16.32
19.75	19.37	19.00	18.65	18.30	17.97	17.66	17.35	17.06	16.77	16.49
20.00	19.61	19.23	18.87	18.52	18.18	17.86	17.54	17.24	16.95	16.67
20.25	19.85	19.46	19.09	18.73	18.39	18.06	17.74	17.43	17.13	16.84
20.50	20.09	19.69	19.31	18.95	18.59	18.25	17.93	17.61	17.31	17.01
20.75	20.33	19.92	19.53	19.16	18.80	18.45	18.12	17.80	17.48	17.18
21.00	20.57	20.15	19.76	19.37	19.00	18.65	18.31	17.98	17.66	17.36
21.25	20.81	20.38	19.98	19.59	19.21	18.85	18.50	18.16	17.84	17.53
21.50	21.05	20.61	20.20	19.80	10.41	19.04	18.69	18.34	18.01	17.70
21.75	21.29	20.84	20.42	20.01	19.62	10.24	18.88	18.53	18.19	17.87

COMPENSATION FOR EFFECT OF VERTEX DISTANCES (USED WHEN PLUS LENS IS MOVED TOWARD THE EYE)

R power (D)	Distance moved (mm)									
	1	2	3	4	5	6	7	8	9	10
7.00	7.05	7.10	7.15	7.20	7.25	7.31	7.36	7.42	7.47	7.53
7.25	7.30	7.36	7.41	7.47	7.52	7.58	7.64	7.70	7.76	7.82
7.50	7.56	7.61	7.67	7.73	7.79	7.85	7.92	7.98	8.04	8.11
7.75	7.81	7.87	7.93	8.00	8.06	8.13	8.19	8.26	8.33	8.40
8.00	8.06	8.13	8.20	8.26	8.33	8.40	8.47	8.55	8.62	8.70
8.25	8.32	8.39	8.46	8.53	8.60	8.68	8.76	8.83	8.91	8.99
8.50	8.57	8.56	8.72	8.80	8.88	8.96	9.04	9.12	9.20	9.29
8.75	8.83	8.91	8.99	9.07	9.15	9.23	9.32	9.41	9.50	9.59
9.00	9.08	9.16	9.25	9.34	9.42	9.51	9.61	9.70	9.79	9.89
9.25	9.34	9.42	9.51	9.61	9.70	9.79	9.89	9.99	10.09	10.19
9.50	9.59	9.68	9.78	9.88	9.97	10.07	10.18	10.28	10.39	10.50
9.75	9.85	9.94	10.04	10.15	10.25	10.36	10.46	10.58	10.69	10.80
10.00	10.10	10.20	10.31	10.42	10.53	10.64	10.75	10.87	10.99	11.11
10.25	10.36	10.46	10.58	10.69	10.80	10.92	11.04	11.17	11.29	11.42
10.50	10.61	10.73	10.84	10.96	11.08	11.21	11.33	11.46	11.60	11.73
10.75	10.87	10.99	11.11	11.23	11.36	11.49	11.62	11.76	11.90	12.04
11.00	11.12	11.25	11.38	11.51	11.64	11.78	11.92	12.06	12.21	12.36
11.25	11.38	11.51	11.64	11.78	11.92	12.06	12.21	12.36	12.52	12.68
11.50	11.63	11.77	11.91	12.05	12.20	12.35	12.51	12.67	12.83	12.99
11.75	11.89	12.03	12.18	12.33	12.48	12.64	12.80	12.97	13.14	13.31
12.00	12.15	12.30	12.45	12.61	12.77	12.93	13.10	13.27	13.45	13.64
12.25	12.40	12.56	12.72	12.88	13.05	13.22	13.40	13.58	13.77	13.96
12.50	12.66	12.82	12.99	13.16	13.33	13.51	13.70	13.89	14.08	14.29
12.75	12.91	13.08	13.26	13.44	13.62	13.81	14.00	14.20	14.40	14.61
13.00	13.17	13.35	13.53	13.71	13.90	14.10	14.30	14.51	14.72	14.94
13.25	13.43	13.61	13.80	13.99	14.19	14.39	14.60	14.82	15.04	15.27
13.50	13.68	13.87	14.07	14.27	14.48	14.69	14.91	15.13	15.37	15.61
13.75	13.94	14.14	14.34	14.55	14.77	14.99	15.21	15.45	15.69	15.94
14.00	14.20	14.40	14.61	14.83	15.05	15.28	15.52	15.77	16.02	16.28
14.25	14.46	14.67	14.89	15.11	15.34	15.58	15.83	16.09	16.35	16.62

R power (D)	Distance moved (mm)									
	1	*2*	*3*	*4*	*5*	*6*	*7*	*8*	*9*	*10*
14.50	14.71	14.93	15.16	15.39	15.63	15.88	16.14	16.41	16.88	16.96
14.75	14.97	15.20	15.43	15.67	15.92	16.18	16.45	16.73	17.01	17.30
15.00	15.23	15.46	15.71	15.96	16.22	16.48	16.76	17.05	17.34	17.65
15.25	15.49	15.73	15.98	16.24	16.51	16.79	17.07	17.37	17.68	18.00
15.50	15.74	16.00	16.26	16.52	16.80	17.09	17.39	17.69	18.01	18.35
15.75	16.00	16.26	16.53	16.81	17.10	17.39	17.70	18.02	18.35	18.70
16.00	16.26	16.53	16.81	17.09	17.39	17.70	18.02	18.35	18.69	19.05
16.25	16.52	16.80	17.08	17.38	17.69	18.01	18.34	18.68	19.03	19.40
16.50	16.78	17.06	17.36	17.67	17.98	18.31	18.65	19.01	19.38	19.76
16.75	17.04	17.33	17.64	17.95	18.28	18.62	18.97	19.34	19.72	20.12
17.00	17.29	17.60	17.91	18.24	18.58	18.93	19.30	19.68	20.07	20.48
17.25	17.55	17.87	18.19	18.53	18.88	19.24	19.62	20.01	20.42	20.85
17.50	17.81	18.13	18.47	18.82	19.18	19.55	19.94	20.35	20.77	21.21
17.75	18.07	18.40	18.75	19.11	19.48	19.86	20.27	20.69	21.12	21.58
18.00	18.33	18.67	19.03	19.40	19.78	20.18	20.59	21.03	21.48	21.95
18.25	18.59	18.94	19.31	19.69	20.08	20.49	20.92	21.37	21.84	22.32
18.50	18.85	19.21	19.59	19.98	20.39	20.81	21.25	27.71	22.20	22.70
18.75	19.11	19.48	19.87	20.27	20.69	21.13	21.58	22.06	22.56	23.08
19.00	19.37	19.75	20.15	20.56	20.99	21.44	21.91	22.41	22.92	23.46
19.25	19.63	20.02	20.43	20.86	21.30	21.76	22.25	22.75	23.28	23.81
19.50	19.89	20.89	20.71	21.15	21.61	22.08	22.58	23.10	23.65	24.22
19.75	20.15	20.56	20.99	21.44	21.91	22.40	22.92	23.46	24.02	24.61
20.00	20.41	20.83	21.28	21.74	22.22	22.73	23.26	23.81	24.39	25.00
20.25	20.67	21.10	21.56	22.03	22.53	23.05	23.59	24.16	24.76	
20.50	20.82	21.38	21.84	22.33	22.84	23.38	23.93	24.52		
20.75	20.91	21.65	22.13	22.63	23.15	23.70	24.28			
21.00	21.45	21.92	22.41	22.93	23.46	24.03				
21.25	21.71	22.19	22.70	23.22	23.78					
21.50	21.97	22.47	22.98	23.52						
21.75	22.23	22.74	23.37							

OPTICAL CONSTANTS OF THE EYE

Optical constants of the eye are summarized as follows:

1. The curvature of the anterior face of the cornea is 7.5 mm.
2. The index of refraction of the corneal tissue, the aqueous humor, and the vitreous equals 1.332.
3. The distance separating the anterior pole of the cornea from the posterior pole of the crystalline lens is 3.6 mm.
4. The curvature of the anterior face of the crystalline lens measures 10.0 mm.
5. The curvature of the posterior face of the crystalline lens is 6.0 mm.
6. The distance separating the anterior pole of the crystalline lens from the posterior pole of the crystalline lens is 4.0 mm.
7. The main refraction index of the crystalline lens equals 1.40.

From Hartstein, J.: Basics of contact lenses manual, Rochester, Minn., 1979, American Academy of Ophthalmology.

8. The dioptric power of the cornea equals 44.26 D.
9. The dioptric power of the crystalline lens alone, when both of its surfaces are immersed in a medium having an index of 1.332, equals 17.82 D.
10. The total power of the eye equals 58.53 D.
11. The distance of the first principal plane of the crystalline lens back of the anterior pole of the crystalline lens is 2.4 mm.
12. The distance of the second principal plane of the crystalline lens ahead of the posterior pole of the crystalline lens is 1.4 mm.
13. The distance separating these two planes is 0.2 mm.
14. The distance of the principal plane of the whole eye behind the anterior pole of the whole cornea is 1.370 mm.
15. The distance of the second principal plane of the whole eye behind the anterior pole of the whole cornea is 1.664 mm.
16. The distance separating these two planes is 0.294 mm.

SAGITTAL RELATIONSHIP OF VARIOUS BASE CURVES AND DIAMETERS

Diameter (mm)	Radius (mm)	Diameter (mm)	Radius (mm)
Flatter			
13.0	8.7	15.0	8.7
13.0	8.4	14.0	7.8
13.5	8.7	14.5	8.1
13.0	8.1	15.0	8.4
13.5	8.4	15.5	8.7
14.0	8.7	13.5	7.2
13.0	7.8	14.0	7.5
13.5	8.1	14.5	7.8
14.0	8.4	15.0	8.1
13.0	7.5	15.5	8.4
14.5	8.7	14.0	7.2
13.5	7.8	14.5	7.5
14.0	8.1	15.0	7.8
13.0	7.2	15.5	8.1
14.5	8.4	15.0	7.5
13.5	7.5	15.5	7.8
		Steeper	

DIOPTRIC CURVES
FOR EXTENDED
RANGE OF
KERATOMETER

High power (with +1.25 D lens over aperture)				*Low power (with −1.00 D lens over aperture)*			
Drum reading (D)	True dioptric curvature (D)	Drum reading (D)	True dioptric curvature (D)	Drum reading (D)	True dioptric curvature (D)	Drum reading (D)	True dioptric curvature (D)
52.00	61.00	46.87	55.87	42.00	36.00	36.87	30.87
51.87	60.87	46.75	55.75	41.87	35.87	36.75	30.75
51.75	60.75	46.62	55.62	41.75	35.75	36.62	30.62
51.62	60.62	46.50	55.50	41.62	35.62	36.50	30.50
51.50	60.50	46.37	55.37	41.50	35.50	36.37	30.37
51.37	60.37	46.25	55.25	41.37	35.37	36.25	30.25
51.25	60.25	46.12	55.12	41.25	35.25	36.12	30.12
51.12	60.12	46.00	55.00	41.12	35.12	36.00	30.00
51.00	60.00			41.00	35.00		
		45.87	54.87				
50.87	59.87	45.75	54.75	40.87	34.87		
50.75	59.75	45.62	54.62	40.75	34.75		
50.62	59.62	45.50	54.50	40.62	34.62		
50.50	59.50	45.37	54.37	40.50	34.50		
50.37	59.37	45.25	54.25	40.37	34.37		
50.25	59.25	45.12	54.12	40.25	34.25		
50.12	59.12	45.00	54.00	40.12	34.12		
50.00	59.00			40.00	34.00		
		44.87	53.87				
49.87	58.87	44.75	53.75	39.87	33.87		
49.75	58.75	44.62	53.62	39.75	33.75		
49.62	58.62	44.50	53.50	39.62	33.62		
49.50	58.50	44.37	53.37	39.50	33.50		

Courtesy Bausch & Lomb, Inc.

High power (with +1.25 D lens over aperture)				Low power (with −1.00 D lens over aperture)			
Drum reading (D)	True dioptric curvature (D)	Drum reading (D)	True dioptric curvature (D)	Drum reading (D)	True dioptric curvature (D)	Drum reading (D)	True dioptric curvature (D)
49.37	58.37	44.25	53.25	39.37	33.37		
49.25	58.25	44.12	53.12	39.25	33.25		
49.12	58.12	44.00	53.00	39.12	33.12		
49.00	58.00			39.00	33.00		
		43.87	52.87				
48.75	57.75	43.75	52.75	38.87	32.87		
48.62	57.62	43.62	52.62	38.75	32.75		
48.50	57.50	43.50	52.50	38.62	32.62		
48.37	57.37	43.37	52.37	38.50	32.50		
48.25	57.25	43.25	52.25	38.37	32.37		
48.12	57.12	43.12	52.12	38.25	32.25		
48.00	57.00	43.00	52.00	38.12	32.12		
				38.00	32.00		
47.87	56.87						
47.75	56.75			37.87	31.87		
47.62	56.62			37.75	31.75		
47.50	56.50			37.62	31.62		
47.37	58.37			37.50	31.50		
47.25	56.25			37.37	31.37		
47.12	56.12			37.25	31.25		
47.00	56.00			37.12	31.12		
				37.00	31.00		

EDGE-THICKNESS*
CHANGES AS A
FUNCTION OF LENS
POWER† (FOR BASE
CURVE 7.6 MM)‡

	Lens diameter (chord diameter in mm)										
Power (D)	6.0	6.5	7.0	7.5	8.0	8.5	9.0	9.5	10.0	10.5	11.0
1.00	0.010	0.013	0.015	0.018	0.021	0.024	0.028	0.033	0.038	0.045	0.052
2.00	0.020	0.025	0.029	0.035	0.041	0.047	0.055	0.064	0.075	0.088	0.102
3.00	0.031	0.037	0.044	0.053	0.062	0.071	0.083	0.097	0.113	0.132	0.153
4.00	0.041	0.049	0.059	0.070	0.081	0.094	0.110	0.128	0.149	0.173	0.201
5.00	0.051	0.062	0.074	0.087	0.102	0.118	0.138	0.160	0.186	0.216	0.251
6.00	0.062	0.074	0.088	0.104	0.122	0.141	0.164	0.191	0.221	0.257	0.298
7.00	0.071	0.086	0.102	0.120	0.141	0.163	0.190	0.220	0.255	0.297	0.344
8.00	0.082	0.099	0.117	0.138	0.161	0.187	0.217	0.252	0.291	0.337	0.390
9.00	0.092	0.110	0.131	0.154	0.180	0.209	0.242	0.281	0.324	0.375	0.433
10.00	0.102	0.122	0.145	0.171	0.199	0.231	0.268	0.310	0.357	0.413	0.476
11.00	0.112	0.134	0.159	0.187	0.218	0.253	0.293	0.339	0.391	0.451	0.520
12.00	0.122	0.146	0.173	0.204	0.238	0.276	0.319	0.369	0.425	0.490	0.564
13.00	0.132	0.158	0.187	0.220	0.257	0.296	0.344	0.397	0.457	0.527	0.605
14.00	0.142	0.170	0.201	0.237	0.276	0.319	0.369	0.426	0.490	0.563	0.647
15.00	0.152	0.181	0.215	0.252	0.294	0.340	0.393	0.453	0.521	0.598	0.687
16.00	0.162	0.193	0.229	0.269	0.313	0.362	0.418	0.482	0.553	0.635	0.728
17.00	0.171	0.205	0.242	0.285	0.331	0.383	0.442	0.509	0.584	0.670	0.767
18.00	0.181	0.216	0.256	0.300	0.349	0.404	0.466	0.536	0.615	0.704	0.806
19.00	0.191	0.228	0.270	0.317	0.368	0.426	0.491	0.564	0.646	0.740	0.846
20.00	0.200	0.239	0.282	0.331	0.385	0.445	0.512	0.589	0.674	0.771	0.881

*Edge thickness is measured perpendicularly to the chord diameter of the lens.

†For minus-powered lenses, values shown serve to increase the edge thickness of the lens over the center thickness. For minus lenses, increase thickness by the following amount for each 0.1 mm of center thickness: 0.002 0.003 0.004 0.005 0.006 0.007 0.008 0.009 0.011 0.013. For plus-powered lenses, values shown serve to decrease the edge thickness of the lens over the center thickness. For plus lenses, do not modify values given for center thickness as is done for minus lenses—this chart for plus lenses is based upon the minimum lens thickness for the powers and diameters shown.

‡This chart was calculated for a base curve of 7.6 mm. However, there is only a small change in values as the base curve is changed; therefore the chart is valid for base curves 7.2 to 8.0 mm. As the base curve is made steeper, the values shown increase; as the base curve is made flatter, the values shown decrease.

ESTIMATING VISUAL LOSS

Loss of central vision in one eye

Visual acuity for distance (Snellen)	Snellen	Meters (D)	Jaeger	Percent visual efficiency*	Percent visual loss
20/20	14/14	0.35	1−	100	0
20/25	14/18	0.44	2−	96	4
20/30	14/21	0.59	—	91	9
20/40	14/28	0.71	3	84	16
20/50	14/35	0.88	6	77	23
20/60	14/42	1.08	—	70	30
20/70	14/49	1.30	7	64	36
20/80	14/56	—	8	59	41
20/100	14/70	1.76	11	49	51
20/160	14/112	—	14−	29	71
20/200	14/140	3.53	—	20	80
20/400	14/280	7.06	—	3	97

*The percentage of visual efficiency of the two eyes may be determined by the following formula:

$$\frac{(3 \times \% \text{ visual efficiency of better eye}) + \% \text{ visual efficiency of poorer eye}}{4} = \% \text{ binocular visual efficiency}$$

Estimating loss of visual field. A visual field test is performed on the perimeter with a 3 mm test object in each of the eight 45-degree meridians. The sum of each of these meridians is added and the percentage of visual efficiency is arrived at when one divides by 485, the total of a normal field. For example:

Normal field	Degrees
Temporally	85
Down and temporally	85
Down	55
Nasally	55
Up and nasally	55
Down and nasally	50
Up	45
Up and temporally	55
TOTAL	485

Constricted field	Degrees
Temporally	45
Down and temporally	25
Down	30
Down and nasally	25
Nasally	25
Up and nasally	25
Up	25
Up and temporally	35
TOTAL	235

% visual efficiency	$\dfrac{235 \times 100}{485} = 46\%$

Estimating loss of muscle function. To determine the degree of visual efficiency lost from diplopia, diplopia fields are measured on the perimeter at 33 cm or on the tangent screen to

From Stein, H.A., and Slatt, B.J.: The opththalmic assistant, ed. 4, St. Louis, 1982, The C.V. Mosby Co.

determine the disability from the double vision.

Diplopia within the central 20 degrees in the straight-ahead position represents 100% loss of visual efficiency of one eye. In the regions beyond 20 degrees the loss of visual efficiency is dependent on the position of gaze. Looking straight down in an area between 20 and 30 degrees would represent a loss of 50%, whereas looking up in the same area between 20 and 30 degrees (a region not commonly used for visual activity) would represent only a 10% loss of visual efficiency. Looking to the sides between 20 and 30 degrees would repesent a 20% loss of visual efficiency of the eye.

In more peripheral zones, where the eyes normally do not function, visual loss from diplopia would be less. For example, looking down between 30 and 40 degrees would represent a 30% loss of visual efficiency, and looking to the sides between 30 and 40 degrees would represent only a 10% loss of visual efficiency.

DRUGS COMMONLY USED IN OPHTHALMOLOGY

Drug	Strength	Container size
Glaucoma medications to improve outflow		
Adsorbocarpine	1%, 2%, 4%	15 ml plastic dropper bottle
Carcholin Powder		0.5 g bottles
Cellucarpine Solution		15 ml bottles
E-Carpine Solution	1%, 2%, 3%, 4%, 6%	15 ml dropper bottle
E-Pilo Solution	1%, 2%, 3%, 4%, 6%	10 ml plastic dropper bottles
Floropryl Solution and Ointment	0.1%	3.5 g tubes
Humorsol Solution	0.125%, 0.25%	5 ml vials with dropper
Isopto Carpine Solution	0.5%, 1%, 2%, 3%, 4%, 6%	15 and 30 ml plastic Drop-Tainer
Isopto Carbachol Solution	0.75%, 1.5%, 2.25%, 3%	15 ml Drop-Tainer
Isopto Eserine Solution	0.25%, 0.5%	15 ml Drop-Tainer
Isopto P-ES Solution		15 ml Drop-Tainer
Miocarpine Solution	0.5%, 1%, 2%, 3%, 4%, 6%	15 and 30 ml plastic bottles
Ocusert Pilo 20		Packages of 8 units
Ocusert Pilo 40		Packages of 8 units
P_2E_1 and P_4E_1 Solutions	2%, 4%	10 and 12.5 ml plastic drops vials
P.V. Carpine Liquifilm Solution	0.5%, 1%, 2%, 3%, 4%, 6%	15 ml plastic dropper
Phospholine Iodide Solution	0.06%, 0.125%, 0.25%	
Pilocar Solution	0.5%, 1%, 2%, 3%, 4%, 6%	15 ml plastic dropper bottles
Pilocel Solution	0.25%, 0.5%, 1%, 2%, 3%, 6%	15 ml plastic container
Pilofrin Solution	0.5%, 1%, 2%, 3%, 4%, 6%	15 ml plastic dropper bottles
Propine	0.1%	10 ml plastic dropper bottles
Glaucoma medications to decrease inflow and improve outflow		
Epifrin Solution	0.25%, 0.5%, 1%, 2%	5 and 15 ml plastic dropper bottles
Epinal Solution	0.25%, 0.5%, 1%	7.5 ml Drop-Tainer
Eppy/N Solution	½%, 1%	7.5 ml dropper bottles
Glaucon Solution	½%, 1%, 2%	10 ml dropper bottles
Propine	0.1%	10 ml dropper bottles
Timoptic	0.25%, 0.5%	5 and 10 ml dispenser
Betagen	0.5%	5 and 10 ml dispenser
Betoptic	0.5%	5 cc

Drug	Strength	Container size
Hyperosmotic agents		
Glycerol (50%)	1 to 1.5 g/kg body weight	
Mannitol (20%)	1 to 2 g/kg body weight	
Urea (30%)	1 to 2 g/kg body weight	
Solutions and ointments to dilate the pupil		
Atropine Sulfate Ointment	0.5%, 1%	3.5 g tubes
Atropine Sulfate Solution	1%, 2%	15 ml plastic dropper bottles
Atropisol Aqueous and Oil Solution	0.5%, 1%, 2%, 3%, 4%	5 ml dropper bottles
Cyclogyl Solution	0.5%, 1%, 2%	15 ml dropper bottles
Cyclomydril Solution	2%	2 and 7.5 ml bottles
Homatropine	2%, 5%	15 ml plastic dropper bottles
Isopto Atropine Solution	0.5%, 1%, 2%	5 and 15 ml Drop-Tainer
Isopto Homatropine Solution	2%, 5%	5 and 15 ml Drop-Tainer
Isopto Hyoscine Solution	0.25%	5 and 15 ml Drop-Tainer
Mydplegic Solution	1%	15 ml plastic dropper bottles
Mydriacyl Solution	0.5%, 1%, 2%	15 ml dropper bottles
Mydfrin	2.5%	5 ml dropper bottles
Neo-Synephrine	2.5%, 10%	30 ml and 5 ml bottles
Paredrine Solution	1%	15 ml dropper bottles
Phenoptic	5%, 10%	5 ml plastic bottles
Scopolamine Ointment	0.2%	⅛ oz tubes
Scopolamine Solution	0.25%	15 ml plastic dropper bottles
Decongestants		
Albalon A		15 ml plastic dropper bottles
Degest 2		15 ml plastic dropper bottles
Isopto Frin Solution	0.12%	15 ml Drop-Tainer
Neo-Propisol Solution		15 ml Steri-Tainer
Neo-Synephrine Solution	0.125%, 2.5%, 10%	15 ml plastic container
Neozin Solution	0.125%	15 ml plastic container
Prefrin-A Solution		15 ml bottle
Prefrin Liquifilm Solution		15 ml plastic dropper bottles
Prefrin-Z Liquifilm		15 ml plastic dropper bottles
Privine Solution	0.1%	15 ml dropper bottles
Soothe Solution	0.125%	15 ml plastic dropper bottle
Tear-Efrin Solution	0.12%	15 ml Lacrivials
Vasoclear		15 ml dropper bottles
Vasocon Regular Solution		15 ml plastic squeeze bottles
Visine Solution	0.05%	15 ml dropper bottles
Zincfrin A Solution	0.25%	15 ml Drop-Tainer
Antihistaminics		
Albalon A		15 ml dropper bottles
Antistine Solution		15 ml dropper bottles
Prefrin-A Solution		15 ml plastic dropper bottles
Vasocon-A Solution		15 ml plastic dropper bottles
Vernacel Solution		15 ml plastic containers
Zincfrin A Solution		15 ml dropper bottles
Steroids		
Cortamed Solution	2.5%	10 ml bottle
Cortril Ointment	0.5%, 2.5%	⅛ oz ophthalmic tipped tubes
Decadron Solution and Ointment		2.5 and 5 ml bottles
Econopred Solution	⅛%, 1%	5 ml bottle
FML Liquifilm Suspension		5, 10, 15 ml plastic dropper bottle
HMS Liquifilm Suspension		5 and 10 ml plastic dropper bottle

Drug	Strength	Container size
Hydeltra Ointment and Solution		Ointment: 3.5 g tubes Solution: 2.5 and 5 ml dropper bottles
Hydrocortone Ointment and Suspension	1.5%, 0.5%, 0.25%	Ointment: 3.5 g tubes Suspension: 5 ml dropper bottles
Inflamase Forte Solution	1%	5 ml dropper bottles
Inflamase Solution	⅛%	5 ml dropper bottles
Isopto Hydrocortisone Suspension	0.5%, 2.5%	5 ml Drop-Tainer
Maxidex Suspension	1%	5 ml plastic Drop-Tainer
Medrysone Solution	1%	5 and 10 ml plastic bottles
Penthasone Solution	0.1%	5 ml bottle
Pred Forte Suspension	1%	5 and 10 ml plastic dropper bottles
Pred Mild Solution	0.12%	5 and 10 ml plastic dropper bottles

Combinations of steroids with sulfonamides or antibiotics

Drug	Strength	Container size
Blephamide Liquifilm Suspension	5 and 10 ml plastic dropper bottles	
Blephamide ointment		3.5 g tubes
Celestone-S		2.5 and 5 ml dropper bottles
Cetapred Ointment		3.5 g tubes
Chloromycetin hydrocortisone suspension		5 ml bottle with droppers
Chloroptic-P ointment		3.5 g tube
Cortisporin ointment and suspension		Ointment: ⅛ oz tubes Suspension: 5 ml dropper bottles
Isopto Cetapred suspension		5 and 15 ml Drop-Tainer
Maxitrol suspension and ointment		Suspension: 5 ml plastic bottles Ointment: 3.5 g tubes
Metimyd with neomycin ointment		⅛ oz tubes
Metimyd suspension		5 ml dropper bottles
Metreton suspension		5 ml dropper bottles
Neo-Aristocort ointment		⅛ oz tubes
Neo-Cortef drops and ointment	0.5%, 1.5%	Drops: 0.5% in 5 ml dropper bottles 1.5% in 2.5 and 5 ml dropper bottles
Neo-Decadron ointment and solution		Ointment: 3.5 g tubes Solution: 2.6 and 5 ml dropper bottles
Neo-Deltef solution		2.5 ml plastic dropper bottles
Neo-Medrol ointment	0.1%	⅛ oz tubes
PolyPred		5 ml plastic dropper bottles
Predmycin solution		5 ml plastic dropper bottles
Sulfapred suspension		5 ml plastic containers
Terra-Cortril suspension		5 ml dropper bottles
Vasocidin solution		5 ml plastic dropper-tipped vials

Sulfonamides

Drug	Strength	Container size
Bleph-10 and Bleph-30 Liquifilm solutions	10%, 30%	5 and 15 ml plastic dropper bottles
Bleph 10 ointment	10%	3.5 g tubes
Cetamide ointment	10%	3.5 g tubes
Gantrisin solution and ointment	4%	Solution: 5 and 15 ml dropper bottles Ointment: ⅛ oz applicator tubes

Drug	Strength	Container size
Isopto Cetamide solution	15%	5 ml dropper bottles and 15 ml Drop-Tainer
Suladrin ointment		3.5 g tubes
Sulamyd ointment and solution	10%, 30%	Solution: 15 ml dropper bottles
		Ointment: ⅛ oz tubes
Sulfacidin solution	10%	7.5 ml Lacrivials
Vasosulf solution	15%	15 ml plastic dropper bottles

Antibiotics

Aureomycin ointment and solution	0.5%, 1%	Ointment: ⅛ oz tubes
		Solution: 5 ml bottles
Achromycin suspension	1.0%	4 ml plastic bottles
Chloromycetin drops and ointment		Solution: 15 ml dropper bottles
		Ointment: ⅛ oz tube
Chloromycetin-polymyxin ointment		⅛ oz tubes
Chloroptic solution and ointment		Solution: 0.5% in 10 ml plastic bottles
		Ointment: 1% in 3.5 g tubes
Fenicol ointment	1%	3.5 g tubes
Garamycin solution and ointment		Solutin: 5 ml dropper bottles
		Ointment: ⅛ oz tubes
Genoptic solution		5 ml plastic dropper bottles
Genoptic ointment		3.5 g tubes
Ilotycin ointment		⅛ oz tubes
Isopto Fenicol solution	0.25%	5 ml dropper bottles
Neo-Polycin ointment and solution		Solution: 10 ml dropper bottles
		Ointment: ⅛ oz tubes
Neosporin ointment and solution		Solution: 10 ml bottle with dropper
		Ointment: ⅛ oz tubes
Pentamycetin solution and ointment		Solution: 10 ml dropper bottle
		Ointment: ⅛ oz tube
Polyspectrin Liquifilm		10 ml dropper bottles
Polyspectrin ointment		⅛ oz tubes
Polysporin ointment		⅛ oz tubes
Spectrocin ointment		⅛ oz tubes
Statrol solution		5 ml dropper bottles
Sulfacidin solution		10 ml Lacrivials and 1 ml Droperettes
Terramycin solution		5 ml dropper vials
Terramycin-polymixin ointment		⅛ oz tubes
Tobrex solution		5 ml dropper vials

Antivirals

Dendrid solution	0.1%	15 ml dropper bottles
Herplex solution and ointment	0.1%	Solution: 15 ml plastic dropper bottles
		Ointment: ⅛ oz tubes
Stoxil solution	0.1%	15 ml dropper bottles
Viroptic (trifluridine)	1%	5 ml dropper bottles

Antifungal

Natacyn	5%	15 ml glass bottles

Antibacterial and steroid combinations

Achromycin ointment		⅛ oz tubes
Blephamide Liquifilm Suspension		5 ml and 10 ml plastic dropper bottles

Drug	Strength	Container size
Belphamide ointments		3.5 g tubes
Celestone-S suspension		5 ml dropper bottles
Chloromycetin hydrocortisone suspension		5 ml dropper bottles and 5 ml vials
Chloroptic-P ointment		3.5 g tubes
Cortisporin ointment and suspension		Ointment: ⅛ oz tubes
		Suspension: 5 ml dropper bottles
Isopto Cetapred suspension		5 and 15 ml Drop-Tainer
Maxitrol suspension and ointment		Suspension: 5 ml plastic bottles
		Ointment: 3.5 g tubes
Metamyd suspension		5 ml dropper bottles
Metimyd with neomycin ointment		⅛ oz tubes
Neo-Aristocort ointment		⅛ oz tubes
Neo-Cortef drops and ointment	0.5%, 1.5%	Drops: 5 ml dropper bottles
		Ointment: ⅛ oz tubes
Neo-Decadron ointment and solution		Ointment: 3.5 g tubes
		Solution: 2.5 and 5 ml dropper bottles
Neo-Deltef solution		2.5 ml plastic dropper bottles
Neo-Hydeltrasol ointment and solution		Ointment: 3.5 g tubes
		Solution: 2.5 and 5 ml dropper bottles
Ophthocort ointment		⅛ oz tubes
Pentamycetin/hydrocortisone solution and ointment		Solution: 10 ml bottle
		Ointment: ⅛ oz tube
Sulfapred suspension		5 ml plastic containers
Terra-Cortril suspension		5 ml dropper bottles
Vasocidin solution		5 ml plastic dropper vials

Anesthetic, topical

Alcaine	0.5%	15 ml plastic bottles
Cocaine	0.25%, 0.5%	Special preparation
Dibucaine	0.1%	15 ml bottles
Ophthaine solution	0.5%	15 ml plastic bottles
Ophthetic solution	0.5%	15 ml plastic bottles
Pontocaine solution	0.5%	15 ml plastic bottles
Proparacaine solution	0.5%	

Carbonic anhydrase inhibitors

Cardrase		125 mg tablets
Daranide		50 mg tablets
Diamox		250 mg tablets
Ethamide		125 mg tablets
Hydrazol		250 mg tablets
Naptazane		50 mg tablets
Oratrol		50 mg tablets

Miscellaneous

Adsorbonac solution	2%, 5%	15 ml plastic dropper bottle
Adsorbotear solution		15 ml plastic dropper bottle
Balanced salt solution		15 ml bottles
Blinx liquid solution		30 ml bottles
Carbachol, intraocular		5 ml bottles
Catarase suspension		3 ml vials
Dacriose irrigating solution		120 ml irrigating bottles
Degest-2		0.5 ml bottles
Duratears		3.5 g tubes
Enuclene solution		15 ml plastic dropper bottles
Estivin solution		¼ oz dropper bottles

Drug	Strength	Container size
Fluorescite solution	5%	10 ml ampules
Fulgo (sodium fluorescein strips)		
Fluress solution		5 ml bottles
Gonio-gel	2.5%	3.5 g tubes
Hypotears		14 ml dropper bottles
Isopto tears	0.5%, 1%	15 ml Drop-Tainer
Lacril artificial tears	0.5%	15 ml plastic dropper bottles
Lacri-Lube ointment		⅛ oz tube
Liquifilm Forte Solution		15 ml dropper bottle
Liquifilm tears	1.4%	15 and 30 ml plastic dropper bottles
Lyteers drops		15 ml dropper bottles
Methisol solution		15 ml plastic bottles
Methulose solution		15 ml plastic bottles
Murocel	1%	15 and 30 ml plastic dropper bottles
Muro 128	5%	15 and 30 ml plastic dropper bottles
Miochol		3 ml vials
Neotears		15 ml bottles
Normal solution		30 ml bottles
Tearisol solution		15 ml Lacrivials
Tears naturale		15 ml plastic dropper bottles
Tears plus		15 ml plastic dropper bottles
Vas-I-Zinc solution		15 ml plastic bottles
Zolyse solution		Unit cartons

SHORT FORMS IN CLINICAL USE

Acc.	accommodation	RH	right hyperphoria
add	addition	LH	left hyperphoria
o.d., OD	right eye *(oculus dexter)*	P.D. or IPD	interpupillary distance
o.s., OS	left eye *(oculus sinister)*	NPA	near point of accommodation
o.u., OU	each eye, both eyes *(oculus uterque)*	NPC	near point of convergence
RE	right eye	MR	medial rectus (muscle)
LE	left eye	LR	lateral rectus (muscle)
NV	near vision	SR	superior rectus (muscle)
PH	pinhole	IR	inferior rectus (muscle)
V	vision or visual acuity	SO	superior oblique (muscle)
mm	millimeter	IO	inferior oblique (muscle)
mg	milligram	BO	base out
SC	without correction	BI	base in
CC	with correction	BD	base down
HM	hand movements	BU	base up
LP	light perception	NRC	normal retinal correspondence
MR	Maddox rod	ARC	abnormal retinal correspondence
L & A	light and accommodation	J1, J2, J3, etc.	test types for reading vision
EOMB	extraocular muscle balance	N5, N6, etc.	test types for near vision
EOM	extraocular movements	b.i.d., b.d.	twice daily
CF	counting fingers	t.i.d., t.d.	three times daily
XP	exophoria	q.i.d.	four times daily
XT	exotropia	a.c.	before meals
W	wearing	p.c.	after meals
IOP	intraocular pressure	i.c.	between meals
T	tension	ne rep. or non rep.	do not repeat
ung	ointment		
A	applanation tensions	oculent	eye ointment
KP	keratitic precipitates	per os	orally, by mouth
PSC	posterior subcapsular cataract	p.r.n.	when required, as necessary
ASC	anterior subcapsular cataract	q.h.	every hour
ET	esotropia	q.2h.	every 2 hours
°	degree	q.s.	quantity sufficient
Δ	prism diopter	stat.	at once
D	diopter		

From Stein, H.A., and Slatt, B.J.: The ophthalmic assistant, ed. 4, St. Louis, 1982, The C.V. Mosby Co.

The following abbreviations may be found on ophthalmic charts:

VA	visual acuity	S or sph	spheric lens
VAc or VAcc	visual acuity with correction	C or cyl	cylinder lens
		$\frown$	combined with
VAs̄ or VAsc	visual acuity without correction	∞	infinity
		E_1	esophoria for distance
VA =	visual acuity with the unaided eye	E^1	esophoria for near range
OT	ocular tension	ET_1	esotropia for distance
AT or Appl	applanation tension	ET^1	esotropia for near range
		X_1	exophoria for distance
ST	Schiøtz tension	X^1	exophoria for near range
EOM	extraocular muscle	E(T)	intermittent esotropia
Pr	presbyopia	X(T)	intermittent exotropia
PRRE	pupils round, regular, and equal	dd	disc diameters

VISION AND DRIVING

Good vision is essential for the proper and safe operation of a motor vehicle. Generally, available vision-testing instruments can be used to ascertain if a person has adequate vision to meet specific standards set by the various state licensing jurisdictions. Because of the increasing injury and death toll resulting from traffic crashes, many of which may be related to visual impairment, physicians should consider it a medical obligation to diagnose visual deficiencies and to inform the patient of potential hazards involved in driving with such deficiencies.

There is no practical way of testing alertness or cerebral perception of what the eye focuses on, but it is important for drivers to have their eyes periodically examined for defects that can be evaluated. This is particularly important for those drivers with significant progressive visual deterioration.

In general, if any doubt exists about a person's visual ability to operate an automobile safely, the physician should not hesitate to recommend road tests for specific evaluation of visual skills.

Visual acuity. Automobile drivers with corrected central visual acuity of 20/40 or better generally read traffic signs and note obstructions, vehicles, and pedestrians while driving at usual speeds, whereas those with optimally corrected vision of 20/70 or less in the better eye have a serious limitation and should not drive.

Adapted from the American Medical Association: Physician's guide for determining driver limitation, Chicago, 1968, The Association.

Drivers with visual acuity between 20/40 and 20/70 should be referred to an ophthalmologist to ascertain if their vision can be improved. The physician, in serving the best interests of patients, should consider the conditions under which each patient drives and the presence or absence of associated defects. The physician is then in a position to advise the patient against driving under certain conditions, such as congested traffic, hazardous road conditions, bad weather, high speed, or at night. It is hoped that continuing research will more exactly define the criteria on which to advise patients.

One-eyed drivers and spectacle-corrected aphakic drivers have visual field limitations and present an increased risk of intersectional crashes. Most postoperative aphakic patients, particularly those in advanced years, also have increased difficulty with night vision and dynamic visual responses. They require special evaluation. Preoperative cataract patients, with early to moderate changes in the lenses of the eye, similarly have night-driving limitations (glare intolerance and reduced night vision) that generally preclude night driving. Patients requiring pupil-constricting medication, as in the control of chronic glaucoma, also have limitation for night operation.

Visual fields. Visual fields are obviously important for safe driving, since a driver must of necessity possess some breadth or lateral awareness to pass approaching vehicles safely and to be aware of vehicles or pedestrians approaching from the side.

Although visual form fields of 140 degrees generally are considered adequate for drivers of private motor vehicles, that figure should be considered as the absolute minimum for drivers of commercial and passenger-carrying vehicles. Such drivers also must have coordinate use of both eyes, as well as a corrected acuity of at least 20/30 in the better eye and no worse than 20/40 in the poorer eye. Persons with lesser fields have driver limitation and must be evaluated for the driving of private vehicles on the basis of the conditions under which they drive, the amount of lateral vision retained, and underlying ocular pathologic condition.

Persons with greatly constricted fields, such as those from advanced glaucoma or retinitis pigmentosa, have distinct driver limitation and should be so advised.

Ocular muscle imbalance. Ocular muscle imbalance (heterophoria) is an indirect cause of automotive crashes in that it may cause driver fatigue. If sudden diplopia occurs, the crash may be directly attributable to the diplopia. Therefore, patients with uncontrolled or intermittent diplopia have definite driver limitation.

Color blindness. Impaired or defective color vision has been considered a potential cause of highway accidents. However, most traffic lights have been standardized, at least regionally; and it is doubtful if this deficiency is too hazardous, except in severe cases. A completely color-blind, or achromatic, individual has very poor vision and should not drive under any circumstance. This also applies to the very limited number of individuals who have severe protanopia, or red deficiency.

Dark adaptation. Dark adaptation and susceptibility to glare are of great importance in night driving, but testing procedures and standards are still largely empiric and not a component of routine eye tests. Dark glasses should never be worn for night driving, and windshield tinting should be limited to the upper one third.

Depth perception. Current testing techniques in the near range do not have significant correlation with distance visual requirements in driving but are adequate for determining visual ability for such tasks as parking. The road test, however, is still the best and most practical guide in this area.

AMERICAN ACADEMY OF OPHTHALMOLOGY'S POLICY REGARDING THE USE OF CONTACT LENSES IN AN INDUSTRIAL ENVIRONMENT

POLICY

Except for unusual situations in which there exists significant risk of ocular damage, individuals should not be disqualified from industrial employment because they wear contact lenses.

BACKGROUND

Patients who wear contact lenses (either for cosmetic or medical reasons) have been disqualified from industrial employment.

Some individuals must wear contact lenses for medical reasons to obtain their best visual performance. An example would be a young monocular aphakic who needs to wear a contact lens in order to obtain binocular vision.

EVALUATION

Recognizing this problem, to assist industry, the Contact Lens Association of Ophthalmologists, and the National Society to Prevent Blindness, have adopted a position paper which defines a reasonable policy, based on current scientific information.

POSITION

Safety and/or medical personnel should not disqualify an employee who can achieve visual rehabilitation by contact lenses, either in job placement or return to a job category. Rather,

Developed by Ophthalmic Contact Lenses Subcommittee, Ophthalmic Instruments and Devices Committee. Approved by Board of Directors, Nov. 1, 1980.

employees whose central and peripheral vision can be increased by the wearing of contact lenses, as contrasted to spectacle lenses, should be encouraged to wear contact lenses in industrial environments, in combination with appropriate industrial safety eyewear,* except where there is likelihood of injury from intense heat, massive chemical splash, highly particulate atmosphere, or where federal regulations‡ prohibit such use. Safety and/or medical personnel should determine on an individual basis the advisability of wearing contact lenses in jobs which require unique visual performance, based on consideration of Occupational Safety and Health Administration (OSHA) and National Institute of Occupational Safety and Health (NIOSH) recommendations.†

Employees who do wear contact lenses should be identified and known to their employer. All first aid personnel should be trained in the proper removal of contact lenses. Employees wearing contact lenses should be required to keep a spare pair of contacts and/or prescription spectacles in their possession on the job to avoid an inability to function if they should damage or lose a contact lens while working.

*ANSI, Z80.1, 1979, or as subsequently amended.
†Federal Register, Vol. 36, No. 106, Part II 1910. 134(e)(5)(ii) page 10591, Saturday, May 29, 1971. NIOSH/OSHA Pocket Guide to Chemical Hazards. (DHEW, Publication No. 78210.)

CLAO POLICY ON EXTENDED WEAR OF CONTACT LENSES (ADOPTED APRIL 1987)

INTRODUCTION

The Contact Lens Association of Ophthalmologists (CLAO) recognizes that there are many patients who desire safe, comfortable and extended wear of contact lenses. Such convenience provides almost "normal" vision at all times. Extended wear lenses are an alternative to refractive surgery. However, the prolonged use of hydrogel contact lenses without a "rest" creates a metabolic stress to the eye, particularly during the closed-eye state of sleep. This stress (from a reduced oxygen supply to the cornea) predisposes the eye to infrequent, but serious, side effects such as corneal infection.

BACKGROUND

Due to technological progress in polymer chemistry and lens manufacturing methods, soft contact lenses can be made to permit sufficient diffusion of oxygen and carbon dioxide to allow lenses to be worn on an extended wear basis. However, none of the presently available hydrogel lenses deliver enough oxygen to the cornea in the closed-eye state to prevent corneal edema and relative hypoxia. There is much physiological variation among patients as to the stress of continuous wear lenses. Unfortunately, it is not possible to avoid all adverse reactions or to predict which patients will have problems.

A significant difficulty with extended wear (or daily wear) contact lenses is deposit formation. Debris from the atmosphere and chemical components from the tear film tend to be deposited on these lenses. The deposits may change the oxygen transmissibility of the lenses, the fitting characteristics, and/or the tendency toward adherence of microorganisms to the lens surface.

PATIENT ADVICE AND MANAGEMENT

Practitioners assuming the responsibility for fitting extended wear contact lenses should do so in carefully selected and monitored patients. Emphatic and thorough instructions, both oral and written, should be given to the patients, namely:

1. Have the patient remove the lenses for an overnight period at reasonable intervals he or she will accept (once a week can be suggested on an experimental basis).
2. Instruct patients to use an approved cleaning system (which should include a surfactant, a sterile saline rinse, an enzymatic cleaner, and lubricating drops), an approved disinfection system (preferably one of the hydrogen peroxide systems with high water content lenses, and heat with low water content contact lenses). **Homemade saline, distilled water, tap water, or saliva must not be used for any step of lens care.**
3. Recommend frequent replacement of lenses. (Recommendations vary from every 3 months to once a year.)
4. Instruct patients to immediately remove the lenses in case of any unusual redness, irritation, blurred vision, or pain.

POLICY

The extended wear contact lens is a major technological development that has fulfilled a need for many patients. In the future, the safety of these lenses may be improved as new lenses with sufficient oxygen transmissibility for the cornea are developed.

The incidence of severe ocular damage from

extended wear lens use is increased by inadequate patient instruction, lack of patient compliance and insufficient professional supervision. The fitting of extended wear lenses and monitoring of patients should be performed by those who have the professional training and experience to recognize and treat the potential complications. Appropriate care of the lenses, according to the practitioner's instructions and within the approved criteria issued by the U.S. Food and Drug Administration, will also lessen the incidence of ocular complications. Any patient experiencing a red, painful eye should seek professional medical care without delay. While extended wear is a useful method of correcting vision, caution and close assessment of the individual patient is essential.

CLAO POLICY ON ARC WELDING AND CONTACT LENSES

POLICY

Exposure to electric arc welding is not associated with an increased risk of ocular damage in individuals who wear contact lenses. To date, no significant risk has been demonstrated by any experimental study. Furthermore, alleged instances of "the cornea fusing to the lens with loss of ocular tissue when the contact lens was removed" have **not** been substantiated.

Individuals exposed to electric arc welding should take the usual precautions, such as wearing goggles. However, individuals who wear contact lenses are not subject to increased risk and should not be subjected to job discrimination.

BACKGROUND

In 1967 there were allegedly two incidents of contact lens wearers being rendered blind due to contact lenses fusing to their corneas after exposure to electric arc welding. Investigation of the two reported incidents has revealed that in one instance the injured employee never worked for AIRCO Welding Products and that in the other instance the patient over-wore contact lenses prior to reporting to work as a welder. The latter incident occurred at the Bethlehem Steel Corp. plant in Baltimore, MD and involved a welder who wore both contact lenses and industrial safety glasses. He had worn his contact lenses for twelve hours prior to reporting to work. At work, while plugging welding units into a 440-volt service line, an electrical switch box exploded. The patient sustained corneal abrasions, which were treated in the usual man-

ner. The contact lenses did not fuse to his corneas. His vision returned to normal within several days. The two ophthalmologists who treated the worker reported that the electrical flash "had no part" in causing the injury. They attributed it to "neglect by the patient, absence of elementary precautions, and overwear of the contact lenses."

In 1983 these cases were cited in several safety bulletins that were widely distributed throughout the United States. Soon thereafter, there appeared a safety bulletin with similar accounts of injuries allegedly sustained by industrial workers in Pittsburgh (at Duquesne Electric, where a worker is said to have thrown an electrical power switch and caused a spark) and at United Parcel Service (where a welder supposedly produced an electrical arc). In both cases, the bulletin claims, the microwaves produced by the electrical arc, or spark, dried up the fluid between the eye and the contact lens, causing the workers' contact lenses to be fused to the corneas of their eyes—resulting in permanent blindness. Spokespersons for Duquesne Electric and United Parcel Service have stated that no such accidents ever occurred at their facilities.

SUMMARY

Electric arc welding is not associated with increased risk to contact lens patients. In an effort to prevent job discrimination, it is in the public interest for CLAO to provide correct information to the national media.

ACANTHAMOEBA KERATITIS

CLAO Policy Statement
Revised May 1989

BACKGROUND

Initially reported in 1974, *Acanthamoeba* keratitis is a potentially blinding disease produced by a free-living amoeba commonly found in water and soil. From 1974 to 1984 approximately 10 cases were reported. None of these patients wore contact lenses, and their infections appear to have been the result of direct minor trauma from a contaminated foreign object. Since 1984 there have been over 100 new cases reported, 90% of which have occurred in contact lens wearers. Although the majority of contact lens wearing patients in whom *Acanthamoeba* keratitis was found wore soft contact lenses, the disease has occurred in wearers of hard lenses, rigid gas-permeable lenses, and combined hard and soft lenses.

The source of *Acanthamoeba* keratitis in contact lens wearers was frequently traced to contamination of contact lens solutions, most often homemade saline solutions prepared from distilled or tap water and salt tablets. These solutions became contaminated with *Acanthamoeba*, which presumably then contaminated the contact lens. It is not known whether *Acanthamoeba* requires a break in the corneal epithelium to establish itself in the eye; however it is known that microtrauma from a contact lens can contribute to other types of corneal infection.

It is presumed that patients who wear hard contact lenses and who rinse their lenses in tap water (which can harbor *Acanthamoeba*) are also at risk for *Acanthamoeba* keratitis.

EVALUATION/CLINICAL CHARACTERISTICS

Acanthamoeba keratitis is a slowly progressive, usually non-suppurative keratitis with a waxing and waning course. It can be very difficult to treat. *Acanthamoeba* keratitis should be considered in the differential diagnosis of any patient with a history of contact lens wear and a keratitis that is unresponsive to the usual treatment. The presence of pseudodendrites in a patient with a non-suppurative keratitis can lead to the most frequent misdiagnosis; herpes simplex keratitis.

Typically, in *Acanthamoeba* infection stromal keratitis will progress to form a ring in the mid-periphery of the cornea. As the disease progresses suppurative keratitis and stromal melting can occur, with ultimate descemetocele formation or perforation of the cornea. Anterior chamber reaction is typically very mild early in the course, although with further progress of the disease hypopyon has been reported.

Extreme eye pain, reported by most *Acanthamoeba* keratitis patients, is one hallmark of the condition. Indeed, the pain, which can be debilitating, may seem out of proportion to the severity of the keratitis. Another hallmark of the condition is the presence of infiltrates along the corneal nerves; these may be seen either early in the disease or later in its course, following the development of a ring infiltrate. The waxing and waning course of the disease may be due to topical steroid therapy that can partially suppress the host response; or it may be due to the natural encystation-excystation cycle. Most often unilateral, *Acanthamoeba* keratitis can also be bilateral. In the earliest reported cases loss of the affected eye was frequent.

LABORATORY DIAGNOSIS

In *Acanthamoeba* keratitis bacterial, viral, and fungal cultures will be negative. This finding should alert the practitioner to the possibility of another etiology for the condition.

To make direct smears from an abnormal corneal epithelium, the cornea may be vigorously scraped and the corneal material placed on alcohol-cleaned glass slides. The slides, which should be immediately fixed with 95% alcohol, can be stained with Gram, Wright's, Giemsa, or trichrome stain. Irrespective of the stain used, the trophozoite will be more difficult to see than the cyst. Experience is required to detect the presence of either form in smears; and both are easily missed by someone who has not seen them before.

For culture, material may be inoculated directly into Page's saline from a swab (premoistened with the saline) that has been used to scrub the cornea. Page's saline will support *Acanthamoeba* organisms during transport to the laboratory for inoculation onto special culture plates.

Acanthamoeba survive by ingesting bacteria, fungi, and unicellular organisms. To grow *Acanthamoeba* in culture, non-nutrient agar plates coated with a layer of *E. coli* or *Enterobacter* spp. are used. (The bacteria provide food for the *Acanthamoeba*. Non-nutrient agar is used to prevent the bacteria from overwhelming the *Acanthamoeba*.) If *Acanthamoeba* are present, the cysts will excyst to become tropozoites; these will move across the surface of the plate, devouring the bacteria that lie in their path and leaving "tracks" that are best seen by phase contrast microscopy. Some investigators have reported seeing these trophozoite "tracks" on blood agar plates.

The preparation and cultivation of *Acanthamoeba* cultures is a difficult process that requires an experienced technician. **Negative cultures and scrapings do NOT rule out the diagnosis of *Acanthamoeba* keratitis.**

If the corneal involvement is deep and the overlying epithelium is normal, diagnosis may require that a corneal biopsy be performed. Additional tests that help support diagnosis include culturing the contact lenses and the saline solution or distilled water used to prepare homemade saline. Large volumes of solution may be passed through a Millipore filter, which can then be inverted into a culture plate.

Viral cultures have in the past been interpreted as positive because of the cytopathic effect of *Acanthamoeba* on cell cultures. Therefore, a "positive" herpes virus culture test does not necessarily prove the presence of a herpes virus keratitis.

THERAPY

Therapy for *Acanthamoeba* keratitis is in the process of evolution. In early reports the diagnosis had been made retrospectively—after enucleation or penetrating keratoplasty had been performed. In the majority of recently reported cases, the diagnosis was not made until 3–6 months after the onset of symptoms, at which time the central cornea was involved. Penetrating keratoplasty was performed in these situations as a debulking and vision restoring procedure.

Recently, heightened awareness of the disease has made possible diagnosis within a few weeks of the onset of symptoms. In some of these cases good results have been obtained using medical treatment alone. Current medical treatment incorporates various combinations of topical propamidine isethionate (Brolene), polymyxin B sulfate-neomycin sulfate-gramicidin (Neosporin), miconazole (Monistat), clotrimazone (Lotrimin), and oral ketoconazole (Nizoral). Because of the persistence of cysts for up to a year in the laboratory (and thus, perhaps, the cornea) medical treatment is continued for at least a year.

The value of penetrating keratoplasty as a debulking procedure and its ideal timing in the course of the disease are unknown at this time. Because recurrences of *Acanthamoeba* keratitis following corneal transplantation can be disastrous, it is necessary to use extreme caution in performing surgery on an eye that has been infected.

POLICY

The Contact Lens Association of Ophthalmologists (CLAO) recognizes that contact lenses are a safe and useful method of correcting vision. However, the increasing recognition of infectious keratitis associated with contact lens wear makes careful handling of contact lenses by patients and practitioners a necessity. With special reference to *Acanthamoeba* keratitis, CLAO suggests the following:

1. Contact lens wearers must be scrupulous in handling, cleaning and disinfecting their lenses. Current contact lens disinfection methods are appropriate for eradicating most pathogens; however, the lens must not be immersed or rinsed in distilled or tap water after the disinfection process is completed and before the lens is inserted in the eye.

Patients who are allergic to preserved saline should use commercially prepared non-preserved saline or preservative-free aerosol saline. **Homemade saline should not be used under any circumstances.**

2. A patient's originally-sterile non-preserved saline may become contaminated after opening. Use of a contaminated solution may expose the patient to a higher risk of developing corneal infection. To reduce this risk, bottled saline solution should be kept refrigerated and should be discarded after 1-2 weeks. Alternatively, patients may use preservative-free aerosol saline, which does not require refrigeration and has a 2-year shelf life. The saline in the contact lens case should be replaced on a daily basis, and the case should be cleaned and stored dry when not in use.

3. The effectiveness of available preservatives for contact lens solutions in eradicating exogenous *Acanthamoeba* trophozoite and cyst contamination has not yet been fully determined and is currently being studied. CLAO supports continuation of this study.

4. Contact lens wearers should avoid wearing their lenses while swimming, soaking in hot tubs, or engaging in water sports. If contact lens are exposed to non-sterile water from these or other sources, they should be appropriately disinfected before further wear.

5. Placing a contact lens in the mouth and then back in the eye is an unsanitary practice that should be avoided. Although it is not known whether contaminating a contact lens with saliva can result in *Acanthamoeba* keratitis, it is known that *Acanthamoeba* can be cultured from the nasopharynx of healthy individuals. Therefore, we advise against placing contact lenses in the mouth.

6. Clinicians who encounter suspected cases of *Acanthamoeba* keratitis should seek the advice of corneal experts familiar with the latest diagnostic and management techniques. (For the names of specialists in your region call the CLAO Hotline at 504/581-4000.)

7. The suggestions in this Policy Statement are based on current information and on the experience of epidemiologists, microbiologists and clinicians. CLAO is exploring the problems posed by *Acanthamoeba* keratitis, including its incidence, pathogenesis, risk factors, treatment, and prevention. The CLAO Hotline (504/581-4000) can be a helpful source of additional information for practitioners.

8. Verified cases of *Acanthamoeba* keratitis should be reported promptly to CLAO (at 504/581-4000) or to G.S. Visvesvara, PhD, at the Centers for Disease Control in Atlanta, GA (404/454-4428).

TRANSLATIONS OF COMMONLY ASKED QUESTIONS AND COMMANDS

English	French
History	
1. What is your name?	1. Quel est votre nom?
2. What is your address?	2. Quelle est votre addresse?
3. When were you born?	3. Quel est votre jour de naissance?
4. What trouble are you having with your eyes?	4. Quel problème avez-vous avec les yeux?
5. Are you having pain?	5. Ça fait mal?
6. Do your eyes itch?	6. Ça pique?
7. Have you had any eye injury?	7. Est-ce que les yeux ont été blessés?
8. Have you had an eye operation?	8. Est-ce que les yeux ont été opérés?
9. Did you get anything in your eye?	9. Y'a-t-il quelque chose dans les yeux?
10. Are you taking any eye drops?	10. Employez-vous des gouttes pour les yeux?
11. Do you have headaches?	11. Avez-vous des maux de têtes?
12. Do you wear glasses?	12. Portez-vous des lunettes?
13. How old are your glasses?	13. Et depuis quand?
14. Do you have trouble reading?	14. Pouvez-vous lire sans difficulté?
15. Do you see double?	15. Voyez-vous double?
16. Do you take pills?	16. Prenez-vous des médicaments?
For: heart	Pour: le coeur
diabetes	le diabète
blood pressure	la tension artérielle
17. Do you have any allergies?	17. Avez-vous des allergies?
To medicine	Aux médicaments?
Others	Ou à des autres choses?
18. Is there a history of diabetes or glaucoma in your family?	18. Y'a-t-il le diabète ou le glaucome dans votre famille?
19. Is there a history of eye problems?	19. Y'a-t-il des problèmes avec les yeux?
Examination	
20. Look straight.	20. Regardez tout droit.
21. Follow my light.	21. Suivez ma lumière.
22. Follow my finger.	22. Suivez mon doigt.
23. Can you count my fingers?	23. Pouvez-vous compter mes doigts?
24. Can you see my hand move?	24. Pouvez-vous voir bouger ma main?
25. Open your eyes. Close your eyes.	25. Ouvrez les yeux. Fermez les yeux.
26. Look at me.	26. Regardez-moi.
27. Is it clear?	27. Est-it clair?
28. Read this.	28. Lisez ça.
29. Which is better, one or two?	29. Le quel est mieux, un ou deux?

Translations of commonly asked questions and commands—**cont'd**

English	German

History

1. What is your name?
2. What is your address?
3. When were you born?
4. What trouble are you having with your eyes?
5. Are you having pain?
6. Do your eyes itch?
7. Have you had any eye injury?
8. Have you had an eye operation?
9. Did you get anything in your eye?
10. Are you taking any eye drops?
11. Do you have headaches?
12. Do you wear glasses?
13. How old are your glasses?
14. Do you have trouble reading?
15. Do you see double?
16. Do you take pills?
    For: heart
    diabetes
    blood pressure
17. Do you have any allergies?
    To medicine
    Others
18. Is there a history of diabetes or glaucoma in your family?
19. Is there a history of eye problems?

Examination

20. Look straight.
21. Follow my light.
22. Follow my finger.
23. Can you count my fingers?
24. Can you see my hand move?
25. Open your eyes. Close your eyes.

26. Look at me.
27. Is it clear?
28. Read this.
29. Which is better, one or two?

---

1. Ihr Name, bitte?
2. Ihre Anschrift, bitte?
3. Ihr Geburtsdatum, bitte?
4. Was für ein Problem haben Sie mit den Augen?
5. Haben Sie Schmerzen?
6. Tun Ihre Augen jucken?
7. Haben Sie mal eine Augenverletzung gehabt?
8. Haben Sie mal eine Augenoperation gehabt?
9. Ist irgendwas in Ihre Augen geraten?
10. Benützen Sie Augentropfen?
11. Haben Sie Kopfschmerzen?
12. Tragen Sie Brillen?
13. Seit wann tragen Sie Brillen?
14. Haben Sie Schwierigkeiten beim Lesen?
15. Sehen Sie doppelt?
16. Nämen Sie Pillen ein?
    Für Herz?
    Zuckerkrankheit
    Blutdruck?
17. Haben Sie irgend Allergien?
    Gegen Medizin?
    Andere Allergien?
18. Laufen Zuckerkrankheit oder Glaucom in Ihre Familie?
19. Laufen Augenkrankheit in Ihre Familie?

20. Schauen Sie gerade aus.
21. Folgen Sie dem Licht.
22. Folgen Sie meinem Finger.
23. Zählen Sie meine Finger.
24. Können Sie Bewegung meiner Hand sehen?
25. Öffnen Sie die Augen. Schliessen Sie die Augen.
26. Schauen Sie mich an.
27. Erscheine ich klar?
28. Lesen Sie dieses.
29. Was ist besser, eins oder zwei?

Continued.

Translations of commonly asked questions and commands—**cont'd**

English	Italian
History	
1. What is your name?	1. Come ti chiami?
2. What is your address?	2. Il tuo indirizzo.
3. When were you born?	3. La tua data di nascita.
4. What trouble are you having with your eyes?	4. Hai qualche problema con i tuoi occhi?
5. Are you having pain?	5. Senti dolore?
6. Do your eyes itch?	6. I tuoi occhi bruciano?
7. Have you had any eye injury?	7. Hai avuto un incidente agli occhi?
8. Have you had an eye operation?	8. Hai mai avuto una operazione agli occhi?
9. Did you get anything in your eye?	9. Cosa e' entrato nel tuo occhio?
10. Are you taking any eye drops?	10. Usi gocce per occhi?
11. Do you have headaches?	11. Hai dolori di testa?
12. Do you wear glasses?	12. Usi occhiali?
13. How old are your glasses?	13. Da quanto tempo usi questi occhiali?
14. Do you have trouble reading?	14. Riesci a leggere?
15. Do you see double?	15. Vedi doppio?
16. Do you take pills?	Per: il cuore
For: heart	il diabete
diabetes	la pressione
blood pressure	
17. Do you have any allergies?	17. Hai allergie?
To medicine	a medicine
Others	di qualsiasi tipo
18. Is there a history of diabetes or glaucoma in your family?	18. C'e' qualche caso di diabete o glaucoma nella tua famiglia?
19. Is there a history of eye problems?	19. Qualcuno in famiglia ha avuto disturbi alla vista?
Examination	
20. Look straight.	20. Guarda diritto.
21. Follow my light.	21. Segui la luce.
22. Follow my finger.	22. Segui il mio dito.
23. Can you count my fingers?	23. Quante dita vedi?
24. Can you see my hand move?	24. Vedi la mia mano muoversi?
25. Open your eyes. Close your eyes.	25. Apri gli occhi. Chiudi gli occhi.
26. Look at me.	26. Guardami.
27. Is it clear?	27. Vedi chiaro?
28. Read this.	28. Leggi.
29. Which is better, one or two?	29. Qual e' meglio, uno o due?

Translations of commonly asked questions and commands—**cont'd**

English	Polish
History	
1. What is your name?	1. Jak się pan (pani) nazywa?
2. What is your address?	2. Jaki jest pana (pani) adres?
3. When were you born?	3. Kiedy się pan urodzil (pani urodzila)?
4. What trouble are you having with your eyes?	4. Jaki pan (pani) ma problem z oczami?
5. Are you having pain?	5. Czy pan (pani) odczuwa ból?
6. Do your eyes itch?	6. Czy pana (pani) swędzą oczy?
7. Have you had any eye injury?	7. Czy oko bylo skaleczone?
8. Have you had an eye operation?	8. Czy mial pan (miata pani) operację na oczy?
9. Did you get anything in your eye?	9. Czy coś się dostalo do oka?
10. Are you taking any eye drops?	10. Czy bierze pan (pani) krople do oczu?
11. Do you have headaches?	11. Czy cierpi pan (pani) na bole glowy?
12. Do you wear glasses?	12. Czy nosi pan (pani) okulary?
13. How old are your glasses?	13. Jak dawno nosi pan (pani) te okulary?
14. Do you have trouble reading?	14. Czy ma pan (pani) problemy z czytaniem?
15. Do you see double?	15. Czy widzi pan (pani) podwójnie?
16. Do you take pills?	16. Czy bierze pan (pani) pastylki?
For: heart	Na: Serce
diabetes	Cukrzyce
blood pressure	Wysokie ciśnienie
17. Do you have any allergies?	17. Czy cierpi pan (pani) na alergie?
To medicine	Na lekarstwa
Others	Inne
18. Is there a history of diabetes or glaucoma in your family?	18. Czy ktoś z rodziny cierpi na cukrzyce lub jaskre?
19. Is there a history of eye problems?	19. Czy ktoś z rodziny ma problemy z oczami?
Examination	
20. Look straight.	20. Proszę patrzeć prosto.
21. Follow my light.	21. Proszę wodzić wzrokiem za światlem.
22. Follow my finger.	22. Proszę wodzić wzrokiem za moim palcem.
23. Can you count my fingers?	23. Czy może pan (pani) policzyć moje palce?
24. Can you see my hand move?	24. Czy widzi pan (pani) jak rusza się moja ręka?
25. Open your eyes. Close your eyes.	25. Proszę otworzyć oczy. Proszę zamknąć oczy.
26. Look at me.	26. Proszę spojrzeć na mnie.
27. Is it clear?	27. Czy to jest dobrze widoczne?
28. Read this.	28. Proszę to przeczytać.
29. Which is better, one or two?	29. Które jest lepsze, pierwsze czy drugie?

Continued.

Translations of commonly asked questions and commands—**cont'd**

English	Spanish
History	
1. What is your name?	1. Su nombre, por favor.
2. What is your address?	2. Su dirección, por favor.
3. When were you born?	3. Su fecha de nacimiento, por favor.
4. What trouble are you having with your eyes?	4. ¿Tiene usted dificultades con la vista?
5. Are you having pain?	5. ¿Le duelen los ojos?
6. Do your eyes itch?	6. ¿Le pican los ojos?
7. Have you had any eye injury?	7. ¿Han recibido daño en alguna forma sus ojos?
8. Have you had an eye operation?	8. ¿Ha sufrido usted alguna operación en los ojos?
9. Did you get anything in your eye?	9. ¿Tiene algo en el ojo?
10. Are you taking any eye drops?	10. ¿Está usted usando gotas para los ojos?
11. Do you have headaches?	11. ¿Sufre usted de dolores de cabeza?
12. Do you wear glasses?	12. ¿Usa usted espejuelos (gafas)?
13. How old are your glasses?	13. ¿Cuántos años tienen sus gafas?
14. Do you have trouble reading?	14. ¿Les molestan cuando lee?
15. Do you see double?	15. ¿Ve doble?
16. Do you take pills?	16. ¿Toma usted medicinas?
For: heart	para: el corazón
diabetes	la diabetes
blood pressure	la presión arterial?
17. Do you have any allergies?	17. ¿Es usted alérgico?
To medicine	a las medicinas
Others	a otras cosas?
18. Is there a history of diabetes or glaucoma in your family?	18. ¿Existen o han existido casos de diabetes o de glaucoma en su familia?
19. Is there a history of eye problems?	19. ¿Existen o han existido problemas de la vista en la familia?
Examination	
20. Look straight.	20. ¡Mire directamente hacia delante!
21. Follow my light.	21. ¡Siga la luz con sus ojos!
22. Follow my finger.	22. ¡Siga mi dedo con sus ojos!
23. Can you count my fingers?	23. ¿Puede contar los dedos?
24. Can you see my hand move?	24. ¿Ve mi mano cuando se mueve?
25. Open your eyes. Close your eyes.	25. ¡Abra los ojos! ¡Cierre los ojos!
26. Look at me.	26. ¡Míreme!
27. Is it clear?	27. ¿Lo ve claramente?
28. Read this.	28. ¡Lea esto!
29. Which is better, one or two?	29. ¿De los dos cuál es el mejor, el uno o el dos?

Index

Materials
    fluorosilicone copolymer, 284
    for gas-permeable lenses, 277
        equivalent oxygen performance of, 267
        silicone-acrylate, 264-266
    for rigid lenses, 18
    for soft lenses, 88
Medical factors in patient selection, 52-55
Medications; *see* Drugs
Meibomian glands, 10-11, 25
    in assessment of anterior lipid layer, 44, 48
Meibomian keratoconjunctivitis, 45
Meibomianitis
    extended-wear lenses and, 374
    low-grade, 45
Menopause as factor in patient selection, 55
Meridian, horizontal, in serial keratometry, 37-38
Metabolism of corneal epithelium, 5-7
Methacrylate added to silicone, 263
Methyl methacrylate, 88
Methylparaben, 128
Microcysts
    epithelial, 221
        soft lens and, 149
    and extended-wear lenses, 384
    intraepithelial, 433, 434
Microscope
    specular, 35
    operating, cameras mounted on, 529-530
Microthin lenses
    rigid
        fitting of, 169-173
        handling of, 184
    spectacle blur and, 223
Microvilli of corneal epithelium, 5
Mineral deposits on extended-wear lenses, 381
Minus and plus tear film, 95
Minus power
    adding, in rigid lens, 199-200
    soft lenses, 109
Minus-carrier lenticular lenses, 360-362
Mires, keratometer, 21, 22
    in rigid lens fitting, 165, 166
    in soft lens with normal fit, 102-103
MMA; *see* Methyl methacrylate
Modification
    of fluorocarbon and silicone acrylate lenses, 294
    of rigid lenses, office, 195-203
        to add minus power, 199-200
        to add plus power, 200
        to adjust peripheral curves, 202
        to blend transition or junction zones, 196-197
        to fenestrate lens, 202-203
        to flatten base curve, 202
        to flatten intermediate curves, 199
        to identify lens, 202
        to polish and refinish edges, 200-202
        polishing compounds for, 196

Modification—cont'd
    of rigid lenses—cont'd
        to reduce optic-zone diameter, 197-198
        to reduce overall lens diameter, 198-199
        to remove scratches, 200
Modulus, 19
Molding of contact lenses, technology of, 62-64
Moll, apocrine glands of, 11
Monocentric bifocal lens, 337
Monocular aphakic myopia, 421
Monocular patient as factor in patient selection, 54-55
Monocurve in peripheral stability of soft lenses, 87-88
Monovision contact lenses for presbyopia, 332-333
    modified, 343
Mooren's corneal ulcer, 411
Morphometric changes, endothelial, 469-471
Mosaic pattern of corneal endothelial cells, 529
Movement
    in evaluating fit of soft lenses, 94
    excessive, of rigid lenses, 216
    in fitting fluorocarbon and silicone acrylate lenses, 288-289
    of soft lens with loose fit, 104, 105
    of soft lens with normal fit, 99-101
Movies, contact lenses in, 142
Mucous layer of tear film, 11
Mucus, formation of, on lenses, 224-225, 226
Multicurve lens, 15
Multifocal rigid lens, 339
Myopia
    induced, soft lens and, 150-151, 154-155
    monocular aphakic, overcorrection of, 421
    reading difficulty in, 234
Myopic refractive errors, 96

N

Nasal and temporal staining, 242-243
Near vision with bifocal lenses
    aspheric, 342
    segmented, 337
Neosporin for corneal ulcer, 480
Neovascularization of cornea, 35, 358
    management of, 477
    after radial keratotomy, 354
    as sign of poor oxygen supply, 423
Nerves, corneal, anatomy of, 9-10
Neutralization of hydrogen peroxide, 431
Newsletters, 515
NIBUT; *see* Noninvasive breakup time
Nicking at edge of soft lens, 153
Ni-Cone lens for keratoconus, 314
Night, ocular change during, 371
Nomogram
    for fitting fluorocarbon and silicone acrylate lenses, 284-285
    Harrison-Stein, 275-276, 287